Invasive Cardiology

Cardiovascular Clinics Series

Brest	1/1	Hypertensive Cardiovascular Disease
Brest	1/2	Coronary Heart Disease
Brest	1/3	Cardiovascular Therapy
Downing	2/1	Congenital Heart Disease
Dreifus	*2/2	Arrhythmias
White	2/3	International Cardiology
Gifford	3/1	Peripheral Vascular Disease
Harken	*3/2	Cardiac Surgery 1
Harken	*3/3	Cardiac Surgery 2
Burch	*4/1	Cardiomyopathy
Edwards	*4/2	Clinical-Pathological Correlations 1
Engle	4/3	Pediatric Cardiology
Edwards	*5/1	Clinical-Pathological Correlations 2
Likoff	*5/2	Valvular Heart Disease
Fisch	*5/3	Complex Electrocardiography 1
Fisch	*6/1	Complex Electrocardiography 2
Melmon	*6/2	Cardiovascular Drug Therapy
Fowler	6/3	Diagnostic Methods in Cardiology
Vidt	7/1	Cleveland Clinic Cardiovascular Consultations
Brest et al.	7/2	Innovations in the Diagnosis and Management of Acute Myocardial Infarction
Spodick	7/3	Pericardial Diseases
Corday	8/1	Controversies in Cardiology
Rahimtoola	8/2	Coronary Bypass Surgery
Rios	8/3	Clinical Electrocardiographic Correlations
Onesti, Brest	9/1	Hypertension
Kotler, Segal	9/2	Clinical Echocardiography
Wenger	*9/3	Exercise and the Heart
Roberts	*10/1	Congenital Heart Disease in Adults
Willerson	*10/2	Nuclear Cardiology
Brandenburg	10/3	Office Cardiology
Castellanos	11/1	Cardiac Arrhythmias: Mechanisms and Management
Engle	11/2	Pediatric Cardiovascular Disease
Rackley	11/3	Critical Care Cardiology
Noble, Rothbaum	12/1	Geriatric Cardiology
Vidt	12/2	Cardiovascular Therapy
McGoon	*12/3	Cardiac Surgery
Rahimtoola	13/1	Controversies in Coronary Artery Disease
Spittell	13/2	Clinical Vascular Disease
Fowler	13/3	Noninvasive Diagnostic Methods in Cardiology
Goldberg	14/1	Coronary Artery Spasm and Thrombosis
Dreifus	14/2	Pacemaker Therapy
Conti	14/3	Cardiac Drug Therapy

*Not Available

Invasive Cardiology

John Speer Schroeder, M.D. | Editor

Associate Professor of Medicine
Stanford University School of Medicine
Stanford, California

CARDIOVASCULAR CLINICS

Albert N. Brest, M.D. | Editor-in-Chief

James C. Wilson Professor of Medicine
Director, Division of Cardiology
Jefferson Medical College
Philadelphia, Pennsylvania

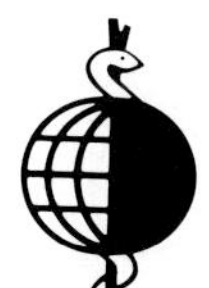

F. A. DAVIS COMPANY, PHILADELPHIA

Cardiovascular Clinics, 15/1, Invasive Cardiology

Printed in the United States of America

NOTE: As new scientific information becomes available through basic and clinical research, recommended treatments and drug therapies undergo changes. The authors and publisher have done everything possible to make this book accurate, up-to-date, and in accord with accepted standards at the time of publication. However, the reader is advised always to check product information (package inserts) for changes and new information regarding dose and contraindications before administering any drug. Caution is especially urged when using new or infrequently ordered drugs.

Library of Congress Cataloging in Publication Data
Cardiovascular clinics. 1-
Philadelphia, F. A. Davis, 1969–

v. ill. 27 cm.

Editor: v. 1– A. N. Brest.
Key title: Cardiovascular clinics, ISSN 0069-0384.
1. Cardiovascular system—Diseases—Collected works. I. Brest, Albert N., ed.
[DNLM: W1 CA77N]
RC681.A1C27 616.1 70-6558
ISBN 0-8036-7756-1 MARC-S

Library of Congress 75[8307]

Preface

Invasive techniques in cardiovascular medicine have provided a veritable explosion in new approaches to both diagnosis and treatment of the known or suspected cardiovascular patient. This issue of CARDIOVASCULAR CLINICS documents the current status of these technologies and provides the reader with a useful and applicable summary. Many of the chapters were written by physicians who pioneered the techniques or who were responsible for their applications in the cardiovascular laboratory today. I am pleased to serve as guest editor for this important volume of CARDIOVASCULAR CLINICS.

During the past five years, our approach to the acute myocardial infarction patient has dramatically changed. Urgent coronary angiography has not only documented the pathophysiologic basis for thrombolytic and angioplastic approaches to the salvage of myocardium, but it has also greatly improved our concepts about the sequence of precipitating events in these patients. Similarly, electrophysiologic evaluation of the arrhythmia patient has provided a better understanding of the etiology of both atrial and ventricular arrhythmias, as well as a new objective measure of antiarrhythmic drug efficacy. Thus, whether the reader leafs through this book or seeks specific answers to questions about invasive cardiology, I believe he or she will be rewarded. It is my hope that not only will the answers be there, but that a sense of the remarkable progress we have made over the past decade will be apparent as well.

I wish to thank each of the individual authors for what I consider to be outstanding contributions that are both thoughtful and to the point. Dr. Albert N. Brest, Editor-in-Chief of CARDIOVASCULAR CLINICS, has been invaluable in his assistance to this volume and patient to the very end.

John Speer Schroeder, M.D.
Guest Editor

Editor's Commentary

The pioneering cardiac catheterization studies by Forssmann, Cournand, and Richards were the forerunners of modern invasive cardiology. Subsequently, stunning advances in invasive methods have opened wide the frontiers of clinical cardiology and cardiac surgery. This issue of CARDIOVASCULAR CLINICS does not attempt to review every aspect of invasive cardiology, but aims instead at examining highlights in the ongoing development of ideas and techniques in this field. The chapters range from discussions of coronary arteriography and coronary blood flow studies to ventriculography, percutaneous transluminal coronary angioplasty, pacing, hemodynamic monitoring, intra-aortic balloon pumping, endomyocardial biopsy, catheter treatment of congenital heart disease, electrophysiologic studies, and so on. I am immensely greatful to John Speer Schroeder for his guidance in the formulation of this volume, and both of us are indebted to the individual authors for their enlightening, scholarly contributions.

Albert N. Brest, M.D.
Editor-in-Chief

Contributors

Edwin L. Alderman, M.D.
Associate Professor of Medicine, Cardiology Division, Stanford University Medical Center, Stanford, California

Donald S. Baim, M.D.
Assistant Professor of Medicine, Harvard Medical School; Co-Director, Hemodynamic Research Laboratory, Beth Israel Hospital, Boston, Massachusetts

Bruce C. Berger, M.D.
Clinical Assistant Professor of Medicine, University of Pennsylvania; Associate Director, Non-Invasive Cardiology, The Graduate Hospital, Philadelphia, Pennsylvania

Arlene B. Bradley, M.D.
Research Fellow in Cardiology, Cardiovascular Division, Department of Medicine, Beth Israel Hospital, Boston, Massachusetts

Richard O. Cannon, III, M.D.
Senior Investigator, Cardiology Branch, National Heart, Lung, and Blood Institute, National Institutes of Health, Bethesda, Maryland

Kanu Chatterjee, M.B., F.R.C.P.
Professor of Medicine; Lucie Stern Professor of Cardiology; Associate Chief, Cardiovascular Division; Director, Coronary Care Unit, Moffitt Hospital, University of California, San Francisco, California

A. Robert Denniss, M.B., B.S., B.Sc. (Med), M.Sc., F.R.A.C.P.
Research Fellow, Cardiology Unit, Westmead Centre, Australia

Lila R. Elveback, Ph.D.
Professor of Biostatistics, Mayo Medical School, Rochester, Minnesota

Mary E. Fontana, M.D.
Associate Professor, Division of Cardiology, The Ohio State University Hospitals, College of Medicine, Columbus, Ohio

Robert E. Fowles, M.D.
Adjunct Associate Professor of Medicine, Division of Cardiology, University of Utah Medical Center, Salt Lake City, Utah

Roger A. Freedman, M.D.
Cardiology Division, Stanford University Medical Center, Stanford, California

Sheldon Goldberg, M.D.
Associate Professor of Medicine; Director, Cardiac Catheterization Laboratory, Thomas Jefferson University Hospital, Philadelphia, Pennsylvania

Lawrence S.C. Griffith, M.D.
Associate Professor of Medicine, Johns Hopkins University School of Medicine, Baltimore, Maryland

Diana F. Guthaner, M.D.
Assistant Professor of Radiology, Cardiovascular Section, Department of Radiology, Stanford University Medical Center, Stanford, California

Geoffrey O. Hartzler, M.D.
Consulting Cardiologist, Mid-America Heart Institute, St. Luke's Hospital; Clinical Associate Professor of Medicine, University of Missouri (Kansas City), Kansas City, Missouri

Graham Jackson, M.B.
Consultant Cardiologist, King's College Hospital, United Kingdom

Harvey G. Kemp, Jr., M.D.
Director, Division of Cardiology, St. Luke's Hospital, St. Luke's-Roosevelt Hospital Center; Professor of Clinical Medicine, Columbia University, College of Physicians and Surgeons, New York, New York

Victoria M. Kusiak, M.D.
Assistant Clinical Professor of Medicine; Co-Director, Cardiac Catheterization Laboratory, Thomas Jefferson University Hospital, Philadelphia, Pennsylvania

Jeffrey A. Laser, M.D.
Cardiology Division, Stanford University Medical Center, Stanford, California

Richard P. Lewis, M.D.
Professor and Director, Division of Cardiology, The Ohio State University College of Medicine, Columbus, Ohio

Philip O. Littleford, M.D.
Attending Cardiologist, Florida Hospital, Orlando, Florida; Clinical Associate Professor of Medicine, University of Florida, Gainesville, Florida

Jay W. Mason, M.D.
Professor of Medicine; Chief, Division of Cardiology, University of Utah Medical Center, Salt Lake City, Utah

Steven G. Meister, M.D.
Professor of Medicine; Director, Cardiovascular Division, The Medical College of Pennsylvania, Philadelphia, Pennsylvania

Michael B. Mock, M.D.
Division of Cardiovascular Diseases and Internal Medicine, Mayo Clinic and Mayo Foundation, Rochester, Minnesota

William J. Rashkind, M.D.
Professor of Pediatrics, University of Pennsylvania School of Medicine; Director, Cardiovascular Laboratories, Children's Hospital of Philadelphia, Philadelphia, Pennsylvania

Guy S. Reeder, M.D.
Division of Cardiovascular Diseases and Internal Medicine, Mayo Clinic and Mayo Foundation, Rochester, Minnesota

Douglas R. Rosing, M.D.
Head, Cardiac Catheterization Laboratory, Cardiology Branch, National Heart, Lung, and Blood Institute, National Institutes of Health, Bethesda, Maryland; Clinical Professor of Medicine, George Washington University Medical Center, Washington, D.C.

David L. Ross, M.B., B.S., F.R.A.C.P.
Staff Specialist, Cardiology, Westmead Centre, Australia

John Speer Schroeder, M.D.
Associate Professor of Medicine, Stanford University School of Medicine, Stanford, California

Hugh C. Smith, M.D.
Director, Cardiac Catheterization Laboratory, Mayo Clinic and Mayo Foundation, Rochester, Minnesota

MaryAngela S. Tait, B.S.
Research Assistant, Children's Hospital of Philadelphia, Department of Cardiology, Philadelphia, Pennsylvania

John B. Uther, B.Sc. (Med), M.D., B.S., F.R.A.C.P.
Senior Staff Specialist, Cardiology, Westmead Centre, Australia

Nelson M. Wolf, M.D.
Associate Professor of Medicine; Director, Cardiac Catheterization Laboratory, The Medical College of Pennsylvania, Philadelphia, Pennsylvania

Contents

Coronary Arteriography: Indications, Techniques, and Morbidity

Harvey G. Kemp, Jr., M.D.

Selective coronary arteriography, once a controversial procedure that stirred heated debates at medical meetings, has now become not only an accepted procedure but almost a standard part of the workup of a patient with suspected coronary heart disease. Such a statement must be qualified, of course; nevertheless, it is quite close to the truth. Twenty years ago coronary arteriography was most frequently performed via the arm through an arteriotomy. In most centers it took several hours, being coupled with classic right and left heart catheterization: It was uncomfortable for both the patient and the physician and was associated with morbidity and mortality rates that will probably never be accurately known. In addition, the end product, the cinearteriogram, was frequently so poor in quality as scarcely to justify all the effort that had gone into obtaining it.

Nowadays, coronary arteriography can be done either from the arm or as a percutaneous procedure from the femoral artery. The usual catheterization consists of obtaining coronary arteriography, intra-aortic and intraventricular pressure tracings, and a ventriculogram. The entire procedure takes 20 to 30 minutes, sometimes less. Complications, discussed later in detail, are rare, and mortality is almost unheard of except in the severely ill. The arteriography that is generated should be of excellent radiographic quality, and the information that it yields is frequently pivotal to determining both diagnosis and management. It is scarcely surprising, therefore, that most authorities have swung toward the view that arteriography should be performed early in the workup of a patient suspected of coronary heart disease and should be repeated as frequently as necessary, depending upon the clinical course.

This would appear to be a good time to review the subject of coronary arteriography and in particular to discuss new information available relating to the reproducibility of coronary arteriographic interpretation and therefore its accuracy; further data that is now available relating to the complication rate associated with coronary arteriography; and, finally, recent attempts to quantify arteriographic lesions.

HISTORICAL PERSPECTIVE

This chapter is too brief to allow for a full development of the history of selective coronary arteriography, but it would be useful to lay a foundation from which to base our further discussion. Beginning with Forssmann's classic experiment in 1929[1] the science and art of cardiac catheterization gradually developed, with progress beginning to accelerate in the 1950s. Prior to selective coronary arteriography, all the attempts to visualize the coronary circulation radiographically had been by bolus injection of 40 to 60 ml of contrast material by a pressure syringe through a catheter placed in the aortic root.[2] A few of these catheters were specially shaped to allow more rapid flow of contrast, in hope that better visualization of the coronary circulation would thereby be obtained. Other methods involved transient decrease of cardiac output either by injection of acetylcholine[3,4] or by increasing intrabronchial pressure.[5]

In 1958, Sones and his colleagues were investigating the use of semiselective coronary arteriography by injecting 20 to 30 ml of contrast medium into each coronary sinus. In the course of these studies it was noted that during an inadvertent power injection of 30 ml of contrast material directly into the right coronary orifice, no serious untoward effects occurred.[6] This observation, coupled with his ongoing interest in opacifying the coronary circulation, stimulated Sones to design a catheter especially suited for selective coronary arteriography. In 1962 he published his account of coronary arteriography in 1020 patients. He had been able to catheterize both coronary arteries in 954 of these patients, and at least one coronary in all of them.[7]

The Sones technique, as the transbrachial approach using the Sones catheter came to be called, requires a moderate amount of training to perform with ease. The brachial artery can be a rather small structure, particularly in women, and undoubtedly there were arterial complications relating to the arteriotomy. Therefore, despite devotion to the procedure, particularly in Sones' own institution, the Cleveland Clinic, there was a considerable impetus to develop a percutaneous femoral technique. Ricketts and Abrams reported such a method in 1962,[8] and others also attempted to develop this technique. It was Judkins, however, in 1967 and 1968, who, in describing his experience with a modified preformed polyurethane catheter,

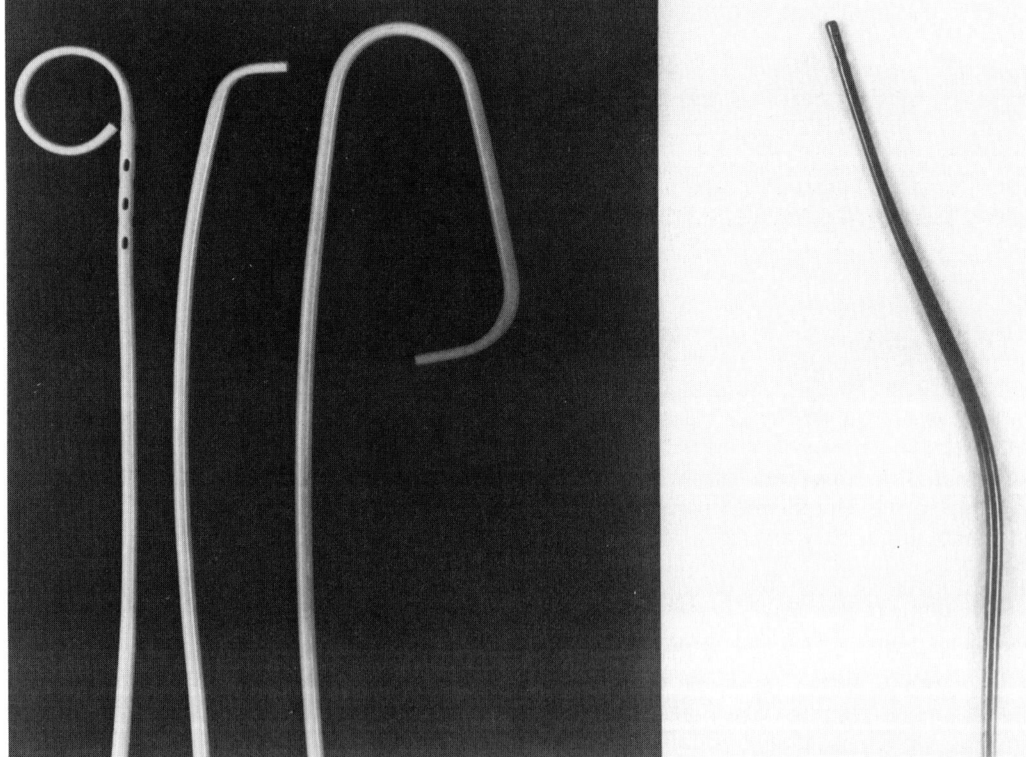

Figure 1. (*Left Panel*) The three Judkins catheters—the pigtail ventriculography catheter, right and left coronary catheters—are shown from left to right. (*Right Panel*) The Sones catheter is shown. (From Randall, AB, and Kemp, HG,[29] with permission.)

came forth with the particular shape for each coronary catheter that enabled it to consistently enter the appropriate coronary ostium.[9,10] Although minor modifications in the tip of the catheters have been made, it is the Judkins technique that predominates in this country today. Catheter tips are shown in Figure 1.

CORONARY ARTERIOGRAPHIC TECHNIQUES

The two predominant techniques for performing coronary arteriography are the brachial technique, as first proposed by Sones, and the percutaneous femoral technique, as proposed by Judkins.

The brachial technique entails a cutdown on the brachial artery in the right antecubital fossa. The artery is isolated, and a small incision is made into it through which the catheter is introduced. The Sones catheter is made of woven Dacron. It comes in the usual 7 to 8 French sizes but tapers over the distal five centimeters to 5 French. There is an open end hole and two very small side holes. Whereas the shaft is stiff, the tip is flexible so as to be manipulated into the coronary ostia. The catheter is advanced through the subclavian and innominate arteries into the aortic arch and then is positioned just above the aortic valve. The catheter can be manipulated in such a way as to guide its tip into each coronary ostium, and arteriography thus performed. The catheter can also be prolapsed into the left ventricle for left ventriculography. In this way the entire procedure can be performed using a single catheter. The catheter is then removed and the arteriotomy closed with fine suture material. The wound is irrigated well and the skin closed.

The percutaneous femoral technique involves the percutaneous puncture of the femoral artery at the level of the right inguinal ligament. A wire guide is advanced through the needle, the needle is removed, and, after appropriate dilatation of the artery, the catheter is passed over the guide wire up through the abdominal aorta into the aortic arch. Three different catheters are ordinarily used for the performance of coronary arteriography: one for the right coronary artery, one for the left, and finally a catheter for ventriculography. The sequence in which the procedures are performed is entirely the option of the arteriographer, but many believe that the coronary arteriography yields the most important information and therefore should be performed first. Others believe that because the contrast material changes the loading characteristics of the myocardium as well as having some direct depressant effects, the ventriculogram should be performed first.

Whichever technique is used, the common denominator is the selective injection of contrast material into the coronary ostium and imaging the coronary circulation. Thirty-five mm cine radiography has proven to be by far the most popular filming technique. Writing about cinearteriography has an inherent problem: You cannot show "movies" on the printed page. The illustrations that follow are offered as the best substitute that this medium can achieve (Figs. 2 to 8).

COMPLICATIONS

A major motivation for the development of noninvasive studies of the coronary circulation is fear of the complications of coronary arteriography. Historically there was a taboo against the selective catheterization of the coronary arteries, probably with the fear that either the catheter would obstruct coronary blood flow and thereby cause a myocardial infarction or that direct injection of the hyperosmolar contrast medium would be injurious to the myocardium. When Sones first presented his initial 1020 patients and reported a mortality rate attributed to the procedure of 0.29 percent, he undoubtedly met some disbelievers.[7] This is particularly true when one realizes that some of these studies were done prior to the availability of external defibrillation.

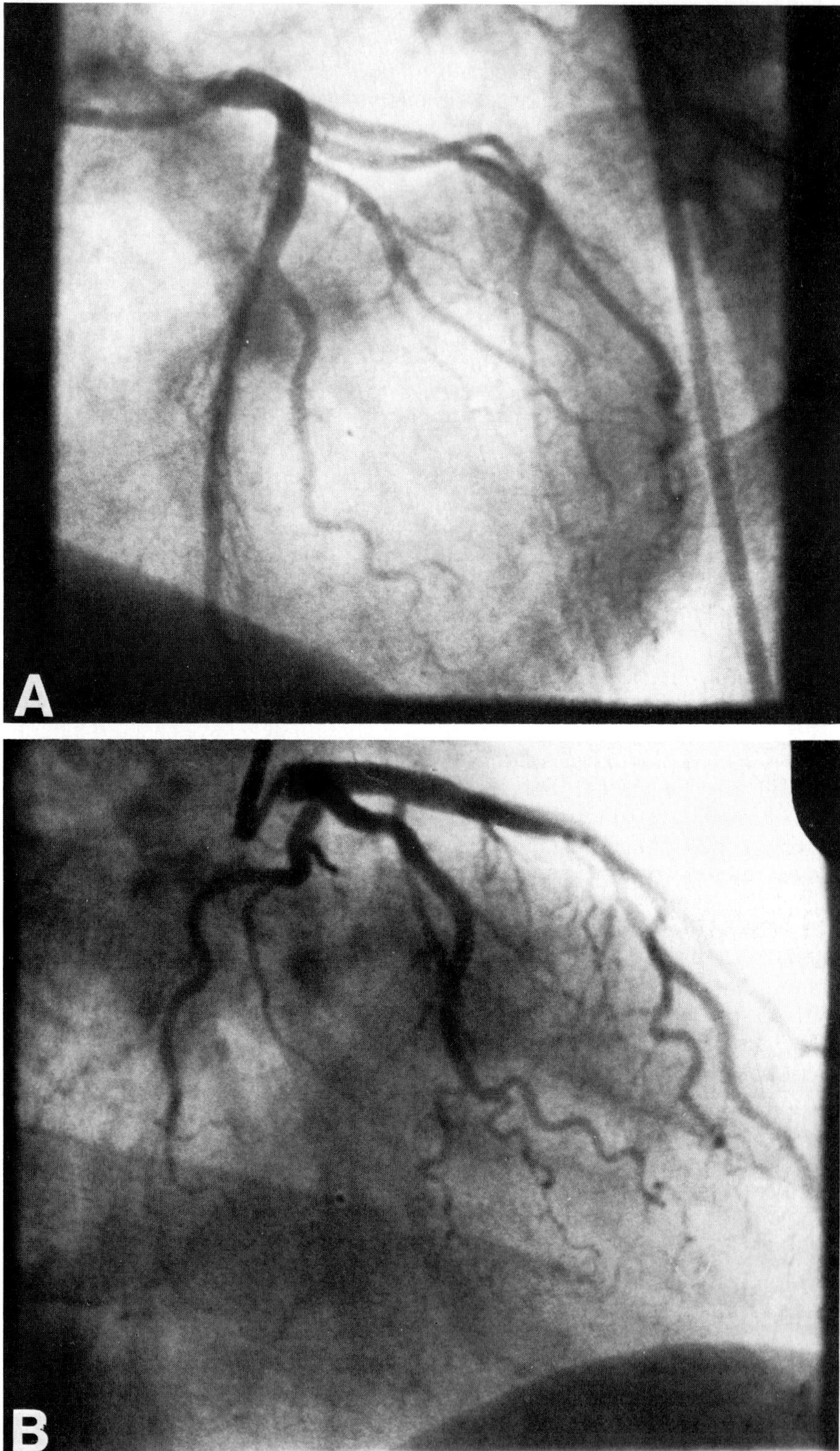

Figure 2. *A*, Here is a normal nondominant left coronary artery viewed in the left anterior oblique (LAO) projection. *B*, Here is the same normal nondominant left coronary artery viewed in the right anterior oblique (RAO) projection.

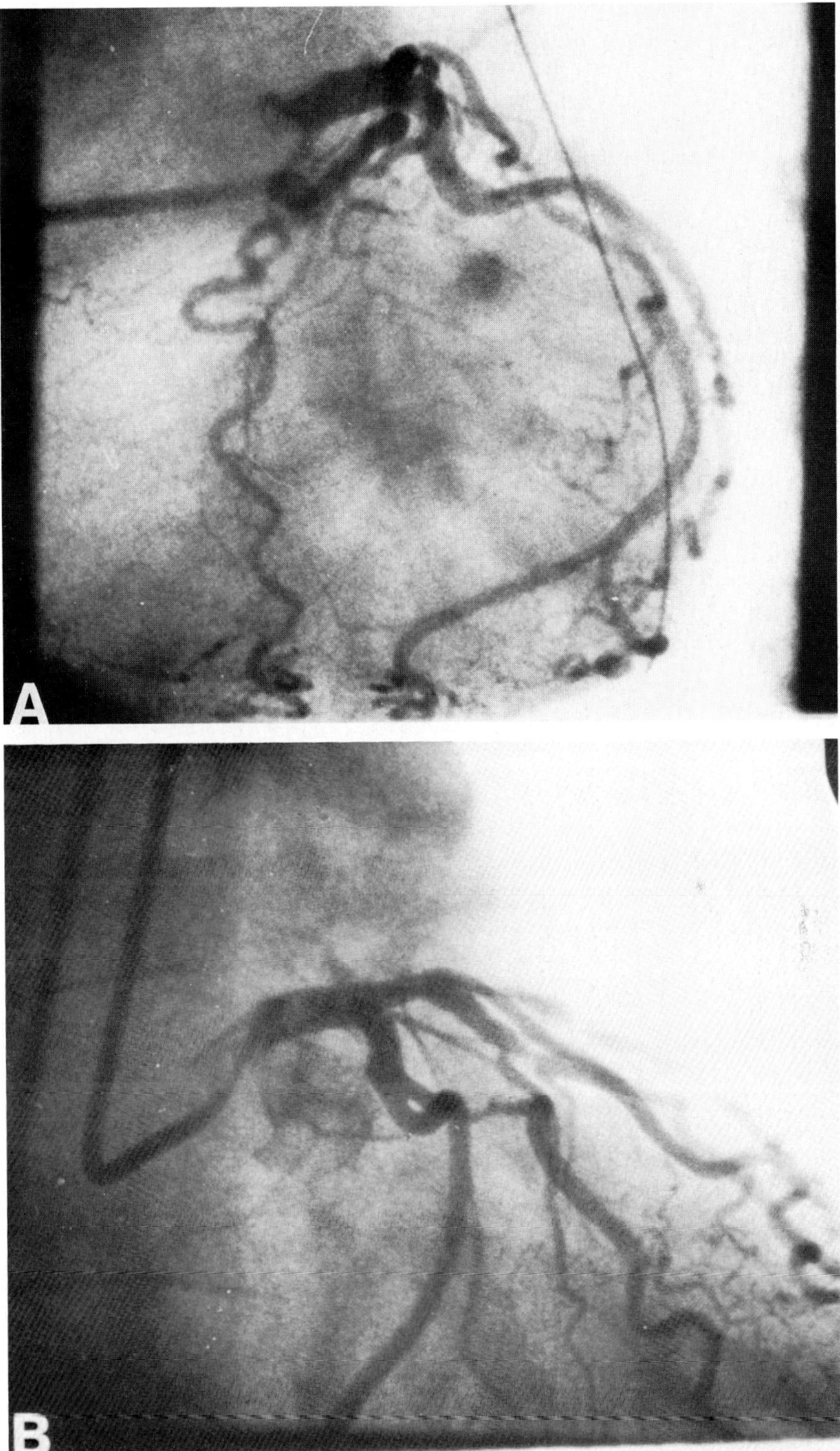

Figure 3. *A,* This is a dominant left coronary artery in the LAO projection. Note extreme tortuosity, particularly of the left anterior descending coronary artery, and overlap of vessels proximally. *B,* An RAO projection of the same vessel is shown. Note stenoses in anterior descending, diagonal, and first obtuse marginal branch of the left circumflex artery brought out in this view.

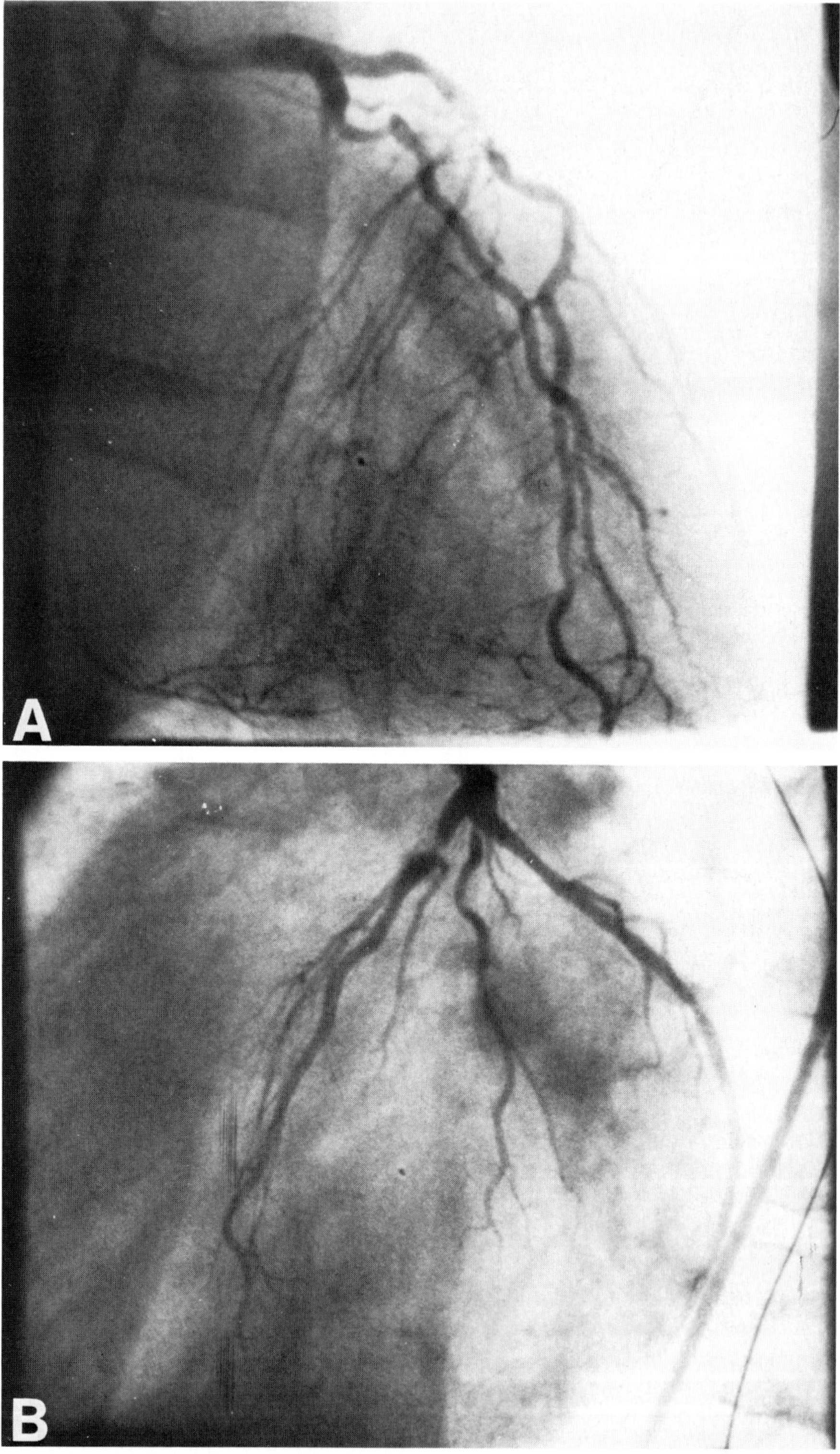

Figure 4. *A,* Left coronary injection in the RAO projection is shown. A severe stenosis is present in the left anterior descending artery, and there is a question of a tubular stenosis in the left circumflex artery. *B,* The LAO projection shows the severe stenosis of the left anterior descending artery and only minimal fusiform narrowing of the circumflex artery.

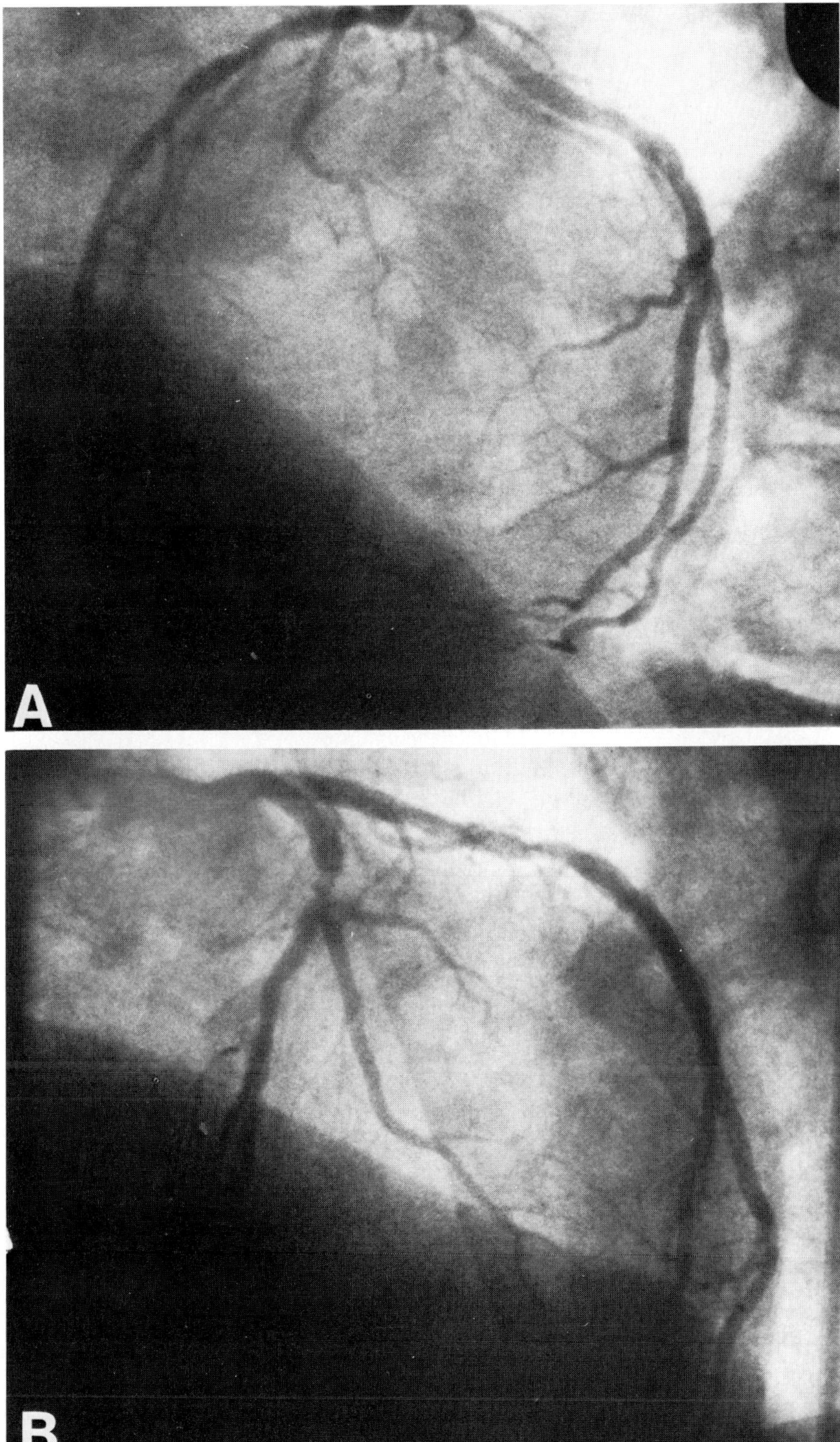

Figure 5. *A,* The LAO projection of this left coronary artery shows no area of significant stenosis. *B,* The LAO axial projection reveals a significant stenosis in the left anterior descending artery just before the first diagonal branch.

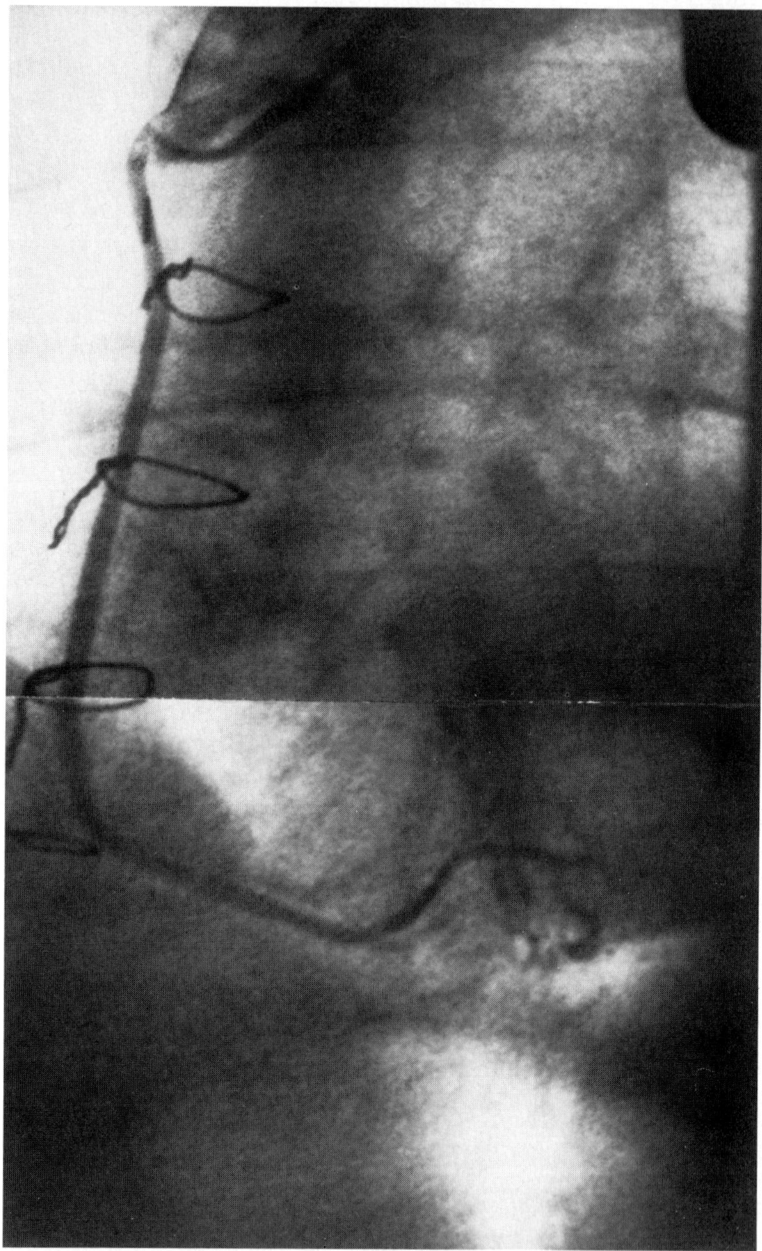

Figure 6. This is a saphenous vein graft to the distal right coronary artery in the LAO projection. (From Randall, AB, and Kemp, HG,[29] with permission.)

The complications associated with coronary arteriography are those associated with any left heart catheterization, including vascular dissection, perforation, or other injury at the site of catheter insertion; arterial embolization (either cerebral or other); arrhythmias; allergic reactions; vasovagal episodes; myocardial infarction; and death. Arteriographers over the years have developed techniques whereby they have markedly reduced the incidence of these complications; however, it is clear that they cannot be avoided altogether. One of the earliest

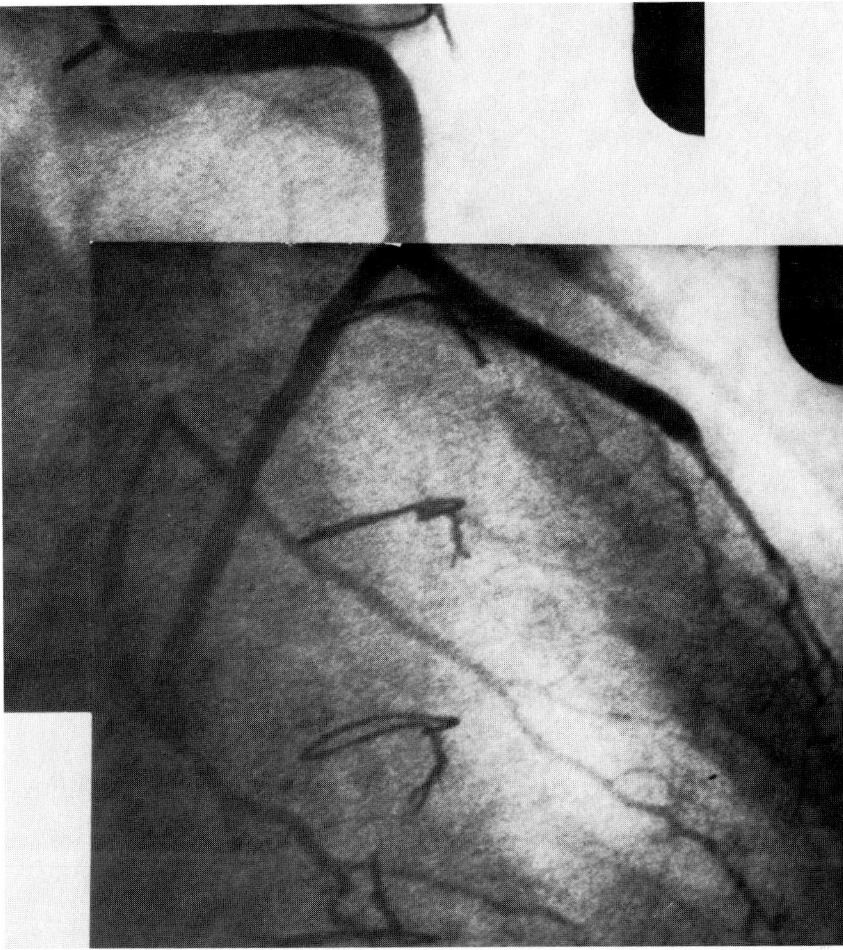

Figure 7. Shown here in the RAO projection is a "Y" saphenous vein graft to a posterolateral branch of the left circumflex artery and a diagonal branch of the left anterior descending artery. (From Randall, AB, and Kemp, HG,[29] with permission.)

reports of the incidence of complications was that of Ross and Gorlin who, in a large cooperative study, reported the complication rate encountered in 3312 procedures, the majority of which were performed at the Cleveland Clinic.[11] The complication rate that they reported was remarkably low, that is, 1.9 percent. Only three deaths occurred, and two of these deaths were associated with severe valvular heart disease. The most frequent complication reported in the study was arrhythmia, occurring in 0.8 percent. The most frequent arrhythmia was ventricular fibrillation, which occurred when contrast was injected into the coronary artery, usually the right coronary artery and usually in women. No patient died from this complication. All responded promptly to defibrillation.

Another well-known study of the complications of coronary arteriography is the report of Adams and coworkers.[12] The methodology of this study was that of a questionnaire survey that was sent to the director of the catheterization laboratory at each of 373 hospitals that were listed as having an open heart surgical team. One hundred and seventy-three responded, or slightly less than half. Analysis of the results of this survey suggested that the risks of mortality or serious morbidity, including myocardial infarction and cerebral embolus, were

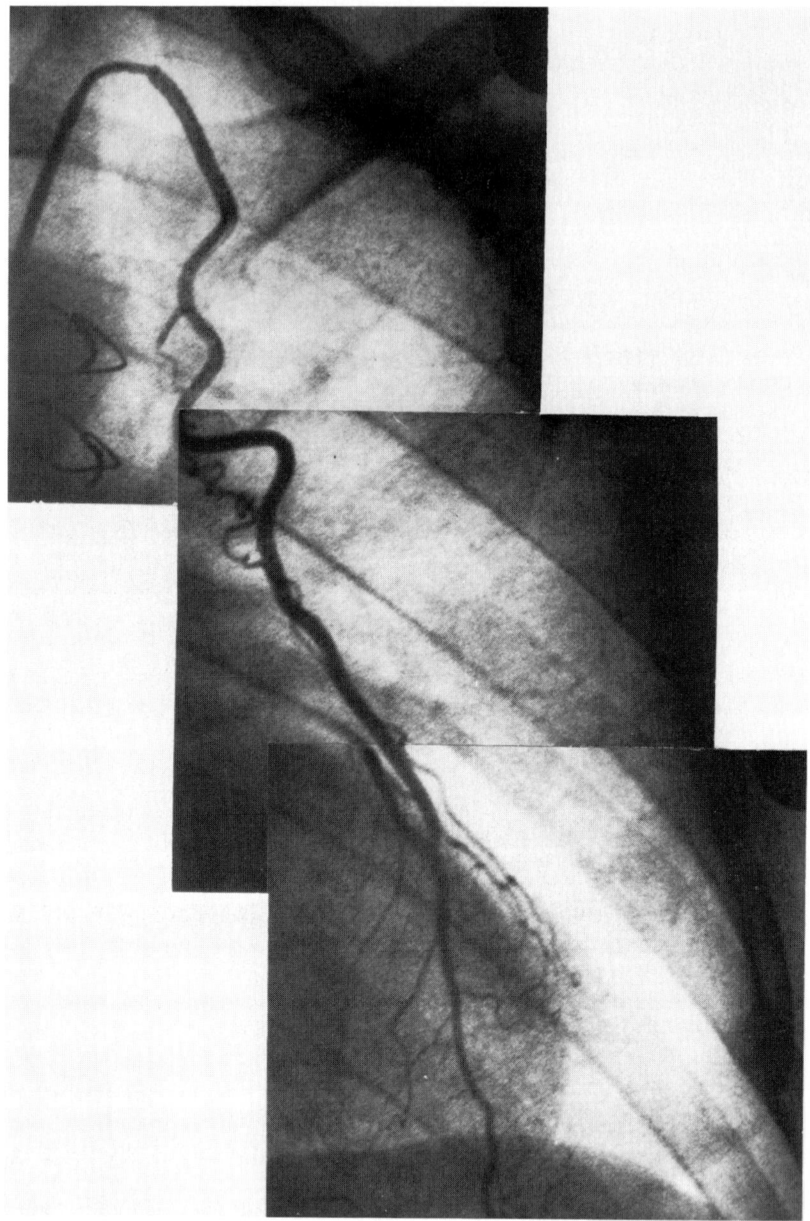

Figure 8. Shown here is a composite photo taken from several frames showing a patent internal mammary artery graft to the left anterior descending artery. (From Randall, AB, and Kemp, HG,[29] with permission.)

greater with the transfemoral technique than with the transbrachial technique. Finally, serious complications were encountered more frequently in those laboratories performing a relatively small number of examinations, irrespective of the technique. The authors realized the limitation of the questionnaire methodology of their study.

The most comprehensive study of complications comes from the American Coronary Artery Surgery Study (CASS), the National Heart, Lung and Blood Institute-supported clinical trial of surgical versus nonsurgical management in the treatment of coronary heart disease.[13] Fifteen major centers in the United States and one in Canada registered consecutive patients who were studied for coronary heart disease. Complications were recorded in a prospective manner. Complications analyzed in this study were restricted to death, nonfatal myocardial infarction, and major vascular complication. Death was defined as procedure-related if it occurred during or following the procedure or on the day after the procedure. Of 7553 patients, 15 deaths occurred on the day of angiography or the day after, with an overall mortality rate of 0.2 percent.

Several interesting findings came from this latter study. As previously noted, it had been suggested that the transfemoral technique might be more hazardous than the transbrachial technique. In fact, this did not prove to be the case. In institutions performing only one technique or the other, the two techniques were equally safe or hazardous, depending upon one's point of view. In institutions doing both, the Judkins technique was actually safer, so that the overall mortality from the femoral technique was less than that of the brachial. The same was true for myocardial infarction, which occurred in 0.25 percent of the total population. The most significant difference between the two techniques, however, was in the incidence of vascular complications. They occurred in 2.8 percent of patients having the brachial technique and in 0.4 percent of patients having the femoral technique. This was true both for institutions performing both techniques and for institutions performing either technique alone.

One of the most tragic complications of left heart catheterization is embolization to the central nervous system. In the CASS study, it was defined as an event that resulted in a residual neurologic deficit. It seems unlikely that such a complication would be underreported. It occurred in only two patients, one catheterized by the femoral technique and one catheterized by the brachial technique. Both patients had received heparin. Five other patients were reported with episodes of arterial embolization, but, again, heparinization did not appear to be protective.

In describing the risks of the procedure to a prospective patient in order to obtain informed consent, it would seem reasonable to say that there are approximately two deaths per thousand, an additional two nonfatal myocardial infarctions per thousand, approximately one episode of arterial embolization per thousand, and seven vascular thrombotic events per thousand. These numbers would have to be modified, of course, for the laboratory's own experience and for the degree of illness of the patient. When 13 of the 15 deaths in the CASS study were analyzed (two were not presented because of lack of informed consent), 11 of the 13 had three-vessel disease, most had impaired ventricular function, and five had significant involvement of the left main coronary artery. Considering this degree of disease, I believe patients can be reassured that they are more at risk from the disease process than from the coronary arteriogram.

ACCURACY OF CORONARY ARTERIOGRAPHY

The coronary arteriogram has been considered to be the most accurate method for assessing the degree of anatomic involvement of the coronary arteries by atherosclerosis. It is frequently referred to as the "gold standard." I participated in one of the earliest studies that appeared to confirm this point of view. We studied the necropsy hearts of 29 patients who had had coronary arteriography premortem.[14] The arteriograms were analyzed by a panel without knowledge of the necropsy findings. A pathologist then carefully examined the coronary arteries of the hearts, both by means of postmortem angiograms and by careful breadloafing of all the involved vessels. We found only 23 errors in the interpretation of the coronary arteriogram as compared with the postmortem data, when defined as a difference in the degree of stenosis of 25 percent or more. We found only two instances in which the error might be of clinical significance. The angiograms were rated for radiographic quality, and all the errors were made in the poorer films. I studied some of the necropsy material with the pathologist and came away with the view that the premortem arteriogram might be at least as accurate as the postmortem examination.

Therefore I was surprised when several studies that appeared in the mid to late 1970s suggested an incredible amount of interobserver and intraobserver variability in the interpretation of coronary arteriography.[15–19] The study of Zir and coworkers[15] showed differences between observers that extended to an artery being assessed as having no disease versus being completely occluded. Subsequent studies confirmed that a considerable amount of interobserver and intraobserver variability existed, although, in general, less than that shown by the Zir study.[16–19] Most studies showed that interobserver variability was considerably greater than intraobserver variability.

A study from CASS was conducted using 30 films and 3 panels of interpreters.[20] Each film was analyzed by all three panels twice so that both interobserver and intraobserver variabilities could be assessed. Interobserver variability was only 60 percent of that of intraobserver, and this difference was statistically significant for the proximal and mid right coronary artery as well as for the proximal left anterior descending artery. There were systematic differences in judgment among the readers in assessing the number of diseased vessels. One reader consistently read less disease. In each case there was significantly less within reader variability than between reader variability.

A particular problem exists with the assessment of the left main coronary artery. This is of importance because disease of the left main coronary artery has been thought to be associated with a grave prognosis unless surgically managed. A separate study of the reliability of interpretation of the left main coronary artery was conducted by Cameron and associates.[21] The severity of stenosis was divided into five grades from normal to totally occluded. Readers agreed on the grade of stenosis only 50 percent of the time. They agreed on whether a stenosis was greater or less than 50 percent (the usual cut-off for significance) 80 percent of the time. The severity of the lesion, its location, or presence of ectasia or calcium did not affect agreement. Segments that were unusually short, diffusely diseased, or obscured by overlapping vessels were especially difficult to interpret.

All the studies cited above demonstrate beyond reasonable doubt that there is a significant variability in the interpretation of percent diameter stenosis by the "eyeballing" method both by the same observer at different times and between observers. Some observers can be identified who systematically read lesions as more or less severe. Interobserver variability is greater than intraobserver variability. The accuracy of the interpretation is undoubtedly related to the quality of the study. It is my opinion that these data do not mean that high-quality arteriography is insufficient for current clinical management. However, more reproducible quantitative methods of assessing the degree and extent of atherosclerotic involvement of the coronary arteries would be of considerable value.

QUANTITATIVE CORONARY ARTERIOGRAPHY

Gensini and coworkers should be credited with the first attempt to take a more quantitative approach to measurements of the coronary arteries, both in the dog and in man.[22] They developed a method whereby coronary angiograms were projected onto a ground glass screen and, by means of the use of a crosshair measuring system, the same number and the X-Y coordinates could be recorded on an IBM punch card. From these data a computer-generated plot of the percentage change of the diameter of the coronary lumen could be obtained. They were able to record relief of catheter-induced spasm and to show the time course of drug action by repeated coronary injections using this technique. They did not, however, attempt to assess stenotic lesions.

Brown and his coworkers reopened the issue of quantitative arteriography in 1977.[23,24] Again the method involved projection of the coronary arterial segment onto a large screen and digitizing by means of an X-Y plotter. Care was taken to introduce corrective methodology for the various distortions introduced by the curvature of the input phosphor of the image intensifier, the magnification distortion, and the distortion introduced by all the optical systems, including that of the projection equipment. Two views of the same lesion were analyzed that were 90° apart and taken during the same instant in the cardiac cycle. This approach allowed the computer to reconstruct the stenosis and, by use of relatively simple and relatively complex hydraulic formulae, the resistance of the stenosis to flow could be calculated. Validation of the technique by comparing the lumen area as predicted from the angiogram with the planimetered area of a histologic section showed close agreement. Reproducibility was greatly enhanced. Nonetheless, such an experiment does not fully simulate the situation in living man. Surrounding soft tissue density is eliminated, motion is not present, and the problem of obtaining views perpendicular to the long axis does not exist. Nevertheless, the approach is very encouraging.

Blankenhorn[25] and Brooks[26] and their colleagues have contributed to our ability to make accurate measurements of atherosclerosis in human vessels. They began their study looking at the femoral artery, which has the advantage of being straight, motionless, and relatively easy to image in perpendicular views. They digitized the image by showing it on the photo cathode surface of an instrument termed an electronic image dissector. This instrument admits electrons proportional to the intensity of the illumination. The electron stream is deflected through a small aperture, and thus the image is scanned and digitized. This eliminates the step of human interaction present in the Brown technique, in which an arteriographer or a technician has to trace the vessel edges. It does introduce the problem of having the computer select the edges, which, of course, means having the investigator tell the computer what difference in density it should consider a vessel edge.

Use of such quantitative techniques has already been important in studies of the coronary circulation. To take the most exciting example, Brown and associates have shown that so-called "fixed" lesions exhibit vasoactivity to vasodilating agents such as nitroglycerin.[27] When one realizes that flow is proportional to the fourth power of the radius, it is apparent that tiny changes in the degree of stenosis can cause marked differences in resistance to flow.[28] These data cause us once again to reverse our thinking about primary action of vasodilators in the treatment of coronary heart disease.

INDICATIONS FOR CORONARY ARTERIOGRAPHY

Customarily a discussion of the indications for coronary arteriography is placed at the beginning rather than at the end of a discussion of this topic. Inasmuch as the indication to do the procedure hinges on the balance between risk and benefit, I have reversed the order. In general, the indications are being liberalized and the reason is the low complication rate and the utility of knowing the coronary anatomy. In a discussion of this topic in a prior review,[29] we divided the indications for coronary arteriography into three broad categories: first, establishing the presence or absence of disease when that is in doubt; second, considering the patient for aggressive management of the coronary disease, either surgical or by transluminal means; and third, establishing the presence or absence of coronary disease when other known forms of heart disease are present. We can add to that list the possible indication of doing an arteriogram during the early hours of acute myocardial infarction.

It is quite clear that the presence of chest pain of an anginal nature can be associated with entirely normal coronary arteries, and very unusual or atypical chest pain may be associated with severe coronary obstructive disease. The incidence of normal coronary arteries in patients who are being studied in good laboratories because of chest pain syndromes is about 20 percent. Identification of patients whose coronary arteries are normal and whose pain is coming from a noncardiac source is of great value. Many of these patients can be rehabilitated, particularly if the correct diagnosis is established early.

Aggressive management of coronary obstructive disease either with surgery or by transluminal angioplasty is discussed in detail elsewhere in this book. Although the mortality question continues relative to surgical versus nonsurgical management of coronary disease, it is clear that at least certain subgroups enjoy a mortality advantage as well as an improved quality of life if their obstruction is relieved. At present, transluminal angioplasty appears to apply to only a relatively small percentage of patients with obstructive disease; however, multivessel disease is now being approached—and quite successfully, according to some investigators.[30] Because the indications for coronary arteriography have always been inextricably related to the benefits of surgical management, it is clear that until the potentials for surgery and for angioplasty are known, it will be impossible to draw any final conclusions.

Patients who are being studied in the cardiac catheterization laboratory because of cardiomyopathy or valvular heart disease should certainly have coronary arteriography as a part of their evaluation. This may be the most important information derived from catheterization. Manchester and coworkers, studying a group of 150 patients with rheumatic valvular heart disease who were free of any signs or symptoms of associated coronary disease, found that whereas only 2 percent of patients less than 50 years old had significant coronary obstruction, approximately 25 percent of patients over 50 years of age had significant coronary disease as well.[31]

Finally, we must now consider whether acute myocardial infarction within the first 6 hours after the onset of symptoms is an indication for coronary arteriography. Elsewhere in this book acute intervention in acute myocardial infarction is discussed in detail. Although I have had only a limited experience with this intervention, it seems clear that it is a safe procedure if it is done with appropriate appreciation for the difference between a therapeutic catheterization and a diagnostic catheterization. The issue of whether thrombolysis changes the course of acute myocardial infarction in a beneficial manner by limiting necrosis remains unknown.

SUMMARY

Coronary arteriography has evolved into a relatively safe and simple procedure, yielding important information about the patient with clinical manifestations of coronary heart disease. The clear trend is to employ arteriography earlier and more frequently in the evaluation. The major therapeutic modality dependent on arteriography at present is bypass surgery, but transluminal angioplasty is rapidly developing and will probably be applicable to an expanding portion of patients. Even newer is thrombolysis in acute myocardial infarction with its promise of limiting myocardial damage in that setting.

REFERENCES

1. Forssmann, W: *Die Sondierung des richten Herzens.* Klin Wochenschr 8:2085, 1929.
2. Paulin, S: *Coronary arteriography.* Acta Radiol (Suppl) (Stockh) 233:1964.
3. Lemmon, WM, Lehman, JS, Kimmel, V, et al: *Use of an artificial pacemaker for acetylcholine-induced cardiac arrest during coronary arteriography.* Circulation 20:726, 1950.
4. Bjork, L, and Hallen, A: *Coronary angiography during acetylcholine-induced cardiac arrest in patients with angina pectoris.* J Cardiovasc Surg 2:9, 1961.
5. Nordenstrom, B: *Contrast examination of the cardiovascular system during increased intrabronchial pressure.* Acta Radiol (Suppl) (Stockh) 200, 1960.
6. Sones, FM: Personal communication.
7. Sones, FM, and Shirey, EK: *Cine coronary arteriography.* Mod Concepts Cardiovasc Dis 31:735, 1962.
8. Ricketts, HJ, and Abrams, HL: *Percutaneous selective coronary cine arteriography.* JAMA 181:620, 1962.
9. Judkins, M: *Selective coronary arteriography. I. A percutaneous transfemoral technique.* Radiology 89:815, 1967.
10. Judkins, M: *Percutaneous transfemoral selective coronary arteriography.* Radiol Clin North Am 6:467, 1968.
11. Ross, RS, and Gorlin, R: *Coronary arteriography.* Circulation 37 (Suppl III):67, 1968.
12. Adams, DF, Fraser, DB, and Abrams, HL: *The complications of coronary arteriography.* Circulation 48:609, 1973.

13. Davis, K, Kennedy, JW, Kemp, HG, et al: *Complications of coronary arteriography from the collaborative study of coronary artery surgery.* Circulation 59:1105, 1979.
14. Kemp, HG, Evans, H, Elliott, WC, et al: *Diagnostic accuracy of selective coronary cinearteriography.* Circulation 36:526, 1967.
15. Zir, LM, Miller, SW, Dinsmore, RE, et al: *Interobservor variability in coronary angiography.* Circulation 53:627, 1976.
16. Detre, KM, Wright, E, Murphy, ML, et al: *Observor agreement in evaluating coronary angiograms.* Circulation 52:979, 1975.
17. DeRouen, TA, Murray, JA, and Owen, W: *Variability in the analysis of coronary angiograms.* Circulation 55:324, 1977.
18. Sanmarco, ME, Brooks, SH, and Blankenhorn, DH: *Reproducibility of a consensus panel in the interpretation of coronary angiograms.* Am Heart J 96:430, 1978.
19. Galbraith, JE, Murphy, ML, and Desoyza, N: *Coronary angiogram interobservor variability.* JAMA 240:2053, 1978.
20. Kemp, HG, Davis, K, Judkins, MP, et al: *Variability within and between readers in the interpretation of coronary arteriograms from the Coronary Artery Surgery Study* (CASS). Submitted for publication to Cathet Cardiovasc Diagn.
21. Cameron, A, Kemp, HG, Fisher, LD, et al: *Left main coronary stenosis. Angiographic determination* (CASS). Circulation 68:484, 1983.
22. Gensini, GG, Kelly, AE, DaCosta, BCB, et al: *Quantitative angiography: The measurement of coronary vasomobility in the intact animal and man.* Chest 60:522, 1971.
23. Brown, BG, Bolson, E, Frimer, M, et al: *Quantitative coronary arteriography.* Circulation 55:329, 1977.
24. McMahon, MM, Brown, BG, Cukingnan, R, et al: *Quantitative coronary angiography: Measurement of the critical stenosis in patients with unstable angina and single vessel disease without collaterals.* Circulation 60:106, 1979.
25. Blankenhorn, DH, and Curry, PJ: *The accuracy of arteriography and ultrasound imaging for atherosclerosis measurement: A review.* Arch Path Lab Med 106:483, 1982.
26. Brooks, SH, Crawford, DW, Selzer, RH, et al: *Discrimination of human arterial pathology by computer processing of angiograms for serial assessment of atherosclerosis change.* Comput Biomed Res 11:469, 1978.
27. Brown, BG, Bolson, E, Peterson, RB, et al: *The mechanisms of nitroglycerin action: Stenosis vasodilatation as a major component of the drug response.* Circulation 64:1089, 1981.
28. Klocke, FJ: *Clinical and experimental evaluation of the functional severity of coronary stenoses.* Council on Clinical Cardiology Newsletter 7 (No 3):1, 1982.
29. Randall, AB, and Kemp, HG: *Coronary arteriography.* In Donoso, E and Gorlin, R (eds): *Current Cardiovascular Topics. III. Angina Pectoris.* Grune & Stratton, New York, 1977, p 100.
30. Hartzler, G: Personal communication.
31. Manchester, JH, Herman, MV, Kemp, HG, et al: *Prevalence of coronary atherosclerosis in valvular heart disease.* Am J Med Sci 263:445, 1972.

The Angiographic Spectrum of Coronary Artery Disease

Guy S. Reeder, M.D., Hugh C. Smith, M.D., Lila R. Elveback, Ph.D., and Michael B. Mock, M.D.

In 1892, William Osler wrote of a relation between angina pectoris and obstructive lesions of the coronary arteries.[1] Clinical knowledge of the coronary anatomy did not attain practical significance, however, until 1959 when Sones demonstrated that high-quality radiographic images of the coronary circulation could be obtained in most patients with an acceptably low risk.[2] This important achievement not only allowed the definitive antemortem diagnosis of coronary artery disease but paved the way for clinical investigations that would establish the natural history of the disease as well as effects of various therapies. Coronary arteriography attained further importance with the development of coronary bypass surgery in 1968. The indications for, and the success of, surgical revascularization are clearly influenced by the severity and location of coronary stenoses as well as other angiographic findings. Knowledge of the detailed coronary angiographic anatomy is also most important in another area of invasive cardiology—that of "catheter therapy." Selection of patients for transluminal coronary angioplasty or intracoronary thrombolysis is made primarily on the basis of the angiographic findings. Nowadays the majority of major clinical management decisions both for patients with unstable angina and for patients with stable angina are based on the results of the coronary and left ventricular angiogram.

Delineation of the coronary anatomy is currently performed for the following reasons: (1) to establish whether coronary artery disease is present; (2) to establish the extent of disease for purposes of risk prognostication; (3) for determination of various treatment options, including medical therapy, coronary revascularization with surgery, angioplasty or thrombolytic therapy; and (4) the evaluation of these therapies. It has been estimated that 400,000 cardiac catheterizations and 110,000 bypass operations are performed yearly.[3] In addition, the application of more recent, catheter therapy procedures is greatly increasing each year. Thus, for these diagnostic and therapeutic considerations, the angiographic spectrum of coronary artery disease will continue to be important in the future.

METHODS

In order to analyze the spectrum of clinical and angiographic findings in patients undergoing coronary arteriography, we turned to our cardiac laboratory data base. This computer data bank stores information on all patients undergoing coronary arteriography at Mayo Clinic. Data is updated quarterly, and the information is stored in a format virtually identical to the Coronary Artery Surgery Study (CASS)[4] in which the Mayo Clinic participated. The CASS registry completed entry of patients in 1979. Clinical data included age, sex, presence and duration of angina pectoris, and angina classification by the Canadian Heart Class.[5] In addition, a Class V angina status was included for angina predominately unrelated to exertion. Angina was classified as unstable if it was of new onset, angina at rest, pain lasting more than 30 minutes, or a changing pattern of intensity or duration. Symptoms of congestive heart failure were assessed as well as information of any recent (1 month) Q wave or non Q wave myocardial infarction.

Angiographic data analyzed for this report included left ventricular ejection fraction as determined by a biplane computer-assisted videometric method.[6] The presence or absence of left ventricular aneurysm, left ventricular mural thrombus, and coexistent valvular disease was also assessed. Coronary arteriographic factors analyzed included coronary vessel dominance, number of vessels diseased (defined as greater than 70 percent luminal diameter narrowing except for the left main coronary artery, which was judged diseased at 50 percent), the maximum stenotic lesion in each patient, results of testing for coronary artery spasm with ergonovine provocation, and the occurrence of less common findings such as myocardial bridging, intracoronary thrombus, and coronary anomalies.

RESULTS

Clinical Data

Our most recent full-year data were assessed. Of 1996 patients undergoing coronary arteriography at the Mayo Clinic in 1982, complete clinical and angiographic data were available on 1628. Four hundred thirty-nine (27 percent) patients were female, and 1189 (73 percent) were male. The median age for females was 62 years and for males 60 years. One hundred thirty-six had coronary arteriography in association with graft angiography; 194 had associ-

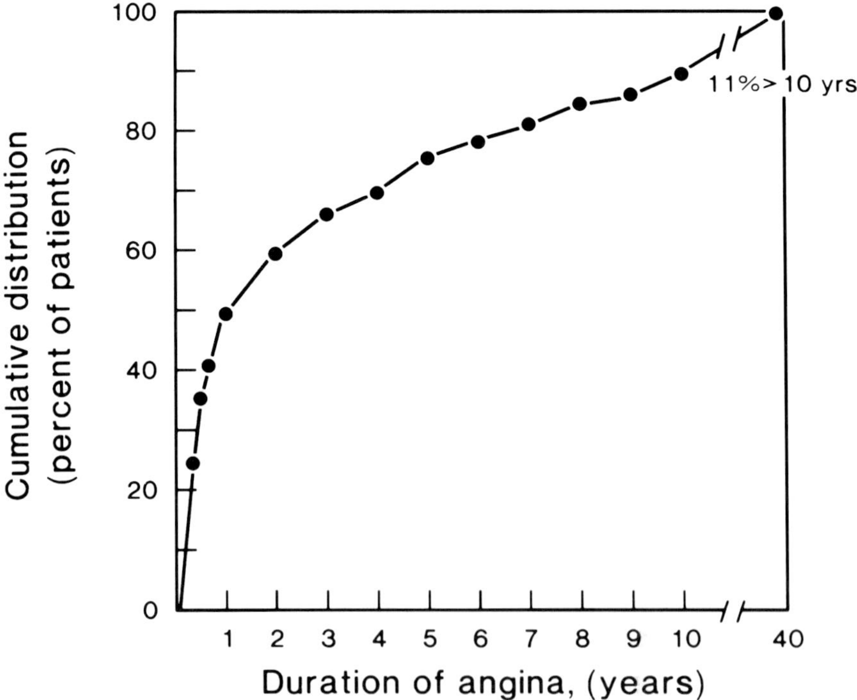

Figure 1. This graph shows the cumulative distribution of duration of angina in 1628 patients undergoing coronary arteriography at the Mayo Clinic during 1982.

Table 1. Angina functional class*

Functional Class	*Patients (%)*
I	5
II	27
III	35
IV	18
Unrelated to exertion	15

*Canadian Cardiovascular Classification

ated ergonovine testing for coronary artery spasm; and in 157 some form of catheter therapy was performed. Of the latter group, 139 underwent transluminal coronary angioplasty, and 18 had intracoronary thrombolysis during acute myocardial infarction.

Definite or probable angina was present in 1303 (80 percent) patients. A median duration of 16 months with a range of less than 1 month to 40 years was observed (Fig. 1). Canadian Heart Association class is demonstrated in Table 1. Ninety-five percent of the patients were Class II or greater. Unstable angina was judged to be present in 397 (37 percent) of the 1303 patients with definite or probable angina.

The classification of congestive heart failure symptoms at the time of catheterization is shown in Table 2. Sixty-two percent of patients had no symptoms of congestive heart failure. Mild symptoms of congestive heart failure were observed in 20 percent of the patients, and moderate to severe symptoms of heart failure occurred in the remaining 18 percent.

The occurrence of previous myocardial infarction was assessed for all patients undergoing coronary angiography. Forty-nine (3 percent) patients had a prior Q wave infarct within 1 month, and 82 (5 percent) patients had a recent (1 month) non Q wave infarct.

A significant number of patients had both prior coronary angiography and coronary artery bypass graft surgery before the current coronary angiogram. Three hundred and thirty-four (20 percent) patients had undergone prior cardiac catheterization. One hundred and sixty (10 percent) had undergone prior coronary bypass grafting. Forty-five (3 percent) had undergone previous valve surgery.

Angiographic Data

The distribution of left ventricular ejection fraction is demonstrated in Figure 2. The mean was 55 percent for patients over age 60 and 57 percent for patients under age 60. Comparison of patients with stable and unstable angina yielded no significant differences. Four hundred and fifty-one (33 percent) patients had an ejection fraction less than 50 percent.

A left ventricular aneurysm was present in 98 (6 percent) patients. The majority of these aneurysms were anteroapical in location.

Left ventricular mural thrombus was seen angiographically in 75 (5 percent) patients. Most often, the thrombus was located within an aneurysm or contiguous to a dyskinetic segment.

Table 2. Congestive heart failure class

Heart Failure	*Patients (%)*
None	62
Mild	20
Moderate	13
Severe	5

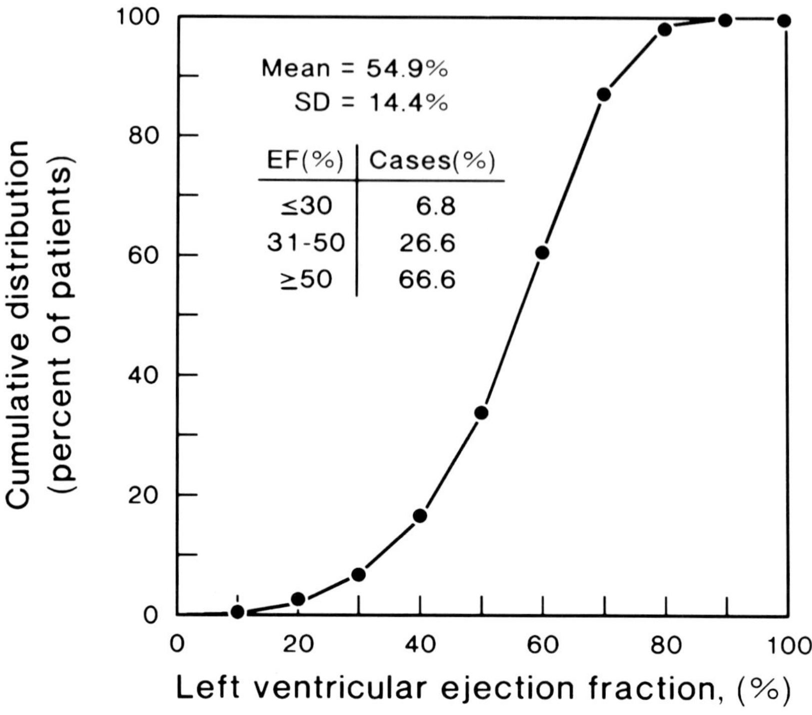

Figure 2. This graph shows the cumulative distribution of ejection fraction in 1628 patients undergoing ventriculography at the Mayo Clinic during 1982.

Coronary artery dominance was left in 9 percent of patients, right in 85 percent of patients, and balanced in 6 percent. Significant left main coronary artery disease (defined as greater than 50 percent diameter obstruction) was present in 138 (8.5 percent) patients. No difference in the prevalence of left main coronary artery disease was present comparing unstable angina pectoris with stable angina pectoris.

Table 3 demonstrates the distribution of diseased vessels. Twenty-seven percent had no significant disease present in any vessel (one half of this subgroup had totally normal coronary

Table 3. Coronary angiographic findings

Extent of Disease	*Mayo* (%)*	*CASS† (%)*
Nonsignificant‡	27§	29
Significant		
one-vessel disease	20	20
two-vessel disease	22	22
three-vessel disease	31	29
Total	100	100
Left main disease	8.5	8

*1982

†1975–1979

‡Significant disease defined as greater than or equal to 70% luminal diameter narrowing in a major epicardial artery and greater than or equal to 50% luminal diameter narrowing of the left main coronary artery.

§Approximately one half (13%) of this group had totally normal coronary arteries.

Table 4. Vessels diseased in stable versus unstable angina*

Vessels Diseased	*Stable (%)*	*Unstable (%)*
0	30	19
1	22	25
2	25	27
3	23	29
Total	100	100

*p <0.01

arteries). Single vessel disease was present in 20 percent, double vessel disease in 22 percent, and three vessel disease in the remaining 31 percent. Table 4 shows the distribution of number of vessels diseased for stable and unstable angina groups. Patients with unstable angina had somewhat more extensive obstructive disease ($p < 0.01$). Table 5 shows the distribution of the maximal stenosis in stable and unstable patient groups. Results are further subdivided into patients over and under the median age of 60. Older patients and patients with unstable angina have a higher mean maximal stenoses ($p < 0.01$).

Ergonovine testing for coronary artery spasm was performed in 194 (12 percent) patients. Most of these patients presented with predominately rest or atypical angina. In 19 (10 percent) of this group, coronary artery spasm was provoked in the laboratory with associated ischemic pain and electrocardiographic ST segment elevation. In 175 patients, the administration of ergonovine resulted in no focal coronary artery narrowings. Ergonovine was administered intravenously, using stepwise doses of 0.1 mg to a total dose of 0.55 mg. No complication attributable to ergonovine testing occurred in this series of patients.

Systolic myocardial bridging was observed in 27 (1.5 percent) patients. The middle portion of the left anterior descending artery was involved in almost all cases. Bridging was not believed to be the cause of myocardial ischemia in any patient in this series.

Congenital anomalies of the coronary circulation were present in 36 (2 percent) patients. The most common coronary anomaly was absence of the left main coronary artery with side-by-side origins of the circumflex and left anterior descending vessels (19 patients). Origin of the circumflex artery from the proximal right coronary artery or near its origin occurred in 9 patients. Four patients had a coronary to pulmonary artery fistula. The remaining 14 patients had a variety of anomalies, including abnormal location of a coronary ostium in 5 cases, a single coronary artery in 1 case, and the right coronary artery arising from the left sinus of Valsalva in 3 cases. Myocardial ischemia was not believed to be due directly to a coronary anomaly in any patient in this series.

Intracoronary arterial thrombus was present in 81 (4 percent) patients. Thrombus occurred more commonly in patients with unstable angina pectoris or prior recent myocardial infarction.

Table 5. Maximum stenosis in stable versus unstable angina*

	Stable Angina		*Unstable Angina*	
Maximum Stenosis	*>Median Age†*	*<Median Age†*	*>Median Age†*	*<Median Age†*
<50%	16%	26%	8%	7%
≥70%	81%	71%	90%	81%
≥90%	72%	64%	86%	75%
Total occlusion	48%	43%	59%	52%

*p <0.02
†60

One hundred and sixty patients underwent saphenous vein bypass graft angiography as part of the coronary arteriography procedure series. In 136 patients this study was clinically indicated, and in the remainder it was a part of a long-term followup study in a graft patency drug intervention trial.

COMMENTS

In patients with clinical suspicion or evidence of coronary artery disease, definition of the coronary anatomy can be useful in a number of ways. First, in the patient with a nonclassical or atypical angina pain pattern, the presence or absence of significant coronary arterial narrowings can be documented. This evaluation may include provocative testing for coronary artery spasm with ergonovine maleate administration. For maximum sensitivity, care must be taken to avoid administration of nitrates or calcium channel blockers prior to ergonovine testing. The low incidence of positive ergonovine responders in our series reflects the rarity of documented coronary artery spasm in proportion to significant fixed lesions as seen in our practice.

Secondly, definition of the coronary angiographic anatomy in patients with stable and unstable angina pectoris allows some estimation of the patient's prognosis. Numerous investigations have defined the natural history of patients with angiographically proven coronary artery lesions.[7–14] In spite of major differences in the design of these studies, which were performed at different times in relation to the evolution of medical and surgical treatment modalities, they report similar conclusions that allow generalizations about prognosis based on the number of diseased vessels and the extent of impairment of ventricular function. The most recent and largest natural history study is the report of the survival of medically treated patients in the Coronary Artery Surgery Study (CASS).[15] This report was based on 20,088 patients without previous coronary artery bypass graft surgery enrolled from 15 centers between 1975 and 1979. The 4-year survival of medically treated patients with no significant obstructive disease was 97 percent. The cumulative survival of patients with one-vessel, two-vessel, and three-vessel disease was 92 percent, 84 percent, and 68 percent, respectively (Fig. 3). This cumulative survival of medically treated patients was better than all previous reports but similar to the experience of the Duke University data bank.[16]

In the CASS study, left ventricular function as determined by ejection fraction had an important effect on survival. Within the traditional one-vessel, two-vessel, and three-vessel disease subgroups, the ejection fraction was a very important and independent predictor of survival. For each ejection fraction category, survival decreased according to the number of vessels obstructed (Fig. 4). Thus with single-vessel or double-vessel disease, patients had in general a good prognosis, but a high-risk subgroup with severely depressed ejection fraction could be identified. Likewise, patients with three-vessel disease and normal ejection fraction were at lower risk of death than those with similar coronary anatomy and reduced left ventricular function.

The natural history of patients with unstable angina pectoris is more difficult to define. One major problem is that the unstable angina group includes many subsets—such as patients with new onset angina, patients with progressive or medically refractory angina, patients presenting primarily with rest angina that may be due to coronary artery spasm, and finally patients presenting with prolonged ischemic pain without evidence of myocardial infarction (the so-called "impending myocardial infarction" or "intermediate syndrome"). Studies reported in the literature differ in their definition of unstable angina, with patient selection performed in many at different times in the evolution of medical and surgical treatment modalities.[17–21] Although these studies had differences, it is generally accepted that patients with prolonged, severe, recurrent rest angina are at significantly increased risk of death, myocardial infarction, and continued severe angina pectoris and should have coronary angiography to define the coronary anatomy and ventricular function.

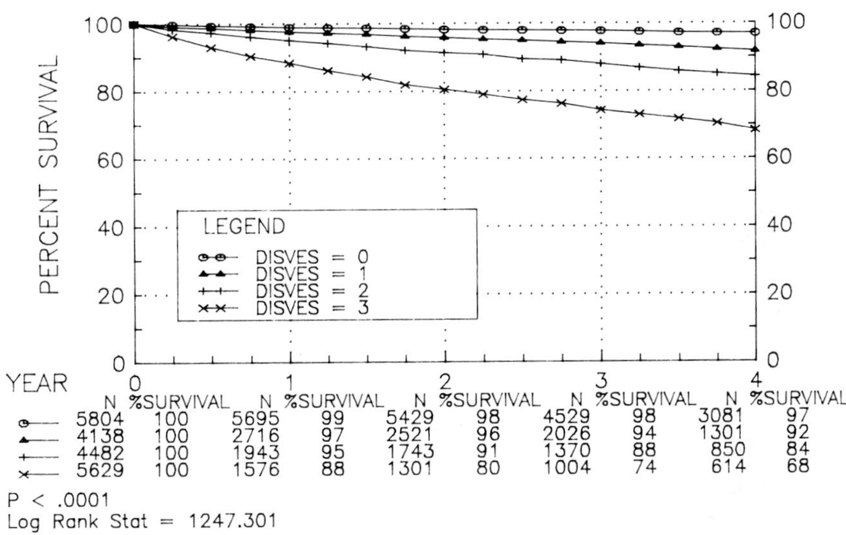

Figure 3. This graph shows the cumulative 4-year survival of all the medically treated CASS registry patients. Four groups are shown on the basis of angiographic extent of coronary obstructive diseases. DISVES = diseased vessels. (From Mock, Ringqvist, Fisher, et al,[15] with permission.)

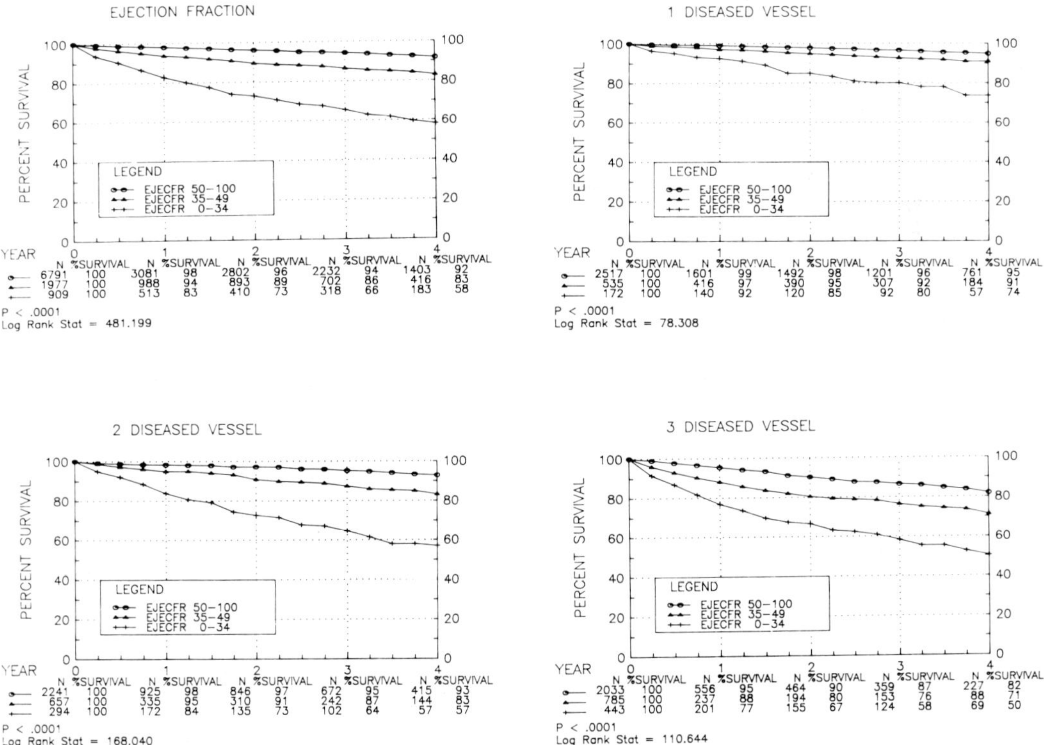

Figure 4. These graphs show the 4-year survival data for patients with at least one-vessel disease, less than 50 percent left main coronary artery obstruction, and a measured ejection fraction (EJECFR). (From Mock, Ringqvist, Fisher, et al,[15] with permission.)

Delineation of the coronary anatomy and ventricular function is useful for selection of treatment modalities in both unstable and stable angina pectoris. The results of four major randomized trials comparing medical therapy versus surgical therapy of patients with symptomatic coronary artery disease are currently available for analysis.[15,22–24] In the NHLBI National Cooperative Unstable Angina Study,[21,22] 288 patients enrolled from 1974 to 1976 with severe prolonged rest angina were randomized to medical or surgical therapy. Patients with left main coronary artery stenoses greater than 50 percent luminal diameter obstruction were excluded. Twenty-four percent of patients in both the medical and surgical groups had single-vessel disease. Thirty-seven percent of the medical patients and 33 percent of the surgical patients had double-vessel disease, and 39 percent of the medical patients and 43 percent of the surgical patients had triple-vessel disease. Figure 5 demonstrates subsequent survival at 48 months. Although no significant difference in survival was observed, 36 percent of the patients assigned to medical therapy crossed over to surgical therapy by 30 months of followup. Although subsequent symptoms and this high rate of medical therapy to surgical therapy cross-over suggest a better long-term symptomatic result with surgical therapy, definite conclusions concerning the efficacy of surgical management with respect to survival are problematic. Myocardial infarction after hospital discharge was comparable in the two treatment groups. Also, no significant differences were found for patients with ST segment elevation as opposed to ST segment depression during pain or in a subset of patients with left anterior descending coronary artery disease.

Currently acceptable medical management for patients presenting with unstable angina includes prompt hospitalization and intensive medical therapy with nitrates, beta blockers and/or calcium channel blockers. On this program, approximately 80 percent will stabilize. In these patients, coronary arteriography should be performed within a few days of hospitalization; and if severe three-vessel disease or left main coronary artery obstruction is present, early coronary bypass surgery is advised. With single- or double-vessel disease and adequate control of symptoms by medical therapy, surgery may be postponed according to the patient's

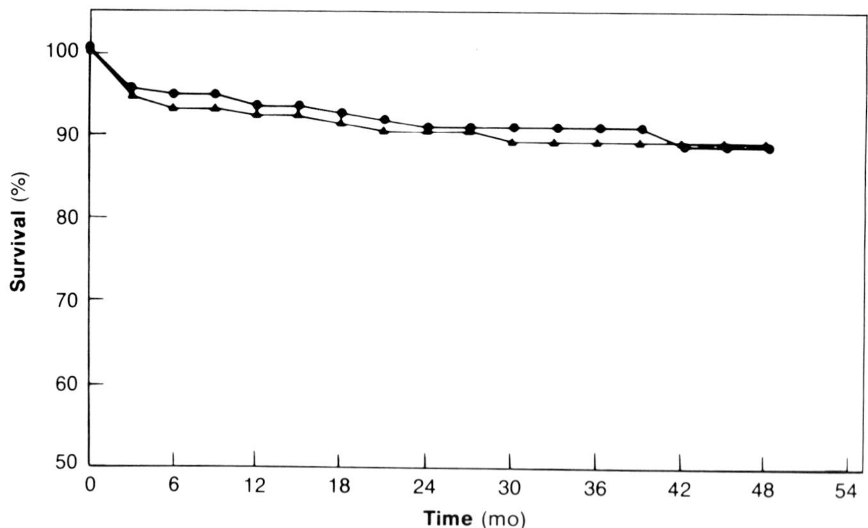

Figure 5. This graph shows survival data of patients having unstable angina. Data from the NHLBI study show that 4-year survival rates are similar for medically and surgically treated patients. However, 36 percent of the medically assigned patients had coronary bypass operations by the second year of the study, so these results should be interpreted cautiously. (Circles = medical treatment; triangles = surgical treatment.) (From Mock, MB, Fisher, LD, Detre, KM, et al: *Bypass surgery or medical therapy? Implications of randomized trials.* Journal of Cardiovascular Medicine 7(9), 1982, with permission.)

symptoms with no increased risk of death or nonfatal myocardial infarction. The role that coronary angioplasty will play in the treatment of patients with unstable angina appears promising but has not been established.

Randomized trials of medical and surgical therapies in chronic stable angina have also been reported. The Veterans Administration (VA) Cooperative Study of Coronary Artery Surgery[23] randomized 686 men with stable angina to medical or surgical therapy. At 5-year followup, the cumulative survival of the patients with left main coronary artery obstruction treated surgically was significantly greater than for those treated medically (90 percent versus 60 percent). This study also reported a probable advantage of surgery in triple-vessel disease without left main coronary artery obstruction, if data from centers with high surgical mortality were excluded from analysis. In a clinically high-risk subgroup of patients, 17 percent of the surgically treated patients died within 5 years, compared with 34 percent of medically treated patients.

In the European Study of Coronary Artery Surgery,[24] 768 men with at least 50 percent luminal diameter obstruction in at least two coronary arteries were randomized to medical or surgical therapy. Again, patients with left main coronary artery obstruction and three-vessel disease randomized to surgery showed better cumulative survival than those treated medically. At 5-year followup, angina relief was significantly better in the surgical group.

Figure 6 shows the comparative survival curves of patients with left main coronary artery disease assigned to medical and surgical therapies for both the VA and European Coronary Artery Surgery studies. Figure 7 shows the survival of patients with three-vessel coronary artery disease for these two studies.

The CASS study[15] also has a randomized study in which patients who presented with mild angina (Class I and Class II) and patients who were asymptomatic following an acute myocardial infarction were randomized to either medical therapy or coronary artery bypass graft surgery. The results of this prospective randomized trial, which enrolled 780 patients, were reported in 1983.*

Knowledge of the detailed coronary anatomy is essential for selection of patients for newer catheter-related therapeutic techniques such as transluminal coronary angioplasty or intracoronary thrombolytic therapy. Initially, coronary angioplasty was limited to symptomatic patients with proximal, concentric, noncalcified stenosis in a single artery. However, with increasing experience and continued improvements in equipment, less stringent angiographic criteria for angioplasty are evolving. Currently, some patients with multiple eccentric lesions in one or more vessels[25] and even patients with recent total occlusion[26] of a coronary artery may benefit from PTCA. However, revascularization with bypass grafting is still considered the optimal treatment for most of these patients.

Intracoronary thrombolytic therapy has been performed in patients with acute or impending myocardial infarction in whom intracoronary thrombus has been demonstrated angiographically at the time of catheterization. Occluding thrombus has been found in a high percentage of patients in the early hours of acute myocardial infarction.[27] In our series, intracoronary thrombus was also seen significantly more frequently in patients with recent (within 1 month) prior myocardial infarction and those patients with severely unstable angina. It is almost never seen in patients with chronic stable angina without prior infarction. In most cases, the thrombus is immediately distal to a high-grade stenosis. In patients with medically refractory unstable angina with associated subtotally obstructing thrombus, selective streptokinase infusion alone or with PTCA is a consideration, but adequate documentation of its efficacy in this clinical setting is not yet available.

One hundred sixty patients in our series (10 percent) were restudied for determination of coronary artery bypass graft patency. Because there is a 5 percent yearly angina recurrence

---

*Coronary Artery Surgery Study (CASS): *A randomized trial of coronary artery bypass surgery.* Circulation 68(5), 939–950, 1983.

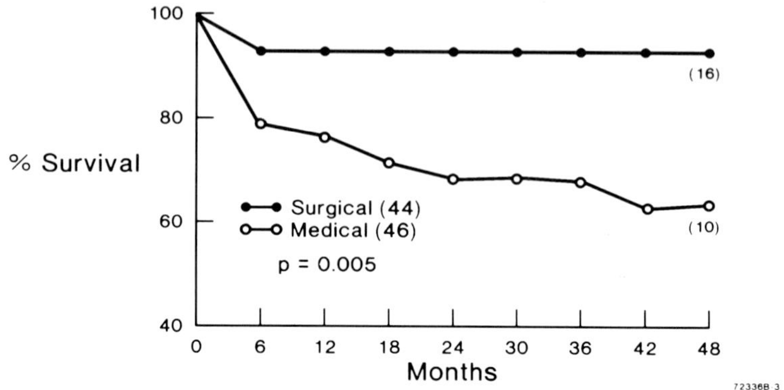

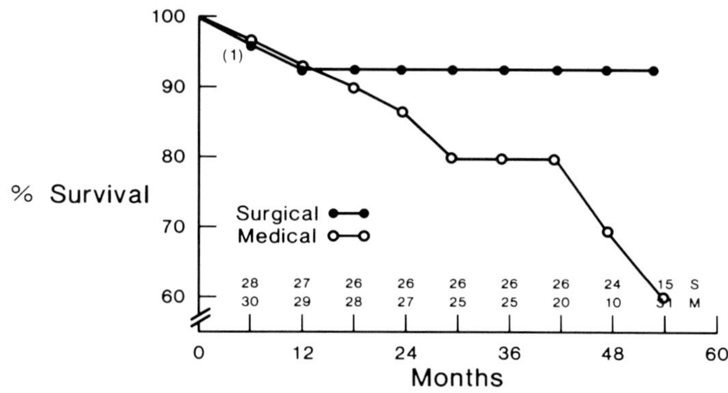

Figure 6. Shown here is a comparison of data on the survival of patients having LMCA obstruction. Comparing surgical treatment with medical treatment of left main coronary obstruction of 50 percent or greater shows that cumulative survival for patients who undergo operation is significantly greater than for those who do not. *Top,* Veterans Administration Study; *bottom,* European Cooperative Study. (Solid circles = surgical treatment; open circles = medical treatment.) (From Mock, MB, Fisher, LD, Detre, KM, et al: *Bypass surgery or medical therapy? Implications of randomized trials.* Journal of Cardiovascular Medicine 7(9), 1982, with permission.)

rate in patients following bypass surgery,[28] we can expect with time a progressively increasing proportion of patients undergoing repeat angiography for angina recurrence after surgery. Analysis of our own annual angiographic data over the past several years has confirmed this trend.[3] Angina recurrence may be due to progression of disease in ungrafted vessels[29] or may be due to vein graft failure. The incidence and severity of this latter problem may be effectively decreased with platelet inhibitors.[30]

Our most recent (1982) clinical, demographic, and catheterization findings, as reported above, do not differ significantly from those reported for CASS, which enrolled patients from 1975 through 1979.[4] Thirteen percent of our patients had totally normal coronary arteries

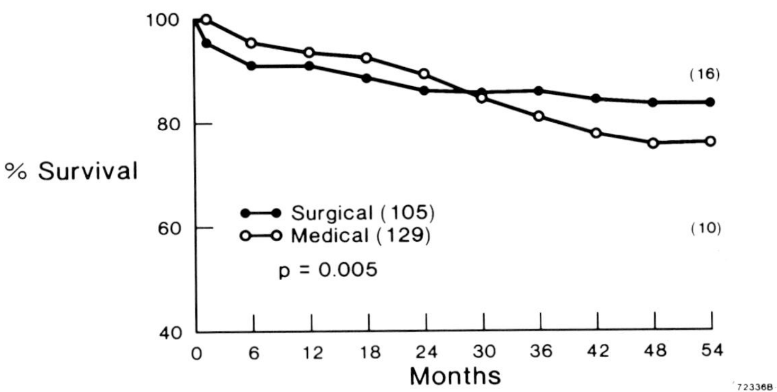

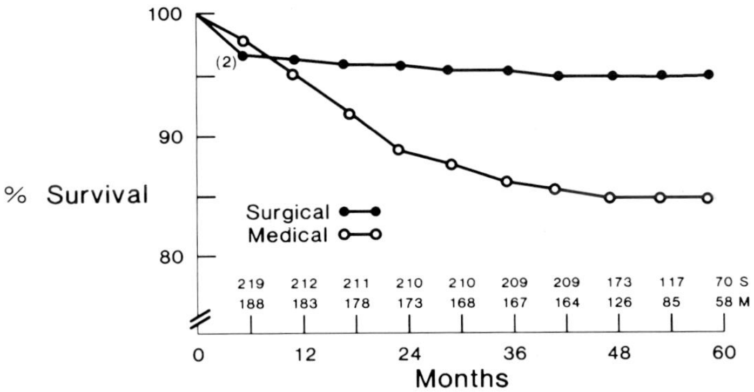

Figure 7. Shown here is a comparison of data on the survival of patients having three-vessel disease. The Veterans Administration Study *(top)* of 105 surgically treated and 129 medically treated patients shows improved cumulative survival rate after operation, but the difference is not statistically significant. In contrast, the European Cooperative Study *(bottom)* shows a distinct improvement in survival rates after operation. (Solid circles = surgical treatment; open circles = medical treatment.) (From Mock, MB, Fisher, LD, Detre, KM, et al: *Bypass surgery or medical therapy? Implications of randomized trials.* Journal of Cardiovascular Medicine 7(9), 1982, with permission.)

compared with 19 percent in the CASS group. Twenty percent of the patients had single-vessel disease, 22 percent had double-vessel disease, and 31 percent had triple-vessel disease; compared with 20 percent, 22 percent, and 29 percent, respectively, in the CASS group. Although patients with unstable angina had an increase in the number of vessels diseased and severity of lesions when compared with the angiographic findings in patients with stable angina, these differences were not large, in agreement with a prior study.[31] Intracoronary thrombus was seen more frequently ($p < 0.01$) in patients with unstable angina than in those with stable angina. However, only a small proportion of those with unstable angina had thrombus found at angiography. The generally accepted management of unstable angina has been previously discussed. In our practice, patients with unstable angina are medically stabilized and undergo angiography with consideration of early revascularization. Those with suitable anatomy may have coronary angioplasty at the time of angiography if cardiac surgical backup is available. It is our experience and that of others[32] that angioplasty is efficacious in patients with unstable angina when there is a high-grade fixed lesion. When rest angina is due to coronary artery spasm with only minor fixed lesions, angioplasty is less helpful.[33]

The prevalence of documented coronary artery spasm was low in our group of patients. As alluded above, this observation most likely represents the preponderance of coronary atherosclerosis as a problem in this and most Western nations. Because of the high rate of restenosis reported with PTCA in patients with coronary spasm and variant angina,[33] this group of patients is not usually considered for PTCA.

Myocardial bridging (muscular systolic arterial compression) was observed in 27 patients. The typical appearance is a symmetric, smooth systolic compression that may be variable in length, ranging from less than one to several centimeters. Occasionally, a beaded-like systolic appearance is present. A wide variety of angiographic prevalence (0.5 percent to 12 percent) and pathologic prevalence (5 percent to 86 percent) has been reported.[34] Pathologic bridging can be of two types: a truly intramyocardial course of an epicardial vessel, or an epicardial course with a few aberrant muscle fibers encircling and tethering the vessels to the epicardium. Myocardial bridging is usually considered to be a benign condition, though occasionally it appears that with high degrees of systolic compression and a long length of bridging segments, myocardial ischemia may result, especially at rapid heart rates.[35,36] Myocardial bridging was not considered to be responsible for ischemic symptoms in any of the patients in our 1-year series.

The frequency and types of congenital coronary arterial anomalies encountered were generally similar to a large series reported by Vlodaver.[37] The most common finding was an absent left main coronary artery with side-by-side origin of the left anterior descending and circumflex arteries from the left coronary cusp. Occasionally, selective catheter engagement of one vessel will totally fail to opacify the other, and it may mistakenly be thought to be occluded. A high index of suspicion and flush injections in the left coronary sinus may be necessary to elucidate the anatomy. The next most common anomaly was origin of the circumflex artery from the right coronary sinus. Frequently, the initial portion of the circumflex artery is small and/or atherosclerotically diseased.

Coronary artery fistulas usually arise from a major epicardial branch and drain to a cardiac chamber, most frequently the right ventricle. We observed four cases of drainage into the pulmonary trunk in this series. Occasionally, when flow through the fistula is large, myocardial ischemia may occur. A fortunately rare anomaly is origin of a coronary artery from the pulmonary artery. In this situation, there is reversed flow in the aberrant artery as it functionally drains into the low-pressure pulmonary circulation. Major myocardial ischemia and necrosis have been demonstrated with this lesion. The occurrence of angina in adolescence with or without myocardial infarction or ischemic left ventricular dysfunction should suggest the possibility of this anatomic variant. Other unusual findings in our series included spontaneous right coronary artery dissection in three cases, which had resulted in myocardial infarction. Spontaneous dissection is extremely rare and must be differentiated from coronary dissection occurring as a complication of the catheterization procedure. In this series, an additional two patients had significant focal aneurysmal coronary artery disease. In both cases, the etiology appeared to be atherosclerotic and not due to Kawasaki's disease.

Delineation of the coronary anatomy should include provocative testing for coronary artery spasm with ergonovine maleate if a patient with ischemic pain has normal or minimally obstructed coronary arteries. It has become increasingly clear that abnormal coronary vasomotion may play a prominent part in predominately rest angina as well as exercise-induced angina and may be superimposed upon variable degrees of underlying fixed coronary artery stenoses. Periodic attacks of rest angina owing to coronary artery spasm may occasionally be encountered in young individuals with little or no fixed obstructive disease. Attacks may be clustered over a period of time (so-called "hot" and "cold" phases). A significant diurnal variation may occur, with peak activity in the early morning hours. Continuous ambulatory monitoring of these patients may show ST segment shifts both during symptoms and at other times in the absence of ischemic pain.[38]

Older patients with coronary risk factors, significant fixed lesions, and exercise angina who become unstable with prolonged episodes of pain represent the other end of the spectrum with lesser degrees of spasm superimposed on their atherosclerotic disease. In these patients, the stimulus for spasm may be related to potent vasoconstrictor substances derived from platelet activation. Still other patients may present with atypical angina in which moderate fixed lesions are made hemodynamically significant by exercise or catecholamine-related vasomotion. Provocative testing with ergonovine maleate may be indicated to document spasm in these groups of patients, though care should be taken in patients with high-grade fixed coronary obstructive lesions. Although death resulting from ergonovine testing has been reported, in our series of over 500 patients spanning several years, we have had rare transient complications (for example, arrhythmia) but no infarctions, deaths, or significant complications.

SUMMARY

A wide spectrum of coronary arteriographic anatomic findings exists in patients presenting with clinically stable and unstable angina pectoris. Although some generalizations about the clinical-angiographic correlations can be made, we are continuously reminded of the frequent individual patient whose findings fall well outside of these generalizations. The majority of patients will have double- or triple-vessel coronary disease, with approximately 10 percent having in addition a left main coronary artery stenosis of at least 50 percent luminal diameter narrowing. Patients with unstable angina tend to have slightly greater vessel involvement in terms of lesion severity, though major differences, in general, are not seen. Intracoronary thrombus is present more frequently in patients with unstable angina and in those with recent myocardial infarction, though the overall incidence of this finding is low. Knowledge of the anatomic extent of coronary atherosclerosis is useful for determining prognosis and for selection from an ever-increasing variety of medical and surgical treatment options.

Cardiac imaging is a continuously evolving field with new techniques such as digital angiography, three-dimensional dynamic imaging (dynamic spatial reconstructor), and nuclear magnetic resonance undergoing preclinical or clinical evaluation. These modalities hold promise for ultimately evaluating the coronary vessels from unlimited angles, assessing regional transmural myocardial perfusion and the cellular metabolic consequences of ischemia. However, current therapies (bypass surgery or coronary angioplasty) are based upon modifications of major epicardial coronary anatomy, and techniques that adequately define this anatomy are required. Moreover, for imaging data to have prognostic application, it must have previously established clinical prognostic correlates and be broadly applicable or widely available for patients. Thus for the present and immediate foreseeable future, coronary angiography will be the primary method for establishing the anatomic abnormalities of the coronary arteries, and these angiographic studies will remain vital for the clinical management of ischemic heart disease.

REFERENCES

1. Osler, W: *The Principles and Practice of Medicine.* Appleton, New York, 1892.
2. Sones, FM Jr: *Acquired heart disease; symposium on present and future of cineangiocardiography.* Am J Cardiol 3:710, 1959.

3. Kennedy, RH, Kennedy, MA, Frye, RL, et al: *Cardiac catheterization and cardiac surgical facilities: Use, trends, and future requirements.* N Engl J Med 307:986, 1982.

4. Killip, T, Fisher, LD, and Mock, MB, (eds): *NHLBI coronary artery surgery study. A multicenter comparison of the effects of randomized medical and surgical treatment of mildly symptomatic patients with coronary artery disease, and a registry of consecutive patients undergoing coronary angiography.* Circulation 63(Part II):1–81, 1981.

5. Campeau, L: *Grading of angina pectoris.* Circulation 54:522, 1976.

6. Ritman, EL, Sturm, RE, and Wood, EH: *Biplane roentgen vidometric system for dynamic (60/sec.) studies of the shape and size of the circulatory structures, particularly the left ventricle.* Am J Cardiol 33:180, 1973.

7. Freisinger, GC, Page, EE, and Ross, RS: *Prognostic significance of coronary arteriography.* Trans Assoc Am Phys 83:78, 1970.

8. Oberman, A, Jones, WB, Riley, CP, et al: *Natural history of coronary artery disease.* Bull New York Acad Med 48:1109, 1972.

9. Moberg, CH, Webster, JS, and Sones, FM Jr: *Natural history of severe proximal coronary disease as defined by cineangiography.* Am J Cardiol 29:283, 1972.

10. Lichtlen, PR and Moccetti, T: *Prognostic aspects of coronary angiography.* Circulation 45(Suppl II): II-7, 1972.

11. Bruschke, AVG, Proudfit, WL, and Sones, FM Jr: *Progress study of 590 consecutive nonsurgical cases of coronary disease followed 5.9 years. I. Arteriographic correlations.* Circulation 47:1147, 1973.

12. Ross, RS, Freisinger, GC, Page, EE, et al: *The natural history of coronary artery disease. Clinical correlation with arteriographic findings.* Med J Australia (Special Suppl) 2:6, 1972.

13. Proudfit, WL, Bruscke, AVG, and Sones, FM Jr: *Natural history of obstructive coronary artery disease: Ten-year study of 602 nonsurgical cases.* Prog Cardiovasc Dis 21:53, 1978.

14. Vlietstra, RE, Assad-Morell, JL, Frye, RL, et al: *Survival predictors in coronary artery disease: Medical and surgical comparisons.* Mayo Clin Proc 52:85, 1977.

15. Mock, MB, Ringqvist, I, Fisher, LD, et al: *Survival of medically treated patients in the Coronary Artery Surgery Study (CASS) registry.* Circulation 66:562, 1982.

16. Harris, PJ, Harrell, FE Jr, Lee, KL, et al: *Survival in medically treated coronary disease.* Circulation 60:1259, 1979.

17. Bertolasi, CA, Trong, JE, Carreno, CA, et al: *Unstable angina—prospective and randomized study of its evolution with and without surgery. Preliminary report.* Am J Cardiol 33:201, 1974.

18. Bertolasi, CA, Trong, JE, Riccitelli, MI, et al: *Natural history of unstable angina with medical or surgical therapy.* Chest 70:596, 1976.

19. Selden, R, Neill, WA, Ritzmann, LW, et al: *Medical versus surgical therapy for acute coronary insufficiency: A randomized study.* N Engl J Med 293:1329, 1975.

20. Pugh, B, Platt, MR, Mills, LJ, et al: *Unstable angina pectoris: A randomized study of patients treated medically and surgically.* Am J Cardiol 41:1291, 1978.

21. *Unstable angina pectoris: National Cooperative Study Group to compare medical and surgical therapy. I. Report of protocol and patient population.* Am J Cardiol 37:896, 1976.

22. *Unstable angina pectoris: National Cooperative Study Group to compare surgical and medical therapy. II. In-hospital experience and initial follow-up results in patients with one, two, and three vessel disease.* Am J Cardiol 42:839, 1978.

23. Murphy, ML, Hultgren, HN, Detre, K, et al: *Treatment of chronic stable angina: A preliminary report of survival data of the randomized Veterans Administration Cooperative Study.* N Engl J Med 297:621, 1977.

24. European Coronary Surgery Study Group: *Prospective randomized study of coronary artery bypass surgery in stable angina pectoris (second interim report).* Lancet 2:491, 1980.

25. Vlietstra, RE, Holmes, DR Jr, Mock, MB, et al: *Balloon angioplasty in multivessel coronary disease: Mayo Clinic experience.* J Am Coll Cardiol 1:656, 1983.

26. Holmes, DR Jr, Vlietstra, RE, Reeder, GS, et al: *Elective percutaneous transluminal coronary angioplasty of total coronary arterial occlusions not associated with acute infarction.* J Am Coll Cardiol 1:656, 1983.

27. DeWood, M, Spores, J, Notske, R, et al: *Prevalence of total coronary occlusion during the early hours of transmural myocardial infarction.* N Engl J Med 303:897, 1980.

28. Bourassa, MG, Campeau, L, Lesperance, J, et al: *Changes in grafts and coronary arteries after saphenous vein aorto-coronary bypass surgery: Results at repeat angiography.* Circulation 65(Suppl II):II-90, 1980.

29. Pasternak, R, Cohn, K, Selzer, A, et al: *Enhanced rate of progression of coronary artery disease following aorto-coronary saphenous vein bypass surgery.* Am J Med 58:166, 1975.

30. Chesebro, JH, Clements, IP, Fuster, V, et al: *A platelet-inhibitor-drug trial in coronary-artery bypass operations: Benefit of perioperative dipyridamole and aspirin therapy on early postoperative vein graft patency.* N Engl J Med 307:73, 1982.

31. Fuster, V, Connolly, DC, Frye, RL, et al: *Angiographic patterns early in the onset of coronary syndrome.* Br Heart J 37:1250, 1975.

32. Faxon, D: Workshop on Percutaneous Transluminal Coronary Angioplasty. Personal communication, May 1983.

33. David, PR, Waters, DD, Scholl, JM, et al: *Percutaneous transluminal coronary angioplasty in patients with variant angina.* Circulation 66:695, 1982.

34. Kramer, JR, Kitazume, H, Proudfit, WL, et al: *Clinical significance of isolated coronary bridges: Benign and frequent conditions involving the left anterior descending artery.* Am Heart J 103:283, 1982.

35. Noble, J, Bourassa, MG, Petitclerc, R, et al: *Myocardial bridging and milking effect on the left anterior descending coronary artery: Normal variant or obstruction?* Am J. Cardiol 37:993, 1976.

36. Ahmad, M, Merry, SL, and Haibach, H: *Evidence of impaired myocardial perfusion and abnormal left ventricular function during exercise in patients with systolic narrowing of the left anterior descending coronary artery.* Am J Cardiol 48:832, 1981.

37. Vlodaver, Z, Neufeld, H, and Edwards, J: *Coronary Arterial Variation in the Normal Heart and in Congenital Heart Disease.* Academic Press, New York, 1975.

38. Maseri, A, Serveri, S, DeNes, M, et al: *"Variant" angina: One aspect of a continuous spectrum of vasospastic myocardial ischemia. Pathogenetic mechanisms, estimated incidence and clinical and coronary arteriographic findings in 138 patients.* Am J Cardiol 42:1019, 1978.

Angiographic Findings after Acute Myocardial Infarction

Lawrence S.C. Griffith, M.D.

Angiographic evaluation of a patient soon after acute myocardial infarction has been done more frequently in recent years. Several reasons for early cardiac catheterization have been given. The postinfarction patient is known to have an increased risk of dying (usually 10 to 12 percent) during the first year after hospital discharge, and some clinicians are concerned that noninvasive techniques are not adequate to identify these high-risk patients. Some centers are proposing early and more vigorous therapeutic intervention that includes intracoronary thrombolysis, angioplasty, and coronary bypass surgery.

This chapter will cover some aspects of early postinfarction angiography and will be in five sections: (1) the extent of coronary artery disease and left ventricular dysfunction; (2) the "infarct" artery and myocardial segment; (3) angiographic findings of patients undergoing a limited exercise electrocardiogram before hospital discharge; (4) contribution of cardiac catheterization findings to predicting outcome after infarction; (5) complications of early coronary arteriography.

EXTENT OF CORONARY ARTERY DISEASE AND LEFT VENTRICULAR DYSFUNCTION

The extent of coronary artery disease in postinfarction patients is shown in Table 1. Multivessel disease is commonly found regardless of whether a significant luminal narrowing is considered to be 50 or 75 percent. Approximately one third of patients will have single-vessel disease, one third double-vessel disease, and one third triple-vessel disease. The prevalence of a 50 percent or greater narrowing in the main left coronary artery is approximately 3 percent. The prevalence of a 50 percent or greater obstruction in the left anterior descending segment before the first septal branch was 57 percent in the Johns Hopkins report[1] and 49 percent in the Gothenburg series.[2,3]

It is very unusual to find a postinfarction patient without a major coronary artery narrowed at least 70 percent. At the time of arteriography, most patients who are initially considered to have normal or insignificant disease of the coronary arteries will have important narrowings identified when special projections are utilized. Coronary segments may be difficult to visualize because of overlapping vessels, and the angiographer would be wise to assume that a significant narrowing will be found in every patient.

Almost all patients recovered from infarction will have on left ventriculography at least one myocardial segment with abnormal wall motion, and most will have an abnormal ejection fraction (EF) on left ventriculography. The frequency distribution of ejection fraction early after infarction is shown in Table 2. The small differences between these three series are likely

Table 1. Extent of coronary artery disease soon after acute myocardial infarction

Artery(s) Narrowed ≥50%	*Baltimore*[1]	*Gothenburg*[2,3]	*Barcelona*[4]	*Amsterdam*[5]	*Total*
One	28 (26%)	36 (29%)	89 (34%)	81 (45%)	234 (35%)
Two	22 (21%)	29 (24%)	86 (33%)	73 (41%)	210 (31%)
Three	56 (53%)	55 (45%)	66 (25%)	25 (14%)	202 (30%)
None	0	3	18 (7%)	0	21 (3%)
	106	123	259	179	667
MLCA	12/106 (11%)	5/123 (4%)	3/259 (1%)	2/179 (1%)	22/667 (3%)

Artery(s) Narrowed ≥70-75%	*Gothenburg*[2,3]	*Alabama*[6]	*Lille*[7]	*Total*
One	48 (39%)	27 (23%)	25 (24%)	100 (29%)
Two	30 (24%)	37 (32%)	46 (43%)	113 (33%)
Three	42 (34%)	51 (44%)	34 (32%)	127 (37%)
None	3 (2%)	22 (2%)	1 (1%)	6 (2%)
	123	117	106	346
MLCA	2/123 (2%)	10/117 (8.5%)	NA	12/240 (5%)

MLCA = main left coronary artery
NA = not available

explained by differing criteria of patient selection for angiography. Less than one third of these patients have an ejection fraction less than 40 percent, and about one half have an EF greater than 50 percent. In the Gothenburg series, the mean EF (± SD) was 53 ± 16 percent. Sixty-seven percent of these patients had at least one akinetic or dyskinetic segment, and 30 percent had evidence of dyskinesis. The dyskinetic segment usually involved the anteroapical segment in the distribution of the left anterior descending artery.[2,3]

The relative contribution of each myocardial segment (left anterior descending—LAD, right—RCA, circumflex—CIRC) can be estimated by comparing the mean ejection fraction of patients with single-vessel coronary disease (see below) who had an infarction prior to angiography (Table 3).[8] If all transmural and nontransmural patients are included, there is little difference in EF among patients with single vessel LAD, RCA, and CIRC disease. Alternatively, if the ejection fractions of patients with transmural infarction (new Q wave) are examined separately, the group with the lowest ejection fraction is comprised of patients with LAD disease, whereas the best ejection fraction is found in patients with circumflex disease. The low EF for the LAD group is due partly to this myocardial segment having the greatest representation in the right anterior oblique (RAO) projection and the circumflex segment the least. A second reason is that the LAD myocardial segment is probably the largest of the three segments. Finally, there is probably more expansion and aneurysmal dil-

Table 2. Frequency distribution of ejection fraction after acute infarction

Ejection Fraction	*Baltimore*[1]	*Barcelona*[4]	*Gothenburg*[2,3]	*Total*
<30%	8 (8%)	44 (17%)	7 (6%)	59 (12%)
30–39%	21 (20%)	51 (20%)	13 (12%)	85 (18%)
40–49%	26 (25%)	71 (27%)	23 (20%)	120 (25%)
≥50%	51 (48%)	93 (36%)	70 (62%)	214 (45%)
	106 pts	259 pts	113 pts	478 pts

Table 3. Ejection fraction in single-vessel infarct patients

	LAD		*RCA*		*CIRC*	
	Pts	*EF*	*Pts*	*EF*	*Pts*	*EF*
All infarct pts	51	53 ± 2*	29	54 ± 2	10	59 ± 5
Q wave infarct pts	31	43 ± 2	26	52 ± 2	10	59 ± 5
		↑ └p <0.005─┘		└p <0.1, ns┘		↑
		└── p <0.001 ──				┘

*Mean ± SEM

atation of the LAD segment (as visualized in RAO projection) than of the other two myocardial segments.

INFARCT ARTERY AND MYOCARDIAL SEGMENT

Prevalence of Total Occlusion

The prevalence of total and subtotal occlusion in the coronary artery responsible for infarction is variable and depends to a considerable extent on the length of time between infarction and subsequent angiography (Fig. 1). In a very large patient series, DeWood and colleagues[9] found 87 percent of infarct arteries to be totally occluded if arteriography was performed within 4 hours of the onset of symptoms. By 24 hours, only 65 percent of patients had total

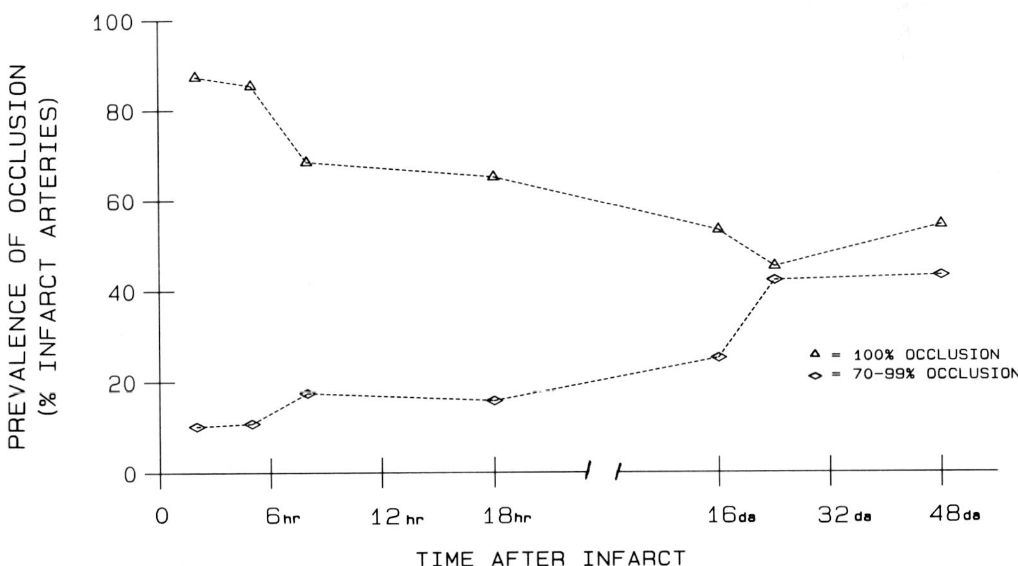

Figure 1. This graph shows the prevalence of total and subtotal occlusion of the coronary artery perfusing the recently infarcted myocardial segment. Data for 0–24 hours after infarction from DeWood;[9] for 16 days, from Bertrand;[7] for 30 days, from Betriu;[4] and for 50 days, from Griffith.[3]

occlusion of the infarct artery. In patient groups undergoing angiography at a mean interval of 16,[6] 30,[7] and 51[2,3] days after admission to the coronary care unit, the prevalence of 100 percent occlusion is 53, 45, and 54 percent, respectively. Not surprisingly, the prevalence of subtotal occlusion (70 to 99 percent narrowing) rises from 10 percent soon after symptoms begin to 43 percent 7 weeks after infarction.

Left Ventriculographic Vascular Territories

Segments of left ventricular silhouettes in both the 30° right anterior oblique projection and 60° left anterior oblique (LAO) projection can be related to specific coronary arteries or major branches.[10] The location of akinetic or dyskinetic segments found in postinfarction patients with single-vessel coronary disease is shown in Figure 2 and in Table 4. Single-vessel disease is defined as one major artery narrowed 70 percent or more while other arteries are narrowed less than 50 percent. For this analysis, an assumption has been made that an akinetic or dyskinetic segment identified on left ventriculography is within the vascular distribution of the single, significantly narrowed coronary artery.

Wall motion of segment 1 is usually preserved in patients with coronary artery disease, regardless of which artery is narrowed or what other myocardial segments are akinetic. Segments 2, 3, 8, and 9 are perfused by the left anterior descending artery. Segment 2 is primarily perfused by LAD diagonal branches, and the apex (segment 3) is almost exclusively perfused by the distal LAD. The proximal and mid portions of the inferior wall (segments 5, 6, 7) are perfused by the right coronary artery in patients with a right dominant or balanced coronary distribution. The more distal inferior wall segments are often perfused by the circumflex marginal coronary artery (segments 4, 5, 6). In the LAO projection, the interventricular septum and apex are perfused by the LAD (segments 8 and 9). The more distal lateral wall (segment 10) is perfused by the left posterior descending artery. The latter is a branch of the RCA if the circulation is right dominant and a branch of the circumflex artery if the circulation is balanced or left dominant. The proximal lateral wall (segment 11) is perfused by the circumflex marginal artery.

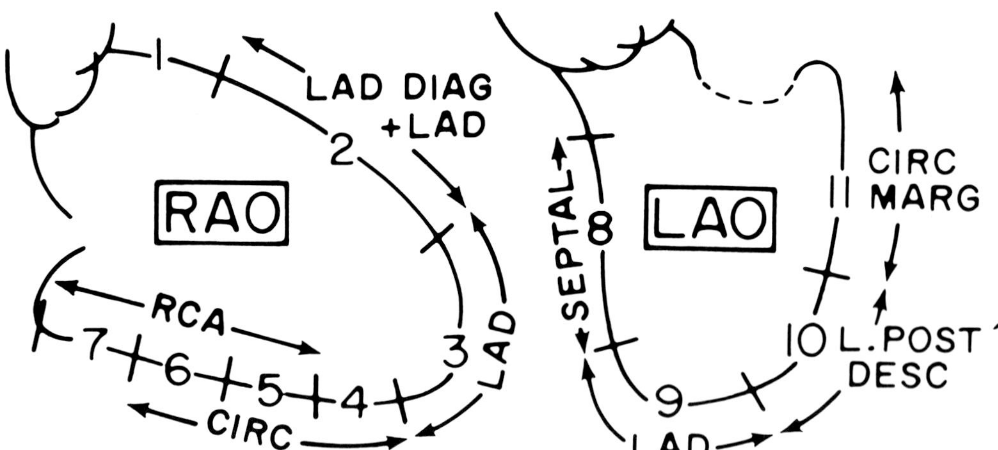

Figure 2. This is a schematic representation of left ventricular vascular segments. (From Griffith, et al,[10] with permission.) Myocardial segments with akinesia or dyskinesia in single vessel coronary disease in 30° RAO and 60° LAO projections are illustrated. LAD = left anterior descending, LAD DIAG = left anterior descending diagonal, CIRC = circumflex, RCA = right coronary artery, L. POST DESC = left posterior descending branch, CIRC MARG = circumflex marginal.

Table 4. Left ventriculographic localization of akinesia or dyskinesia after infarction in patients with single-vessel disease*

		LV Segments (RAO Projection)†						
	Pts	*1*	*2*	*3*	*4*	*5*	*6*	*7*
LAD	28	1‡	23	21	0	0	0	0
RCA	21	0	0	0	6	13	18	19
CIRC	7	0	0	0	2	6	6	0
		LV Segments (LAO Projection)†						
	Pts	*8*	*9*	*10*	*11*			
LAD	22	10‡	21	0	0			
RCA	12	0	0	0	0			
CIRC	7	0	0	4	4			

*From Griffith, et al,[10] with permission.
†See Figure 2
‡Number of patients with akinesia or dyskinesia of segment

Infarct ECG Changes in Single-Vessel Disease

The electrocardiographic changes at the time of infarction in patients with single-vessel disease are shown in Table 5.[11] The appearance of Q waves and ST segment elevation in leads I, AVL, and V1-V4 is characteristic of infarction in the left anterior descending vascular territory, whereas changes in leads II, III, and AVF are found in infarctions in right and circumflex territories. Although it is possible to distinguish LAD-related from right-related or circumflex-related infarctions, there are no ECG changes that permit recognition of right-related from circumflex-related infarctions because both myocardial segments are reflected in the inferior ECG leads.

Because of the high prevalence of "reciprocal" ST segment depression found in some leads at the same time other leads have ST segment elevation, ST segment depression in acute infarct patients cannot be utilized to identify which vascular territory is ischemic or infarcted. Among infarct patients with single-vessel LAD disease, 39 percent had ST segment depression in inferior leads at the same time there was ST segment elevation in anterior leads. In

Table 5. Electrocardiographic changes during acute infarction in single-vessel disease*

Artery Narrowed ≥70%	*ECG Change*	*Pts*	*Patients with ECG Change*										
			I	*AVL*	*V1*	*V2*	*V3*	*V4*	*V5*	*V6*	*II*	*III*	*AVF*
LAD	Q wave	29	10	15	24	27	26	23	11	7	1	1	1
	ST ↑	36	15	17	24	34	31	29	25	15	6	6	6
RCA	Q wave	25	0	0	0	0	0	0	1	4	18	25	24
	ST ↑	16	0	0	3	3	3	2	2	2	12	16	16
CIRC	Q wave	6	0	0	0	0	0	1	3	4	3	5	5
	ST ↑	5	1	0	0	0	0	1	2	2	4	4	5

*From Fuchs, et al,[11] with permission.

patients with right-related and circumflex-related infarctions, 80 and 89 percent, respectively, had ST segment depression in the anterior leads at a time when ST segment elevation was present in the inferior leads. Because reciprocal ST segment depression is so frequent and more than two thirds of infarct patients subsequently are found to have multivessel disease, it is difficult to determine whether ST depression reflects a reciprocal ECG change or subendocardial ischemia in a different noninfarcted vascular territory ("ischemia at a distance"). It is probable that most ST segment depression that occurs simultaneously with ST segment elevation is due to reciprocal changes rather than to ischemia in a different, noninfarcted segment.

Viable and Scarred Myocardium

To determine whether a myocardial segment might be identified on left ventriculography as viable or scarred, Griffith and colleagues[12] examined the clinical findings of 43 patients with single-vessel coronary disease who had an exercise electrocardiogram and thallium-201 perfusion scan. The cardiac catheterization findings were interpreted without knowledge of the exercise test results. Each patient was classified into one of two angiographic groups—either normal or hypokinetic wall motion was present in the distribution of the narrowed artery, or the myocardial segment perfused by the obstructed artery was judged to be entirely akinetic or dyskinetic. Each patient had both rest and postexercise thallium-201 perfusion scans. The occurrence of angina pectoris and 1 mm or more ST segment depression during or after the exercise test was noted.

Most patients with normal or hypokinetic wall motion in the distribution of the narrowed coronary artery developed angina and 1 mm or more ST segment depression during exercise and had a new Tl-201 perfusion defect after exercise (Table 6). The majority of these patients had a normal rest Tl-201 perfusion scan. Conversely, patients with akinesia or dyskinesia of the myocardial segment perfused by the narrowed artery had no angina, no significant ST segment depression, and no new Tl-201 perfusion defect with exercise. Most patients in this second group had a Tl-201 defect at rest. This study suggests that myocardial segments with normal or hypokinetic wall motion are "viable," but akinetic or dyskinetic segments are "scarred."

Table 6. Angina, electrocardiographic, and thallium-201 perfusion findings at exercise test in single-vessel disease patients*

		LV Wall Motion in Territory of Obstructed Coronary Artery		
		Normal or Hypokinetic	*Entirely Akinetic or Dyskinetic*	*p*
Angina during exercise test	Yes	19	3	<0.001
	No	3	18	
ST ↓ during exercise test	Yes	15	1	<0.001
	No	6	19	
Rest ^{201}Tl perfusion defect	Yes	7	16	<0.01
	No	15	5	
New ^{201}Tl perfusion defect after exercise	Yes	17	3	<0.001
	No	5	18	

*From Griffith, et al,[12] with permission.

Postinfarction Angina in Single-Vessel Disease

In patients with single-vessel disease, angina pectoris after acute infarction may depend on the "completeness" of the infarction of the myocardial segment that is perfused by the narrowed coronary artery. Kalus and colleagues[13] examined the left ventriculographic findings of patients recovered from acute infarction who at angiography had single-vessel right or left anterior descending coronary disease. Each patient included in this study had the significant coronary narrowing proximal to all major branches. Utilizing a modification of the method of Feild and colleagues,[14] the length of the akinetic segment was measured at end-diastole in the RAO projection and was expressed as a percentage of the left ventricular silhouette (minus the aortic valve length). All patients had maximal exercise ECG tests, and the presence or absence of angina pectoris and ST segment depression during this test was noted. When the left ventriculographic findings of patients with and without angina were compared, patients without angina were found to have large akinetic or dyskinetic segments, whereas patients with angina had smaller akinetic segments (Fig. 3). The two LAD patients with angina and large akinetic segments on RAO ventriculogram had preserved septal wall motion noted on the LAO ventriculogram. Eleven of 15 patients who had angina during exercise testing also had 1 mm or more ST segment depression on their ECGs. None of the 15 patients without angina had significant ST segment depression.

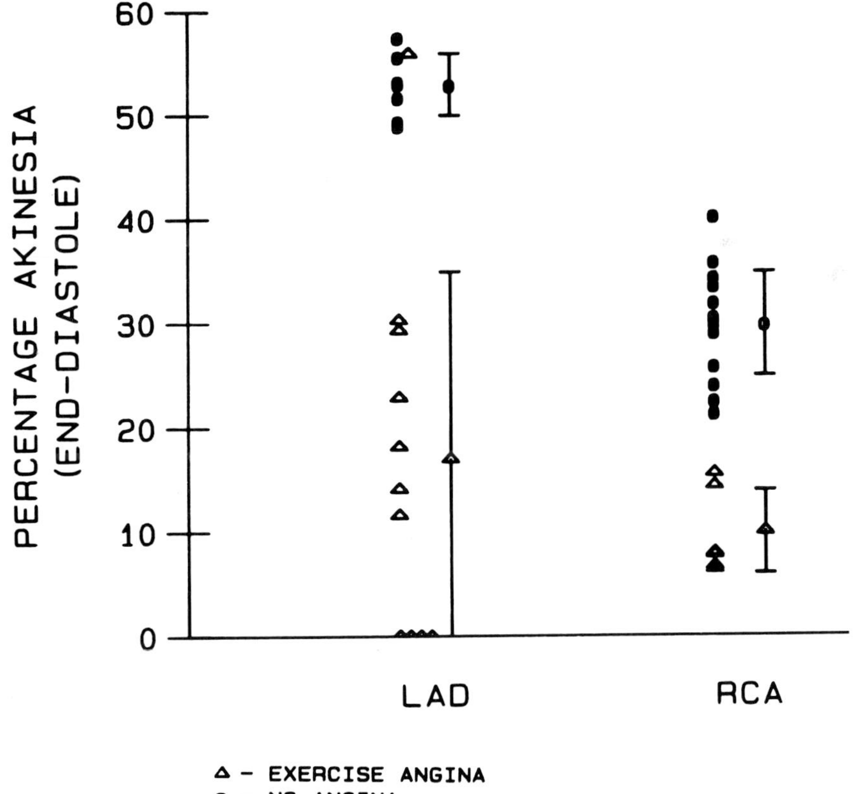

Figure 3. This graph shows the length of an akinetic or dyskinetic myocardial segment, expressed as a percentage of RAO left ventricular silhouette, in patients with single-vessel disease with or without angina pectoris. LAD = left anterior descending, RCA = right coronary artery. (m ± SD)

Table 7. Segmental LV wall motion and fibrosis replacement

Wall Motion	*Segments (no.)*	*Fibrosis Present*	*No Fibrosis*
Akinesis/Dyskinesis	30	26	4
Hypokinesis	51	24	27
Normal	19	1	18

Thus, most patients with single-vessel disease and small akinetic segments had both angina and ST segment depression. It is likely that these patients had an "incomplete" infarction in the territory of the narrowed coronary artery. Conversely, patients with large akinetic segments had neither angina nor ST segment depression. These patients likely had a "completed" infarction in the vascular territory of the narrowed artery. There appear to be finite limits of the LAD and RCA myocardial segments on the RAO ventriculogram that can be quantified as a percentage of the left ventricular silhouette. If a border zone of viable and potentially ischemic myocardium exists at the periphery of a completely infarcted segment, it is not sizeable enough to cause either angina or ST segment depression.

Correlation Between Ventriculographic and Pathologic Findings

Segmental left ventricular wall motion on left ventriculogram and the extent of fibrosis replacement at postmortem examination have been compared by Hutchins and colleagues.[15] The study included 27 patients who had coronary arteriography shortly before death and subsequently came to autopsy. Segmental wall motion in the distribution of each major coronary artery was judged to be normal, hypokinetic, or akinetic/dyskinetic (Table 7). Segments with normal wall motion had little or no fibrosis, whereas most akinetic or dyskinetic segments had fibrosis replacement. Fibrosis replacement was present in approximately half of hypokinetic segments. Only 16 of 30 akinetic segments had extensive scar replacement. These findings are in agreement with Bodenheimer and colleagues,[16] who demonstrated by operative biopsy that most dyskinetic segments had at least 75 percent muscle loss, whereas fibrosis replacement in akinetic segments could vary from 10 percent to more than 75 percent.

POSTINFARCTION EXERCISE TESTS AND ANGIOGRAPHIC FINDINGS

Recently, investigators in Gothenburg[2,3] have compared the angiographic findings of infarct survivors who had a limited exercise ECG test prior to hospital discharge. Patients were grouped according to whether they had a positive or negative electrocardiographic response during or after this test. A positive test response was defined as depression of the ST segment by 1 mm or more 60 msec after the J point during or after exercise. ST segment elevation or less than 1 mm depression was considered a negative response. The limited exercise test was performed on an upright bicycle ergometer and was stopped if any of the following endpoints were reached: (a) target heart rate of 70 percent predicted maximal rate for age; (b) a target work load of 80 watts (5 metabolic equivalents); (c) angina pectoris; (d) profound dyspnea or fatigue; (e) claudication; or (f) the appearance of frequent (more than 10 per minute), multifocal, or paired ventricular extrasystoles or ventricular tachycardia.[17] One hundred twenty-three patients (83 percent of those exercised) were readmitted to hospital for coronary arteriography 50 $\pm$ 20 days (m $\pm$ SD) after the index infarction.

The angiographic findings of these patients are shown in Table 8. Patients with a positive exercise ECG response more often had multivessel disease (two or three arteries narrowed by 75 percent or more) and more commonly had significant narrowings in the left anterior descending and circumflex arteries and in the LAD segment proximal to the first septal

Table 8. Coronary artery disease and left ventricular ejection fraction in patients with predischarge limited exercise tests*

	Exercise ECG Response		
Artery(s) Narrowed ≥75%	*Positive (45 pts)*	*Negative (78 pts)*	*p*
One	9 (20%)	39 (50%)	<0.01
Two	14 (31%)	16 (21%)	NS
Three	22 (49%)	20 (26%)	NS
None	0	3 (4%)	NS
LAD (n)	39 (87%)	48 (62%)	<0.003
RCA (n)	32 (71%)	44 (56%)	NS
CIRC (n)	32 (71%)	29 (37%)	<0.001
LAD before first septal br (n)	26 (58%)	23 (29%)	<0.002
EF (mean ± SD)	54 ± 15%	54 ± 16%	NS

*From Ejdebäck, et al,[2] and Griffith, et al,[3] with permission.

branch. There was no difference between the mean ejection fraction of positive and negative ECG responders.

Segmental left ventricular wall motion in the vascular distribution of each major coronary artery was judged to be either present (that is, normal or hypokinetic and presumably viable) or absent (that is, entirely akinetic or dyskinetic and presumably scarred). Thus, if wall motion of each myocardial segment is combined with the presence or absence of a 75 percent or greater narrowing in the perfusing artery, it is possible to group myocardial segments into one of three categories: (a) there is viable but potentially ischemic myocardium in the distribution of a significantly narrowed artery; (b) the segment is scarred and less likely to result in ischemic findings; or (c) the segment is viable, but there is no significant narrowing in the perfusing coronary artery. Postinfarction exercise patients were then analyzed according to these findings. Among patients with a positive exercise response, a greater proportion had both a significant coronary narrowing in the left anterior descending and circumflex arteries and in the proximal LAD segment *and* normal or hypokinetic wall motion of the myocardial segment, compared to patients with a negative exercise response (Table 9).

A positive limited exercise ECG response before hospital discharge helped identify patients with a 75 percent or greater narrowing before the first LAD septal branch. This was the case regardless of whether the index infarction was anterior or inferior by ECG criteria. Among anterior infarctions, a positive response identified 10 of 26 patients with a 75 percent or greater narrowing before the first LAD septal branch, and a negative response identified 24 of 26 patients with no significant narrowing in this LAD segment ($p < 0.05$). Among patients

Table 9. Coronary artery disease and segmental LV wall motion in patients with limited predischarge exercise test*

	Exercise ECG Response		
Artery Narrowed ≥75% and Normal or Hypokinetic Wall Motion	*Positive (45 pts)*	*Negative (78 pts)*	*p*
Left anterior descending (n)	38 (84%)	32 (41%)	<0.001
Right coronary artery (n)	13 (29%)	18 (23%)	NS
Circumflex coronary artery (n)	23 (51%)	20 (26%)	<0.004
Proximal LAD before first septal (n)	25 (56%)	9 (12%)	<0.001

*From Ejdebäck, et al,[2] and Griffith, et al,[3] with permission.

with an inferior infarction, a positive response identified 15 of 18 patients with significant proximal LAD disease, while a negative response identified 31 of 45 patients without important proximal LAD disease ($p < 0.001$).

ANGIOGRAPHIC PREDICTORS OF OUTCOME AFTER MYOCARDIAL INFARCTION

During a 25-month period, Taylor and colleagues[1] at Johns Hopkins enrolled 106 patients in a prospective study in which clinical, electrocardiographic, and angiographic findings obtained before hospital discharge were assessed as outcome predictors over a 30-month followup period. All patients were less than age 66 years and had no other life-threatening disease. No patient had cardiogenic shock, a ventricular septal defect, or papillary muscle rupture. Coronary angiography and left ventriculography were performed at a mean interval of 12.5 days after admission to the coronary care unit. Nineteen patients (18 percent) subsequently underwent coronary bypass surgery because of unstable or disabling angina (17 patients) or high-grade narrowing of the left main coronary artery (2 patients) and were not included in the assessment of outcome predictors of medically treated patients.

More than 80 variables were evaluated separately and in combination. A univariate analysis of all variables against the dichotomous outcome of death identified eight clinical and angiographic variables that were predictive of increased mortality at 30 months ($p < 0.05$) (Table 10). All variables that correlated significantly with mortality after infarction ($p < 0.1$) were included in a multivariate stepwise discriminant function analysis of death among 87 medically treated patients. This analysis included the eight variables listed in Table 10 and 22 other variables such as obesity, cigarette smoking, duration of angina before infarction, and so on. Two variables, a history of prior infarction and an ejection fraction of less than 40 percent, were significant independent predictors of mortality. Using these two variables, 51 of 74 (69 percent) living patients were correctly identified as being alive, and all 13 dead patients were identified as being dead. Once history of prior infarction and the ejection fraction were known, no other variable provided a significant additional contribution to prediction of mortality. Taylor and colleagues[1] concluded that routine cardiac catheterization after myocardial infarction is not needed because the risk of dying within a 2.5 year followup could be judged using history, physical examination, and noninvasive assessment of left ventricular function. The authors emphasized that their study was not a controlled trial of therapy, and the effect of bypass surgery or other new therapy such as thrombolysis or angioplasty is unknown.

Sixty-five of the 87 medically treated patients had at least one left ventricular "risk segment," defined as a contracting (that is, normal or hypokinetic wall motion) and presumably

Table 10. Clinical and angiographic variables predictive of increased mortality (univariate analysis)*

History of angina pectoris before index infarction
Previous myocardial infarction†
Advanced Killip class II or III
Three coronary arteries narrowed by 50% or more
Proximal LAD narrowed by 50% or more before first septal branch
Ejection fraction less than 40%†
Left ventricular "risk segment" present (artery narrowed 50% or more perfusing contracting, presumably viable, myocardium)
Complicated late hospital-phase ventricular arrhythmia

*Based on the data of Taylor, et al,[1] with permission.

†Independent predictor of increased mortality by multivariate stepwise discriminant function analysis

viable myocardial segment that was perfused by a coronary artery narrowed by at least 50 percent. Twenty-two patients had no ventricular "risk segments." Only 3 of the 22 (14 percent) patients without a risk segment had postinfarction angina, compared with a 75 percent prevalence of angina among those with risk segments ($p < 0.01$). All 13 deaths and 12 subsequent infarctions were in patients with one or more risk segments.

DeFeyter and colleagues[5] in Amsterdam have done a similar analysis of subsequent death after recovery from infarction. Their study assessed variables obtained at maximal exercise ECG testing and cardiac catheterization from 179 patients studied 6 to 8 weeks after infarction. Clinical and electrocardiographic variables were not included in this same analysis. In their study, an ejection fraction less than 30 percent and presence of three-vessel coronary disease were significant predictors of increased mortality ($p < 0.001$).

COMPLICATIONS OF CORONARY ARTERIOGRAPHY

The reported complications of early coronary arteriography performed soon after myocardial infarction are shown in Table 11. Because the type of problem encountered by the angiographer may be different at varying intervals after infarction, the studies have been grouped into those done within 24 hours of admission, those done 2 to 3 weeks after infarction before hospital discharge, and those done 6 to 8 weeks after infarction when recovery is probably complete.

Several comments concerning these complications might be made. First, although the prevalence of serious permanent complications (death, infarct, or stroke) is relatively low in these patients, the complication rate is nevertheless several times higher than that reported for stable angina patients.[18,19] Second, patients are more likely to have ventricular tachycardia/fibrillation soon after infarction, and this risk diminishes with time. Third, because systemic emboli can occur as a spontaneous complication of infarction, it is not clear whether catheterization enhances this adverse development. Both patients in the Johns Hopkins study with cerebral emboli experienced this complication 2 and 24 hours after an uneventful arteriogram.

Until controlled trials demonstrate a measureable benefit from very early therapeutic intervention (for example, bypass surgery, balloon angioplasty, or intracoronary thrombolysis), there appears to be little clinical benefit for a patient to undergo coronary arteriography until infarct recovery is complete. At this later time, selection of patients for angiography and possible bypass surgery can be made on the basis of more certain criteria, such as congestive heart failure or disabling angina pectoris.

Table 11. Complications of coronary arteriography soon after myocardial infarction

	Pts	*Mean Interval After CCU Admission (Days)*	*Complications (no. pts)*
Acute Phase			
Spokane[9]	322	Less than 1	Death, 2; plaque disruption, 2; myocardial stain, 1; VT/VF, 30
Predischarge			
Johns Hopkins[1]	109	13	Infarct, 1; stroke, 2; femoral thrombosis, 2
Alabama[6]	92	22	Infarct, 1; VT/VF, 2
Mayo Clinic[20]	50	24	None
Lille[7]	106	16	Pulmonary edema, 1
Recovered			
Gothenburg[2,3]	123	51	Femoral thrombosis, 1
Amsterdam[5]	179	42–56	Stroke, 1; VT/VF, 2

REFERENCES

1. Taylor, GJ, Humphries, JO, Mellits, ED, et al: *Predictors of clinical course, coronary anatomy and left ventricular function after recovery from acute myocardial infarction.* Circulation 62:960, 1980.
2. Ejdebäck, J, Varnauskas, E, Wallin, J, et al: *Angiographic findings of infarct survivors with positive or negative predischarge exercise test.* Circulation 66(Suppl II): II-342, 1982.
3. Griffith, LSC, Varnauskas, E, Wallin, J, et al: *Cardiac angiography in postinfarction patients. Correlation with predischarge limited exercise testing.* (Submitted for publication.)
4. Betriu, A, Castaner, A, Sanz, GA, et al: *Angiographic findings one month after myocardial infarction: A prospective study of 259 survivors.* Circulation 65:1099, 1982.
5. DeFeyter, PJ, van Eenige, MJ, Dighton, DH, et al: *Prognostic value of exercise testing, coronary angiography and left ventriculography 6–8 weeks after myocardial infarction.* Circulation 66:527, 1982.
6. Turner, JD, Rogers, WJ, Mantle, JA, et al: *Coronary angiography soon after myocardial infarction.* Chest 77:58, 1980.
7. Bertrand, ME, Lefebvre, JM, Laisne, CL, et al: *Coronary arteriography in acute transmural myocardial infarction.* Am Heart J 97:61, 1979.
8. Dodge, HT, Sandler, H, Bellew, DW, et al: *The use of biplane angiography for the measurement of left ventricular volume in man.* Am Heart J 60:762, 1960.
9. DeWood, MA, Spores, J, Notske, R, et al: *Prevalence of total coronary occlusion during the early hours of transmural myocardial infarction.* N Engl J Med 303:897, 1980.
10. Griffith, L, Grunwald, L, Gerry, J, et al: *Segmental left ventricular akinesis in single vessel coronary disease.* Am J Cardiol 41:414, 1978.
11. Fuchs, RM, Achuff, SC, Grunwald, L, et al: *Electrocardiographic localization of coronary artery narrowings: Studies during myocardial ischemia and infarction in patients with one-vessel disease.* Circulation 66:1168, 1982.
12. Griffith, LSC, Bailey, I, Strauss, HW, et al: *Significance of segmental wall motion in the development of angina pectoris.* Circulation 54(Suppl II): II–6, 1976.
13. Kalus, ME, Grunwald, L, and Griffith, LSC: *Postinfarction angina in single vessel disease. The "incomplete" infarction.* Unpublished data, 1982.
14. Feild, BJ, Russell, RO, Dowling, JT, et al: *Regional left ventricular performance in the year following myocardial infarction.* Circulation 46:679, 1972.
15. Hutchins, GM, Bulkley, BH, Ridolfi, RL, et al: *Correlation of coronary arteriograms and left ventriculograms with postmortem studies.* Circulation 56:32, 1977.
16. Bodenheimer, MM, Banka, VS, Hermann, GA, et al: *Histopathologic and electrographic correlations in patients with coronary artery disease.* Circulation 53:792, 1976.
17. Théroux, P, Water, DD, Halphen C, et al: *Prognostic value of exercise testing soon after myocardial infarction.* N Engl J Med 301:341, 1979.
18. Abrams, HL and Adams, DF: *The complications of coronary arteriography.* Personal communication. In Julian, DG (ed): *Angina Pectoris.* Churchill Livingstone, New York, 1977, p 172.
19. Bourassa, MG and Noble, J: *Complication rate of coronary arteriography. A review of 5250 cases studied by percutaneous femoral technique.* Circulation 53:106, 1976.
20. Madigan, NP, Rutherford, BD, and Frye, RL: *The clinical course, early prognosis and coronary anatomy of subendocardial infarction.* Am J Med 60:634, 1976.

Laboratory Diagnosis of Myocardial Ischemia

Graham Jackson, M.B.

In the evaluation of the patient with ischemia, studies of myocardial metabolism reflect the functional significance of the anatomic lesion. It is now most unlikely that anyone involved in the angiographic evaluation of patients with chest pain would accept metabolic studies as a diagnostic substitute for high-quality arteriography,[1] but a complimentary role exists with regard both to judging the effects of therapy as well as to basic research.

In this chapter I will concentrate on placing myocardial metabolic studies in the clinical context with regard to ischemia. Many excellent and detailed accounts of myocardial metabolism exist,[2–4] but a brief review of the normal pathways and the effects of ischemia is appropriate.

MYOCARDIAL METABOLISM

Normal Metabolism

The myocardium requires adenosine triphosphate (ATP) for its contractile process. Under physiological aerobic conditions, cardiac muscle utilizes a variety of substances for generating ATP, the proportions being as follows: free fatty acids (FFA), 65 percent; glucose, 15 percent; lactate and pyruvate, 12 percent; and amino acids, 5 percent.[5] These substrates are extracted by the myocardium in proportion to their arterial concentration.[6] When mitochondrial oxidative phosphorylation is active, surplus ATP may be stored as creatinine phosphate (CP).

Under aerobic conditions, the myocardium derives most of its energy supply from oxidation of FFAs (Figs. 1 and 2). Fatty acids in the plasma are bound to albumin and enter the cell via cellular binding sites. Short chain FFAs are activated to acyl CoA, a fatty acid complex with coenzyme A, prior to transportation into the mitochondria; but long chain FFAs need to be coupled to carnitine prior to transportation.[7] They are then broken down to acetyl coenzyme A (acetyl CoA), which is metabolized via the Krebs cycle. FFAs metabolized in the presence of adequate oxygen result in a high yield of ATP.

Glycolysis plays only a minor role in myocardial metabolism under aerobic conditions, to a large extent being inhibited by FFA oxidation as well as the Pasteur effect, that is, the inhibition of anaerobic glycolysis by oxygen. Glycolysis is extramitochondrial, occurring in the cytoplasm of the cell (see Figures 1 and 2). Glucose is either transported actively across the cell membrane or derived from endogenous glycogenolysis and metabolized via the gly-

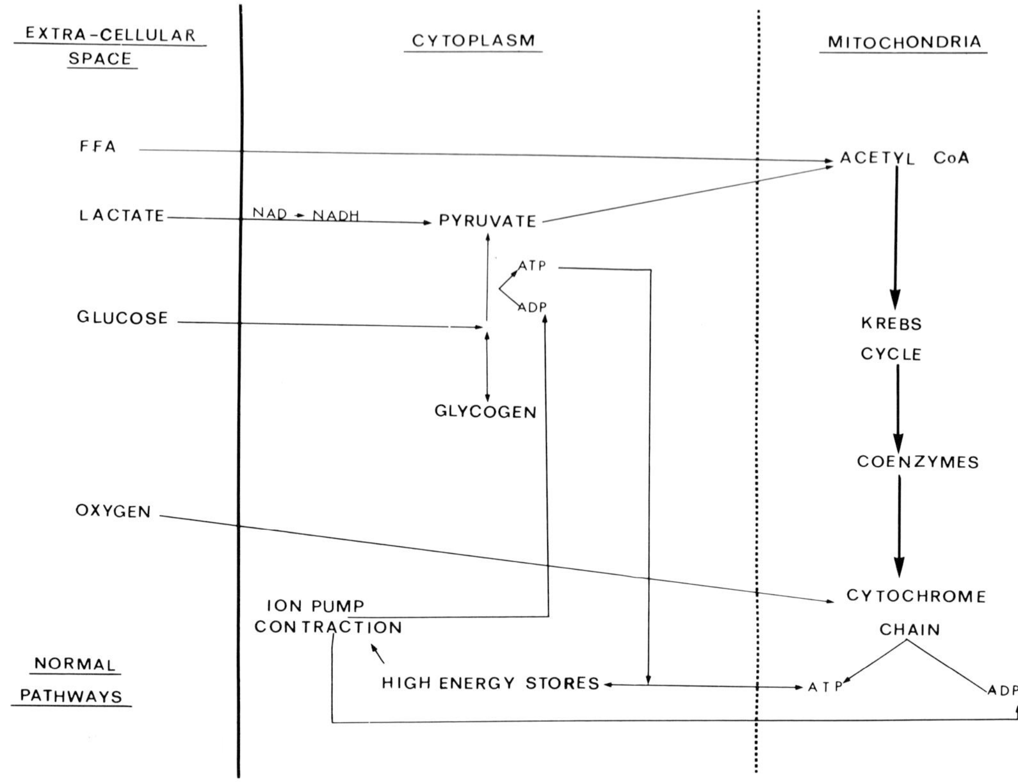

Figure 1. Normal metabolism. Shown here is a simplified account of myocardial metabolism. Note that lactate is extracted and converted to pyruvate and that the majority of fatty acid is converted to acetyl CoA.

colytic pathway to pyruvate. The initial irreversible phosphorylation of glucose in the presence of hexokinase to glucose-6-phosphate leads, however, to feedback inhibition of phosphorylase and hence protection of glycogen stores. The conversion of fructose-6-phosphate to fructose 1,6-diphosphate is catalyzed by phosphofructokinase (PFK), a regulatory enzyme that is inhibited by ATP, its own substrate, and citrate, a product of FFA oxidation. The sole oxidative reaction of the glycolytic pathway is the conversion of glyceraldehyde-3-phosphate (GAP) to 1,3-diphosphoglycerate. This reaction is dependent on the coenzyme nicotinamide-adenine dinucleotide (NAD); and unless reoxidization of NADH occurs, the activity of the whole pathway will be terminated. There is only a net yield of 2 moles of ATP during glycolytic degradation, in marked contrast to the 36 moles of ATP produced per molecule of glucose during mitochondrial (that is, aerobic) metabolism. Under conditions of adequate oxygen supply, pyruvate is converted to acetyl CoA and is further metabolized in the Krebs cycle.[8] Lactate is not normally produced by the heart because in the presence of adequate oxygen it is extracted from the circulation, converted to pyruvate, and metabolized either via the Krebs cycle or converted to glycogen.

It is worth emphasizing the important interactions between FFAs and carbohydrate metabolism. Oxidation of FFAs leads to accumulation of citrate, which inhibits PFK, thereby slowing glycolysis. Furthermore, the increase in acetyl CoA decreases glycolytic flux by inhibiting pyruvate dehydrogenase.[9] Fatty acid oxidation is further dependent on transport into mitochondria via carnitine and on the continued utilization of acetyl CoA.

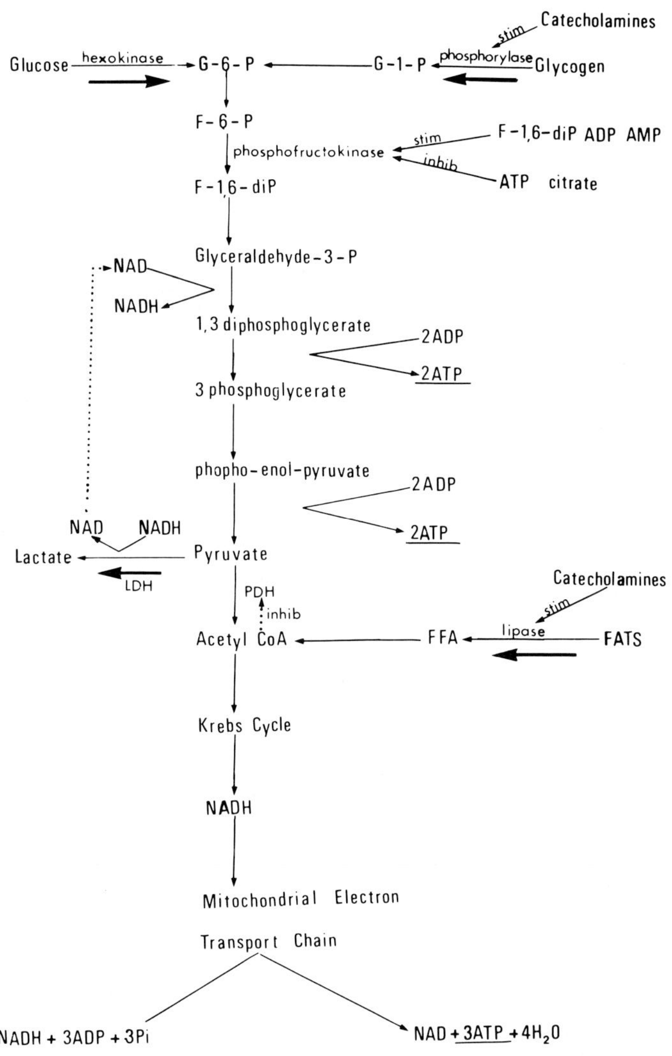

Figure 2. Normal and abnormal metabolism. The detailed normal pathways are indicated by the fine arrows. The changes during ischemia are indicated by the thick black arrows. The utilization of glucose or glycogen increases and pyruvate accumulates. The lactate-pyruvate reaction reverses, and lactate accumulates. Increased glycolysis is an inadequate compensatory mechanism for the formation of ATP.

Abnormal Metabolism

Under conditions of decreased oxygen availability, major alterations occur in myocardial metabolism (Figs. 2 and 3).[10] Oxidative phosphorylation and hence ATP production cannot proceed at their normal rates because of the absolute requirement for oxygen of the cytochrome oxidases. Acetyl CoA can no longer be oxidized at the normal rate by the Krebs cycle, and therefore FFAs may accumulate within the myocardial cell.[11] It has been suspected for

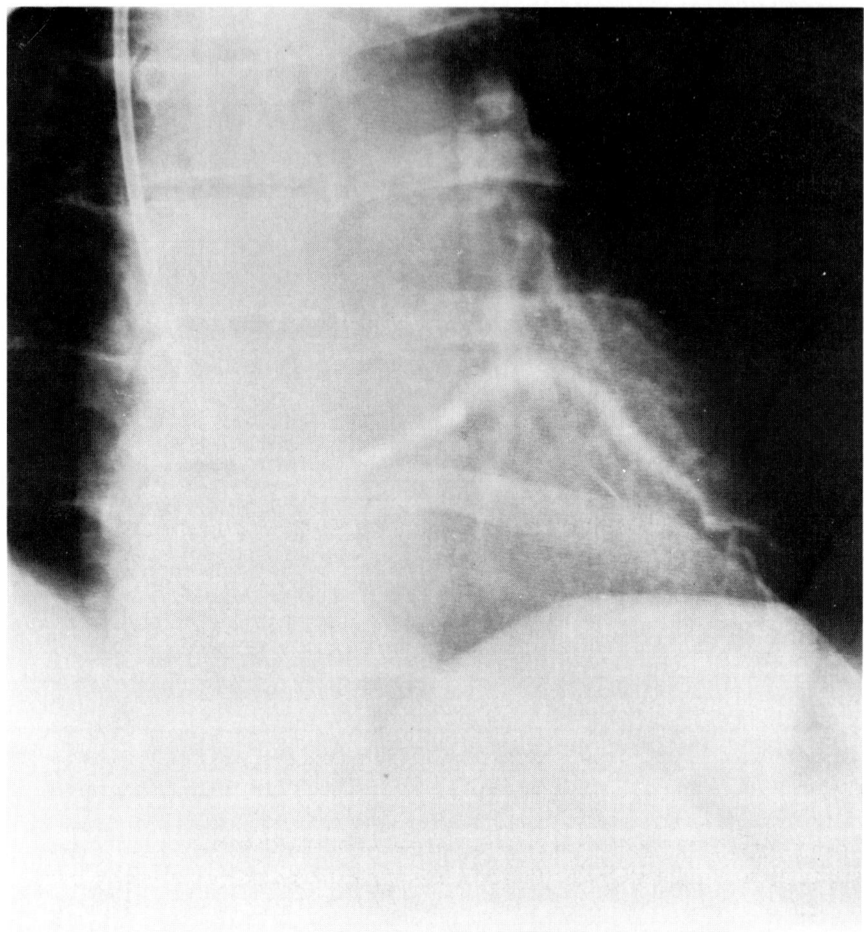

Figure 3. Shown here is a Zucker pacing and sampling catheter positioned in the main coronary sinus.

some time that FFAs, particularly those bound to protein, exert toxic effects on the myocardium, including depression of contractility, derangement of mitochondrial function, and precipitation of arrhythmias.[12,13]

In contrast, glycolytic flux increases as a result of increasing ADP and AMP in response to ischemia.[14] There is increased glucose transport into the cell, and G-6-P inhibition of hexokinase is reduced by an increase in orthophosphate (Pi) concentration, leading to enhanced phosphorylation. Glycogen does not normally meet myocardial substrate requirements, though it is the endogenous carbohydrate store of the heart. In the absence of other sources of oxidizable substrate, it may account for up to 25 percent of myocardial oxygen consumption. Glycogenolysis is markedly accelerated by the transformation of phosphorylase "b" (inactive) to "a" (active) and, soon after, because of stimulation of phosphorylase "b" by phosphate and decreasing inhibition by G-6-P. Conversion of phosphorylase "b" to "a" may be facilitated by local release of catecholamines, leading to stimulation of adenyl cyclase and accumulation of cyclic-AMP in the ischemic myocardium.[15]

At the time that glycolysis is generating increased pyruvate, hypoxia is also decreasing the rate of pyruvate conversion to acetyl CoA. The pyruvate–lactate equilibrium shifts toward lactate formation, which freely diffuses out of the cell and appears in the coronary sinus.

NADH, which was previously oxidized by the mitochondrial electron-transport chain under aerobic conditions, is now oxidized by linked reactions, of which the conversion

$$\underset{\text{pyruvic acid}}{CH_3-\underset{\underset{O}{\|}}{C}-COOH} + NADH + H^+ \rightleftharpoons \underset{\text{lactic acid}}{CH_3-\underset{\underset{OH}{|}}{C}OOH} + NAD^+$$

is by far the most important. The NAD/NADH redox potential of the mitochondrion is indirectly coupled to the cytoplasmic NAD/NADH ratio, and this is grossly reflected in lactate concentration. The measurement of this accumulation of lactic acid in the coronary sinus as a result of anaerobic metabolism forms the basis of the biochemical detection of myocardial ischemia.

THE HISTORY OF MYOCARDIAL METABOLIC STUDIES IN MAN

Investigation of myocardial metabolism by measurement of coronary arteriovenous (AV) substrate differences in man is feasible because drainage of the major mass of left ventricular muscle occurs through the coronary sinus. Since the introduction of coronary sinus catheterization by Bing and coworkers in 1947,[16] it has been possible to measure AV differences of various substrates across the myocardium.

The advantages and disadvantages of various metabolic measurements were first reviewed by Gorlin in 1969.[3] Hypoxia has been demonstrated to be associated with increased oxygen extraction,[17] but along with coronary venous pH the oxygen saturation measurements in human patients have proved too variable to be of any clinical use. Similar negative studies have excluded the usefulness of increased glucose extraction,[18,19] increased potassium loss,[19–21] and decreased FFA extraction[22,23] associated with ischemia. Other metabolic markers of ischemia that have been utilized are amino acids,[24] prostaglandins,[25] and ATP catabolites.[19,26] At present it appears that only the additional measurement of hypoxanthine[19] may confer advantages over lactate, which is still the most sensitive index of ischemia that is readily available.[4,23,27]

In the ischemic heart, lactate abnormalities can be elicited by any stress that increases cardiac effort to a degree that nutrient demand exceeds supply. In man, however, biochemical evidence of myocardial ischemia has not always been convincingly demonstrated. Early valuable work showed a reasonable correlation between angina and abnormal lactate metabolism but was unsatisfactory because the modes of stress were exercise and isoprenaline. Exercise (usually supine leg raising) significantly raises arterial lactate, thereby preventing proper interpretation of the metabolic state of the myocardium.[28] Isoprenaline infusions have been employed in doses sufficiently small to stress the heart and to precipitate anaerobic metabolism without obvious hemodynamic and metabolic effects, but lactate uptake by the myocardial cell could be decreased by the FFA mobilizing effect of isoprenaline via a mechanism of preferential substrate utilization.[29]

The introduction of atrial pacing by Sowton and associates in 1967[30] facilitated more precise metabolic evaluation of myocardial ischemia inasmuch as arterial lactate concentrations remained relatively unchanged by atrial pacing. Furthermore, it was possible to detect the onset and course of anaerobic metabolism by obtaining accurately timed samples.

It is surprising, therefore, that little published data exists regarding atrial pacing and myocardial lactate extraction in patients with and without obstructive coronary arterial disease. Cohen and colleagues[28] found abnormal lactate metabolism in only 73 percent of patients with coronary artery disease, but their method of stress was supine leg raising or isoprenaline. The important regional sampling work of Herman and coworkers[31] again incorporated the limitations of catecholamine stress, and neither Herman nor Cohen's studies provided data of stress heart rates or defined stress end points. Neill[32] reported 13 patients who underwent atrial pacing at an average rate of 105 beats per minute, and only 4 patients exhibited lactate production. The latter level of stress is clearly submaximal. Parker and colleagues in 1969[33] then provided a well-constructed atrial pacing study involving myocardial metabolic studies. In this study of only 21 patients, the pacing rate was 20 beats per minute greater than that achieved during supine bicycle leg exercise. Pacing rates ranged from 132 to 160 beats per minute for a 10-minute pacing period. It is unusual for a patient with angina and significant coronary artery disease (CAD) to be able to sustain a rapid maximal heart rate for 10 minutes without developing severe chest pain and therefore forcing the study to be discontinued. This fact alone casts doubts on the adequacy and methodology of pacing in this study. In addition, four patients with severe CAD failed to develop anaerobic metabolism (20 percent). Parker's study, however, provided important objective information regarding myocardial metabolic studies and clearly showed the advantages of atrial pacing. Thus, the possibility of improving technique by changing the pacing protocol to provide a sudden maximal stress, thereby precipitating ischemia rapidly, might be expected to improve sensitivity. The work of Livesley and Oram[1] provided a maximal stress or continuous pacing protocol, and, in addition, the accuracy of estimation of lactate in whole blood was improved by the use of a Tris-hydrazine buffer.[34] Subsequently the concept of continuous pacing has been established as the method of choice.[35]

Coronary artery disease is most often segmental and may involve one or more vessels with various degrees of severity. The absence of biochemical evidence of ischemia after atrial pacing may occur, therefore, as a result of mixing problems when drainage from ischemic zones is diluted by normal blood from aerobic zones. Furthermore, if the venous drainage from the ischemic zone is proximal to the position of the catheter tip within the coronary sinus, it will not be sampled.[36] Most of the previous studies have incorporated sampling from only the main coronary sinus, and therefore their reliability may be suspect because of anatomic limitations.

Although the most obvious limitations on the predictive value of coronary sinus lactate studies for coronary artery disease are inadequate stress techniques and failure to assess the regional nature of myocardial ischemia, several other factors may influence the AV lactate difference. The most important practical limitation is starvation-induced increases in FFAs. Studies therefore should be done in the nonfasting state. Also, phosphofructokinase activity can be increased by alkalosis and hyperventilation. It should be clear from Table 1 that myocardial lactate may be disturbed by factors other than ischemia.

Coronary Blood Flow

Interpretation of metabolic changes should include the assessment of changes in coronary blood flow. A valid measurement of blood flow would enable conversion of AV differences to

Table 1. Effects of certain conditions on lactate extraction*

Condition	*Mechanism*	*A-V lactate*
Exercise	Arterial lactate↑	↑
Shock	Arterial lactate↑	↑
Diabetes	Insulin ↓, FFA↑	↓
Starvation	Glycolysis, FFA↑	↓
Hyperventilation	Phosphofructokinase↑	↓
Catecholamines	FFA, glycogenolysis↑	↓
Heparin	FFA↑	↓

*Adapted from Moret, et al.[4]

absolute uptake and discharge of metabolites, but techniques available have limitations. Deep layers of the myocardium are extremely susceptible to a reduction in perfusion pressure such as that which occurs distal to fixed obstructive CAD.[37] Measurement of radioisotope tracer washout is open to criticism because of the regional, and at times small areas of, ischemia. Cohen and coworkers,[28] using Krypton to measure coronary flow, found no means of distinguishing patients with and without CAD, either at rest or during stress, and concluded that a measurement of lactate extraction was the most useful laboratory test in addition to morphologic evaluation of the coronary arteries.

Thermodilution techniques[38] rely on mean flow over time and do not provide information on redistribution of flow when the heart is rendered ischemic. When regional flow is not measured, we are really looking at arteriocoronary sinus differences at a new steady state, limiting the quantitative value of the method. In short, it seems at present that attention to the detail and methodology of AV lactate sampling provides the backbone of the laboratory studies of myocardial ischemia,[39] but, where available, coronary flow techniques may provide useful, additional, though not quantitatively essential, information.

CORONARY SINUS PACING: METHODOLOGY

I perform coronary sinus pacing on a separate occasion from coronary arteriography to avoid any effects of contrast media. My patients are studied in the nonfasting state.

After the patient has rested for 45 minutes, a Zucker[40] bipolar electrode catheter is inserted into a left antecubital vein and positioned fluoroscopically 2 cm within the coronary sinus (as viewed in the anterior-posterior projection) for a main sampling procedure (see Figure 3). During a regional lactate study the catheter is positioned at three sites in the coronary sinus. Animal experimentation has shown that it is possible to relate the ischemia induced by coronary artery ligation with a specific zone of lactate abnormality, by selective sampling within the coronary sinus.[11] The three sites in the study are designated (1) "distal," designed to reflect drainage of the great cardiac vein and hence left anterior descending artery (LAD) territory; (2) "mid," reflecting ischemia from the bulk of the left ventricle and in particular the addition of circumflex drainage to LAD drainage; and (3) "proximal," which is located as close to the ostium as possible in an attempt to sample blood from right coronary artery territory (Fig. 4). Catheter position is checked throughout the study by fluoroscopy and injections of small amounts of contrast media. Arterial samples are obtained from a two-way tap attached to manometer tubing and a 2-inch No. 19G needle that is inserted into the femoral artery under local anesthesia. Femoral artery pressure is recorded throughout the study on a Mingograph 81 recorder. Both the venous catheter and the arterial needle are intermittently flushed with heparinized saline except when FFAs are being measured, at which time saline alone is used. Before pacing, at least two control samples are taken simultaneously from the coronary sinus and from the femoral artery. No medication at all (that is, analgesics or sedatives) is given to the patient on the day of the study, to avoid any effects on myocardial metabolism and to standardize the procedure.

Using a battery-powered pacemaker (Devices) the heart rate is increased at 5-second intervals by increments of 10 beats per minute and then held constant at 10 beats per minute above the peak exercise heart rate or the maximum predicted heart rate, whichever is the greater. Pacing is discontinued when the patient experiences the usual chest discomfort or pain of a severity that would stop him or her in normal daily life. Blood samples are taken at peak pacing and at 2.5 and 10 minutes after cessation of pacing.

Electrocardiographic (leads II and V5) recordings are taken throughout the study. The amount of ST segment depression in V5 is measured before and after pacing, disregarding the first two post-pacing beats;[33] and lactate studies are performed by Livesley's[34] modification of Hohorst's method using a Tris-hydrazine buffer (pH 9.6), thereby producing more accurate and reproducible results. Myocardial lactate extraction ratio is defined as the dif-

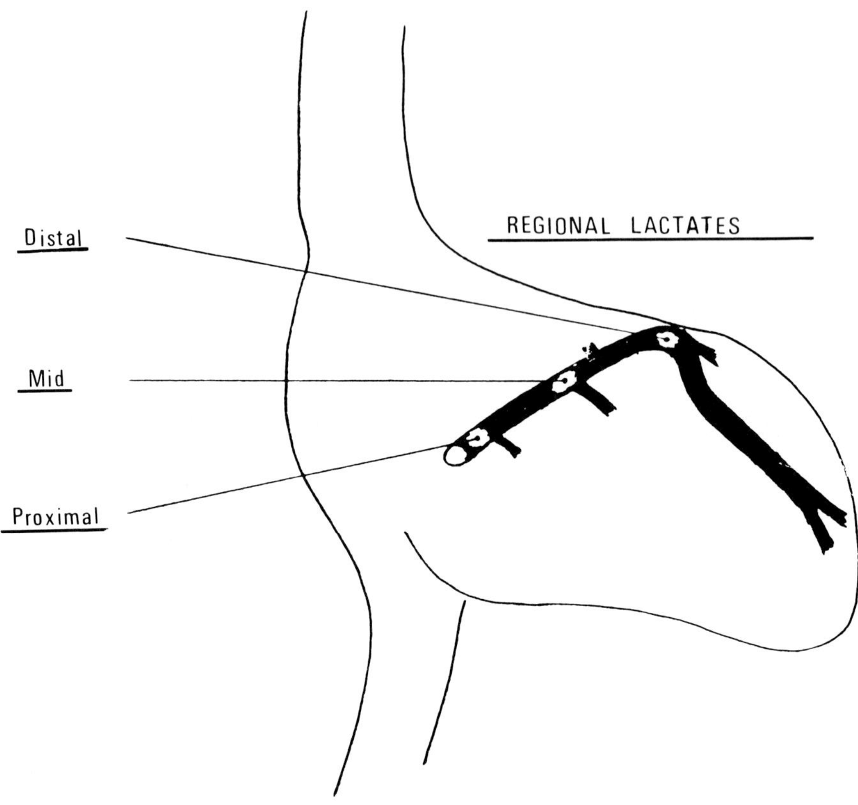

Figure 4. Shown here are regional sampling points. The distal sample reflects left anterior descending disease; the mid sample, circumflex disease; and the proximal sample, right coronary disease.

ference between arterial and coronary sinus lactate, divided by arterial lactate and expressed as a percentage:

$$\frac{A - V}{A} \times 100\%$$

A lactate extraction ratio of less than 10 percent or a coronary sinus lactate greater than arterial lactate (production) is believed to reflect myocardial ischemia.[28] A change in AV lactate difference of greater than 0.8 mg percent has previously been considered more sensitive for ischemia.[39] We express the lactate changes by both methods and compare them with the angiographic results.

CLINICAL CONTEXT OF CORONARY SINUS LACTATE STUDIES

Diagnosis of Coronary Disease

Looking specifically at the relationship between abnormal lactate metabolism and the extent of coronary artery disease, we prospectively evaluated 100 patients with chest pain.

A change in coronary AV lactate difference of less than 0.8 mg percent with atrial pacing was associated with normal coronary arteries in all but one patient, who had a single distal lesion of the circumflex artery (Table 2). No patient with normal coronary arteries had a

Table 2. Correlation between abnormal lactate metabolism with atrial pacing and the degree of coronary artery disease

Control Minus Peak Pacing Lactate A-V Difference (mg%)	Number of Diseased Arteries				
	0 (N = 45)	1 (LAD) (N = 7)	1 (RCA/CIRC) (N= 6)	2 (N = 18)	3 (N = 24)
0–0.8	22	0	1	0	0
0.8–2.0	23	3	4	5	4
>2.0 or frank production	0	4	1	13	20

N = Number of patients

change in AV lactate difference of more than 2.0 mg percent. In the range between 0.8 mg percent and 2.0 mg percent there were patients with both normal and abnormal coronary arteriograms. A change in AV lactate difference greater than 2.0 mg percent or lactate production was diagnostic of advanced coronary artery disease (Table 3). Thus the severity of coronary artery disease paralleled the degree of change in AV lactate difference with pacing (Fig. 5) ($p < 0.01$). Only in the presence of coronary artery disease did lactate production with atrial pacing result in coronary sinus levels greater than arterial levels. The arterial levels of lactate were stable throughout the pacing stress, thereby increasing the reliability of the study. Expressing lactate abnormalities in terms of an extraction ratio of less than 10 percent was a less sensitive means of predicting coronary artery disease. Eight patients (17 percent) with normal coronary arteries, and only 39 (71 percent) with coronary artery disease had a ratio of less than 10 percent on peak pacing. Therefore, expressing lactate abnormalities in terms of AV difference is more sensitive for the detection of coronary artery disease.

To try to improve the specificity and sensitivity of lactate metabolic studies, 31 patients were evaluated using our regional sampling protocol. Normal coronary arteries were present in 7 patients and coronary artery disease in 24. The relationship between the location of regional coronary artery disease and regional lactate abnormalities is illustrated in Table 4. The mean arterial lactate before pacing was 7.63 ± 0.06 mg percent and 7.75 ± 0.52 mg percent after pacing. This difference is not significant, reflecting stable arterial levels during pacing.

Abnormal regional lactate metabolism is believed to reflect ischemia of anteroseptal, anterolateral, and anterolateral plus inferior regions. The left anterior descending artery drains into the anteroseptal region. The circumflex artery drainage is added at the lateral point, and the right coronary artery drainage at the inferior/posterior site.

A series of representative results shows examples of abnormal regional lactate metabolism (Table 5).

Table 3. Lactate measurements

	NCA N=45	CAD N=55	p
Mean C–P A/V difference (mg%)	0.73 ± 0.04	3.3 ± 0.6	<0.001
Mean lactate extraction ratio (%)	23.25 ± 2.4	−12.4 ± 8.5	<0.001
Lactate production	0	29 (53)	<0.001
Abnormal lactates 2 min post pacing	2	28 (51)	<0.001

NCA = normal coronary arteries
CAD = coronary artery disease

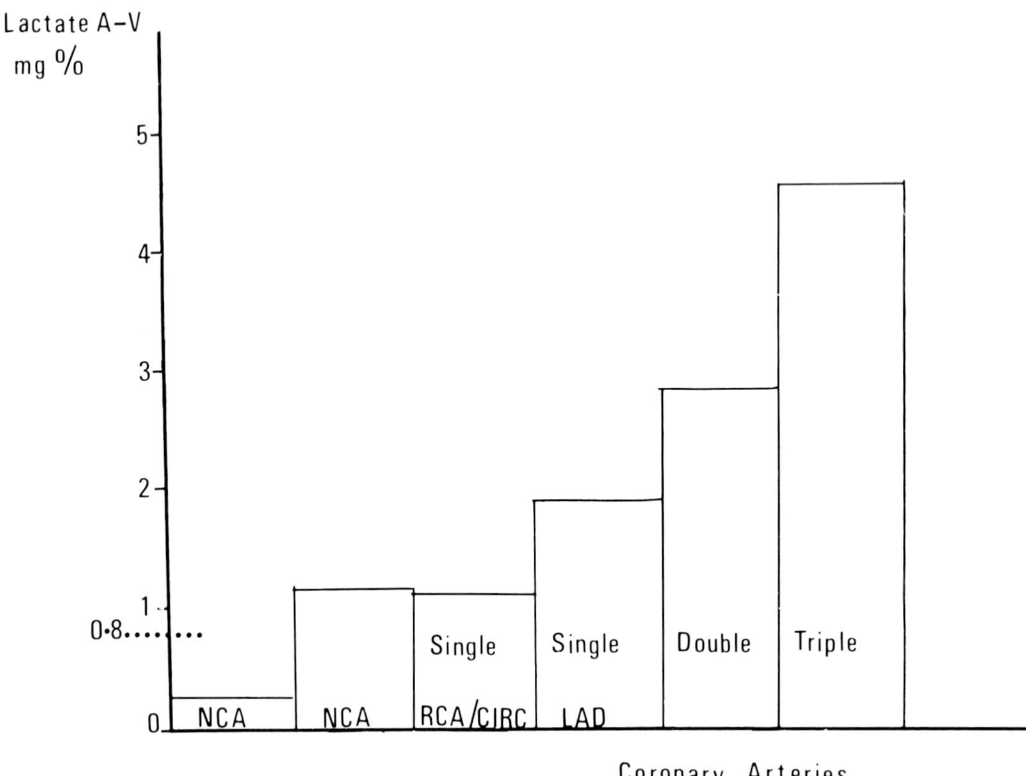

Figure 5. Increasing severity of coronary artery disease leads to increasing abnormalities of lactate extraction.

Lactate AV differences were normal from all three sampling positions in 4 of 7 patients with normal coronary arteries, suggesting normal myocardial lactate metabolism in response to pacing. Three patients with normal coronary arteries had a change in AV lactate difference in the anterolateral region on pacing (of between 0.8 and 2 mg percent), suggesting regional ischemia.

All 24 patients with coronary artery disease had abnormal lactate metabolism with atrial pacing. The ischemic zone could be accurately predicted in 19 (79 percent) by regional sampling. In those patients with coronary artery disease, regional lactate sampling did not overpredict the extent of the coronary artery disease.

Incorrect prediction was associated with right coronary artery lesions in four cases and left anterior descending artery disease in one. The right coronary artery drains proximally into the sinus, and lactate gradients at that position are the most easy to miss inasmuch as the

Table 4. Regional lactates (N = 31)

	NCA *N = 7*	*CAD* *N = 24*
Abnormal lactates	3 (42%)	24 (100%)
Regional accuracy		19 (79%)

NCA = normal coronary arteries
CAD = coronary artery disease

Table 5. Examples of abnormal regional lactate metabolism

Patient 10			
Vessel disease:	RCA 0	LAD 0	Circ 70%
Lactate change mg%:	Proximal 1.3	Distal 0.7	Mid 1.4
Comment			
AV lactate differences are normal from the distal sampling point, suggesting a normal left anterior descending artery. The mid portion is abnormal, suggesting circumflex artery disease; and there is no further increase at the proximal point, suggesting a normal right coronary artery.			
Patient 16			
Vessel disease:	RCA 0	LAD 100%	Circ 0
Lactate change mg%:	No sample	Distal 2.0	Mid 2.2
Comment			
Left anterior descending artery disease is inferred from the distal sample. The minimal step-up in the mid portion suggests no significant circumflex artery lesion. Right coronary artery disease cannot be interpreted owing to lack of sample.			
Patient 20			
Vessel disease:	RCA 100	LAD 90	Circ 90
Lactate change mg%:	Proximal 3.7	Distal 1.6	Mid 2.0
Comment			
There is disease of all three vessels, indicated by the significant increase in lactates as the catheter is withdrawn from the sinus.			

catheter may be sampling distally. This problem is not easily solved. A double lumen catheter may be the answer and warrants further study.

The estimation of main coronary sinus lactate after a maximal atrial pacing stress had been used in this study in an attempt to define its specificity and sensitivity in screening for coronary artery disease. The procedure is conducted on an outpatient basis and takes less than 30 minutes. It is invasive, but in this study it was not associated with any significant morbidity. The coronary sinus has been catheterized with ease in 98 percent of patients referred for investigation. This study represents the first large series comparing coronary sinus lactate sampling after atrial pacing at maximal heart rates with coronary arteriography. First of all, it shows that the use of a lactate extraction ratio of less than 10 percent as an indication of coronary artery disease is more specific but less sensitive in comparison with results expressed as AV difference. The exact reason for this is not clear, but it could reflect a more reliable lactate assay, or it may be that a new ratio of abnormality needs to be defined inasmuch as the 10 percent figure has until now no adequate correlative support.

All patients with a change in AV lactate difference of less than 0.8 mg percent with pacing had normal coronary arteries, with the exception of one who had localized distal disease (70 percent) of the circumflex artery. This finding illustrates the limitation of sampling from the main coronary sinus in the presence of localized regional ischemia;[31] the normal result in the presence of distal disease in a small vessel probably reflects dilution of the lactate from the ischemic area by the venous blood from larger aerobic zones. All patients with a change in AV lactate difference of greater than 2.0 mg percent with pacing had coronary artery disease, but a change between 0.8 and 2.0 mg percent did not distinguish between those with normal coronary arteries and those with coronary artery disease. A total of 39 patients (39 percent) fell into this overlap group, and all varieties of coronary artery disease were present, thus significantly limiting the usefulness of main coronary sinus lactates as an isolated test for coronary artery disease. Nevertheless, two important groups emerge: one with a lactate change of less than 0.8 mg percent (23 percent) when it is highly likely that the patient has normal coronary arteries, and another with a lactate change greater than 2.0 mg percent (38 percent) when it is highly likely that the patient has coronary artery disease. Patients with isolated left anterior descending artery lesions had a greater change than those with isolated right coronary artery or circumflex artery lesions, reflecting the fact that in most people the left anterior descending artery probably supplies the major part of the left ventricle. This study of atrial pacing with main coronary sinus sampling of lactate shows the advantages and disadvantages of this technique in screening patients with atypical or typical anginal pain for coronary artery disease. Its specificity for coronary artery disease is 77 percent and its sensitivity, 98 percent; but, like exercise electrocardiography, it has the similar limitation that patients may need to proceed to coronary angiography to establish the diagnosis.

Regional sampling fails to clarify the group of patients whose changes were between 0.8 and 2.0 mg percent but adds greater authority to the claim that normal coronary arteries are present when the change in AV lactate difference is less than 0.8 mg percent. Although regional lactates provide no greater specificity for coronary artery disease, they more accurately reflect the metabolism of the left ventricle than main sinus lactates.

Thus, the role of coronary sinus lactates is limited in a diagnostic capacity, and although there is enough evidence to suggest it has a part to play in the diagnosis of coronary artery disease, there is insufficient evidence to justify widespread usage if diagnosis is the only objective.

LACTATES AND INTERVENTIONS

Reproducibility

In order to judge the effect of any therapeutic maneuver, the same baseline stimulus for the same duration in the same patient must be associated with the same degree of abnormality. Serial pacing studies at varying time intervals resulted in variable lactate results (Fig. 6). When pacing was repeated after a 45-minute resting period, accurate results were obtained. We named this period the myocardial recovery time.[41] Protocols for the evaluation of drugs in particular must take into account a minimum resting period of 45 minutes. Recovery times of less than 45 minutes can either give a false impression of the value of a drug or unfairly suggest adverse myocardial effects.

Drugs

In varying protocols, several agents—including nitrates,[42] perhexiline,[43] and verapamil[44]—have now been shown to benefit myocardial metabolism during atrial pacing when the heart rate is fixed. The improvement with verapamil resulted from decreased demand from lower arterial pressure. In contrast, the calcium channel blocker nifedipine did not improve metabolism when given as monotherapy, but when combined with beta blockade there was a significant improvement,[45] again reflecting peripheral effects on arterial pressure.

Perhaps the most interesting drugs to evaluate are the beta blocking agents.[46] After myocardial infarction beta blocking drugs have been shown to improve myocardial metabolism at rest.[47] However, in patients with angina it was believed that an atrial pacing stress test, in which the effect of the drug on heart rate is eliminated, might fail to show any beneficial effect of the beta blocker.[48] Our group showed that when the heart was paced at the same rate in individual patients before and after administration of beta blocker, pacing time to angina increased and myocardial lactate extraction significantly improved (Fig. 7). This improvement occurred with both selective and nonselective beta blockade. Subsequent studies from our department and others[49] have shown that the improvement in metabolism is independent of changes in overall coronary flow, leading to the concept of redistribution of flow from nonischemic to ischemic zones, as first documented by Pitt and Craven in 1970.[50]

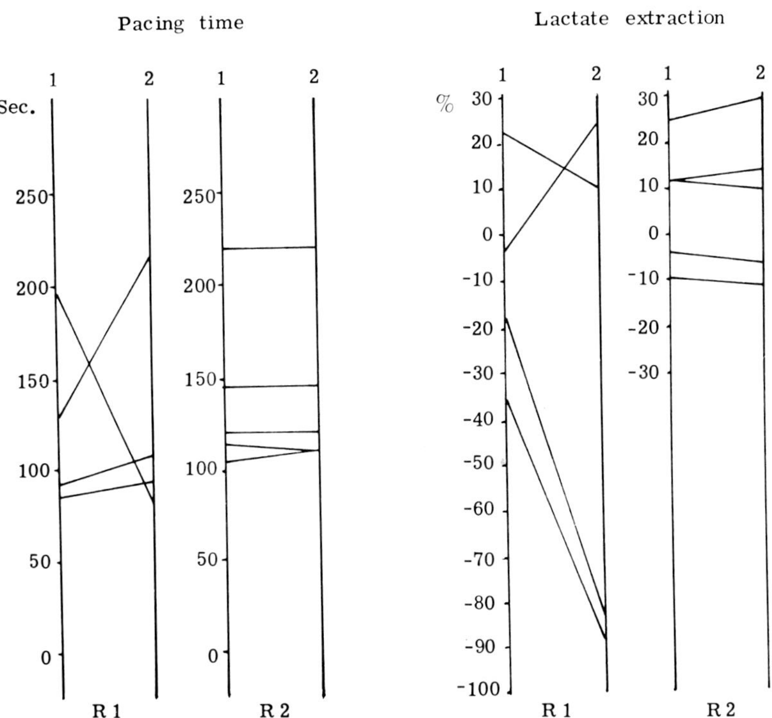

Figure 6. Demonstrated here is the effect of atrial pacing on pacing time and lactate extraction. R1, interval between atrial pacing tests 1 and 2 less than 45 minutes; R2, interval greater than 45 minutes. Measurements of pacing time and lactate extraction are reproducible when the second pacing test follows 45 minutes after the initial pacing test.

In 1977[46] we believed that the improvement of metabolism secondary to beta blockade might explain the beneficial effects on mortality post infarction, first reported with practolol[51] and subsequently with alprenolol,[52] timolol,[53] metoprolol,[54] and propranolol.[55] The addition of beta blockade acts both to delay the onset of pain and to decrease the rate at which anaerobic metabolism develops (see Fig. 7). The response resembles the classic dose response curves of isoprenaline and beta blockers, with the degree of ischemia being moved to the right. Thus by extending atrial pacing time to a fixed point, it may be possible to identify the early development of ischemia before the pain threshold is reached (Fig. 8).

If we assume all beta blockers exert similar metabolic effects, a so-called protective effect can be envisaged if the rate of development as well as the degree of ischemia holds the key to subsequent events. Evidence from sudden death studies in patients with significant coronary disease but without infarction, and documented cases of out-of-hospital ventricular fibrillation, support the concept of a sudden ischemic etiology.[56] Corday and coworkers,[57] performing coronary occlusion studies in dogs, documented a more severe metabolic disorder of the coronary-occluded segment prior to the onset of ventricular fibrillation in comparison with the occluded segments of dogs who did not fibrillate. In five animals studied within 5 minutes of the onset of fibrillation, there was a sudden massive lactate production, potassium loss, and increased acidosis. It is therefore possible that beta blockers exert their beneficial effects by decreasing the incidence of ventricular fibrillation secondary to a reduction in the rate of

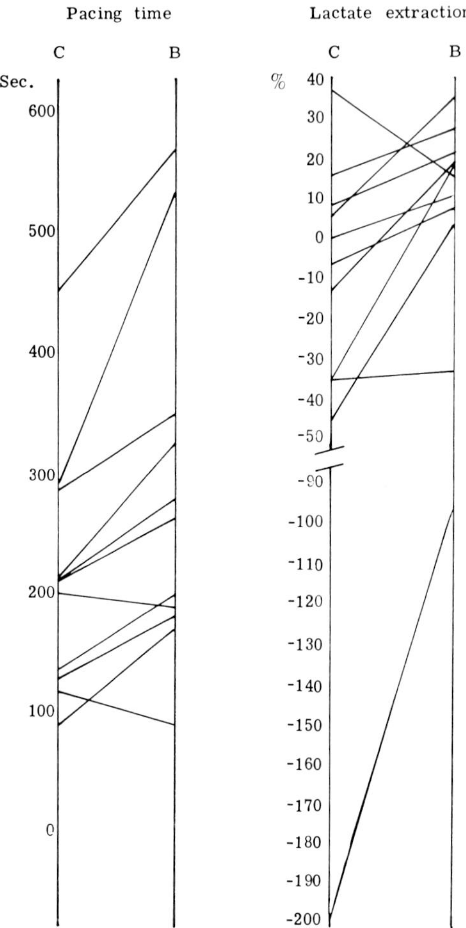

Figure 7. Illustrated here is atrial pacing stress before and after beta blockade. Improvement in pacing time and lactate extraction was exhibited by beta blockade (B) when compared with control (C).

developing ischemia. In Figure 9, already proven observations are summarized, leading us also to note that beta blockade in addition to coronary artery bypass grafting provides additional protection from developing ischemia.

Surgery

Several studies have now shown improved myocardial metabolism following coronary artery bypass surgery.[58,59] The exact preoperative protocol must be repeated postoperatively for meaningful results to be obtained. As shown in Figures 8 and 9, abnormal metabolism may still occur if paced long enough, but the degree of change and speed of developing ischemia are substantially modified. If paced for an identical time the improvement may be impressive (Fig. 10), but by extending the pacing time to the new end point (Fig. 11) the improvement may not be sustained, in a sense like a dose response curve. It is also of interest that those with and without occluded grafts may develop ischemia, still reflecting areas of the myocardium that are not completely revascularized. It is perhaps in this group that regional

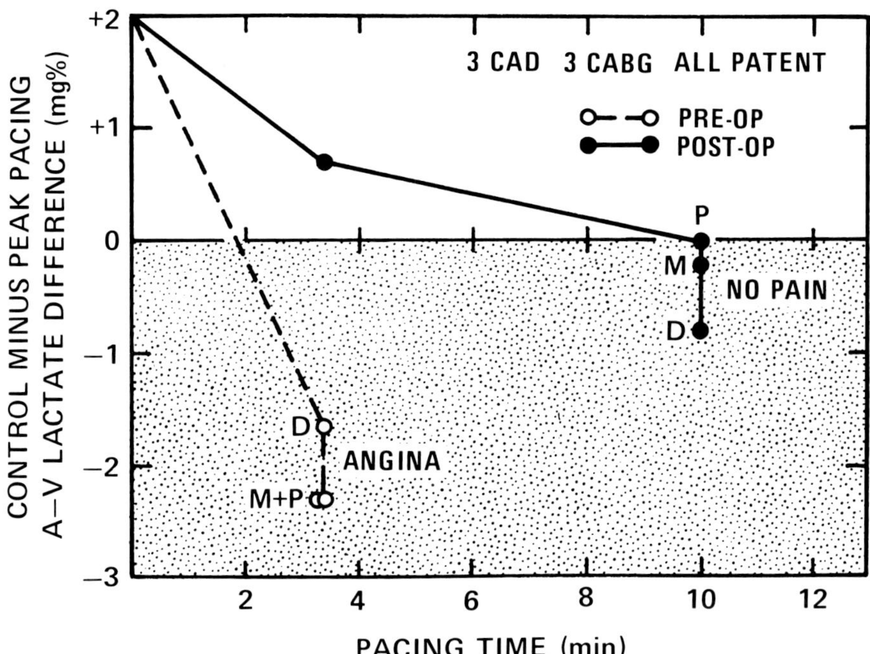

Figure 8. This graph pertains to a patient studied after successful coronary artery surgery. Pacing to a fixed time beyond the preoperative time reveals the delayed onset of ischemia. P, M, and D reflect sampling points in the coronary sinus.

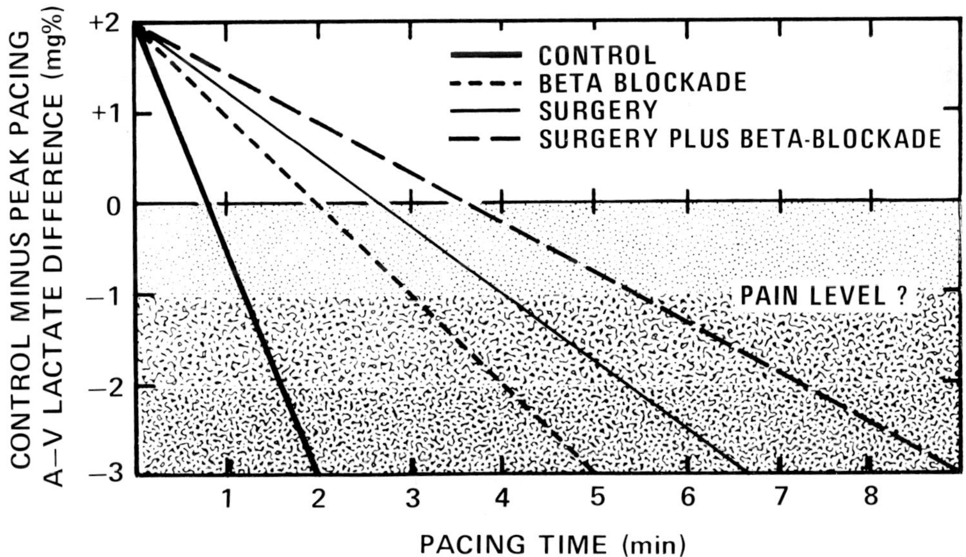

Figure 9. The rate of development of myocardial ischemia may be modified by various therapeutic maneuvers. Depending on each patient, the pain level—and speed in reaching this level—will vary.

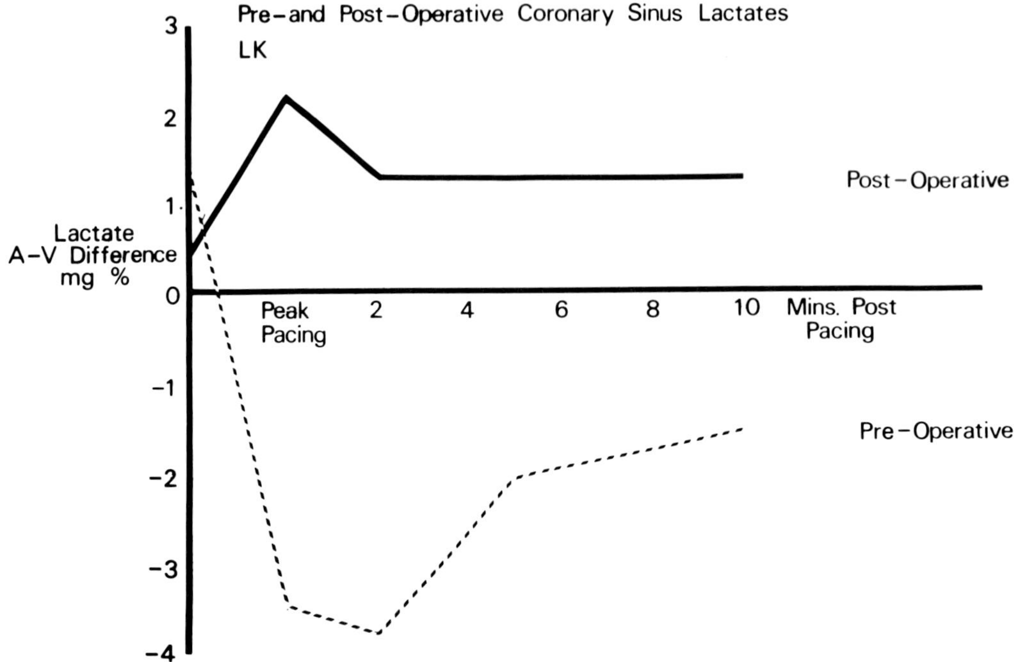

Figure 10. This graph represents the substantial metabolic improvement at identical pacing times pre- and post-coronary bypass surgery.

studies (see Figure 8) may identify patent grafts that are not sufficiently improving flow to an ischemic area. In Figure 8 the distal sampling point (D) reflects localized left anterior descending artery segment ischemia, but overall metabolism is improved, as reflected in a normal main sinus (P) sample—an example of the dilution effect of overall coronary sinus blood on local ischemic samples.

Angioplasty

Angioplasty can be evaluated in the same way as surgery or drugs.[60] It may be possible thereby to follow the functional significance of the procedure with time.

Heart Transplantation

Accelerated coronary artery disease may develop in the transplanted heart; and with the absence of pain as a signal of ischemia, it can be difficult to judge the functional significance of the lesions and the need for retransplantation. We performed atrial pacing and lactate studies in patients with and without coronary artery disease in their transplanted hearts. We could not induce abnormal metabolism (Fig. 12) in any patient despite pacing at 160 beats per minute for a minimum of 15 minutes, even when extensive disease was present (Fig. 13). These surprising observations suggest that the intact nervous system is essential for the evaluation of myocardial metabolic changes and sadly shed no light on the evaluation of coronary artery disease in the transplanted heart.

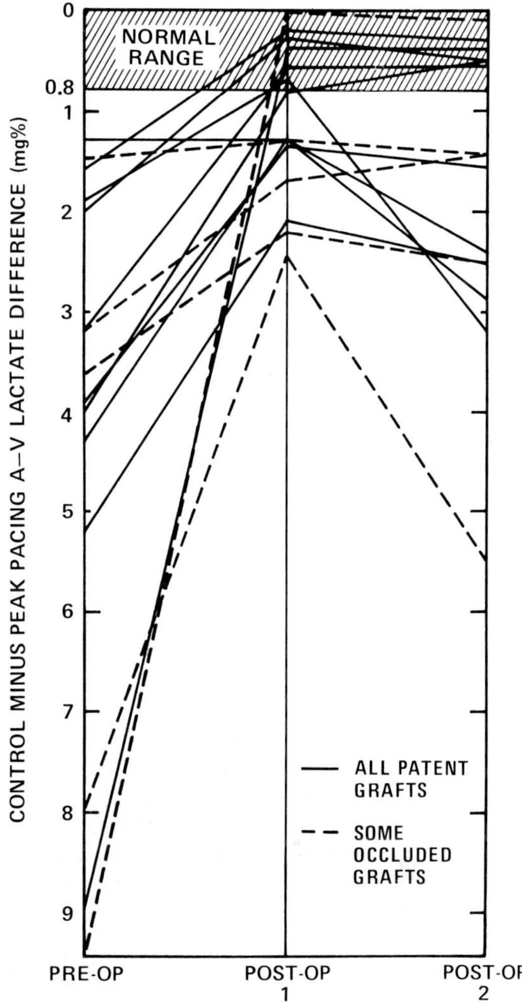

Figure 11. Illustrated here are the effects of coronary artery bypass grafts on myocardial lactate metabolism. It is important to sample at the same end-point as preoperatively (post-op 1) for direct comparisons. The new end-point (post-op 2) is used to judge the extent of improvement.

SUMMARY

The evaluation of myocardial metabolic changes in ischemic heart disease remains centered on the coronary sinus pacing and sampling techniques established over the last 25 years. Lactate remains the marker of choice for most institutions, though centers with more sophisticated laboratories will always be trying to improve on the sensitivity and specificity for ischemia, perhaps using ATP catabolites and nucleotides and measuring coronary sinus flow. The diagnostic value of lactate changes is limited and probably not superior to a well-conducted 12-lead treadmill exercise electrocardiogram test, but it does provide an objective marker for reliable further study and evaluation of interventions. It is almost certainly in the research context that metabolic studies have their place—evaluating drugs, surgery, or angioplasty and perhaps shedding light on obscure entities, such as chest pain with normal coronary arteries and cardiomyopathies. Attention to detail and simplicity of study are more likely to lead to valuable results rather than concentrating on the complexities. Each laboratory should establish the reproducibility of its results before commencing any procedures.

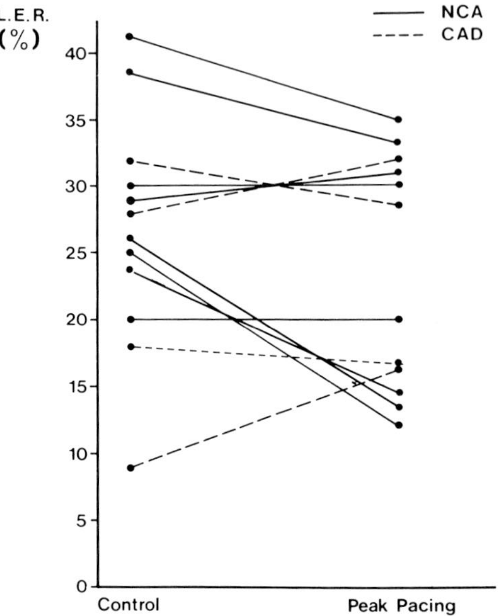

Figure 12. After heart transplantation, patients with significant coronary disease (CAD) and those with normal arteries (NCA) could not be differentiated by lactate studies.

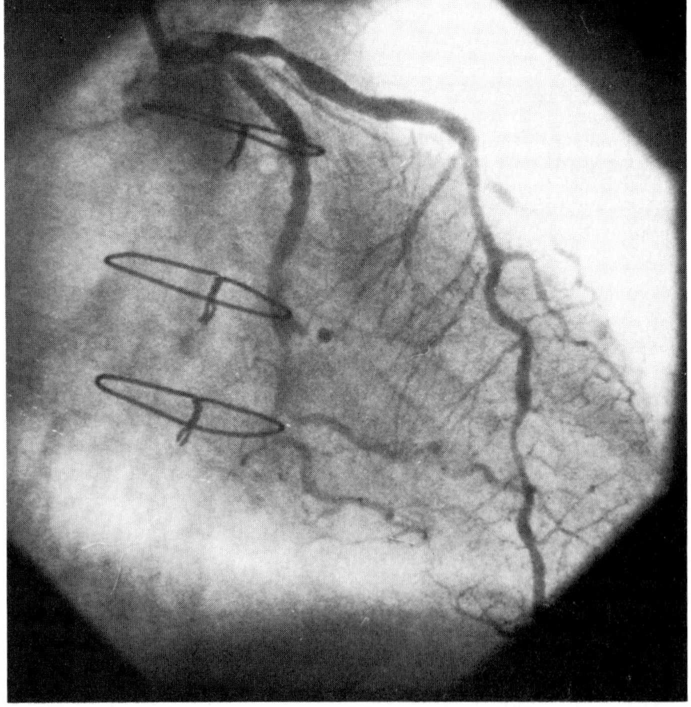

Figure 13. Pictured here is extensive coronary disease in a transplanted heart.

REFERENCES

1. Livesley, B, and Oram, S: *Diagnosis of doubtful angina.* Lancet 1:1461, 1973.
2. Opie, LH: *Metabolism of the heart in health and disease.* Am Heart J Part I 76:685, 1968; Part II 77:100, 1969; Part III 77:383, 1969.
3. Gorlin, R: *Evaluation of myocardial metabolism in ischemic heart disease.* Circulation Suppl IV:155, 1969.
4. Moret, PR, Weber, J, Haissly, J-CI, et al: *Lactate: Physiologic, Methodologic and Pathologic Approach.* Springer-Verlag, Berlin, 1980.
5. Lassers, BW, Carlson, LA, Kaijser, L, et al: *The nature and control of myocardial substrate metabolism in healthy man.* In Oliver, MF (ed): *Effect of Acute Ischemia on Myocardial Infarction.* Churchill Livingstone, Edinburgh, 200, 1972.
6. Bing, RJ: *The metabolism of the heart.* Harvey Lecture 50:27, 1954.
7. Evans, JR: *Cellular transport of long chain fatty acids.* Canad J Biochem Physiol 42:955, 1964.
8. Krasnow, N, Neill, WA, Messer, JV, et al: *Myocardial lactate and pyruvate metabolism.* J Clin Invest 41:2075, 1962.
9. Crass, MF III, McCaskill, ES, and Shipp, JC: *Glucose-free fatty acid interactions in the working heart.* J Appl Physiol 29:87, 1970.
10. Sobel, BE: *Salient biochemical features in ischemic myocardium.* Circ Res Suppl III:173, 1974.
11. Owen, P, Thomas, M, Young, V, et al: *Comparison between metabolic changes in local venous and coronary sinus blood after acute experimental coronary artery occlusion.* Am J Cardiol 25:562, 1970.
12. Henderson, AH, Craig, RJ, Gorlin, R, et al: *Free fatty acids and myocardial function in perfused rat hearts.* Cardiovasc Res 4:466, 1970.
13. Kurien, VA, and Oliver, MF: *Metabolic cause for arrhythmias during acute myocardial infarction.* Lancet 1:813, 1970.
14. Brachfeld, N and Sheuer, J: *Uptake and metabolism of glucose by the ischemic myocardium.* J Clin Invest 43:1301, 1964.
15. Wollenberger, A and Kraise, EG: *Metabolic control characteristics of the acutely ischemic myocardium.* Am J Cardiol 20:349, 1968.
16. Bing, RJ, Vandam, LD, Gregoire, F, et al: *Catheterization of coronary sinus and middle cardiac vein in man.* Proc Soc Exp Biol Med 66:239, 1947.
17. Messer, JV, Wagman, RJ, Levine, HJ, et al: *Patterns of human myocardial oxygen extraction during rest and exercise.* J Clin Invest 41:725, 1962.
18. Most, AS, Gorlin, R, and Soeldner, JS: *Glucose extraction by the human myocardium during pacing stress.* Circulation 45:92, 1972.
19. Remme, WJ, De Jong, JW, and Verdouw, PD: *Effects of pacing-induced myocardial ischemia on hypoxanthine efflux from the human heart.* Am J Cardiol 40:55, 1977.
20. Case, RB, Nasser, MG, and Crampton, RS: *Biochemical aspects of early myocardial ischemia.* Am J Cardiol 24:766, 1969.
21. Parker, JO, Chiong, MA, West, RO, et al: *The effect of ischemia and alterations of heart rate on myocardial potassium balance in man.* Circulation 62:205, 1970.
22. Sheuer, J and Brachfeld, N: *Myocardial uptake and fractional distribution of palmitate-1-6[14] by the ischemic dog heart.* Metabolism 15:945, 1966.
23. Gorlin, R: *Assessment of hypoxia in the human heart.* Cardiology 57:24, 1972.
24. Mudge, GH Jr, Mills, RM Jr, Taegtmeyer, H, et al: *Alterations in myocardial amino acid metabolism in chronic heart disease.* J Clin Invest 58:1185, 1976.
25. Berger, HJ, Zaret, BL, Speroff, L, et al: *Cardiac prostaglandin release during myocardial ischemia induced atrial pacing in patients with coronary artery disease.* Am J Cardiol 39:481, 1977.
26. Fox, AL, Reed, GE, and Glassman, E: *Release of adenosine from human hearts during angina induced by rapid atrial pacing.* J Clin Invest 53:1447, 1974.
27. Opie, LH, Owen, P, Thomas, M, et al: *Coronary sinus lactate measurements in the assessment of myocardial ischemia.* Am J Cardiol 32:295, 1973.
28. Cohen, LS, Elliott, WC, Klein, MD, et al: *Coronary heart disease: Clinical cinearteriographic and metabolic correlations.* Am J Cardiol 17:153, 1966.
29. Mueller, PS and Horwitz, D: *Plasma free fatty acids and blood glucose responses to analogues of norepinephrine in man.* J Lipid Res 3:251, 1962.

30. SOWTON, GE, BALCON, R, CROSS, D, ET AL: *Measurement of the angina threshold using atrial pacing: New technique for the study of angina pectoris.* Cardiovasc Res 1: 301, 1967.

31. HERMAN, MV, ELLIOTT, WC, AND GORLIN, R: *An electrocardiographic, anatomic and metabolic study of zonal myocardial ischemia in coronary heart disease.* Circulation 35:834, 1967.

32. NEILL, WA: *Myocardial hypoxia and anaerobic metabolism in coronary heart disease.* Am J Cardiol 22:507, 1968.

33. PARKER, JO, CHIONG, MA, WEST RO, ET AL: *Sequential alterations in myocardial lactate metabolism, ST-T segments, and left ventricular function during angina induced by atrial pacing.* Circulation 60:113, 1969.

34. LIVESLEY, B AND ATKINSON, L: *Accurate quantitative estimation of lactate in whole blood.* Clin Chem 20:1478, 1974.

35. THADANI, U, LEWIS, JR, MATTHEW, JM, ET AL: *Reproducibility of clinical and hemodynamic parameters during pacing stress testing in patients with angina pectoris.* Circulation 60:1036, 1979.

36. BRACHFELD, N: *Characterization of the ischemic process by regional metabolism.* Am J Cardiol 37:467, 1976.

37. MOIR, TW AND DEBRA, W: *Effects of left ventricular hypertension, ischemia and vasoactive drugs on the myocardial distribution of coronary flow.* Circ Res 21:65, 1967.

38. GANZ, W, TAMURA, K, MARAUS, HS, ET AL: *Measurement of coronary sinus blood flow by continuous thermodilution in man.* Circulation 61:181, 1971.

39. JACKSON, G, ATKINSON, L, CLARK, M, ET AL: *Diagnosis of coronary artery disease by estimation of coronary sinus lactate.* Br Heart J 60:979, 1978.

40. ZUCKER, IR, ROTHFIELD, EL, AND BERNSTEIN, A: *A new multipurpose cardiac catheter.* Am J Cardiol 15:45, 1965.

41. JACKSON, G, ATKINSON, L, AND ORAM, S: *Improvement of myocardial metabolism in coronary arterial disease by beta blockade.* Br Heart J 39:829, 1977.

42. CHIONG, MA, WEST, RO, AND PARKER, JO: *Influence of nitroglycerin on myocardial metabolism and hemodynamics during angina induced by atrial pacing.* Circulation 45:1044, 1972.

43. PEPINE, CJ, SCHANG, SJ, AND BEMILLER, CR: *Effects of perhexilene on coronary hemodynamics and myocardial metabolic responses to tachycardia.* Circulation 49:887, 1974.

44. ROULEAU, JL, CHATTERJEE, K, PORTS, TA, ET AL: *Mechanism of relief of pacing induced angina with oral verapamil: Reduced oxygen demand.* Circulation 67:94, 1983.

45. DALY, K, BERGMAN, G, ROTHMAN, M, ET AL: *Beneficial effect of adding nifedipine to beta-adrenergic blocking therapy in angina pectoris.* Eur Heart J 3:42, 1982.

46. JACKSON, G, ATKINSON, L, AND CRAM, S: *Improvement of myocardial metabolism in coronary artery disease by beta blockade.* Br Heart J 39:829, 1977.

47. MUELLER, HS, AYRES, SM, RELIGA, A, ET AL: *Propranolol in the treatment of acute myocardial infarction: Effect on myocardial oxygenation and hemodynamics.* Circulation 49:1078, 1974.

48. BALCON, R: *Assessment of drugs in angina pectoris.* Postgrad Med J 47 (Suppl Advances in Adenergic Beta-Receptor Therapy): 53, 1971.

49. KUPPER, W, HAMM, CW, AND BLEIFELD, W: *The effect of pindolol on myocardial blood flow, metabolism and function during rest and pacing in patients with coronary heart disease.* Br J Clin Pharmacol 13:3095, 1982.

50. PITT, B AND CRAVEN, P: *Effect of propranolol on regional myocardial blood flow in acute ischemia.* Cardiovasc Res 4:176, 1970.

51. *A multicentre study: Improvement in prognosis of myocardial infarction by long-term beta adrenoceptor blockade using practolol.* Br Med J 3:735, 1975.

52. ANDERSEN, MP, BECHSGAARD, P, FREDERIKSEN, J, ET AL: *Effect of alprenolol on mortality among patients with definite or suspected acute myocardial infarction: Preliminary results.* Lancet 2:865, 1979.

53. THE NORWEGIAN MULTICENTER STUDY GROUP: *Timolol-induced reduction in mortality and reinfarction in patients surviving acute myocardial infarction.* N Engl J Med 304:801, 1981.

54. HJALMARSON, A, ELMFELDT, D, HERLITZ, J, ET AL: *Effect on mortality of metoprolol in acute myocardial infarction: A double blind randomized trial.* Lancet 2:823, 1981.

55. NATIONAL HEART, LUNG AND BLOOD INSTITUTE: *The beta blocker heart trial.* JAMA 246:2073, 1981.

56. PRINEAS, RJ AND BLACKBURN, H (EDS): *Sudden cardiac deaths outside hospital.* Circulation 52 (Suppl 3):1, 1975.

57. CORDAY, E, HENG, MK, MEERBAUM, S, ET AL: *Derangements of myocardial metabolism preceding onset of ventricular fibrillation after coronary occlusion.* Am J Cardiol 39:880, 1977.

58. Chatterjee, K, Matloff, JM, Swan, HJC, et al: *Abnormal regional metabolism and mechanical function in patients with ischemic heart disease: Improvement after successful regional revascularization by aortocoronary bypass.* Circulation 52:390, 1975.

59. Carlson, RG, Kline, S, Apstein, C, et al: *Lactate metabolism after aorto-coronary artery vein bypass grafts.* Ann Surg 176:680, 1975.

60. Williams, DO, Riley, RS, Singh, AK, et al: *Restoration of normal coronary hemodynamics and myocardial metabolism after percutaneous transluminal coronary angioplasty.* Circulation 62:653, 1980.

Measurement of Coronary Blood Flow in Man: Methods and Implications for Clinical Practice

Arlene B. Bradley, M.D., and Donald S. Baim, M.D.*

During the past 25 years, a variety of techniques have been developed for the measurement of coronary blood flow in man. An ideal method would be reproducible, repeatable, and capable of detecting brief alterations in regional (anterior versus inferior) and transmural (endocardial versus epicardial) perfusion and relating these alterations to instantaneous myocardial oxygen consumption and the mass of myocardium perfused. Although no method currently available for use in man meets all these criteria, several techniques have contributed importantly to our understanding of coronary physiology.

This chapter will review the basic physiology of coronary regulation, the methods currently used to measure coronary flow in man, and the results of such measurements in a variety of disease states.

REGULATION OF CORONARY BLOOD FLOW

Coronary blood flow (CBF) is determined by the ratio between the transmyocardial perfusion pressure (ΔP) and the instantaneous coronary vascular resistance (R). Klocke has separated the total resistance into three physiologically distinct components: R_1, the epicardial coronary artery resistance, contributes only 3 to 10 percent of the total resistance in the absence of epicardial coronary stenosis or spasm; R_2, the arteriolar resistance, is the major resistance and responds predominantly to local metabolic demands; and R_3, the compressive resistance, results from compression of the intramyocardial vessels during systole and accounts for the fact that resting CBF occurs predominantly during diastole.[1,2]

Inasmuch as the myocardium is essentially obligated to aerobic metabolism, and myocardial oxygen extraction is already nearly maximal at rest,[3] autoregulation must maintain adequate blood flow in the face of changes in perfusion pressure or alterations in instantaneous myocardial oxygen demand.[4,5] These autoregulatory functions require the availability of coronary vascular reserve—the ability to increase coronary blood flow by reduction of the arteriolar resistance, R_2.[6] In the normal coronary circulation, coronary vascular reserve is adequate to raise coronary flow four to six times above resting levels.[2,6] As atherosclerosis or disorders in coronary tone supervene, this vasodilatory reserve (and correspondingly the patient's exercise tolerance) is progressively eroded.

In examining changes in coronary blood flow, it is important to distinguish "primary" vasomotion (alteration in coronary flow despite constant myocardial oxygen demand, $M\dot{V}O_2$)

*Supported in part by Grant NIH-07374 from the National Heart, Lung, and Blood Institute

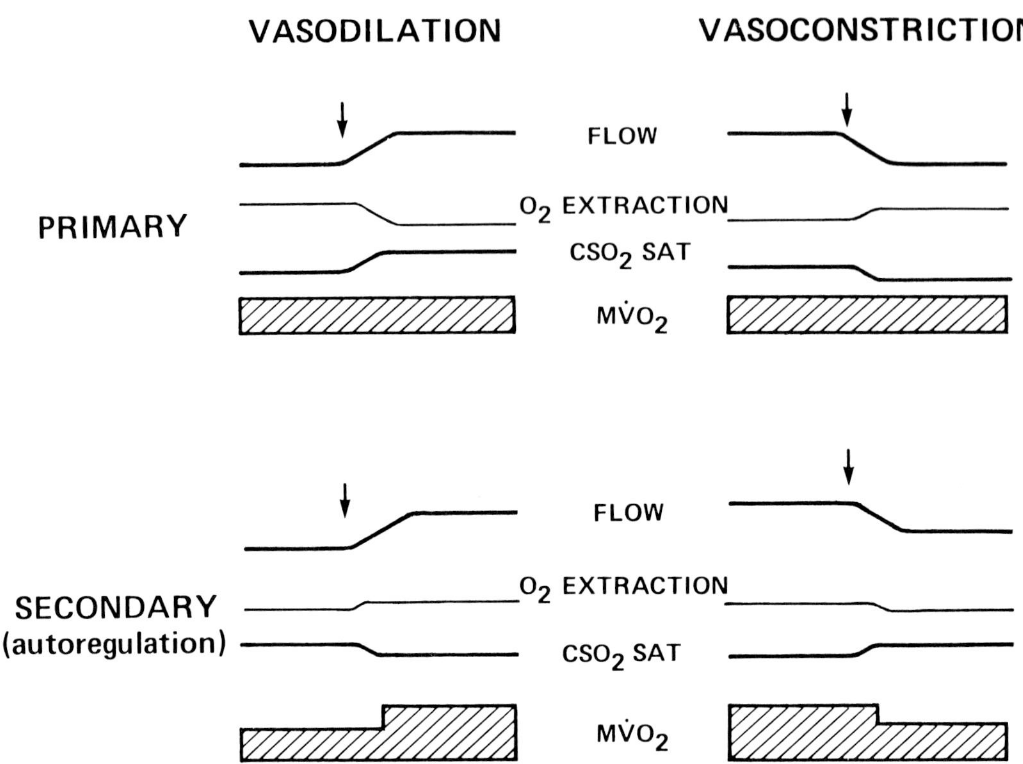

Figure 1. Primary and secondary coronary vasomotion as reflected by coronary blood flow (FLOW) and coronary sinus oxygen saturation (CSO_2 SAT). In primary vasodilation, flow increases at a constant myocardial oxygen consumption ($M\dot{V}O_2$), so that myocardial oxygen extraction (O_2 extraction) falls and coronary sinus oxygen saturation rises. In secondary, or autoregulatory, vasodilation, however, flow increases owing to an increase in myocardial oxygen consumption, leading to either a constant or slightly reduced coronary sinus saturation. Similar analysis can be applied to distinguish primary from secondary coronary vasoconstriction. (From Baim, DS, Rothman, MT, and Harrison, DC,[7] with permission.)

from "secondary" vasomotion (alteration in flow in response to a change in oxygen demand)[7] (Fig. 1), and to distinguish between vasomotion of the large (epicardial or R_1) and small (arteriolar or R_2) vessels.[8,9] Differences in the response of large and small vessels determine the net coronary hemodynamic effect of vasoactive drugs on myocardial perfusion in patients with coronary artery disease or focal coronary spasm. Thus, agents that selectively decrease arteriolar tone may worsen ischemia by causing coronary "steal," that is, diversion of blood flow away from the ischemic territory and the subendocardial layer.[10] In contrast, agents that reduce large vessel tone may enlarge the stenotic lumen and increase collateral blood flow to the ischemic territory.[11,12]

CORONARY BLOOD FLOW MEASUREMENT TECHNIQUES

Compared with the modalities available in the animal laboratory, the techniques that are applicable to the measurement of coronary blood flow in man are relatively limited.

Electromagnetic Flowmeters

The electromagnetic flowmeter is based on Faraday's induction law, according to which a conductor (blood) moving in a magnetic field produces an electric field perpendicular to both the magnetic field and to the conductor's movement.[13] If an electromagnet is energized by an alternating sinusoidal or square wave current, gated sampling can be used to monitor the resulting electric field.[14] Because such flow probes must be applied directly to the coronary artery, they can be used in man only at the time of cardiac surgery, where they are routinely used to monitor aortocoronary bypass graft flow.[15] Although similar electromagnetic flow velocity sensors can be affixed to a cardiac catheter to assess aortic blood flow velocity, they have not yet been employed to measure coronary blood flow.[16]

Electromagnetic flow measurement has numerous advantages, including a high-frequency response that permits monitoring of phasic changes in coronary blood flow, linearity over the physiologic range of coronary blood flow, and the ability to measure both antegrade and retrograde flow. Its disadvantages, however, include limited applicability to human studies, the requirement for repeated confirmation of the zero flow point by vessel occlusion, and the inability to distinguish subendocardial from subepicardial flow.

Doppler Velocity Probes

The Doppler probe is based on the principle that sound waves reflected from a medium containing moving particles (red blood cells) undergo a shift in sound frequency that is linearly proportional to the velocity of the medium.[17,18] Piezoelectric crystals applied to the vessel wall are used to transmit and to receive high-frequency sound waves, and electronic circuits determine the magnitude of Doppler shift and thus the instantaneous blood flow velocity. The use of pulsed emission of high-frequency sound allows velocity measurement by a single crystal and discrimination between forward and backward flow.[19,20] A human velocity probe has recently been developed for use at the time of open heart surgery: the ultrasonic transducer (containing a 1 to 2 mm piezoelectric cystal) is mounted on a silicone suction cup applied to either a native coronary vessel or a coronary graft for measurement of flow velocity.[21,22]

The Doppler flow sensor has also been modified for intracoronary use in conscious humans by mounting the crystal on the tip of a catheter that can be positioned at the orifice of either the right or left coronary artery to record instantaneous coronary flow velocity. Benchimol and coworkers used a continuous wave Doppler system that could not distinguish between forward and backward flow,[23,24] but Cole and Hartley subsequently developed a pulsed Doppler system that allows directional velocity measurements and simultaneous pressure recording during intracoronary injections of radiographic contrast or other vasoactive agents.[25]

Advantages of the Doppler velocity meter include a high-frequency response, a stable zero velocity point without the need for repeated occlusive measurements, sensitivity to flow direction, and catheter tip mounting for the study of coronary velocity in conscious humans. Disadvantages of Doppler flow probes include the fact that the technique measures blood velocity rather than volume flow (which must then be obtained by multiplying flow velocity by vessel cross-sectional area). Because epicardial coronary diameter changes up to 5 percent during a single cardiac cycle,[26] and interventions that increase coronary flow may substantially change epicardial coronary cross-sectional area, reliance on flow velocity alone may underestimate coronary volume flow by up to 40 percent.[27] The catheter-tip Doppler flow technique has a limited (70 percent) success rate in man owing to difficulties in correct catheter positioning within the coronary arteries.[23] Velocity measurements performed at the left coronary ostium are insensitive to distal stenoses because of the interposition of major branch vessels,[25] and Doppler measurements cannot differentiate between subendocardial and subepicardial perfusion.

Videodensitometry

Videodensitometry evaluates epicardial coronary flow velocity by measuring the transit time of radiographic contrast between two preselected points along the vessel length. Coronary cross-sectional area is simultaneously determined from biplane cineangiography, so that volume flow can be calculated.[28–30]

Positive aspects of this method include its applicability to conscious humans and the ability to monitor multiple interventions and to measure volume flow, albeit with the assumption that epicardial diameter remains unchanged during a cardiac cycle.

Negative aspects of this measurement technique include the following: First, expensive technology is required for background subtraction and compensation for alterations in density resulting from cardiac and respiratory cycles. Secondly, coronary flow measurement may be distorted by high-pressure selective intracoronary injection or by the vasodilator properties of currently available contrast agents.[31] Thirdly, the frequency response of videodensitometry is too slow to demonstrate phasic coronary flow, and this method does not discriminate between subendocardial and subepicardial blood flow.

Microspheres

Microsphere animal studies have been the cornerstone of our current understanding of perfusion of the left and right ventricles and the subendocardium relative to the subepicardium.[1] Because they measure myocardial perfusion directly, microspheres are not influenced by the capacitance effects of the epicardial and intramural vessels.[32,33] Light plastic microspheres (typically 9 to 15 μm in diameter) are labelled with a radioactive isotope. Up to nine different isotope labels can be employed to allow flow determinations during serial interventions. When injected into the left atrium, these microspheres are trapped within body tissue in direct proportion to local blood flow. If a peripheral arterial sample is withdrawn at a known rate during injection of each set of microspheres, absolute local myocardial blood flow can be determined by comparison of the radioactivity in the myocardial tissue with that in the reference blood sample.[34]

Microsphere studies clearly have numerous advantages in animal studies: They allow repeated accurate measurements of transmural distribution of blood flow in different parts of the heart but do not disturb regional hemodynamics.[35] The obviously serious shortcomings of this method are that the subject must be sacrificed for isolation and counting of myocardial sections, that the frequency response of this measurement is slow (about 30 seconds), and that a maximum of nine interventions can be studied.

Some adaptations of microsphere studies have, however, been employed in conscious human beings. Human studies use degradable particles consisting of either albumin or dextran.[36] These microspheres, labelled with ^{99m}Tc or ^{113m}In, are injected intra-arterially before and after coronary vasodilation,[37] allowing quantitation of microsphere distribution by precordial imaging. Clearly this method of microsphere administration allows only for qualitative assessment of blood flow, does not distinguish subendocardial from subepicardial perfusion, and allows study of only a limited number of interventions. Moreover, it is not clear that the spatial resolution achieved by precordial imaging after the injection of microspheres is superior to that obtained following intravenous administration of the potassium congener ^{201}Tl, [38] described below.

Myocardial Perfusion with Potassium Congeners

This method is based on myocardial uptake and concentration of potassium congeners via Na^+-K^+ ATPase activity.[39] The monovalent cations $^{43}K^+$, $^{81}Rb^+$, ^{129}Cs, and particularly ^{201}Tl have biologic and physical properties that are best suited for myocardial imaging.[40] Following intravenous injection, 2 to 5 percent of the radionuclide reaches the coronary circulation, where its distribution and cellular uptake parallel regional myocardial blood flow. Advantages of this method include its easy and safe applicability to studies in conscious humans, its sensitivity to regional transmural perfusion defects, and its ability to differentiate between transient defects caused by hypoperfusion and chronic defects caused by focal myocardial destruction or replacement.[36]

This method has numerous shortcomings: The relationship between thallium distribution and coronary blood flow is not linear: cellular thallium extraction tends to increase at low myocardial flow rates and to decrease at high flow rates.[40] Thallium perfusion provides only an index of relative coronary blood flow—true quantitation of coronary flow is generally not possible. Global left ventricular ischemia (owing to severe multivessel or left main coronary disease) or nontransmural (subendocardial) perfusion defects are difficult to detect, and current resolution is limited to one to two centimeters. Only two states of the coronary circulation may be evaluated during a given study: a coronary hemodynamic stress (physical exercise, spasm, pharmacologic arteriolar dilation) and subsequent thallium equilibration during the redistribution phase. This method provides no information on either phasic coronary flow or rapid transient flow changes.[36,38,39]

Positron Emission Tomography

Positron emission tomography is an adaptation of the microsphere and diffusible indicator techniques that allows repeated quantitative measurements of regional and subendocardial blood flow in conscious man. Studies employ the short-lived positron-emitting radionuclides ^{15}O, ^{13}N, and ^{11}C as well as a ring of cameras to detect coincidence radiation emitted by positron-electron annihilation. Sophisticated computers then reconstruct transverse myocardial sections. These studies require an on-site cyclotron for the generation of isotopes and are still in very limited use. Although resolution is limited to one to two square centimeters and the frequency response ranges from seconds to minutes, the ability to synthesize specific metabolic tracers raises the possibility of simultaneously studying myocardial blood flow and metabolism.[36,38,41–44]

Clearance Methods

The clearance methods were initially applied by Kety and Schmidt[45] to the measurement of central nervous system blood flow, but were adapted subsequently to measure coronary blood flow.[46] The indicators used are diffusible substances that (a) are physiologically inert, (b) are rapidly diffusible across the capillary endothelium to allow full myocardial tissue saturation and desaturation, (c) have a known tissue-blood partition coefficient, (d) allow for accurate determination of indicator concentration by either coronary sinus blood sampling or precordial imaging, and (e) do not recirculate.[47] Diffusible indicators can be subdivided into substances that behave like water ($H_2{}^{15}O$ and ^{131}I-antipyrine) and gases (N_2O, H_2, N_2, He, Ar, ^{85}Kr, ^{133}Xe).[36] They may be administered by inhalation or injection, with determination of myocardial saturation or desaturation by repeated arterial and coronary sinus sampling, or by precordial imaging in the case of radioactive tracers.[48–52] Such measurements allow for the calculation of the myocardial blood flow per 100 grams of left ventricular mass.

The advantages of clearance techniques include their applicability to conscious humans, and their abilities to relate coronary blood flow to left ventricular mass and to detect regional left ventricular perfusion abnormalities by precordial scintillation imaging or selective great cardiac vein tracer sampling.

Some of the disadvantages of the clearance method for coronary blood flow determination include slow frequency response, limitation in the number of determinations that can be made, and inability to quantitate transmural blood flow distribution.

Coronary Venous Flow

Direct measurement of cardiac venous outflow provides one of the most sensitive and useful determinations of regional left ventricular coronary blood flow in conscious human beings.

In contrast to coronary arterial inflow, coronary venous outflow occurs primarily in systole. Approximately 80 percent of left ventricular blood flow drains into the coronary sinus (CS), 15 percent of left ventricular venous flow enters the right ventricle via Thebesian veins, and a small percentage enters the left ventricle directly. Coronary sinus outflow thus represents the bulk of left ventricular myocardial perfusion.[47,53]

In the dog, venous drainage of the left anterior descending coronary artery (LAD) occurs principally (63 ± 8 percent) via the great cardiac vein (GCV) (Fig. 2), which begins at the point where the anterior interventricular vein enters the atrioventricular groove. The remainder of left anterior descending coronary blood flow reaches the coronary sinus via alternate

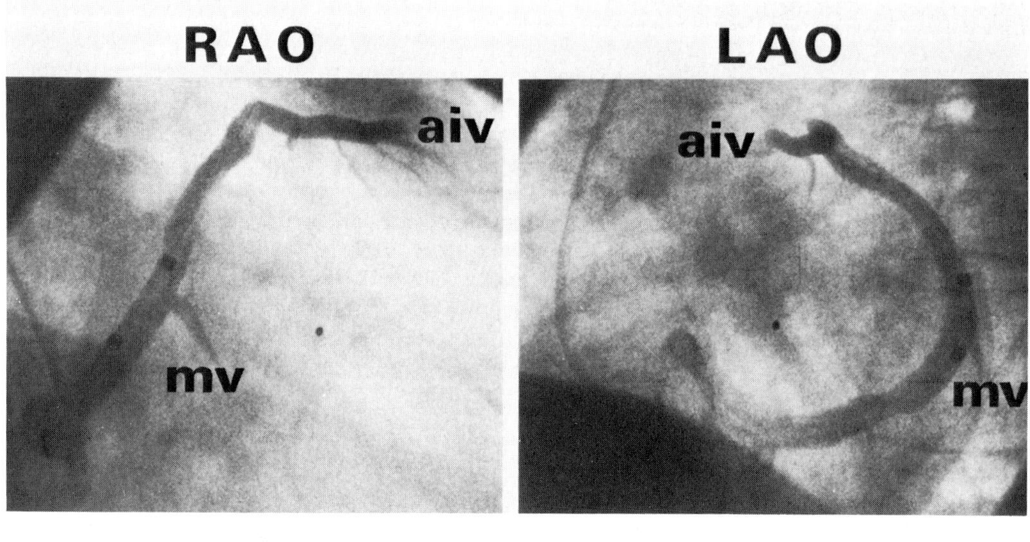

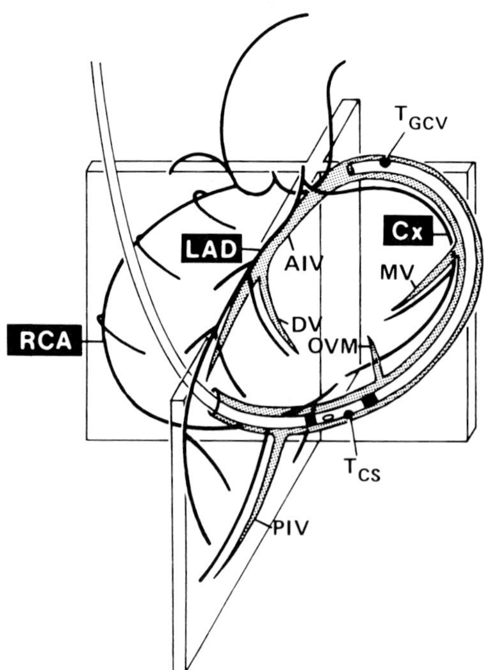

Figure 2. Coronary venous anatomy. (*Top*) Contrast injection through the tip of a coronary sinus flow catheter in the right anterior oblique (RAO) and left anterior oblique (LAO) projections shows the anterior interventricular vein (aiv) and a single marginal vein (mv). (*Bottom*) A representation of the LAO anatomy shows the relationship between the coronary venous and coronary arterial structures: diagonal vein (DV), posterior interventricular vein (PIV), and the left anterior descending, circumflex, and right coronary arteries (LAD, Cx, RCA, respectively).

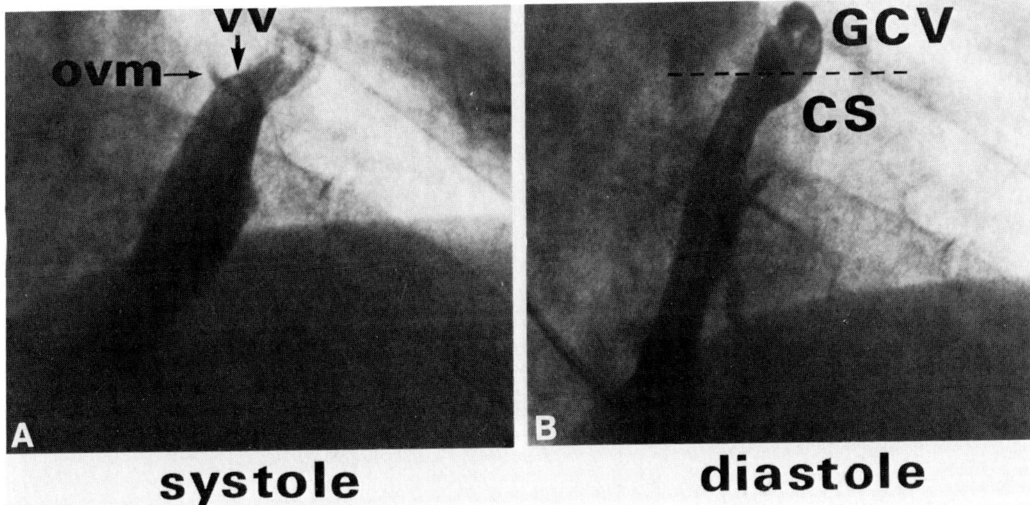

Figure 3. Anatomic structures delimiting the great cardiac vein-coronary sinus junction. Coronary venogram performed in the RAO projection with the catheter tip at the great cardiac vein (GCV)-coronary sinus (CS) junction. (*A*) During ventricular systole, outflow of unopacified blood from the great cardiac vein has silhouetted the domed valve of Vieussens (vv), while contrast has refluxed into the small left atrial oblique vein of Marshall (ovm), the remnant of the embryonic left-sided superior vena cava. (*B*) With the onset of ventricular diastole, contrast refluxes beyond the valve of Vieussens and into the great cardiac vein. Retrograde filling of several small marginal veins is also seen. Unless the valve of Vieussens makes retrograde passage into the great cardiac vein difficult, the great cardiac vein-coronary sinus transition is usually not evident.

epicardial venous pathways.[54] The transition between the great cardiac vein and the coronary sinus occurs at the valve of Vieussens and the oblique vein of Marshall, a left atrial vein that is the remnant of the embryonic left-sided superior vena cava (Fig. 3). Most venous drainage from the left circumflex territory enters the coronary sinus via the left marginal vein and circumflex venous branches, but only 3 percent of left circumflex drainage reaches the great cardiac vein.[54,55] Thus, great cardiac vein flow represents predominantly left anterior descending coronary artery outflow, whereas coronary sinus flow represents an admixture of both left anterior descending and left circumflex coronary artery venous drainage.

Measurement of coronary venous flow is based on the thermodilution principle: Fluid at room temperature is infused upstream into the coronary sinus for 30 to 60 seconds, where it mixes with coronary venous blood. The temperature of this mixture is related to instantaneous venous blood flow according to the formula first introduced by Ganz,[56] and recently modified by Baim[57] (Fig. 4):

$$Q = F \times C \times (Tm - Ti)/(Tb - Tm)$$

where

Q is coronary venous flow
F is the rate of injection of thermodilution indicator
T is temperature
- i = injectate
- b = blood
- m = mixture

C is the ratio of the specific heats of blood and injectate equal to
- 1.08 for 5% dextrose injection
- 1.19 for normal saline injection

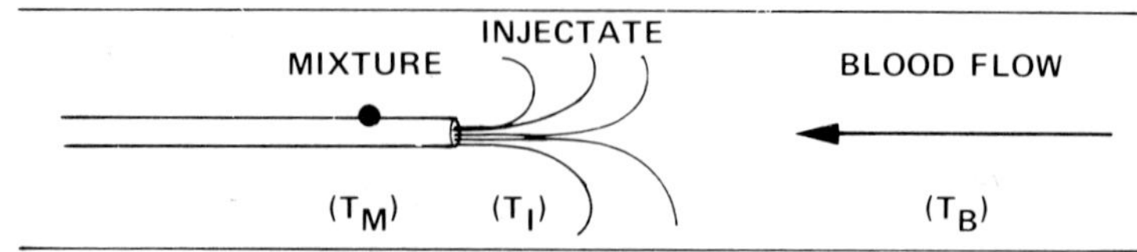

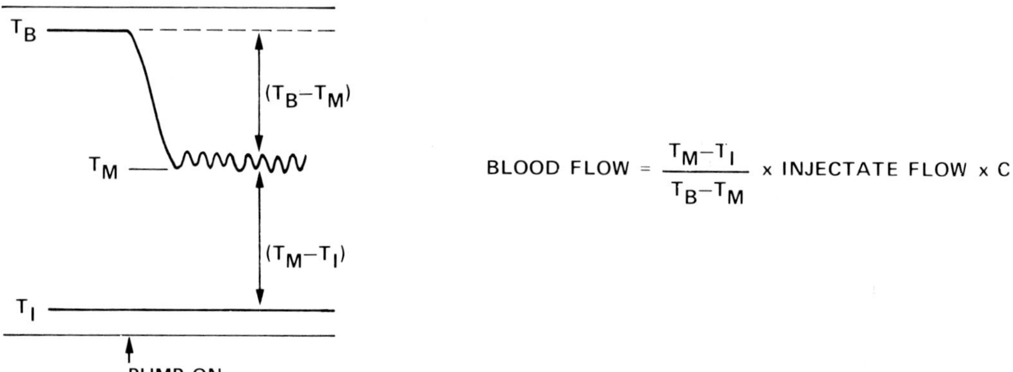

Figure 4. Calculation of coronary venous blood flow by thermodilution. In this schematic recording of a coronary venous flow measurement, the temperatures sensed by the catheter-tip thermistor and injectate thermistor are recorded on a uniform temperature scale. Before the continuous infusion of room temperature indicator, the catheter-tip thermistor records baseline blood temperature (T_B), while the injectate thermistor records injectate temperature (T_I). During continuous infusion at a flow rate F (usually 50 ml per minute), turbulence generated by rapid upstream injection causes complete mixing of the injectate and the coronary venous blood. As this mixture washes down the shaft of the catheter, temperature (T_M) is sensed by the catheter thermistor. Because the heat lost by the blood is equal to the heat gained by the injectate, it is possible to calculate the coronary venous flow from the respective temperatures, the injectate flow rate, and the constant C, which reflects the relative specific heat of blood and injectate.

In order to ensure turbulent mixing, the thermal indicator must be infused through a small orifice at a rate of 35 to 50 ml per minute, using a catheter that possesses adequate thermal insulation to prevent heat exchange between the indicator lumen and the sensing thermistor.[55]

Although the basic principle of coronary venous thermodilution has been maintained, modifications have enhanced the ease of catheter insertion. A recently designed coronary sinus catheter includes the following features: a more flexible catheter shaft, an end-hole to allow use of a guide wire in cases where coronary venous branches or valves complicate insertion into the great cardiac vein, and the incorporation of optical fibers to permit continuous reflectance measurement of great cardiac vein oxygen saturation (Fig. 5). Simultaneous thermodilution measurement of great cardiac vein and coronary sinus flow during continuous reflectance measurement of great cardiac vein oxygen saturation allows calculation of myocardial oxygen consumption and differentiation between "primary" regional (oxygen demand-independent) and "secondary" (autoregulatory) vasomotion[7] (Fig. 6).

Coronary sinus thermodilution has numerous other strong points. It can be safely employed in conscious human beings and correlates well with electromagnetic flow measurements.[58] Prolonged or multiple serial measurements can be performed easily, and the frequency response is adequate to detect transient changes in blood flow and oxygen tension.

Shortcomings of the technique include the following: If the catheter is not in a secure position, motion may lead to unpredictable incorporation or exclusion of the flow contributions from branches located near the thermistors. Complete left coronary venous drainage cannot

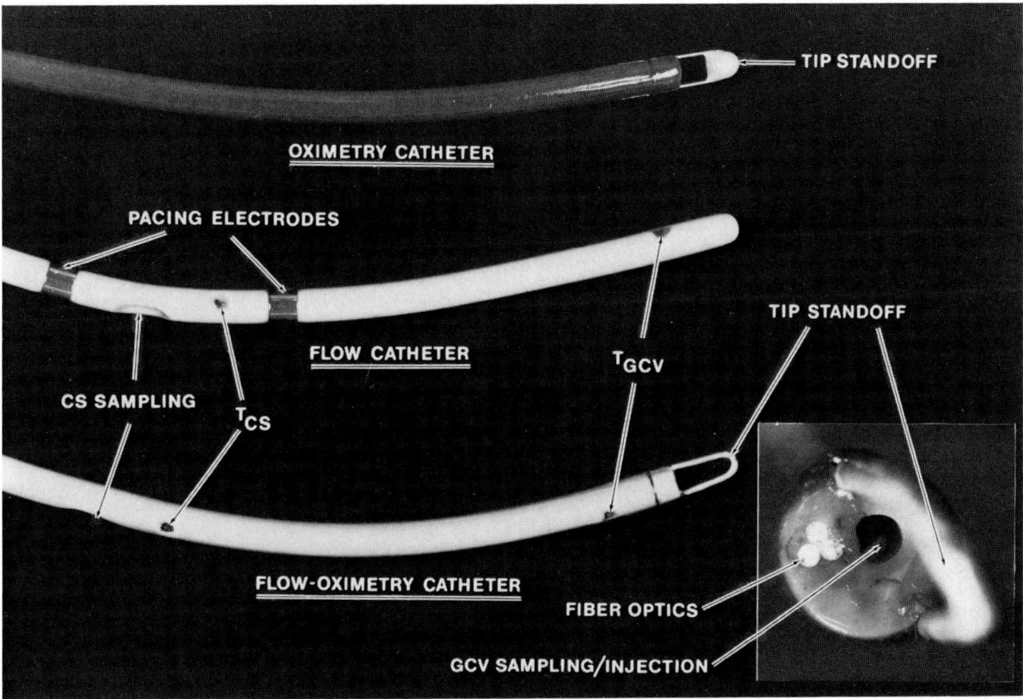

Figure 5. Coronary venous catheters (*top to bottom*): Oximetry catheter, regional thermodilution flow catheter, and combined flow-oximetry catheter. Both the flow and flow-oximetry catheters have sampling thermistors positioned to measure temperature in the great cardiac vein (T_{GCV}) and coronary sinus (T_{CS}), a lumen for sampling and injecting indicator in the great cardic vein (see insert), and a lumen for sampling blood from the coronary sinus. Both the oximetry and flow-oximetry catheters are fitted with a fiberoptic bundle to permit reflectance measurements of great cardiac venous saturation. (From Baim, DS, Rothman, MT, and Harrison, DC,[7] with permission.)

be assessed, because the posterior interventricular vein enters the coronary sinus too close to the right atrium to allow measurement without contamination of the temperature profile by right atrial blood reflux. Finally, coronary venous measurements do not reflect phasic coronary flow and do not discriminate between subendocardial and subepicardial coronary perfusion.

In summary, no method for measuring CBF in conscious human beings is ideal in all respects, but several methods possess sufficient capabilities to allow their use in ongoing studies of coronary physiology in a variety of disease states.

CORONARY FLOW MEASUREMENTS IN VARIOUS CLINICAL SITUATIONS

Coronary blood flow determinations have been used primarily to study the coronary hemodynamics of epicardial stenoses, in order to relate the degree of stenosis to its effect on coronary flow. In vitro and animal models have demonstrated that resting myocardial blood flow is not altered until a critical (90+ percent diameter reduction) stenosis is produced.[59,60] During reactive hyperemia following brief (20-second) coronary occlusions, however, stenoses as mild as 50 to 60 percent may limit available coronary flow reserve. Thus, resting coronary blood flow should be normal in all but the most severe stenoses, whereas flow reserve (obtained by comparing the resting and maximally hyperemic flow) should reflect the hemodynamic importance of any given stenosis.[6]

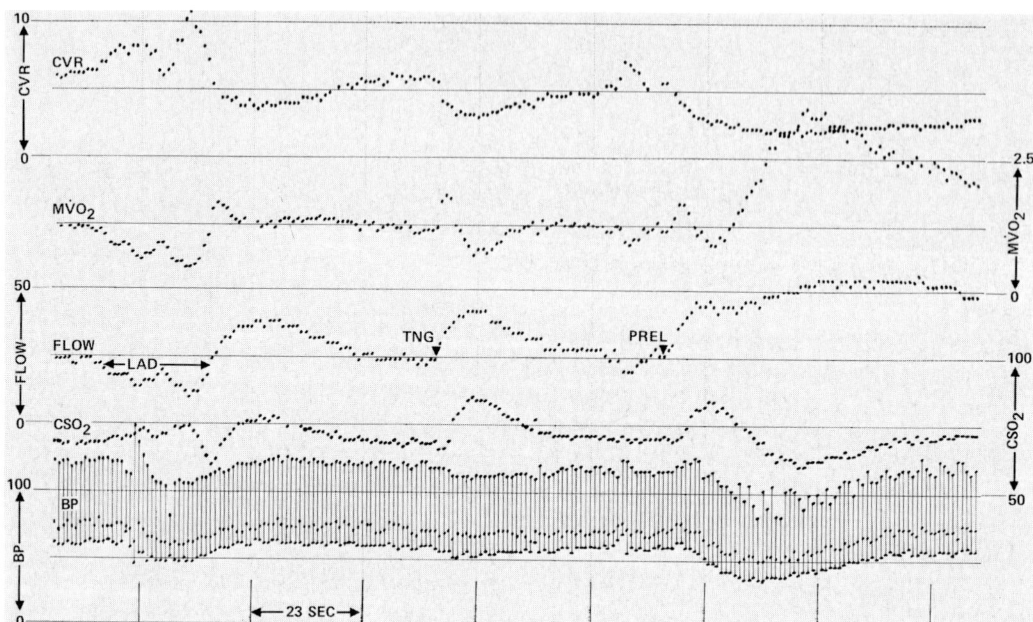

Figure 6. On-line computer processing of coronary venous flow (FLOW) and coronary venous oxygen saturation (CSO_2) permits differentiation between primary and secondary coronary vasodilation in an open chest dog model subjected to three vasodilatory interventions: transient occlusion of the mid-left anterior descending coronary artery (LAD) with reactive hyperemia, intracoronary administration of nitroglycerin (TNG), and intracoronary administration of isoproterenol (PREL). The arterial blood pressure (BP), calculated myocardial oxygen consumption ($M\dot{V}O_2$) and coronary vascular resistance (CVR) are shown. Nitroglycerin causes primary vasodilation with an increase in flow at constant $M\dot{V}O_2$ (note the increase in CSO_2). Isoproterenol, on the other hand, causes brief primary coronary vasodilation (owing to stimulation of vasodilatory beta-2 receptors) that rapidly progresses to prolonged secondary coronary vasodilation (continued increased flow associated with an increase in myocardial oxygen consumption and a fall in CSO_2). The distinction between these two types of vasodilation would not have been possible using measurement of coronary flow alone, thus highlighting the value of combined flow and oximetry measurements. (From Baim, DS, Rothman, MT, and Harrison, DC,[7] with permission.)

Coronary Artery Disease

A variety of techniques have been employed to measure coronary flow in patients with arteriographically documented coronary disease. Klocke, using the inert gas clearance method, found a systematic decrease in resting coronary flow in patients with significant multivessel coronary disease compared with normals, that is, 54 ± 11 ml per min per 100 g versus 70 ± 13 ml per min per 100 g, respectively.[61] Using ^{133}Xe as radioactive tracer, Cannon found discrete regional underperfusion in severe single-vessel coronary disease and diffuse hypoperfusion in significant multivessel disease.[62,63] During rapid atrial pacing, patients developed chest pain and electrocardiographic signs of ischemia while showing significantly smaller rises in coronary blood flow than observed in normals.[63] Selwyn, using intra-arterial ^{81}Kr during pacing, observed abnormal regional perfusion prior to the development of symptoms and electrocardiographic signs of ischemia. Tracer activity in the ischemic area not only failed to increase under the stress of pacing but actually diminished, suggesting coronary steal by adjacent territories during physiologic stress.[64]

These results obtained via the inert gas clearance methods contrast with those obtained via thermodilution studies. Yoshida and coworkers and subsequently Fuchs and associates have observed normal resting great cardiac vein flows in patients with moderate left anterior descending coronary artery stenoses. During pacing, flow increased appropriately until coronary vascular reserve was exhausted, and then it remained constant as signs of ischemia ensued.[65,66] Only left anterior descending coronary artery stenoses of greater than 90 percent severity were associated with a diminution of resting coronary blood flow.

This apparent conflict in resting flow measurements by the clearance and thermodilution methods may be partially explained by the data of Chen and coworkers.[67] Using ^{133}Xe, they demonstrated that patients with severe coronary artery disease have greater left ventricular wall thickness and mass and decreased calculated left ventricular wall stress. The lower measured blood flow per 100 grams might thus be appropriate for the reduced left ventricular wall stress and myocardial oxygen demand,[67] while total resting coronary blood flow would remain normal.[68]

Patients with significant epicardial stenoses have also been reported to show marked attenuation of the phasic coronary velocity profile during Doppler measurements.[23]

Because patients with severe coronary artery disease may be forced to utilize a significant portion of their arteriolar vasodilatory reserve to maintain normal resting flow, they may be more vulnerable than normals to arteriolar vasoconstrictor stimuli such as the cold pressor test and inhibition of prostaglandin synthesis by indomethacin.[69–71]

Coronary Artery Spasm

Coronary blood flow determinations have been used to elucidate the pathophysiology of rest angina. Chierchia and Maseri employed fiberoptic reflectance measurements of coronary sinus oxygen saturation to investigate patients with angina at rest. Episodes of chest pain or of silent ischemia involving the anterior wall were preceded by a fall in great cardiac vein oxygen saturation, which persisted as conventional signs of ischemia (diminished systolic left ventricular function, ST segment shifts, and chest pain) developed.[72,73] Given the lack of change in heart rate and blood pressure, these investigators inferred that myocardial oxygen consumption was initially constant, and that the fall in coronary sinus oxygen saturation (widening of arterial-coronary sinus oxygen saturation difference) was the result of a primary reduction in myocardial blood flow. This primary reduction in coronary blood flow during episodes of chest pain at rest has also been documented directly by coronary sinus thermodilution measurements and by thallium perfusion scanning.[36,74,75]

Chest Pain Syndromes

Coronary blood flow measurements have been used occasionally to investigate the etiology of anginal chest pains in patients with normal coronary anatomy and no evidence of left ventricular hypertrophy. Using coronary sinus thermodilution, R. O. Cannon and coworkers demonstrated an inappropriately high arteriolar vasoconstrictor tone in selected patients, which limited the available coronary vasodilator reserve during increased myocardial oxygen demand.[76] These findings were accentuated following ergonovine administration.[77] Similarly, Strauer and associates found evidence suggesting impaired arteriolar dilatory reserve in patients with systemic lupus erythematosus.[78]

Ventricular Hypertrophy

Patients with severe left ventricular hypertrophy and normal coronary arteries may have chest pain syndromes of uncertain etiology. Using ^{133}Xe scintigraphy, P. J. Cannon and coworkers documented diminished resting coronary blood flow per left ventricular unit weight.[63] Employing thermodilution measurements to evaluate coronary reserve during contrast-induced hyperemia, Pichard and associates found that patients with aortic stenosis or insufficiency and severe left ventricular hypertrophy have increased resting coronary blood flow but diminished coronary reserve.[79,80] These findings were also confirmed by Marcus and colleagues, employing an extravascular Doppler probe at the time of open heart surgery.[81,82]

Coronary Vasodilator Agents

NITROGLYCERIN. The systemic administration of nitroglycerin has been found to evoke transient significant increases in coronary blood flow as measured by intravascular Doppler,[23] ^{133}Xe,[38] and coronary sinus thermodilution.[11] Ganz and subsequently Fuchs and their colleagues evaluated the effects of intracoronary and systemic nitroglycerin on the relief of pacing-induced angina: Low-dose intracoronary nitroglycerin increased great cardiac vein and coronary sinus flow transiently but did not relieve pacing-induced angina, whereas systemic administration of larger doses of nitroglycerin resulted in a fall in the determinants of myocardial oxygen consumption and relief of chest pain.[83,84] This does not, however, exclude a concomitant vasodilatory effect of nitroglycerin on the epicardial coronary vessels or collaterals.

NIFEDIPINE. The calcium channel blocker nifedipine is effective in the control of both effort-related and resting angina pectoris. Several clinical investigators have sought to determine the coronary hemodynamic effects responsible for this antianginal action. Using sequential precordial imaging with ^{133}Xe, Malacoff and coworkers found that sublingual nifedipine caused an improvement in the perfusion of previously abnormal regions.[85] Using coronary sinus thermodilution measurements, Schanzenbaecher and associates found that intracoronary nifedipine administration produced "primary" coronary vasodilation, that is, increased myocardial blood flow in the setting of diminished myocardial oxygen consumption.[86] Kaltenbach and colleagues demonstrated (with coronary sinus oximetry) that this "primary" vasodilation following systemic or intracoronary nifedipine was of brief duration (minutes), compared with prolonged improvement in exercise tolerance.[87] Using coronary sinus oximetry and angiographic determination of epicardial coronary artery diameters in patients with coronary artery disease, Serruys and coworkers observed brief "primary" arteriolar vasodilation, followed by sustained dilation of the epicardial coronary arteries associated with a prolonged reduction of stenosis severity.[88] Thus, one major antianginal effect of nifedipine may result from prolonged epicardial arterial dilation rather than transient arteriolar dilation.

Monitoring of Therapeutic Interventions

Standard electromagnetic or Doppler flowprobes have been used to assess graft patency and flow during aortocoronary bypass surgery. Coronary sinus thermodilution has played a similar, albeit investigative, role during percutaneous transluminal coronary angioplasty (PTCA). Rothman and associates[89] followed the incremental efficacy of repeated balloon inflations during angioplasty procedures. An improvement in the degree of reactive hyperemia following repetitive, 10-second balloon inflations suggested that coronary reserve was being progressively restored as the percent stenosis of the epicardial coronary lesion decreased. Williams and coworkers studied the coronary hemodynamic effect of pacing before and after angioplasty of a coronary stenotic lesion, noting no change in resting coronary blood flow but an improved response during pacing (higher myocardial oxygen consumption, higher peak great cardiac vein flow, normalization of lactate extraction, and absence of angina) after successful angioplasty.[90]

Other Cardiac Medications

Inotropic drugs may increase coronary blood flow by "secondary" vasodilation in response to increased myocardial oxygen demand. Although a rise in myocardial contractility should increase myocardial oxygen consumption, this effect may be partially offset by a reduction in ventricular chamber diameter and consequently wall stress. In patients with congestive heart failure and coronary artery disease, the net effect on myocardial oxygen demand is therefore difficult to predict. Using coronary sinus thermodilution and oximetry in the evaluation of the effect of amrinone on myocardial oxygen demand and blood flow, Benotti and associates found that even though the acute administration of amrinone was associated with a rise in cardiac index and left ventricular stroke work, coronary blood flow and oxygen consumption actually fell, suggesting that the oxygen cost of increased contractility was more than offset by the reduction in left ventricular wall stress.[91]

FUTURE APPLICATIONS OF CORONARY BLOOD FLOW MEASUREMENTS

In summary, no current method of coronary blood flow measurement applicable to conscious man can match the sophistication possible in the animal laboratory. The techniques that are available, however, have provided important information about normal and abnormal human coronary physiology in the following situations:

a. determination of the hemodynamic severity of coronary stenoses,
b. evaluation of the adequacy of collateral blood flow,
c. evaluation of anginal syndromes in patients with normal coronary arteries,
d. assessment of coronary vascular reserve in left ventricular hypertrophy,
e. determination of the mechanism of action of antianginal agents,
f. early and late follow-up of patients undergoing interventional angiographic procedures or aortocoronary bypass surgery,
g. investigation of the myocardial oxygen cost of inotropic agents in patients with known coronary artery disease.

Although coronary blood flow measurements are unlikely to become part of routine clinical cardiologic practice in the near future, the insights into human coronary pathophysiology that they continue to provide should further enhance the diagnosis and treatment of cardiac disorders.

REFERENCES

1. Bache, R, McHale, PA, and Greenfield, JC Jr: *Transmural myocardial perfusion during restricted coronary inflow in the awake dog.* Am J Physiol 232:H645, 1977.
2. Klocke, FJ: *Coronary blood flow in man.* Prog Cardiovasc Dis 19:117, 1976.
3. Weber, KT and Janicki, JS: *The metabolic demand and supply of the heart: Physiologic and clinical considerations.* Am J Cardiol, 44:722, 1979.
4. Dole, WP and Bishop, VS: *Influence of autoregulation and capacitance on diastolic coronary artery pressure-flow relationships in the dog.* Circ Res 51:261, 1982.
5. Dole, WP and Bishop, VS: *Regulation of coronary blood flow during individual diastoles in the dog.* Circ Res 50:377, 1982.
6. Gould, KL and Lipscomb, K: *Effects of coronary stenoses on coronary flow reserve and resistance.* Am J Cardiol 34:48, 1974.
7. Baim, DS, Rothman, MT, and Harrison, DC: *Simultaneous measurement of coronary venous blood flow and oxygen saturation during transient alterations in myocardial oxygen supply and demand.* Am J Cardiol 49:743, 1982.
8. Macho, P and Vatner, SF: *Effects of nitroglycerin and nitroprusside on large and small coronary vessels in conscious dogs.* Circulation 64:1101, 1981.
9. Vatner, SF and Hintze, TH: *Effects of a calcium-channel antagonist on large and small coronary arteries in conscious dogs.* Circulation 66:579, 1982.
10. Cohen, MV: *Coronary steal in awake dogs: A real phenomenon.* Cardiovasc Res 16:339, 1982.
11. Mehta, J and Pepine, CJ: *Effect of sublingual nitroglycerin on regional flow in patients with and without coronary disease.* Circulation 58:803, 1978.

12. FELDMAN, RL, PEPINE, CJ, AND CONTI, CR: *Magnitude of dilatation of large and small coronary arteries by nitroglycerin.* Circulation 64:324, 1981.

13. MARSTON, EL, BAREFOOT, CA, AND SPENCER, MP: *Non-cannulating measurements of coronary blood flow.* Surg Forum 10:636, 1959.

14. KHOURI, EM AND GREGG, DE: *Miniature electromagnetic flowmeter applicable to coronary arteries.* J Appl Physiol 18:224, 1963.

15. GREENFIELD, JC JR, REMBERT, JC, YOUNG, WG JR, ET AL: *Studies of blood flow in aorto-to-coronary venous bypass grafts in man.* J Clin Invest 51:2724, 1972.

16. KLINKE, WP, CHRISTIE, LG, NICHOLS, WW, ET AL: *Use of catheter-tip velocity-pressure transducer to evaluate left ventricular function in man: Effects of intravenous propranolol.* Circulation 61:946, 1980.

17. KALMUS, HP, HEDRICH, AL, AND PARDUE, DR: *The acoustic flowmeter using electronic switching.* IRE Trans Ultrasonics Eng UE-1:49, 1954.

18. WOODCOCK, JP: *Theory and Practice of Blood Flow Measurement.* Butterworth, Woburn, Mass, 1975.

19. HARTLEY, CJ AND COLE, JS: *An ultrasonic pulsed Doppler system for measuring blood flow in small vessels.* J Appl Physiol 37:626, 1974.

20. FRANKLIN, D, PATRICK, T, KEMPER, S, ET AL: *A system for radiotelemetry of blood pressure, blood flow and ventricular dimensions from animals: A summary report.* Proceedings of the International Telemetry Conference, Washington, DC, 1971, p 244.

21. MARCUS, M, WRIGHT, C, DOTY, D, ET AL: *Measurements of coronary velocity and reactive hyperemia in the coronary circulation of humans.* Circ Res 49:877, 1981.

22. WRIGHT, CB, EASTHAM, CL, DOTY, DB, ET AL: *Intraoperative evaluation of the functional significance of coronary obstructions.* In RAPAPORT, E (ED): *Cardiology Update.* Elsevier Biomedical, New York, 1983.

23. BENCHIMOL, A, STEGALL, HF, AND GARTLAN, JL: *New method to measure phasic coronary blood velocity in man.* Am Heart J 81:93, 1971.

24. BENCHIMOL, A AND DESSER, KB: *Measurement of phasic aortocoronary bypass graft blood flow velocity in conscious man.* Am J Cardiol 32:895, 1973.

25. COLE, JS AND HARTLEY, CJ: *The pulsed Doppler coronary artery catheter: Preliminary report of a new technique for measuring rapid changes in coronary artery flow velocity in man.* Circulation 56:18, 1977.

26. MACHO, P, HINTZE, TH, AND VATNER, SF: *Regulation of large coronary arteries by increases in myocardial metabolic demands in conscious dogs.* Circ Res 49:594, 1981.

27. GOULD, KL AND KELLEY, KO: *Physiological significance of coronary flow velocity and changing stenosis geometry during coronary vasodilation in awake dogs.* Circ Res 50:695, 1982.

28. RUTISHAUSER, W, SIMON, H, STACKY, JP, ET AL: *Evaluation of roentgen cinedensitometry for flow measurements in models and in the intact circulation.* Circulation 36:951, 1967.

29. GENSINI, GG, KELLY, AE, DA COSTA, BCB, ET AL: *Quantitative angiography: The measurement of coronary vasomobility in the intact animal and man.* Chest 60:522, 1971.

30. SMITH, HC, STRUM, RE, AND WOOD, EH: *Videodensitometric system for measurement of vessel blood flow, particularly in the coronary arteries, in man.* Am J Cardiol 32:144, 1973.

31. GOULD, KL, LIPSCOMB, K, AND CALVERT, C: *Compensatory changes of the distal coronary vascular bed during progressive coronary constriction.* Circulation 51:1085, 1975.

32. ENG, C, JENTZER, JH, AND KIRK, ES: *The effects of the coronary capacitance on the interpretation of diastolic pressure-flow relationships.* Circ Res 50:334, 1982.

33. CHILIAN, WM AND MARCUS, ML: *Phasic coronary blood flow velocity in intramural and epicardial coronary arteries.* Circ Res 50:775, 1982.

34. HEYMANN, MA, PAYNE, BD, HOFFMAN, JIE, ET AL: *Blood flow measurements with radionuclide-labeled particles.* Prog Cardiovasc Dis 20:55, 1977.

35. GRAMES, GM, JANSEN, C, GANDER, MP, ET AL: *Safety of the direct injection of radiolabeled particles.* J Nucl Med 15:2, 1974.

36. ADELSTEIN, SJ AND MASERI, A: *Radioindicators for the study of the heart: Principles and applications.* Prog Cardiovasc Dis 20:3, 1977.

37. RITCHIE, JL, HAMILTON, GW, GOULD, KL, ET AL: *Myocardial imaging with indium-113m and technetium-99m-macroaggregated albumin: New procedure for identification of stress-induced regional ischemia.* Am J Cardiol 35:380, 1975.

38. HOLMAN, BL: *Radioisotopic examination of the cardiovascular system.* In BRAUNWALD, E (ED): *Heart Disease.* WB Saunders, Philadelphia, 1980.

39. PROKOP, EK, STRAUSS, HW, AND SHAW, J: *Comparison of regional myocardial perfusion determined by ionic potassium-43 to that determined by microspheres.* Circulation 50:978, 1974.

40. PITT, B AND STRAUSS, HW: *Myocardial imaging in the noninvasive evaluation of patients with suspected ischemic heart disease.* Am J Cardiol 37:797, 1976.

41. PHELPS, ME, HOFFMAN, EJ, HUANG, SC, ET AL: *ECAT: A new computerized tomographic imaging system for positron-emitting radiopharmaceuticals.* J Nucl Med 19:635, 1978.

42. GOULD, KL, SCHELBERT, H, PHELPS, M, ET AL: *Non-invasive assessment of coronary stenosis with myocardial perfusion imaging during pharmacologic coronary vasodilation: Detection of 47 percent diameter coronary stenosis with intravenous nitrogen-13 ammonia and emission-computed tomography in intact dogs.* Am J Cardiol 43:200, 1979.

43. TER-POGOSSIAN, MM, RAICHLE, ME, AND SOBEL, BE: *Positron-emission tomography.* Scientific American 243:139, 1980.

44. TER-POGOSSIAN, MM, KLEIN, MS, AND MARKHAM, J: *Regional assessment of myocardial metabolic integrity in vivo by positron-emission tomography with ^{11}C-labeled palmitate.* Circulation 61:357, 1980.

45. KETY, SS AND SCHMIDT, CF: *The determination of cerebral blood flow in man by the use of nitrous oxide in low concentrations.* Am J Physiol 143:53, 1945.

46. ECKENHOFF, JE, HAFKENSCHIEL, JH, HARMEL, MH, ET AL: *Measurement of coronary blood flow by the nitrous oxide method.* Am J Physiol 152:356, 1948.

47. BERNE, RM AND RUBIO, R: *Coronary circulation.* In *Handbook of Physiology. Section 2: The Cardiovascular System—The Heart, Vol. I.* American Physiological Society, Bethesda, MD, 1979.

48. KLEIN, MD, COHEN, LS, AND GORLIN, R: *Krypton-85 myocardial blood flow: Precordial scintillation versus coronary sinus sampling.* Am J Physiol 209:705, 1965.

49. BASSINGTHWAIGHTE, JB, STRANDELL, T, AND DONALD, DE: *Estimation of coronary blood flow by washout of diffusible indicators.* Circ Res 23:259, 1968.

50. CANNON, PJ, DELL, RB, AND DWYER, EM JR: *Measurements of regional myocardial perfusion in man with ^{133}xenon and a scintillation camera.* J Clin Invest 51:964, 1972.

51. HIRZEL, HO AND KRAYENBUEHL, HP: *Validity of the ^{133}xenon method for measuring coronary blood flow.* Pfluegers Arch Ges Physiol 349:159, 1974.

52. KLOCKE, FJ, BUNNELL, IL, GREENE, DG, ET AL: *Average coronary blood flow per unit weight of left ventricle in patients with and without coronary artery disease.* Circulation 50:547, 1974.

53. HOOD, WB, JR: *Regional venous drainage of the human heart.* Br Heart J 30:105, 1968.

54. NAKAZAWA, HK, ROBERTS, DL, AND KLOCKE, FJ: *Quantitation of anterior descending vs circumflex venous drainage in the canine great cardiac vein and coronary sinus.* Am J Physiol 234:H163, 1978.

55. ROBERTS, DL, NAKAZAWA, HK, AND KLOCKE, FJ: *Origin of great cardiac vein and coronary sinus drainage within the left ventricle.* Am J Physiol 230:486, 1976.

56. GANZ, W, TAMURA, K, MARCUS, HS, ET AL: *Measurement of coronary sinus blood flow by continuous thermodilution in man.* Circulation 44:181, 1971.

57. BAIM, DS, ROTHMAN, MT, AND HARRISON, DC: *Improved catheter for regional coronary sinus flow and metabolic studies.* Am J Cardiol 46:997, 1980.

58. PEPINE, CJ, MEHTA, J, WEBSTER, WW, ET AL: *In vivo validation of a thermodilution method to determine regional left ventricular blood flow in patients with coronary disease.* Circulation 58:795, 1978.

59. GOULD, KL, LIPSCOMB, K, AND HAMILTON, GW: *Physiologic basis for assessing critical coronary stenosis.* Am J Cardiol 33:87, 1974.

60. LIPSCOMB, K AND GOULD, KL: *Mechanism of the effect of coronary artery stenosis on coronary flow in the dog.* Am Heart J 89:60, 1975.

61. KLOCKE, FJ, BUNNELL, IL, GREENE, DG, ET AL: *Average coronary blood flow per unit weight of left ventricle in patients with and without coronary artery disease.* Circulation 50:547, 1974.

62. CANNON, PJ, DELL, RB, AND DWYER, EM, JR: *Regional myocardial perfusion rates in patients with coronary artery disease.* J Clin Invest 51:978, 1972.

63. CANNON, PJ, WEISS, MB, AND SCIACCA, RR: *Myocardial blood flow in coronary artery disease: Studies at rest and during stress with inert gas washout techniques.* Prog Cardiovasc Dis 200:95, 1977.

64. SELWYN, AP, STEINER, R, KIVISAARI, A, ET AL: *Krypton-81 in the physiologic assessment of coronary arterial stenosis in man.* Am J Cardiol 43:547, 1979.

65. YOSHIDA, S, GANZ, W, DONOSO, R, ET AL: *Coronary hemodynamics during successive elevation of heart rate by pacing in subjects with angina pectoris.* Circulation 44:1062, 1971.

66. FUCHS, RM, BRINKER, JA, MAUGHAN, WL, ET AL: *Coronary flow limitation during the development of ischemia: Effect of atrial pacing in patients with left anterior descending coronary artery disease.* Am J Cardiol 48:1029, 1981.

67. CHEN, PH, NICHOLS, AB, WEISS, MB, ET AL: *Left ventricular myocardial blood flow in multivessel coronary artery disease.* Circulation 66:537, 1982.

68. KLOCKE, FJ: *Measurements of coronary blood flow and degree of stenosis: Current clinical implications and continuing uncertainties.* J Am Coll Cardiol 1:31, 1983.

69. MUDGE, GH, GROSSMAN, W, MILLS, RM, ET AL: *Reflex increase in coronary vascular resistance in patients with ischemic heart disease.* N Engl J Med 295:1333, 1976.

70. MUDGE, GH, GOLDBERG, S, GUNTHER, S, ET AL: *Comparison of metabolic and vasoconstrictor stimuli on coronary vascular resistance in man.* Circulation 59:544, 1979.

71. FRIEDMAN, PL, BROWN, EJ, GUNTHER, S, ET AL: *Coronary vasoconstrictor effect of indomethacin in patients with coronary-artery disease.* N Engl J Med 305:1171, 1981.

72. CHIERCHIA, S, BRUNELLI, C, SIMONETTI, I, ET AL: *Sequence of events in angina at rest: Primary reduction in coronary flow.* Circulation 61:759, 1980.

73. MASERI, A AND CHIERCHIA, S: *Coronary artery spasm: Demonstration, definition, diagnosis, and consequences.* Prog Cardiovasc Dis 25:169, 1982.

74. MASERI, A, PAROTI, O, AND SEVERI, S: *Transient transmural reduction of myocardial blood flow, demonstrated by thallium-201 scintigraphy, as a cause of variant angina.* Circulation 54:280, 1976.

75. RICCI, DR, ORLICK, AE, DOHERTY, PW, ET AL: *Reduction of coronary blood flow during coronary artery spasm occurring spontaneously and after provocation by ergonovine maleate.* Circulation 57:392, 1978.

76. CANNON, RO, WATSON, RM, ROSING, DR, ET AL: *Angina caused by abnormal coronary arteriolar vasoconstriction in patients with insignificant fixed coronary artery disease.* Circulation 66 (II):174, 1982.

77. CANNON, RO, WATSON, RM, ROSING, DR, ET AL: *Small vessel coronary constriction as a cause of atypical angina: Pitfalls of ergonovine testing.* Circulation 66(II):993, 1982.

78. STRAUER, BE, BRUNE, I, SCHENK, H, ET AL: *Lupus cardiomyopathy: Cardiac mechanics, hemodynamics, and coronary blood flow in uncomplicated systemic lupus erythematosus.* Am Heart J 92:715, 1976.

79. PICHARD, AD, GORLIN, R, SMITH, H, ET AL: *Coronary flow studies in patients with left ventricular hypertrophy of the hypertensive type. Evidence for an impaired coronary vascular reserve.* Am J Cardiol 47:547, 1981.

80. PICHARD, AD, SMITH, H, HOLT, J, ET AL: *Coronary vascular reserve in left ventricular hypertrophy secondary to chronic aortic regurgitation.* Am J Cardiol 51:315, 1983.

81. MARCUS, ML, DOTY, DB, WRIGHT, CB, ET AL: *Limitations of coronary vasodilator reserve in pressure-induced left ventricular hypertrophy in man.* Clin Res 28:194A, 1980.

82. EASTHAM, CL, DOTY, DB, HIRATZKA, LF, ET AL: *Volume-overload left ventricular hypertrophy impairs coronary reserve in humans.* Circulation 64 (Suppl IV):26, 1981.

83. GANZ, W AND MARCUS, HS: *Failure of intracoronary nitroglycerin to alleviate pacing-induced angina.* Circulation 46:880, 1972.

84. FUCHS, RM, BRINKER, JA, GUZMAN, PA, ET AL: *Regional coronary blood flow during relief of pacing-induced angina by nitroglycerin.* Am J Cardiol 51:19, 1983.

85. MALACOFF, RF, LORELL, BH, MUDGE, GH, ET AL: *Beneficial effects of nifedipine on regional myocardial blood flow in patients with coronary artery disease.* Circulation 65 (Suppl I): I-32, 1982.

86. SCHANZENBAECHER, P, LIEBAU, G, DEEG, P, ET AL: *Effect of intravenous and intracoronary nifedipine on coronary blood flow and myocardial oxygen consumption.* Am J Cardiol 51:712, 1983.

87. KALTENBACH, M, SCHULZ, W, AND KOBER, G: *Effects of nifedipine after intravenous and intracoronary administration.* Am J Cardiol 44:832, 1979.

88. SERRUYS, PW, STEWARD, R, BOOMAN, F, ET AL: *Effects of intracoronary nifedipine on coronary vasomobility and left ventricular hemodynamics.* Circulation 62:86, 1980.

89. ROTHMAN, MT, BAIM, DS, SIMPSON, JB, ET AL: *Coronary hemodynamics during percutaneous transluminal coronary angioplasty.* Am J Cardiol 49:1615, 1982.

90. WILLIAMS, DO, RILEY, RS, SINGH, AK, ET AL: *Restoration of normal coronary hemodynamics and myocardial metabolism after percutaneous transluminal coronary angioplasty.* Circulation 62:653, 1980.

91. BENOTTI, JR, GROSSMAN, W, BRAUNWALD, E, ET AL: *Effects of amrinone on myocardial energy metabolism and hemodynamics in patients with severe congestive heart failure due to coronary artery disease.* Circulation 62:28, 1980.

Provocative Testing for Coronary Artery Spasm

John Speer Schroeder, M.D.

The growing appreciation that myocardial ischemia can be caused by temporary, focal vasoconstriction or spasm of the coronary artery has helped us understand the etiology of unprovoked angina in patients with stable, unstable, or Prinzmetal's angina. Despite this growing appreciation, the establishment of a significant role of coronary artery spasm in spontaneous angina states has been difficult because of the lack of a standard for documenting spasm during electrocardiographic or coronary arteriographic monitoring. Since the introduction of standardized ergonovine provocative testing for coronary artery spasm during cardiac catheterization, the diagnosis of coronary artery spasm has been easier to establish.[1] The purpose of this chapter is to address the clinical applications and methods of provocative testing for coronary artery spasm in the cardiac catheterization laboratory.

BACKGROUND

When a patient presents with rest or nocturnal angina, it may be difficult to ascertain whether the patient has severe occlusive coronary artery disease, presenting as crescendo and rest angina, or whether the patient has primarily focal spasm superimposed upon mild or even relatively normal coronary artery segments. Studies reporting coronary arteriographic results in patients presenting with symptoms of crescendo angina indicate that as many as 10 percent of such patients may have hemodynamically insignificant occlusive coronary disease.[2,3] In the past, these patients were relegated to diagnoses consisting of nonanginal syndromes, and they frequently underwent gastrointestinal workup or were even referred for psychotherapy. In the 1970s, however, a number of isolated case reports documented spontaneous episodes of focal coronary spasm occurring during coronary arteriography, primarily in patients with Prinzmetal's angina.[4,5] As the importance of these observations was realized, investigators began to search for a provocative agent that could be used to stimulate focal coronary artery spasm in patients in whom occlusive coronary artery disease was insufficiently severe to explain their symptoms. The use of ergot alkaloids to induce angina pectoris had been reported in the 1950s, utilizing electrocardiogram (ECG) monitoring and reporting of symptoms to establish angina. Stein reported that angina pectoris was produced in 14 of 15 patients with angina pectoris within 12 minutes of administration of 0.2 to 0.6 mg of ergonovine maleate.[6,7] He also observed that nine of these patients had ST segment depression on the electrocardiogram. Moreover, he reported that there were no complications from this study, and he postulated that coronary artery spasm was the etiology of the pain. Scherf and associates performed similar provocative testing with ergonovine or dihydro-ergotamine in 19 patients with coronary artery disease.[8] During the testing, five of their patients developed prolonged episodes of coronary insufficiency, and one patient died. Because of this and other reported complications, and the lack of the ability to monitor the degree of vasoconstriction, provocative testing lost favor until the advent of routine coronary arteriography in the 1970s. On the basis of controlled clinical trials, with carefully administered ergonovine maleate, the use of this test has now become established for patients in whom the etiology of angina pectoris is not clear after completion of routine coronary arteriography.[9,10]

PRELIMINARY EVALUATION

One current approach to patients who may have coronary artery spasm is to attempt to document electrocardiographic ST segment shifts during episodes of chest pain, prior to scheduling coronary arteriography. For example, the patient who presents with rest or unprovoked angina, particularly if it occurs at night or in the early morning hours, should be suspected of having focal coronary artery spasm until proven otherwise. It is important to emphasize that the chest pain should be typical of myocardial ischemia; that is, a band-like or constricting pressure sensation in the chest that may radiate to the inner aspects of the arms, to the neck, or to the jaw and is usually relieved by nitroglycerin. Absence of exertional angina is not mandatory inasmuch as approximately 50 percent of the patients in the Stanford series with documented focal coronary artery spasm also reported some exertional angina.[11] A high index of suspicion is necessary to identify these patients because many do not have the typical risk factors for coronary artery disease. In fact, in our experience, the patients most likely to have documented coronary artery spasm as the predominant component of their angina pectoris syndrome are women between the ages of 30 and 50 who are cigarette smokers, who may be under unusual emotional stress, and who may have other symptoms of vascular spasm such as a past history of migraine headaches or Raynaud's phenomenon. On the other hand,

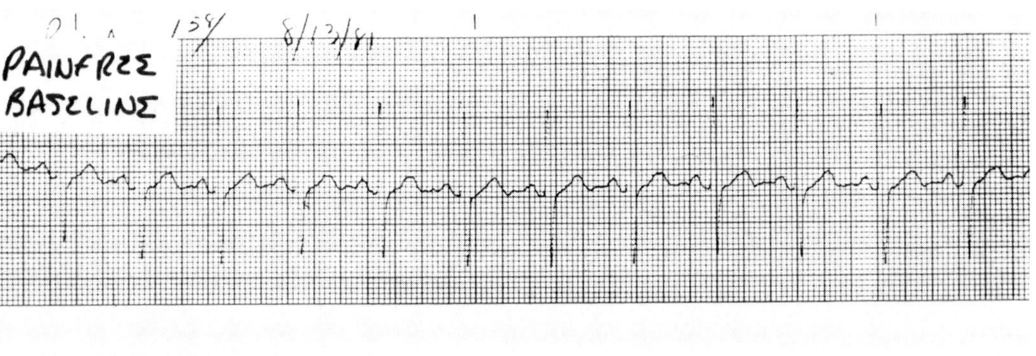

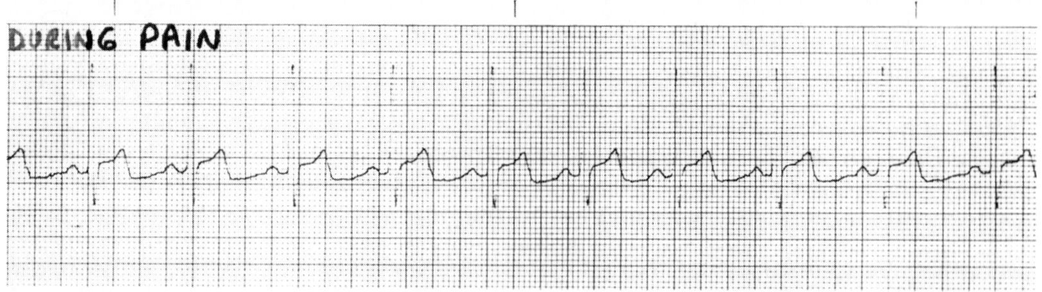

Figure 1. Shown here is ST segment elevation compared with baseline, documented by transtelephonic ECG transmission during chest pain.

it should be noted that changes in vasomotor tone may play an important role in the wide day-to-day variability of precipitating factors or exercise tolerance in patients with angina owing to fixed occlusive coronary artery disease. However, for the purposes of this chapter, I will focus on the patient in whom it is important to document coronary artery spasm at the time of coronary arteriography.

Once the diagnosis of coronary artery spasm is suspected, the patient is given nitroglycerin tablets for sublingual use to ascertain whether the pain is relieved by this agent. Prior to using the nitroglycerin, patients are asked to transmit their electrocardiogram by transtelephonic monitoring (Cardiobeeper, Survival Technology, Inc.). Because the patients present with episodic angina pectoris, they are simply asked to transmit the electrocardiogram during a period of pain, whether it occurs at day or night. The transmitter is small and can be carried throughout the day, and the only requirement is the availability of a phone. The purpose of this ECG monitoring and transmission is to document ST segment shifts during an episode of pain. Experience reported by Ginsburg and coworkers has suggested that this approach is useful and can document ST segment shifts in as many as 50 percent of patients (Fig. 1).[12]

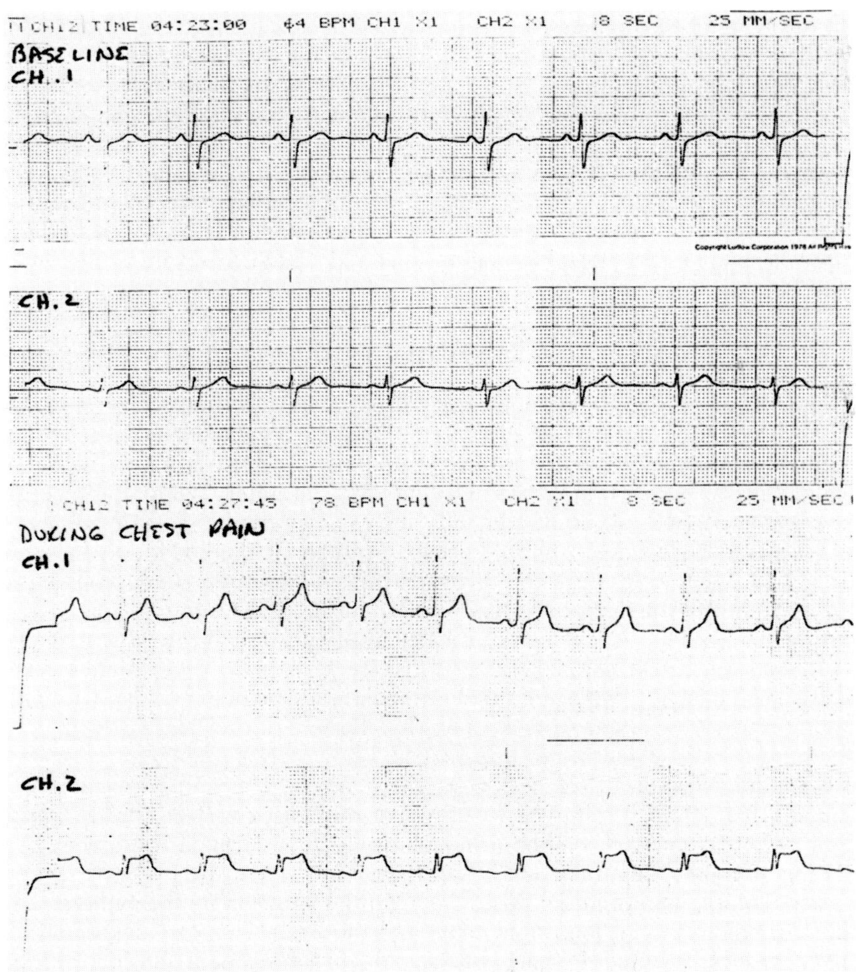

Figure 2. Shown here are two-channel ambulatory ECG recordings during pain-free period *(upper panel)* and during angina *(lower panel)*.

Either underarm or precordial electrodes can be utilized, and these can be shifted to various lead placements in an effort to document where the ischemia is occurring. If the patient is having frequent episodes of angina on a daily basis, ambulatory ECG (Holter) monitoring may also be useful in documenting ST segment shifts during pain. Preferably, patients should be having one or two episodes of pain daily so that the utilization of ECG monitoring will be cost effective. Studies by our group and others have documented that these patients may also be having silent episodes of ST segment depression or pain; however, if the patient does not have at least one symptomatic episode of angina during the 24-hour recording, there will be some question whether any ST segment shift reflects true myocardial ischemia or simply false-positive movement of the ST segment. We utilize the ICR Model 6201 and the ambulatory 2-channel ECG recorder, which has been documented to have excellent frequency response for ST segment shifts and has been useful in our experience in documenting spasm.[13] Figure 2 shows a 2-channel baseline recording when the patient was asymptomatic. The lower panel demonstrates marked ST segment shift in one lead, whereas the other lead shows no change at all. This type of documentation may preclude the necessity for subsequent provocative testing with ergonovine maleate, as discussed below.

Depending upon the frequency and severity of the patient's symptoms, the patient is then admitted to the hospital for further evaluation, including coronary arteriography. Because it may not be clear whether the patient has very severe occlusive coronary artery disease with fixed occlusions or less severe disease with superimposed spasm, all patients undergoing cardiac catheterization at Stanford University Medical Center sign an informed consent which includes the statement, "If the coronary arteriographic findings do not explain your chest pain, the drug ergonovine may be given to induce temporary constriction of the artery in an effort to reproduce your pain." The routine use of this consent form therefore allows the arteriographer to proceed with ergonovine testing immediately if the arteriographic findings do not support a diagnosis of unstable angina pectoris related to severe occlusive coronary artery disease.

TECHNIQUE

In the United States the ergot alkaloid ergonovine maleate has been the most commonly used provocative agent for coronary artery spasm. How the ergonovine maleate induces focal spasm is still not completely understood. It may produce vasoconstriction via alpha receptors in the vascular smooth muscle wall or via stimulation of serotonin membrane receptors. It is important to remember that all ergot alkaloids such as ergonovine maleate will cause some constriction of all vascular smooth muscle groups throughout the body, and therefore carefully applied ECG monitoring must be utilized during the testing procedure. The procedure that is used at Stanford University Medical Center for administration of ergonovine provocation is outlined in Table 1. At the end of routine arteriography, if the patient has not demonstrated sufficient occlusive coronary artery disease to explain the patient's rest angina symptoms, ergonovine testing can be initiated immediately. The patient should not have taken any long-acting nitrates or calcium blockers on the morning of provocative testing, and preferably not sublingual nitroglycerin for at least 1 to 2 hours prior to the test.

Prior to the administration of the first dose of ergonovine maleate (Ergotrate), a 12-lead standard electrocardiogram is obtained by applying radioluscent electrodes to the patient's chest (Hayes pediatric electrodes). The protocol sequence is outlined in Table 1. An initial dose of 0.05 mg of ergonovine maleate is administered intravenously. If the patient is having frequent episodes of angina, an initial dose of 0.025 mg may be administered instead. At the end of 3 minutes an electrocardiogram is taken and the coronary artery suspected of having focal coronary spasm is injected. If there is no significant ST segment shift on the electrocardiogram and no focal spasm, the next dose of 0.1 mg of ergonovine is administered. The same sequence is followed with a 12-lead electrocardiogram and coronary injections at 3 minutes.

Table 1. Stanford protocol for ergonovine provocation

Preparation

1. Stop all antianginal medications
2. Minimal premedication
3. Informed consent
4. Prepare ergonovine
5. Prepare IV nitroglycerin
6. Place electrodes for 12-lead ECG.

Protocol sequence

Minimal time interval (min)	*Dose of IV ergonovine*	*12-lead ECG*	*Coronary Injection*
0	0.05 mg	√	R and L
1.5		√	Inject R or L at onset of chest pain or ST shift
3.0	0.1 mg	√	
4.5		√	
6.0	0.25 mg	√	
7.5		√	
9.0		√	
11.0		√	R and L before completing procedure

At onset of pain or ST segment shift:

1. Inject suspicious coronary artery. If no spasm, inject other coronary artery. If no spasm, proceed to next dose if pain mild to moderate.
2. As soon as focal spasm documented, reverse spasm with IV or IC nitroglycerin 100–200 μg.

R = right
IV = intravenous
min = minutes
L = left
μg = micrograms
IC = intracoronary

Again, if there is no significant abnormality and if the patient is not having chest pain, the final dose of 0.25 mg of ergonovine is administered. Three to five minutes after the last dose of ergonovine, a 12-lead electrocardiogram is performed and both right and left coronary arteries are injected. Whether or not the patient has demonstrated focal coronary artery spasm at that point, an IV bolus of 100 to 200 μg nitroglycerin is administered to reverse any diffuse vasoconstriction that may be present. If the patient develops chest pain with ST segment shift on ECG at any time during the procedure, both coronary arteries should be injected because it is highly likely that focal spasm will be documented at that time. Once documented, it is important to proceed immediately to reversing the focal coronary spasm with intravenous or intracoronary nitroglycerin to limit the time of myocardial ischemia. Once reversed, a final injection in the involved coronary artery is performed to document reversal of the spasm, and the procedure is completed. In cardiac catheterization laboratories where the Judkins' technique is used, it is acceptable to inject only one coronary artery as long as the patient remains asymptomatic and there is no ST segment shift on the electrocardiogram. However, at the end of all ergonovine injections, it is essential to inject both coronary arteries inasmuch as severe but nonocclusive focal spasm can occur prior to producing symptoms of myocardial ischemia. In addition, if the patient is having typical angina, an effort to identify the etiology by injecting the right and left coronary arteries is mandatory.

Inasmuch as most of the complications of ergonovine provocation have been reported in patients during procedures where myocardial ischemia has been allowed to continue without quick reversal, it is absolutely essential to reverse the spasm as quickly as possible after it has been documented. Intravenous nitroglycerin in a dose of 100 to 200 μg is usually administered; but if there is severe spasm, a similar dose can be administered intracoronary with repeated doses as necessary unless the patient becomes severely hypotensive.

COMPLICATIONS

Adverse side effects related to ergonovine maleate provocation include nausea, but it is usually of mild degree. Some investigators have reported a slight rise in blood pressure, but generally there are minimal hemodynamic abnormalities as long as severe focal spasm and myocardial ischemia have not occurred. In 1980, Heupler reported on a collected experience in 862 patients who had undergone ergonovine testing.[14] There were 110 positive tests in this particular series, without a death or a myocardial infarction. Heupler did comment on episodes of prolonged angina, and he emphasized the need to reverse the spasm quickly with either intravenous or intracoronary nitroglycerin. The only collected series of deaths and major complications was reported by Buxton and associates, who described five patients who were "refractory to sublingual nitroglycerin" and had prolonged episodes of ergonovine-induced coronary artery spasm.[15] Four of the patients actually developed cardiac arrest caused by prolonged myocardial ischemia, and three patients died during the procedure. In our review of these reported adverse experiences, it appeared that the patients had a large initial dose of ergonovine maleate, particularly in circumstances where the patient was having frequent episodes of angina. In other cases the patient did not appear to receive adequate nitroglycerin in either an intravenous or intracoronary form to reverse the focal spasm. In one case, it appeared that the myocardial ischemia was allowed to persist for a significant period of time before attempts were made to reverse it. Since publication of these complications, it appears that there has been a stricter adherence to a protocol involving graduated doses of ergonovine, such as the Stanford protocol.

Crevey and associates reported on a patient with variant angina and moderately severe underlying three-vessel coronary atherosclerosis who developed an inferior myocardial infarction during provocative testing.[16] After administration of 0.05 mg of ergonovine, the patient developed total occlusion of the right coronary artery, which was previously obstructed 90 percent by fixed atherosclerotic disease. The patient was given 0.8 mg of sublingual nitroglycerin without any change in the spasm. For the next 50 minutes he received an additional 3.6 mg of sublingual nitroglycerin without reversal of the occlusion. It should be noted that the patient never received intravenous or intracoronary nitroglycerin and went on to develop ECG and enzyme changes consistent with acute transmural inferior infarction. This case points up the necessity of having intravenous nitroglycerin immediately available at the time of ergonovine testing because in our experience intravenous or at times intracoronary administration has always reversed spasm in resistant cases.

INTERPRETATION

In our original report in 1977, 13 of the 57 patients who underwent provocative testing were considered to have positive tests.[1] Spasm, in most circumstances, was occlusive or nearly occlusive in nine patients, with reproduction of chest pain and ST segment elevation that was similar to the spontaneous episodes. An additional patient had ST segment depression rather

Figure 3. *A*, Shown here is the arteriogram before ergonovine administration. *B*, Focal, nearly occlusive spasm of the proximal left anterior descending artery in response to 0.1 mg ergonovine maleate. Note especially the focal nature of the spasm.

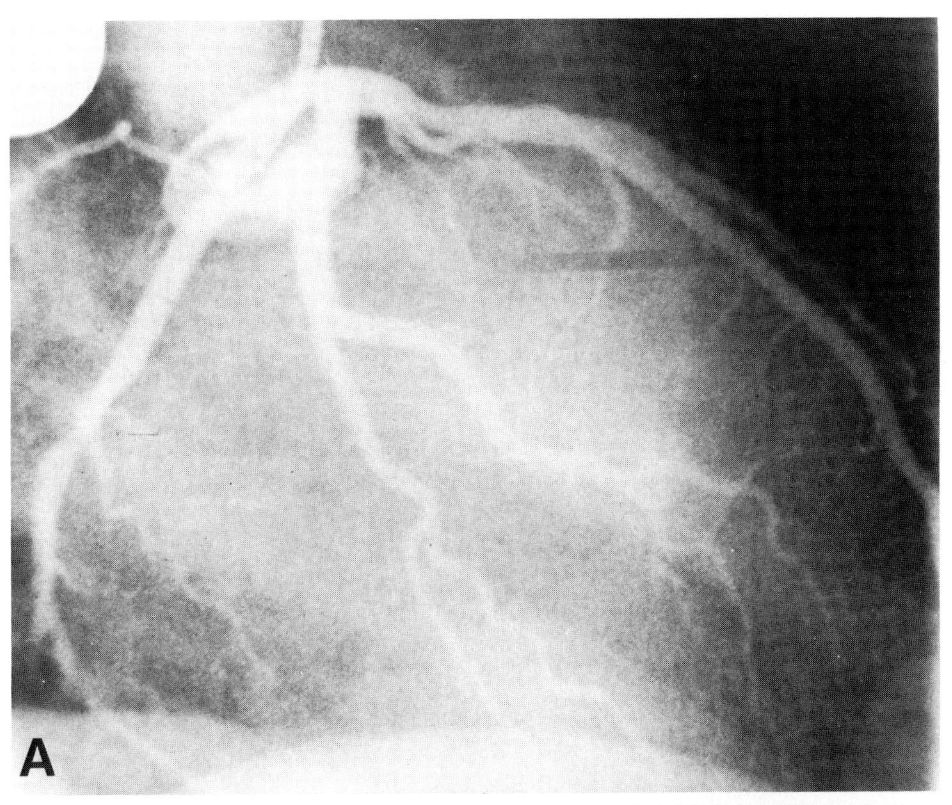
A

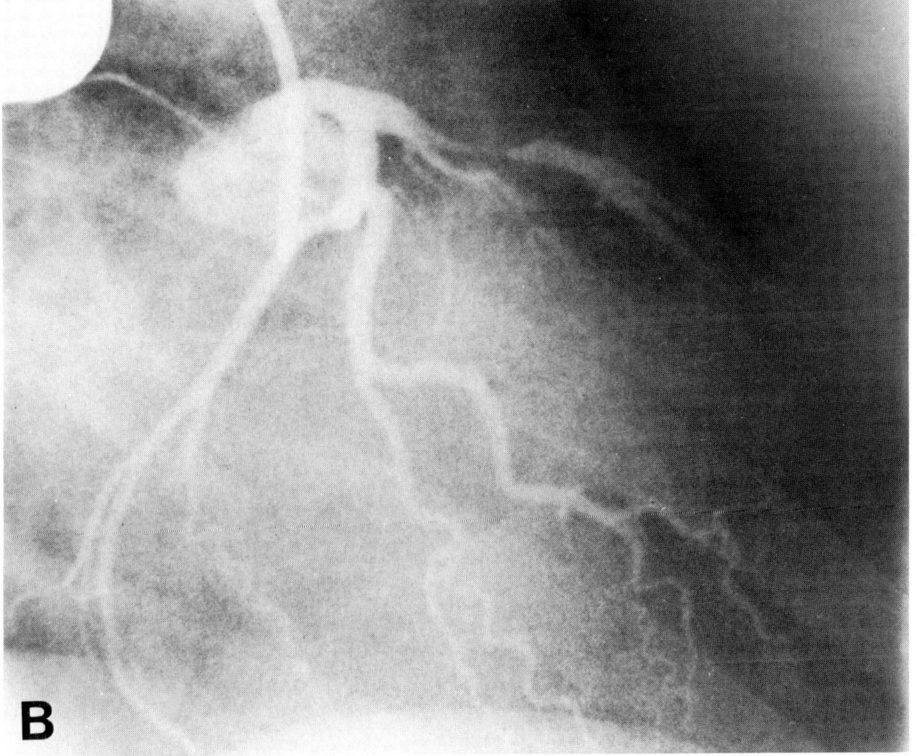
B

than elevation associated with the chest pain. The final three patients had focal narrowing that was severe but without complete occlusion, or reproduction of the chest pain, or electrocardiographic changes. In the other 44 patients who did not demonstrate coronary artery spasm, approximately two thirds had normal coronary arteries, and one third had various degrees of underlying disease. In these patients there was mild narrowing of up to 20 percent but no focal spasm.

Based on this experience and subsequent experience with more than 400 patients as of 1983, I believe that the patient should develop either symptomatic or electrocardiographic evidence of myocardial ischemia, as well as focal spasm, at the time of arteriography. It is the reproduction of the patient's symptoms and signs of myocardial ischemia, in addition to the pathophysiologic provocation of focal spasm, that is important in relating the spasm

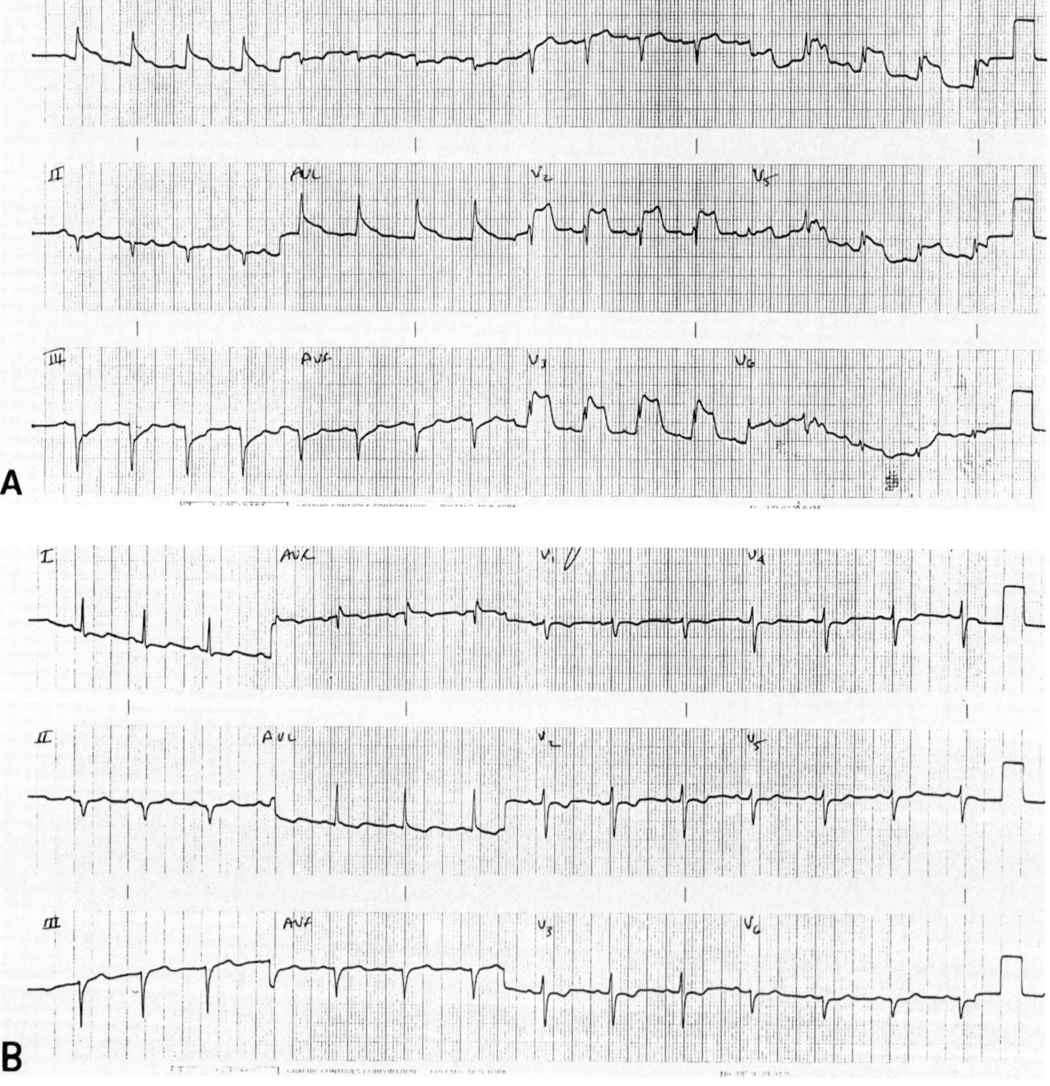

Figure 4. Shown here is marked ST segment elevation in the anterior leads of 12-lead ECG during angina caused by spasm of left anterior descending artery induced by 0.1 mg ergonovine maleate (*A*) and after nitroglycerin (*B*).

to the patient's symptoms. We require that the spasm be *focal* and that it further occlude a coronary artery by at least 50 percent. In many circumstances this occurs in the area of an atherosclerotic plaque or an irregularity in a coronary artery. Figure 3 shows an example of the type of focal spasm that can be provoked by ergonovine testing in appropriate patients. In the control panel (see Figure 3A) there is minimal irregularity and the coronary arteries were considered normal. After provocation with 0.10 mg of ergonovine maleate, there is discrete, severe focal narrowing, which is easily seen and was associated with evidence of myocardial ischemia (see Figure 3B). The associated electrocardiograms are shown in Figure 4A and Figure 4B.

How much narrowing can be related to a normal physiologic response to 0.4 mg of ergonovine maleate? Cipriano and coauthors have reported that the narrowing that occurs as a physiologic response to ergonovine maleate is always of a diffuse nature and that it usually narrows the coronary arteries less than 20 percent.[17] The authors reported a dose-response curve demonstrating an approximately 10 percent diffuse narrowing with a dose of 0.05 mg of ergonovine, 16 percent narrowing with 0.1 mg, and 20 percent with a cumulative total dose of 0.4 mg. It was also noted in this study that the cardiac transplant patients had exactly the same degree of narrowing, despite lack of autonomic innervation to their hearts. An example of physiologic narrowing is shown in Figures 5A and 5B.

How similar are the episodes of coronary artery spasm induced by ergonovine to spontaneous attacks of pain? Curry and collegues studied this question by analyzing seven patients who developed transient episodes of spontaneous rest pain during arteriography and compared these with ergonovine-induced episodes.[18] They compared clinical, electrocardiographic, left ventricular hemodynamic, as well as coronary arteriographic changes during the spontaneous episodes and after ergonovine testing with 0.2 to 0.5 mg ergonovine maleate intravenously. The ST segment elevation occurred in the inferior leads in three patients and anteriorly in three, and in both leads in one patient during both episodes. There were similar rises in left ventricular end-diastolic pressure during both spontaneous and ergonovine-induced episodes. Most importantly, they noted subtotal or total dynamic obstruction in the left anterior descending coronary artery in the three patients with anterior ECG changes, in the right coronary artery in the three patients with inferior changes, and in both arteries in the one with both anterior and inferior ECG changes. The location of the spasm was similar during both spontaneous and ergonovine-induced episodes. The authors therefore concluded that ergonovine stimulation does produce spontaneous episodes of pain and is useful in identifying patients with variant angina.

How frequently is focal coronary artery spasm seen in patients having undergone routine coronary arteriography? Bertrand and coworkers reported on a large group of 1089 consecutive patients undergoing coronary arteriography who also underwent provocative testing with 0.4 mg of methyl ergonovine maleate after routine arteriography.[19] Patients who had spontaneous coronary spasm, left main coronary artery narrowing, or severe vessel disease were excluded. The authors reported that 134 patients experienced focal spasm. It was observed most frequently in patients who reported angina at rest and less often when exercise-induced angina as well as angina at rest were reported. It should be noted that spasm was observed in 20 percent of patients who had a recent myocardial infarction. The authors reported that spasm was superimposed on fixed atherosclerotic lesions in 60 percent of their patients. Thus, overall, 15 percent of patients who complained of chest pain had focal coronary spasm during consecutive testing in patients undergoing routine arteriography. This relatively high percentage of patients may reflect the fact that the patients were not pretreated with nitrates or any other drugs prior to angiography owing to routine use of provocative testing in the arteriographic laboratory. The authors reported no serious irreversible complications; however, four patients did develop ventricular fibrillation and several others exhibited bradycardia or transient atrioventricular (AV) block. All the complications occurred in patients who developed coronary artery spasm and myocardial ischemia during testing. They

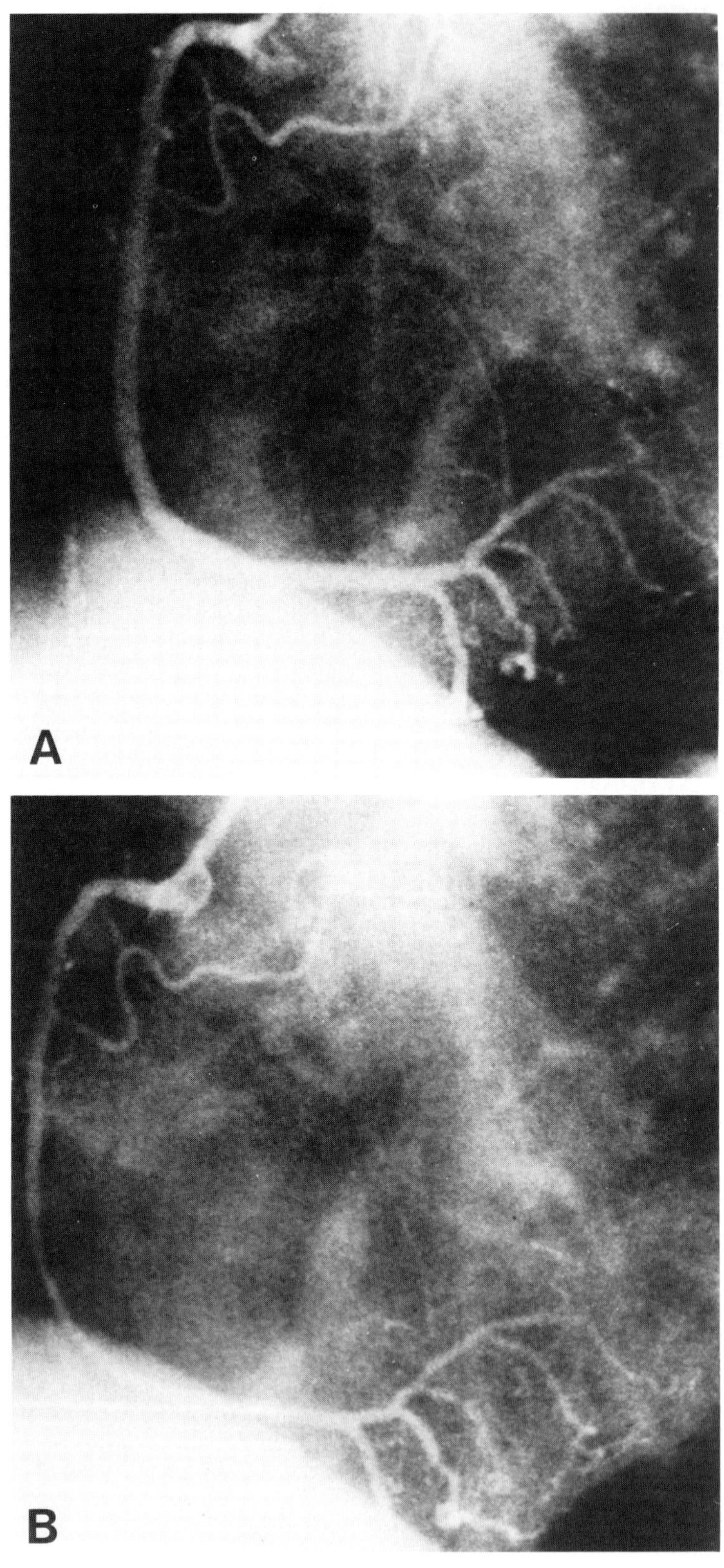
A
B

observed that it is essential to reverse the coronary spasm as quickly as possible once it has been documented, and they emphasized the importance of electrocardiographic monitoring as well as serial arteriographic observations.

ESOPHAGEAL SPASM VERSUS CORONARY SPASM

Eastwood and associates reported in 1981 on the use of ergonovine to identify esophageal spasm in patients with chest pain.[20] They studied 14 patients who had chest pain believed to represent angina pectoris and four healthy volunteers. During ergonovine testing, five of the patients developed typical chest pain and esophageal manometric signs of esophageal spasm. The remaining nine patients and four volunteers did not develop chest pain typical of their spontaneous episodes of pain. It is of interest that two of the nine patients and one of the four normal volunteers also developed manometric signs of esophageal spasm during ergonovine testing but denied any angina or chest pain. Of most importance is that two of their five positive responders to ergonovine developed simultaneous abnormal electrocardiograms showing marked ST segment elevations. After sublingual nitroglycerin the symptoms of chest pain and ST segment changes returned to normal. These two patients had previous negative ergonovine testing at the time of coronary arteriography; however, the authors noted that both these patients had received nitrates at the time of arteriography that may have prevented a positive ergonovine test from occurring.

Gravino and coworkers reported on a 62-year-old man with suspected coronary artery spasm who was subsequently shown to have marked esophageal spasm during ergonovine testing.[21] These authors concluded that the chest pain associated with esophageal spasm could be similar to angina, and they recommended that ergonovine tests not be considered positive unless there is simultaneous arteriographic or electrocardiographic proof of myocardial ischemia.

On the basis of these reports and on the basis of our own experience at Stanford, it has not been particularly useful to do esophageal manometry during ergonovine testing owing to the frequency of "false positives" and the difficulty in correlating chest pain symptoms with the observed abnormalities. We continue to believe that rigid adherence to proof of myocardial ischemia by electrocardiographic monitoring is necessary to determine a true positive response of coronary artery spasm to ergonovine stimulation.

PROVOCATIVE TESTING TO ASSESS THE EFFICACY OF THERAPY FOR VARIANT ANGINA

Waters and colleagues at the Montreal Heart Institute in Canada have reported extensively on the utilization of provocative testing to assess response to therapy, primarily with calcium channel blocking agents, of variant angina patients. They reported on 27 patients who all had a positive ergonovine test during the control period while on no medication.[22] During therapy with nifedipine, 20 mg every 6 hours, ergonovine testing up to 0.4 mg total dose resulted in a negative response in 11 patients, improvement in five patients, and requirement for a higher dosage in two patients. Similar results were obtained during treatment with diltiazem. However, during treatment with verapamil the test result was negative in only eight patients and positive at a dose similar to that of the control group in the remaining nine patients. The authors then attempted to correlate the responsiveness to ergonovine testing with a clinical response. They noted that during a 7-month period of followup, 14 of 15 patients who were treated with a calcium channel blocker that converted their ergonovine test to negative

←

Figure 5. *A*, Shown here is the baseline right coronary artery. *B*, There is a normal physiologic narrowing affecting the right coronary artery in response to a total 0.4 mg ergonovine maleate.

remained angina-free, whereas only 4 of 12 patients remained pain-free with a persistently positive test. They concluded that ergonovine testing was useful during active calcium channel blocker therapy as a semiobjective method of testing drug efficacy. It should be noted, however, that this testing was done in the coronary care unit without coronary arteriographic monitoring of the degree or extent of coronary artery spasm. Although no complications were reported in this particular group of patients, complications have been reported elsewhere during testing in the coronary care unit in this type of situation, and it is recommended that such testing be limited to clinical research protocols.

PROVOCATIVE TESTING WITH METHACHOLINE

Endo and coworkers reported in 1976 that methacholine may produce coronary artery spasm.[23] The commonly accepted theory regarding mechanism has been that excessive parasympathetic activity stimulates the sympathetic nerves which then cause severe vasoconstriction by activating alpha receptors. More recently, Stang and associates reported on 13 patients with unequivocal variant angina. Five of these patients underwent methacholine testing with 10 mg administered subcutaneously.[24] Three of the five patients developed subsequent delayed appearance of chest pain with ECG changes and coronary artery spasm. These authors proposed that the coronary artery spasm resulted from the direct stimulation of cholinergic muscarinic receptors on vascular smooth muscle peripherally, which resulted in abrupt relative hypotension with reflex-mediated increases in sympathetic tone (as manifested by reflex tachycardia) and increase in alpha tone to the coronary arteries precipitating coronary artery spasm. In view of these observations and the fact that hypotension may be a required component of the methacholine testing, it does not appear to be as reliable or as safe as ergonovine testing.

HYPERVENTILATION TESTING

Yasue and associates first reported that hyperventilation, particularly in combination with Tris-buffer infusion sufficient to raise the arterial pH to 7.65, precipitated variant angina attacks in eight of nine patients so tested.[25] More recently, Girotti reported on ten cases of Prinzmetal's angina in whom repeated episodes of myocardial ischemia were reproducibly induced by hyperventilation.[26] They performed the test a total of 111 times, 41 times during control conditions and 70 times during treatment with multiple antianginal agents. The authors observed that the ECG changes and chest pain tended not to occur during the time that alkalosis was maximal but when the arterial pH was returning toward normal. The ten patients reported were screened from among 143 patients who were admitted to their coronary care unit during two years. The hyperventilation test was positive in a total of 19 patients, and the ten patients selected for study were available and suitable for repeated testing. The authors also noted that calcium channel blocker therapy or nitrate therapy tended to prevent recurrent episodes of coronary artery spasm during hyperventilation in this particular patient group. They admitted, however, that hyperventilation seemed to be less sensitive than ergonovine testing and not necessarily positive in all patients with Prinzmetal's variant angina.

COLD PRESSOR TESTING

The observation that cold pressor stimulation could induce coronary artery spasm in selected patients has led to further interest in this provocative test because of its presumed ease of administration and safety. Raizner and colleagues reported on a total of 35 patients who were undergoing coronary arteriography for evaluation of chest pain syndromes.[27] The patients were exposed to 1 minute of cold pressor stimulation during which time heart rate did not change but systolic blood pressure increased by 17 mm Hg. Focal spasm was induced in seven patients, but only two had ischemic manifestations on ECG. A total of six patients were believed to have possible angina prior to coronary arteriography, compared with 14 patients who had more typical exertional angina and negative cold pressor tests. Quantitative angiography demonstrated increased luminal narrowing of coronary segments in both groups; however, it was more pronounced in the variant angina group (-12.7 ± 11.5 percent compared with the control group -5.1 ± 1.2 percent). More recently, Waters and coworkers compared the sensitivity of exercise, ergonovine, and cold pressor testing in patients with documented variant angina.[28] They compared the sensitivity of the three tests performed serially in 34 patients, by exercise testing in 17 patients, and by cold pressor testing in only 5 patients ($p < 0.005$). Evidence of myocardial ischemia as manifested by ST segment elevation developed during ergonovine testing in 94 percent of patients, during exercise testing in 29 percent, and during cold pressor testing in only 9 percent of patients. On the basis of these observations, the authors concluded that the sensitivity of cold pressor testing was far too low to be of much clinical value when one is trying to identify variant angina patients. These impressions agree with the observations at Stanford and elsewhere. However, regardless of the mechanism used to stimulate spasm in myocardial ischemia, it can be equally dangerous when similar degrees of focal spasm in susceptible patients are provoked.

OTHER PROVOCATIVE AGENTS

Ginsburg and associates recently reported on the use of histamine provocation in 12 patients who had suspected coronary artery spasm.[29] Histamine was infused at a dose of 0.05 to 0.1 μg/kg per minute in the presence of large doses of selective H_2 blocker (cimetidine).[29] Coronary artery spasm was provoked in 4 of these 12 patients. Side effects included headaches and nausea and limited the usefulness of this test.

CONCLUSION

Provocative testing with ergonovine maleate remains the most sensitive and specific test to identify patients who are having angina pectoris caused primarily by coronary artery spasm. This patient group represents between 5 and 15 percent of patients who are undergoing coronary arteriography for chest pain syndromes, thus emphasizing the need to obtain routine permission to perform ergonovine testing prior to the time of arteriography. Although these patients can frequently be identified on the basis of their symptoms of unprovoked rest or nocturnal angina, ergonovine testing remains a highly reliable way to confirm focal spasm in patients in whom the diagnosis has not become clarified during outpatient or inpatient electrocardiographic monitoring during episodes of spontaneous pain. The test has now been performed on thousands of patients and appears to be safe if suitable precautions are made for immediate reversal of focal spasm as soon as it is observed at the time of arteriography. Provocative testing with other agents appears to be less sensitive and predictable in patients who have clear-cut variant angina pectoris. Finally, provocative testing to determine clinical efficacy of antianginal medications should be reserved for clinical research protocols owing to the occasional complications that may occur.

REFERENCES

1. Schroeder, JS, Bolen, JL, Quint, RA, et al: *Provocation of coronary spasm with ergonovine maleate. New test with results in 57 patients undergoing coronary arteriography.* Am J Cardiol 40:487, 1977.
2. Scanlon, PJ, Niemickas, R, Moran, JF, et al: *Accelerated angina pectoris: Clinical, hemodynamic, arteriographic and therapeutic experience in 85 patients.* Circulation 47:19, 1973.

3. Trenouth, RS, Rosch, J, Antonovic, R, et al: *Ventriculography and coronary arteriography in the acutely ill patient: Complications, extent of coronary artery disease and abnormalities of left ventricular function.* Chest 69:647, 1976.
4. Schroeder, JS, Silverman, JF, and Harrison, DC: *Right coronary artery spasm causing Prinzmetal's variant angina.* Chest 65:573, 1974.
5. Oliva, PB, Potts, DE, and Pluss, RG: *Coronary arterial spasm in Prinzmetal angina: Documentation by coronary arteriography.* N Engl J Med 288:745, 1973.
6. Stein, I: *The ergonovine test for coronary insufficiency.* Angiology 14:23, 1963.
7. Stein, I and Weinstein, J: *Further studies of the effect of ergonovine on the coronary circulation.* J Lab Clin Med 36:66, 1950.
8. Scherf, D, Perlman, A, and Schlackman, M: *Effect of dihydroergotamine on heart.* Proc Soc Exp Biol Med 71:420, 1949.
9. Heupler, FA, Proudfit, WL, Razavi, M, et al: *Ergonovine maleate provocative test for coronary artery spasm.* Am J Cardiol 41:631, 1978.
10. Pepine, CP, Feldman, RL, and Conti, CR: *Recommendations for use of ergonovine to provoke coronary artery spasm.* Cathet Cardiovasc Diagn 6:423, 1980.
11. Allaire, BI and Schroeder, JS: *Prinzmetal's angina. Clinical and anatomic aspects.* West J Med 122:187, 1975.
12. Ginsburg, R, Lamb, IH, Schroeder, JS, et al: *Long-term transtelephonic monitoring in variant angina.* Am Heart J 102:196, 1981.
13. Ginsburg, R and Schroeder, JS: *Coronary artery spasm: Approach to diagnosis and treatment.* Practical Cardiology 6:August, 1980.
14. Heupler, FA: *Provocative testing for coronary arterial spasm: Risk, method and rationale.* Am J Cardiol 46:335, 1980.
15. Buxton, A, Goldberg, S, Hirshfeld, JW, et al: *Refractory ergonovine-induced coronary vasospasm: Importance of intracoronary nitroglycerin.* Am J Cardiol 46:329, 1980.
16. Crevey, BJ, Owen, SF, and Pitt, B: *Irreversible coronary occlusion related to administration of ergonovine.* Circulation 64:853, 1981.
17. Cipriano, PR, Guthaner, DF, Orlick, AE, et al: *The effects of ergonovine maleate on coronary arterial size.* Circulation 59:82, 1979.
18. Curry, RC, Pepine, CJ, Sabom, MB, et al: *Similarities of ergonovine-induced and spontaneous attacks of variant angina.* Circulation 59:307, 1979.
19. Bertrand, ME, LaBlanche, JM, Tilmant, PY, et al: *Frequency of provoked coronary arterial spasm in 1089 consecutive patients undergoing coronary arteriography.* Circulation 65:1299, 1982.
20. Eastwood, GL, Weiner, BH, Dickerson, WJ, et al: *Use of ergonovine to identify esophageal spasm in patients with chest pain.* Ann Intern Med 94:768, 1981.
21. Gravino, FN, Perloff, JK, Yeatman, LA, et al: *Coronary arterial spasm versus esophageal spasm: Response to ergonovine.* Am J Med 70:1293, 1981.
22. Waters, DD, Szlachcic, J, Theroux, P, et al: *Ergonovine testing to detect spontaneous remissions of variant angina during long-term treatment with calcium antagonist drugs.* Am J Cardiol 47:179, 1981.
23. Endo, M, Hirosawa, K, Kancko, N, et al: *Prinzmetal's variant angina: Coronary arteriogram and left ventriculogram during angina attack induced by methacholine.* N Engl J Med 294:250, 1976.
24. Stang, JM, Kolibash, AJ, Schorling, JB, et al: *Methacholine provocation of Prinzmetal's variant angina pectoris: A revised perspective.* Clin Cardiol 5:393, 1982.
25. Yasue, H, Nagao, M, Omote, S, et al: *Coronary arterial spasm and Prinzmetal's variant form of angina induced by hyperventilation and tris-buffer infusion.* Circulation 56:56, 1978.
26. Girotti, LA, Crosatto, JR, Messuti, H, et al: *The hyperventilation test as a method for developing successful therapy in Prinzmetal's angina.* Am J Cardiol 49:834, 1982.
27. Raizner, AE, Chahine, RA, Ishimorei, T, et al: *Provocation of coronary artery spasm by the cold pressor test.* Circulation 62:925, 1980.
28. Waters, DD, Szlachcic, J, and Bonan, R: *Comparative sensitivity of exercise, cold pressor and ergonovine testing in provoking attacks of variant angina in patients with active disease.* Circulation 67:310, 1983.
29. Ginsburg, R, Bristow, MR, Kantrowitzh, N, et al: *Histamine provocation of clinical coronary artery spasm. Implications concerning pathogenesis of variant angina pectoris.* Am Heart J 102:819, 1981.

Coronary Angioplasty: Indications and Results

Geoffrey O. Hartzler, M.D.

Since its clinical introduction in 1978,[1] the practice and application of percutaneous transluminal coronary angioplasty (PTCA) have undergone rapid evolution. Initial concepts and results suggested that the procedure would have limited application, being appropriate for 5 percent or fewer patients with symptomatic coronary artery disease.[2,3] However, continued experience indicates that PTCA can reduce the morbidity and mortality resulting from coronary atherosclerosis by effectively restoring coronary flow in an increasing number of patients, including those with complex coronary artery disease.[4-7] PTCA can potentially reduce the frequency of coronary artery bypass surgery performed yearly, with consequent reduction in health care costs.[8]

At present, the indications, contraindications, success, and complications of the procedure vary greatly from institution to institution, largely dependent upon the technical skills and number of procedures performed by the dilator. As with all technical and manipulative procedures, it is not unexpected that *experience* has emerged as the single most important factor in predicting a successful, uncomplicated PTCA outcome. The National Heart, Lung and Blood Institute's voluntary registry has clearly documented the presence of a "learning curve" for the beginning dilator.[9]

The performance of successful PTCA has been facilitated by many technical improvements of the dilating and guiding catheter systems. Lower balloon catheter profiles in the deflated state allow tighter and longer stenoses to be passed. Improved balloon materials allow higher expansion pressures for dilatation of rigid lesions. Greater x-ray opacity has improved visualization of the balloon catheters and guide wires. The availability of a variety of balloon sizes allows matching of the inflated balloon diameter with native coronary arterial size, reducing the likelihood of arterial wall disruption. The more recent introduction of "steerable," or, more accurately, "directionally changeable," balloon catheters has increased the safety of the technique and has facilitated dilatation of more complex coronary lesions. The refinement of guide wires, with some being more torqueable or directionally changeable and others being less rigid or extremely "floppy," has improved the approach to eccentric, distal, diffuse, and previously nondilatable coronary stenoses.

WHO SHOULD PERFORM CORONARY ANGIOPLASTY?

In many respects, PTCA has become a more complex procedure as a result of movable guide wire systems. At the same time, these modifications have increased the inherent safety of the technique, particularly in skilled and experienced hands. However, the performance of coronary angioplasty is *not* analogous to the performance of routine coronary angiography.

Procedural differences are substantial, as are the technical skills, attitude, and approach required of the invasive cardiologist. The potential for major complications, including myocardial infarction and death, is greater, as are the emotional stresses experienced by the catheterization laboratory support personnel. Clearly, consistently successful PTCA is enhanced by a high-volume catheterization laboratory with experienced technical staff, better fluoroscopic imaging systems, and cardiologists who perform angioplasty on a frequent basis.

My personal view is that the training and performance of PTCA should be limited to cardiologists with experience performing routine coronary angiography frequently for at least one year following completion of a formal training program. The prospective dilator should have demonstrated superb technical abilities with routine and complex catheterization cases, good judgment in the management of complications, and have personal strengths and attitudes allowing for self-criticism, introspection, and change. A reasonable initial approach would include attendance at major symposia dealing with all aspects of coronary intervention, observation in a high-volume angioplasty center, cautious patient selection designed to facilitate success and minimize complications while allowing familiarization with catheter systems, and assistance by an experienced dilator during initial procedures. Failure to achieve or to better the NHLBI success rates by the first 30 to 50 procedures should prompt reevaluation of the cardiologist's commitment to perform PTCA.

INDICATIONS FOR PTCA

The initial guidelines for identifying PTCA candidates were intended to facilitate a successful, uncomplicated outcome utilizing relatively crude equipment, at a time when technical skills were minimal and results uncertain. Presently, experiences accumulated at higher-volume angioplasty centers, including our own, support the aggressive application of PTCA to patient subgroups with complex coronary artery disease and clinical circumstances previously believed to represent contraindications for the procedure.[4–6,10] The "ideal" patient rarely exists, that is, one with recent onset of angina pectoris caused by a single, proximal, concentric, noncalcified, subtotal obstructive coronary stenosis in the setting of normal left ventricular function and failed medical management, yet in the absence of contraindication to coronary bypass surgery. Rigid adherence to such "criteria" would unreasonably limit the benefit of coronary angioplasty to a minority of patients with coronary artery disease.

Increased Experience and Technologic Improvement Have Changed Indications and Contraindications

PTCA need no longer be restricted to single-vessel and single-lesion coronary anatomy. Utilizing newer catheter designs, it is now possible to cross and to dilate successfully diffuse lesions, those that are heavily calcified or eccentric, and those that are located distally or in branches of major vessels.

The presence of poor left ventricular function cannot be considered a contraindication to the procedure but may instead support a decision for angioplasty in certain circumstances. In experienced centers, the risks of attempted single- or multiple-lesion angioplasty may be less than or comparable to those associated with coronary bypass surgery in the setting of a highly compromised left ventricle. Similarly, advanced age may favor a decision for PTCA when anatomically appropriate lesions are present, as opposed to coronary bypass surgery, which carries increased risk in this population, characterized by less recuperative vigor and with associated medical problems potentially complicating recovery from a major operation.

The requirement that all patients be candidates for coronary bypass surgery can no longer be accepted as an absolute dictum. In some cases, diffuse and severe "inoperable" coronary artery disease may be effectively palliated by judicious PTCA performed with "acceptable" risk relative to alternatives. Dilatation of selected lesions such as an isolated right coronary, diagonal or marginal branch stenosis in a vessel of modest size can be performed reasonably without commitment to operation should acute obstruction occur. The morbidity associated with infarction in this circumstance is generally equivalent to or less than that associated with coronary bypass surgery.

It is no longer reasonable to insist that angioplasty candidates should have failed to respond to maximal medical therapy prior to a decision for PTCA. In experienced hands, a high primary success rate combined with low morbidity supports a decision for early dilatation. Successful PTCA can thereby avoid a commitment to long-term beta blocker and calcium channel blocker therapy, especially inasmuch as both groups of drugs have the potential for significant side effects.

The indication for coronary angioplasty might be described as the presence of anatomically appropriate obstructive coronary lesions in a symptomatic patient or in a patient judged at risk of a major cardiovascular problem should a high-grade obstruction progress to total occlusion. A majority of patients presently considered candidates for coronary bypass surgery might also be considered candidates for coronary angioplasty, depending upon the skills of the dilating team. In this context, it needs to be repeatedly emphasized that *experience* is the major factor allowing aggressive application of coronary angioplasty and that these comments are not intended to be support for PTCA in higher-risk patients by inexperienced dilators.

PROCEDURAL ASPECTS OF CORONARY ANGIOPLASTY

Our protocol for pharmacologic management of patients undergoing PTCA includes the administration of aspirin, 300 mg bid, and dipyridamole, 75 mg tid, commencing 48 hours prior to the procedure. Additionally, patients receive a calcium channel blocker, and beta blockers are discontinued prior to PTCA in an attempt to decrease the likelihood of coronary artery spasm during the procedure. Premedication includes meperidine, 50 to 75 mg; promethazine hydrochloride, 25 mg; and atropine, 0.6 mg intramuscularly.

In the catheterization laboratory, a rapid infusion of low molecular weight dextran is commenced. Although it is controversial, I believe that dextran administration allows greater manipulation of and less trauma to the arterial wall without resultant acute occlusion, and at present there is no conclusive study providing evidence to the contrary. Additionally, patients are given verapamil, 5 mg intravenously; lidocaine, 75 to 100 mg intravenously as a single bolus; isosorbide dinitrate, 5 mg sublingually; and diazepam intravenously as needed for sedation. Immediately upon introduction of a sheath into the femoral artery, patients receive 10,000 units of heparin intravenously.

Following the procedure, the patient is returned to his room with the femoral sheath in place for withdrawal following spontaneous heparin dissipation at approximately 4 hours. If the coronary artery has been extensively traumatized or if the zone dilated was particularly diffuse or disrupted, an intravenous heparin infusion is commenced and continued for 12 to 24 hours followed by sheath withdrawal. Long-acting nitrates are continued for 24 hours. Treatment with aspirin, dipyridamole, and a calcium channel blocker is resumed. Beta blockers are not continued, assuming the patient has no remaining significant obstructive coronary lesions producing myocardial ischemia.

RESULTS

At the Mid-America Heart Institute of St. Luke's Hospital in Kansas City, Missouri, aggressive coronary angioplasty has been performed since the summer of 1980. By February 1983, three cardiologists had performed 1000 consecutive procedures, attempting to dilate 1502 stenoses. There were 769 males and 231 females, with ages ranging from 30 to 83 years (mean 58 years). Numerous "high-risk" subgroups were included in this series, with 123 patients being 70 years of age or older. Seventy-eight procedures were attempted during acute

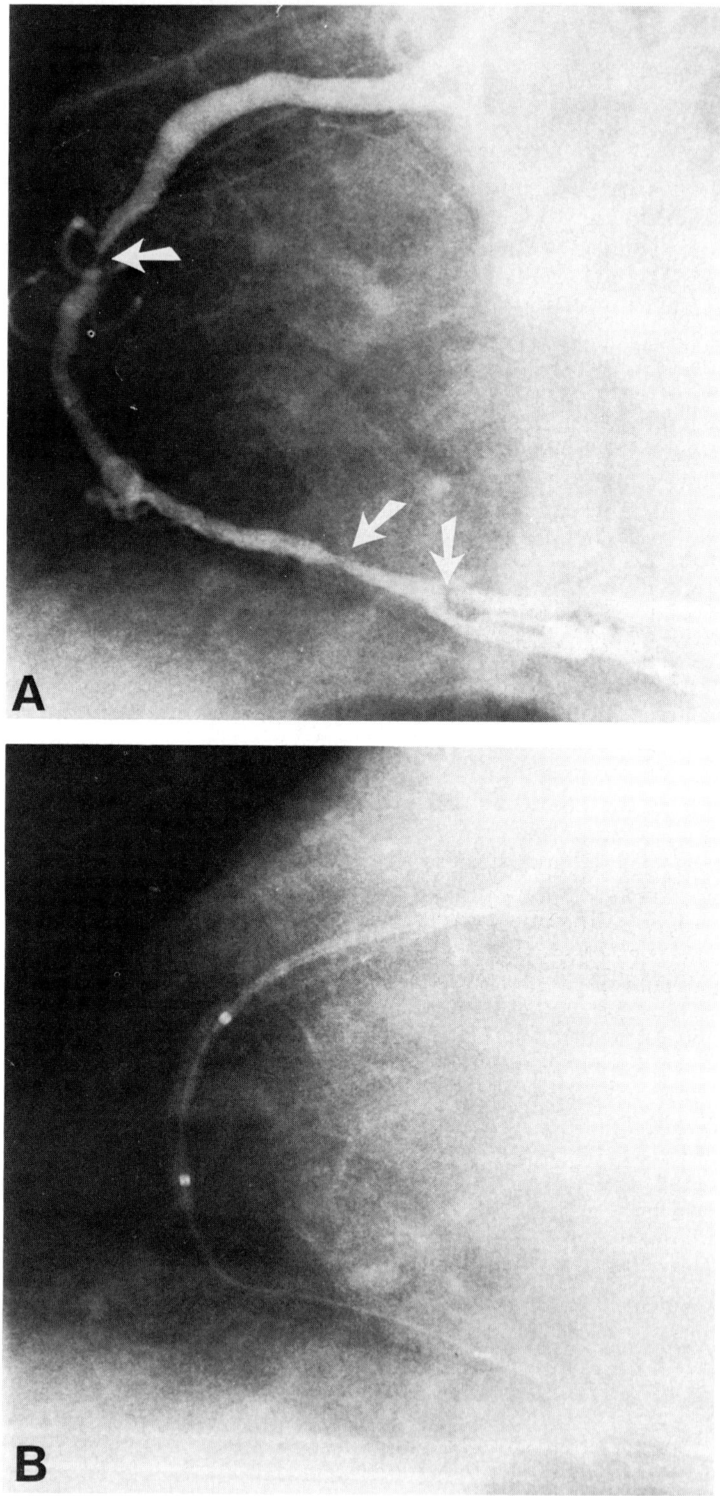

Figure 1. Multiple lesion and vessel angioplasty in a 69-year-old woman with Class IV angina. (*A*) Diffuse disease of the right coronary artery is evident. Arrows indicate sites of higher-grade stenoses. Mid-RCA is 90 percent obstructed by a discrete lesion, distal RCA is 70 to 80 percent narrowed by diffuse disease, and origin of postero-lateral segment is subtotally occluded.

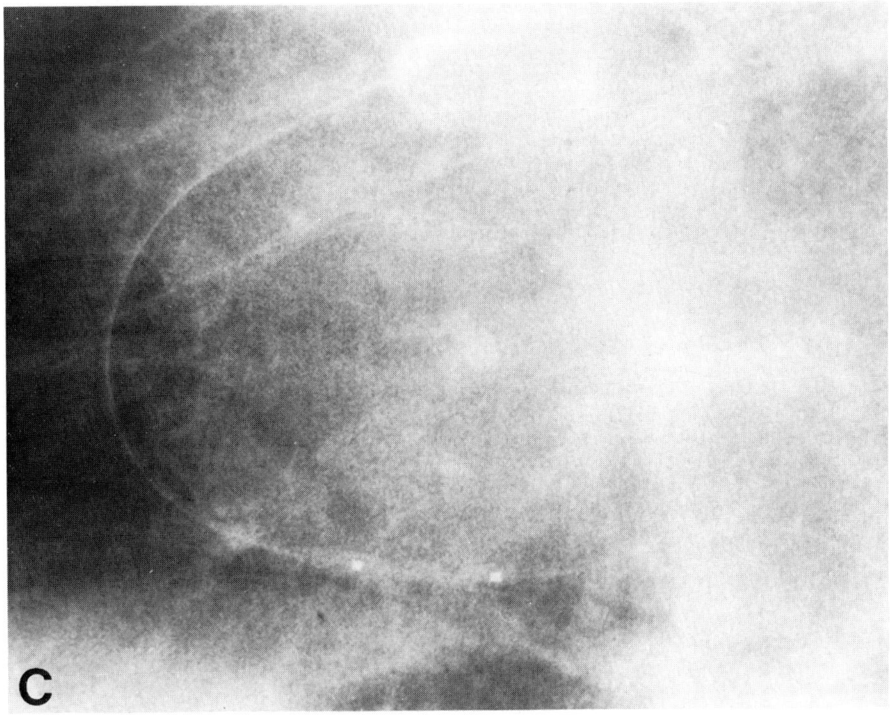

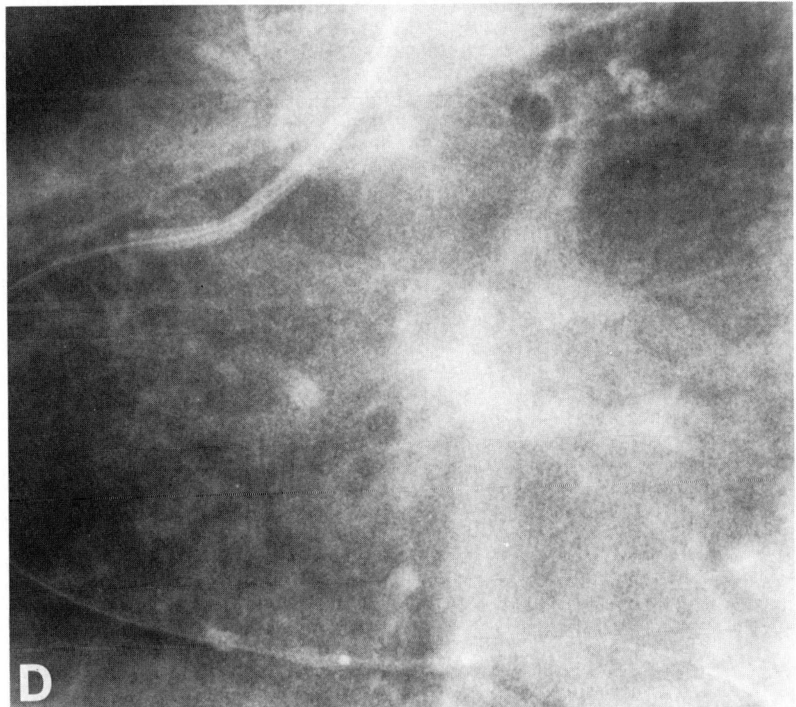

Figure 1. *Continued.* (*B, C, D*) A 3-mm balloon catheter was passed over a floppy guide wire for dilatation of the mid and distal lesions. A 2.5-mm balloon (*C*) was utilized for the smaller posterolateral branch.

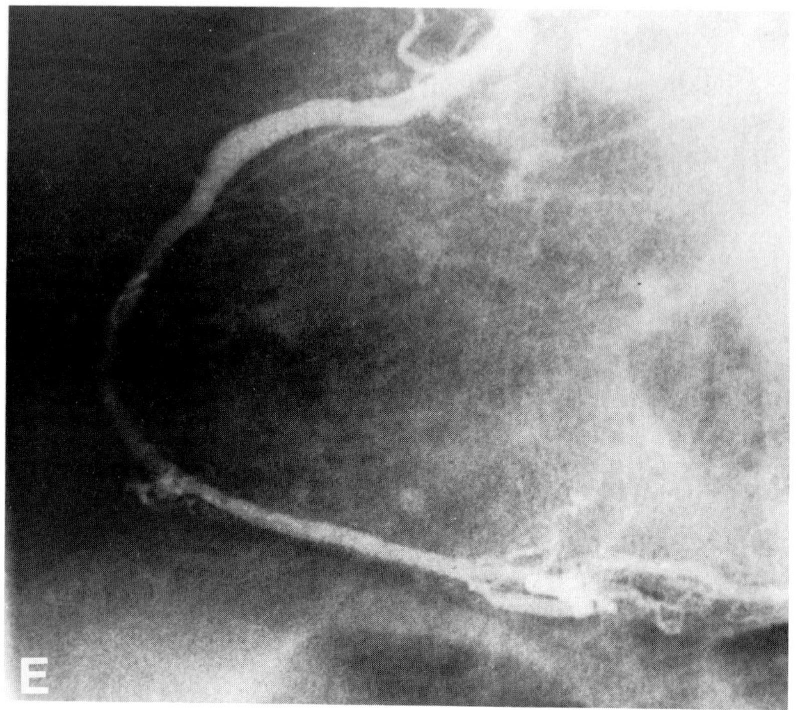

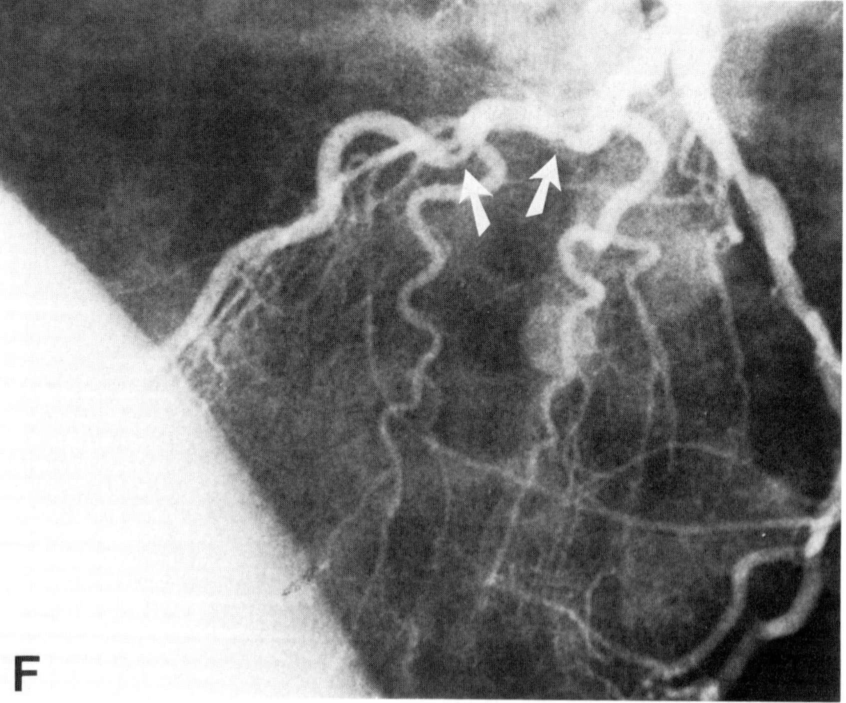

Figure 1. *Continued.* (*E*) Shown is the final result of right coronary dilatation. (*F*) LAO projection demonstrating 70 to 80 percent obstructions of the proximal and mid-LAD (*arrows*).

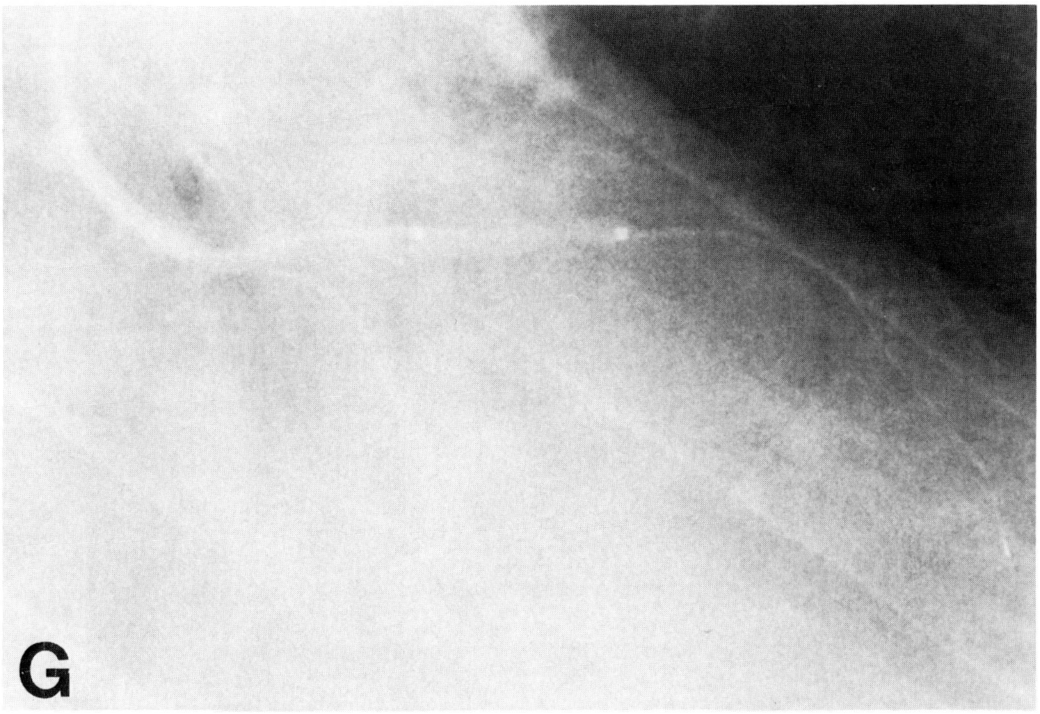

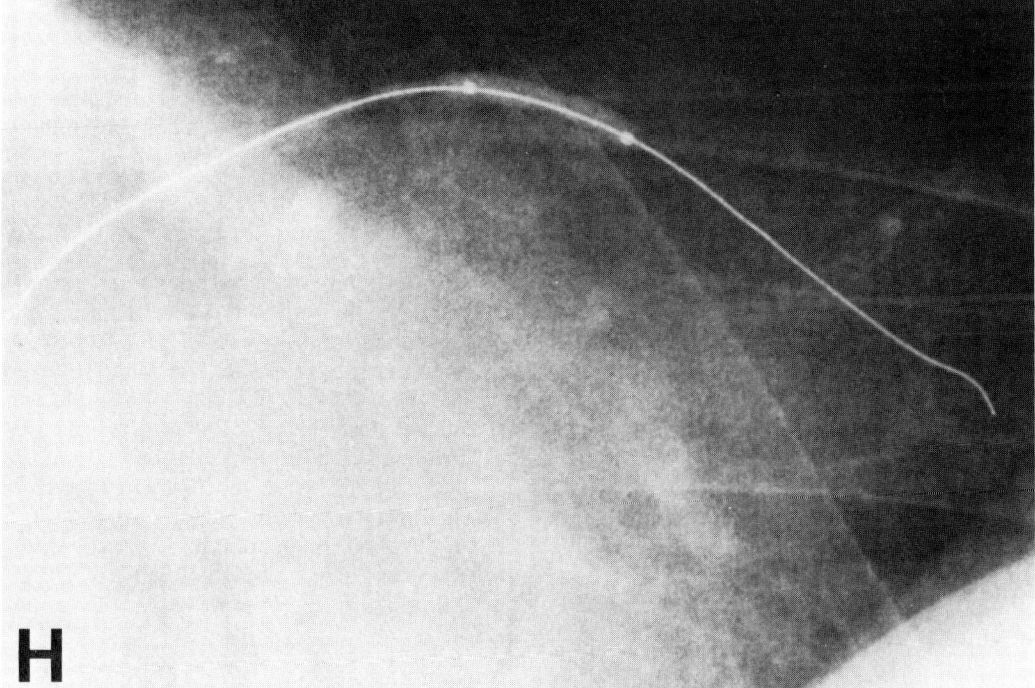

Figure 1. *Continued.* (*G*) A 3-mm balloon was passed over a floppy wire for dilatation of the proximal lesion in an RAO projection. (*H*) A 3-mm balloon combined with a platinum guide wire was used for dilatation of the mid-LAD lesion.

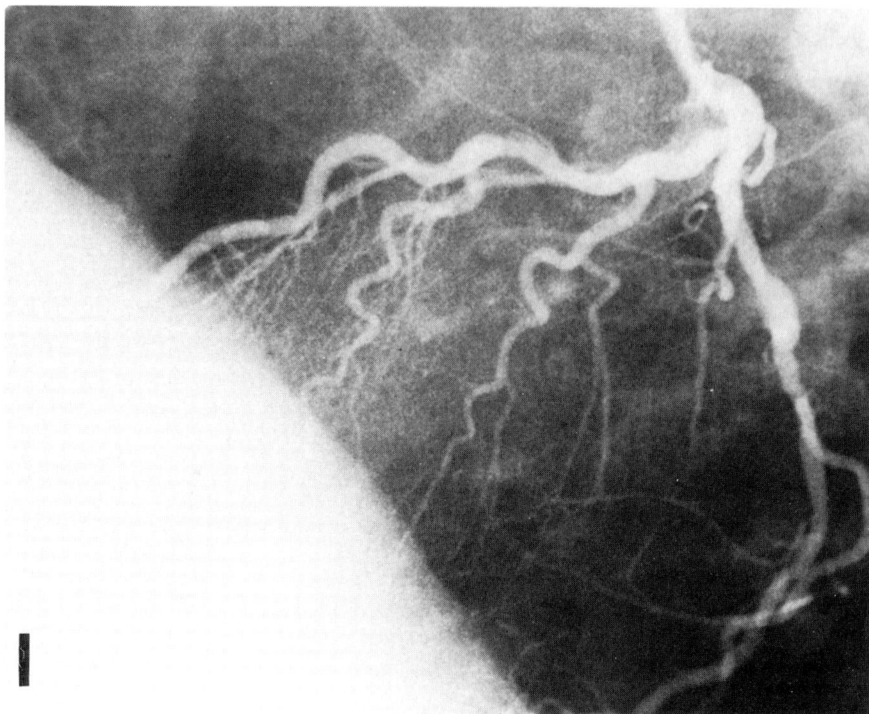

Figure 1. *Continued.* (*I*) Shown is the final result of LAD PTCA.

myocardial infarction. Over 120 patients had undergone prior coronary bypass surgery. One hundred nine had "poor" left ventricular function defined as an ejection fraction equal to or less than 45 percent, not in the setting of an acute myocardial infarction. Three hundred twelve procedures were multiple-vessel or multiple-lesion dilatation attempts (Fig. 1), including 185 double-lesion, 80 triple-lesion, 24 quadruple-lesion, 14 quintuple-lesion and 5 six-lesion dilatation procedures.

Successful PTCA

In this series, "successful" dilatation was defined as 40 percent or greater angiographic improvement and, when measured, included the hemodynamic criterion of a reduction in the resting gradient. Virtually no patient was left with a residual stenosis greater than 40 percent obstructive, and most had residual lesions judged less than 20 to 30 percent obstructive based upon two angiographic views. Few patients had residual gradients exceeding 10 mm Hg.

Eighty-eight percent of stenoses within the left anterior descending coronary artery and its branches were successfully dilated. Similarly, 87 percent of right coronary lesions attempted and 86 percent of circumflex coronary artery lesions attempted were successfully dilated. It is noteworthy that distal vessels and septal, diagonal, posterior descending, posterolateral, conus, anomalous circumflex, acute marginal, and obtuse marginal branches were included. Eighty-six percent of 51 saphenous vein grafts were successfully dilated, as were 8 of 10 left main coronary artery stenoses. Thirteen hundred eight, or 87 percent, of 1502 lesions attempted were successfully dilated (Table 1).

Complications

Major complications of the procedure included 18 transmural myocardial infarctions (1.8 percent), 26 emergency coronary bypass graft procedures (2.6 percent), and 12 deaths (1.2

Table 1. Percutaneous transluminal coronary angioplasty at Mid-America Heart Institute: Distribution of coronary arterial segments with individual and total success rates

Arteries dilated (2-83)		
	Number	*Success*
RCA		
Proximal	120	109 (91%)
Mid	167	147 (88%)
Distal	108	88 (81%)
PDA-PLAT	36	31 (86%)
Conus	1	1
Acute Marginal	2	2
	434 (29%)	378 (87%)
CIRC		
Proximal	98	88 (90%)
Distal	75	54 (72%)
Marginal	121	110 (91%)
	294 (20%)	252 (86%)
LAD		
Proximal	358	317 (89%)
Mid	259	222 (86%)
Distal	38	36 (95%)
Septal	2	2 (100%)
Diagonal	56	49 (88%)
	713 (47%)	626 (88%)
Grafts	51 (3.4%)	44 (86%)
Left Main	10 (0.67%)	8 (80%)

RCA = right coronary artery
CIRC = circumflex coronary artery
LAD = left anterior descending coronary artery

percent). Six of the 12 deaths occurred in patients presenting with acute myocardial infarction, all of whom were in shock at the time of attempted PTCA.

Post-Procedure Followup

Ambulatory patients have had repeat treadmill exercise testing immediately prior to hospital dismissal 24 to 48 hours following the PTCA procedure. The subsequent drug protocol included continued aspirin, one tablet bid; dipyridamole, 75 mg tid; and low-dose calcium channel blocker. At 8 weeks, repeat exercise testing was performed and drug regimen reduced to either aspirin alone or aspirin and dipyridamole in combination. A repeat exercise test was obtained at one year.

One hundred twenty patients undergoing successful PTCA were followed from 12 to 23 months (mean 18 months). Sixty percent of this population underwent elective repeat late angiography. One hundred two patients (85 percent) remained asymptomatic or without objective evidence of coronary restenosis when restudied. Sixteen patients (13 percent) had unequivocal restenosis at the site of previous PTCA. Eleven patients underwent successful repeat dilatation. Consequently, at a mean of 18 months followup, 113 patients (94 percent) were asymptomatic, although a second dilatation procedure was required in 9 percent.

During the past two years it has not been our policy to perform "routine" late coronary angiography. However, patients have been followed clinically and assessed by noninvasive techniques in a manner analogous to "routine" followup of those patients who have had coronary artery bypass surgery. Should anginal symptoms recur or a change in functional class or treadmill exercise test be demonstrated, repeat coronary angiography has been recommended with the assumption that a restenosis or new lesion has occurred.

OBSERVATIONS

Simultaneous multiple-lesion or multiple-vessel dilatation procedures now account for 50 percent of patients undergoing PTCA in our institution. Similarly, changes have occurred in our technical approach to the patient. Of the first 700 procedures, virtually all were performed with "standard" and available fixed-wire balloon catheters (United States Catheter and Instrument, Billerica, Massachusetts). However, in the subsequent 300 patients and our continued experience, a majority of patients are now initially approached with movable wire or directionally changeable catheter systems (Advanced Catheter Systems, Inc., Mountainview, California). This technical change reflects a response to the continued and increasing complexity of coronary lesions attempted and our conviction that guide wire systems offer increased flexibility yet greater inherent safety.

The incidence of coronary restenosis may be as high as 30 percent,[11–13] dependent upon factors of definition and interpretation. In this regard, many important questions remain unanswered. Can the patient with a tendency for rapid restenosis be identified? Is restenosis exacerbated by mechanical or other technical factors operative at the time of PTCA? Can pharmacologic manipulations reduce the incidence of restenosis? What is the proper treatment for a patient with coronary restenosis? What is the "natural" history of a lesion or arterial segment that has been successfully dilated on two, three, or more occasions?

Because of an impression that the lesion which restenoses vigorously may be one that was inadequately dilated, we presently average five to six 20- to 30-second balloon inflations at each lesion site and attempt to produce an optimal angiographic or "cosmetic" result. Less importance is attached to the initial and residual gradient, with emphasis being placed instead upon achieving a good angiographic result and a relative reduction in gradient.

Although high balloon inflation pressures (7 to 15 atmospheres) may be required to fully expand the balloon, a majority of lesions open with 4 to 6 atmospheres pressure. We believe that, in general, "routine" use of pressures greater than those required to achieve full balloon expansion is associated with increased arterial wall disruption and should be avoided.

On some occasions, full balloon expansion will occur and wide angiographic patency will be demonstrated despite persistence of a 10 to 15 mm gradient. This result should be considered acceptable. Repeated attempts to further reduce the residual gradient by high-pressure balloon expansion may lead to complications.

Many of these observations reflect an evolving philosophy, changing technical approach, and a departure from previous beliefs concerning PTCA. Consequently, these comments cannot be accepted as dogma but must be considered as opinions that are subject to change.

Future Implications

Coronary artery bypass graft surgery is clearly established as a "definitive" procedure for the relief of pain and prolongation of life in certain subsets of patients with coronary artery disease. Still, PTCA has increased attractiveness because of its simplicity, lesser patient trauma, and reduced cost.

A multicenter study compared similar groups of patients undergoing PTCA and coronary bypass surgery.[8] The mean hospital stay for PTCA patients was 4 $\pm$ 1 days compared with

12 ± 3 days for those undergoing bypass surgery. Assuming that only 15 percent of coronary artery bypass graft patients are suitable candidates for angioplasty and assuming an 80 percent primary success rate, PTCA was estimated to save over $7000 per case, with potential savings over 189 million dollars per year. At present, our own experience suggests that over 50 percent of coronary artery bypass graft patients are suitable candidates for PTCA. Consequently, the potential savings for the health care industry resulting from the successful performance of PTCA are enormous and cannot be ignored by patients, physicians, third-party health care insurers, and policy makers within the federal government.

At present, the limiting factor in aggressive application of PTCA is the widespread lack of technical skills and experience necessary to offer PTCA to larger and more complex patient subgroups. However, there is little doubt that time will modify these restricting circumstances and that a major change in the treatment of symptomatic coronary artery disease will evolve.

Neither the squeeze of a balloon nor the placement of a saphenous vein bypass graft will cure coronary artery disease. Symptomatic relief may be obtained with PTCA, coronary bypass surgery, and medical management, but no therapy can be considered truly definitive. Each treatment has unique limitations and advantages that need to be considered as they apply throughout the course of a patient's disease.

CONCLUSIONS

Coronary angioplasty can be performed with early results comparable to those of coronary bypass surgery. The procedure can be performed effectively and safely in patients with prior coronary bypass surgery, multiple-vessel disease, acute myocardial infarction, and "complex" coronary artery disease, including the elderly and those with poor left ventricular function. Coronary angioplasty is no longer an investigational procedure but an accepted alternative to coronary bypass surgery and continued medical management in patients with anatomically appropriate disease.

REFERENCES

1. Gruentzig, A: *Transluminal dilatation of coronary artery stenosis.* Lancet 1:263, 1978.
2. Berger, SM and Gorfinkle, HJ: *Candidates for transluminal coronary angioplasty.* Am J Cardiol 48:810, 1981.
3. Gruentzig, A, Senning, A, and Siegenthaler, WE: *Nonoperative dilatation of coronary-artery stenosis: Percutaneous transluminal coronary angioplasty.* N Engl J Med 301:61, 1979.
4. McCallister, BD, Hartzler, GO, Rutherford, BD, et al: *Palliative percutaneous transluminal angioplasty for unstable angina in patients over 70 years of age.* Circulation 64 (Suppl IV):IV-255, 1981.
5. Hartzler, GO, Rutherford, BD, McConahay, DR, et al: *Simultaneous multiple lesion coronary angioplasty. A preferred therapy for patients with multiple vessel disease.* Circulation 66 (Suppl II):II-5, 1982.
6. McConahay, D, Hartzler, G, and Rutherford, B: *Percutaneous transluminal coronary angioplasty: Use in management of symptomatic patients with recent myocardial infarction.* Circulation 66 (Suppl II):II-329, 1982.
7. Vlietstra, RE, Holmes, DR Jr, Mock, MB, et al: *Balloon angioplasty and multivessel coronary disease: Mayo Clinic experience.* J Am Coll Cardiol 1:656, 1983.
8. Jang, GC, Block, PC, Cowley, MJ, et al: *Comparative cost analysis of coronary angioplasty and coronary bypass surgery: Results from a nationally cooperative study.* Circulation 66 (Suppl II):II-124, 1982.
9. *Proceedings of the NHLBI PTCA registry, percutaneous coronary angioplasty workshop.* June 11-12, 1982. Bethesda, Maryland.
10. Hartzler, GO, Rutherford, BD, and McConahay, DR: *Percutaneous coronary angioplasty with and without prior streptokinase infusion for treatment of acute myocardial infarction.* Am J Cardiol 49:1033, 1982.
11. Dangoisse, V, Val, PG, David, PR, et al: *Recurrence of stenosis after successful percutaneous transluminal coronary angioplasty (PTCA).* Circulation 66 (Suppl II):II-331, 1982.
12. Holmes, DR, Vlietstra, RE, Smith, HC, et al: *Restenosis following percutaneous transluminal coronary angioplasty (PTCA): A report from the NHLBI PTCA registry.* Am J Cardiol 49:905, 1982.
13. Jutzy, KR, Berte, LE, Alderman, EL, et al: *Coronary restenosis rates in a consecutive patient series one year post-successful angioplasty.* Circulation 66 (Suppl II):II-331, 1982.

Thrombolysis in Acute Myocardial Infarction

Steven G. Meister, M.D., and Nelson M. Wolf, M.D.

In the past two decades major advances have been made in prevention and treatment of the fatal arrhythmias that may complicate acute myocardial infarction (MI). In fact, primary arrhythmic death is now infrequent in MI patients who are receiving adequate medical care. Much less progress has been made in preventing death or disability from congestive heart failure, cardiogenic shock, and other complications of extensive myocardial necrosis. During the past several years, a great deal of research effort has been targeted toward finding practical means of limiting myocardial necrosis during acute infarction. Until recently, most researchers concentrated on pharmacologic or mechanical interventions designed to influence the hemodynamic determinants of myocardial oxygen demand.[1-3] Despite considerable early optimism for several modalities, results to date have not been impressive enough to justify widespread clinical application.

Recent developments have raised the exciting prospect of rapidly restoring myocardial oxygen supply to normal or near normal resting levels and thus effectively aborting an ongoing infarction before necrosis is complete.

OCCLUSIVE INTRACORONARY THROMBUS IN ACUTE MYOCARDIAL INFARCTION

The exact sequence of events involved in the genesis of an acute transmural myocardial infarction has not been fully elucidated. However, it is now generally agreed that a common event in most patients is total or nearly total occlusion of a coronary artery or major branch.[4] Moreover, after years of controversy, it now seems clear that this occlusion is usually due to thrombosis at a site of pre-existing atherosclerotic narrowing. This was formerly a generally accepted concept. However, it was called into serious question in the late 1960s and early 1970s by pathologists who noted infrequent intracoronary thrombi in sudden death victims and a somewhat higher incidence in patients dying several days or weeks after an acute MI.[5-7] Roberts and Buja[5] proposed that intracoronary thrombi were a consequence of MI, rather than a cause, attributable to stasis of blood in vessels supplying a recently infarcted myocardium.

More recent studies employing postmortem coronary angiography and meticulous preparation of sections have demonstrated intracoronary thrombi in over 90 percent of patients dying of acute transmural MI.[8,9] DeWood and coworkers[4] performed coronary angiography within 24 hours of onset of acute MI in 322 patients being prepared for emergency coronary bypass surgery. They found total occlusion of the coronary artery supplying the infarct zone in 87 percent of patients studied within 4 hours of the onset of symptoms. The incidence of total occlusion declined to 66 percent in patients studied 12 to 24 hours after onset of the infarction. These investigators also retrieved intracoronary thrombus at the time of surgery from 72 percent of patients in whom this was attempted.

Findings such as these have revitalized the concept of intracoronary thrombus as a cause of acute myocardial infarction. They also form the basis for a renewal of efforts to re-establish coronary blood flow by thrombolysis. In retrospect, the paucity of intracoronary thrombi in sudden death patients may be explained by a relatively high incidence of primary arrhythmic death, rather than acute myocardial infarction, in such patients.

MECHANISM OF ACTION OF THROMBOLYTIC AGENTS

As intravascular thrombi are formed, the developing fibrin network entraps molecules of the circulating proenzyme plasminogen. In the presence of enzymatic activators, plasminogen is converted to its active form, plasmin. The latter is a proteolytic enzyme of low specificity capable of lysing fibrin (and thereby dissolving thrombi) and other plasma proteins including fibrinogen and clotting factors V and VIII.[10] Ordinarily, plasminogen is converted to plasmin by a specific activator, found in vascular endothelial cells, which requires fibrin as a cofactor. Thus, this naturally occurring plasminogen activator works only within or upon thrombi and can be considered clot selective. Moreover, any excess plasmin spilling into the general circulation is inactivated by circulating alpha-antiplasmin.

Currently, there are two available thrombolytic drugs—streptokinase and urokinase. Streptokinase is extracted from cultures of Type C streptococci.[10] In plasma it combines with plasminogen to form a potent plasminogen activator. Urokinase is derived from human urine or renal cell cultures and is a direct plasminogen activator. Neither agent is clot selective because neither requires fibrin as a cofactor. Furthermore, in dosages used for thrombolysis, both release plasmin into the circulation in quantities sufficient to overwhelm the antiplasmin system. Accordingly, large quantities of fibrinogen and other clotting factors are destroyed, and a bleeding tendency results. Streptokinase is highly antigenic. Most patients have some level of circulating antibodies capable of reacting with it because of prior streptococcus infections. Accordingly, loading doses are frequently used. Also because use of streptokinase for thrombolysis promotes an anamnestic response, it cannot be used a second time, at least not within a 6-month interval.[11,12] Urokinase is extremely expensive, and so a majority of studies to date have employed streptokinase.

EARLY THROMBOLYTIC TRIALS

Thrombolytic therapy for acute myocardial infarction was first attempted in man in the late 1950s and early 1960s.[13–15] These initial studies were either uncontrolled or examined too few patients to permit definitive conclusions. Interestingly, Boucek and Murphy[14] in 1959 performed semiselective coronary infusion of a thrombolytic agent. These authors positioned cardiac catheters in the aortic root near the coronary orifices and infused fibrinolysin, a streptokinase-plasminogen complex, in early diastole (via an electrocardiogram [ECG]-gated infusion pump) to coincide with the period of maximal coronary filling. They noted rapid evolution of electrocardiographic and cardiac enzyme patterns, as well as ventricular arrhythmias, occurring during the infusions. We now know that these are reperfusion events that are to be expected when an occluded coronary artery reopens during an acute MI.

Although these early studies established the safety and feasibility of administering thrombolytic agents during acute myocardial infarction in man, they provided little if any information regarding efficacy. In order to learn more about this approach, several large randomized controlled studies were performed in Europe and the United States in the late 1960s and 1970s.[16–23] These trials most often employed intravenous streptokinase. Typical dosages were 250,000 to 500,000 units initially as a loading dose, followed by 100,000 to 150,000 units per hour for 12 to 24 hours. Notably, thrombolytic treatment was begun at any time up to 12 to 24 hours from the onset of infarction symptoms. Angiography was not performed, either prior to or after thrombolysis. Mortality and clinically detectable congestive heart failure were the usual endpoints used to assess efficacy. A statistically significant reduction in mortality in the streptokinase-treated group was reported in some of the earlier controlled trials.[24] However, subsequent studies, which in some respects were better designed, noted no important differences between treated and control groups. These disappointing results, coupled with growing skepticism of the role of intracoronary thrombosis in genesis of acute myocardial infarction, led to abandonment of thrombolysis in all but a few centers in Europe.

In retrospect, some important flaws in the design of these studies are evident. First of all, there is now evidence from animal studies that with occlusion of a coronary artery, irreversible necrosis begins within 30 minutes and is largely completed by 4 to 6 hours.[25,26] The practice of beginning thrombolytic therapy 12 or 24 hours after onset of infarction symptoms probably resulted in study of many patients who were well past the point at which any benefit from thrombolysis could reasonably have been expected. Any beneficial effects in patients studied earlier would very likely have been masked. Secondly, with the exception of death, other endpoints, such as congestive heart failure, were relatively "soft" and subject to considerable subjective interpretation by the investigators. Since angiography was not performed, it was not known whether, or how quickly, reopening of coronary arteries was being achieved in treated patients. Also, at that time there were no suitable technical means for establishing whether appreciable amounts of myocardium were being salvaged.

In spite of these very considerable drawbacks, Stampfer and associates[27] pooled the results of eight of the most consistent intravenous streptokinase trials and found a 20 percent reduction of mortality in the treated groups ($p < 0.01$).

INTRACORONARY INFUSION OF THROMBOLYTIC AGENTS

In the years since most major intravenous thrombolytic trials were performed, selective coronary catheterization has evolved from a rather heroic and dangerous adventure to a routine procedure of low mortality and low morbidity. Studies in peripheral arteries have shown that selective local infusion of thrombolytic agents results in more rapid clot lysis at lower doses than are required with systemic infusions.[28] Thus, it was a logical next step to investigate the effects of selective intracoronary infusion of thrombolytic agents during acute myocardial infarction. The first recorded successful use of intracoronary thrombolysis was by Rentrop[29] in a patient who developed occlusion of a coronary artery during diagnostic catheterization. There have been several reports of intracoronary thrombolysis in patients presenting in the early hours of acute myocardial infarction.[30–33] In most patients, therapy was begun within 6 hours of the onset of infarction, but in one study streptokinase was begun up to 18 hours afterward.[33] Ganz and associates[30] advocated subselective streptokinase infusion, using a specially designed catheter threaded down the coronary artery as close to the site of thrombotic occlusion as possible. These authors reported reopening of a totally or subtotally occluded coronary artery supplying the site of ongoing infarction (infarct-related vessel) in 19 of 20 patients within 8 to 80 minutes after beginning the infusion. Similarly, Mathey and coworkers[32] reported reperfusion in 73 percent of patients within 1 hour, and Rentrop and associates[31] in 75 percent within 15 to 90 minutes. These authors used selective infusion into the left or right coronary orifices rather than subselective infusion. In most of these patients, previously administered intracoronary nitroglycerin had failed to reopen the occluded infarct-related vessels. A few investigators[31–33] have also utilized mechanical perforation of the obstructing thrombus with a guide wire as an adjunct to streptokinase in a few cases. However, this approach has generally been abandoned because of the risk of vessel perforation or dissection. Figure 1, from our laboratory, illustrates reopening of a totally occluded artery in a patient with acute MI receiving intracoronary streptokinase.

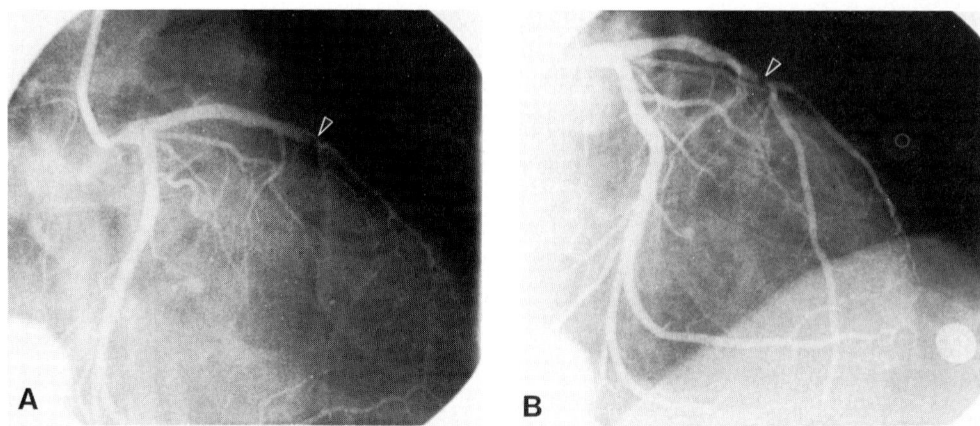

Figure 1. *A,* This is a totally occluded left anterior descending artery *(arrow)* in a patient having an acute anteroseptal MI. *B,* After 20 minutes of intracoronary streptokinase the artery has reopened, leaving a very severe residual stenosis *(arrow).* Coronary bypass surgery was subsequently performed.

Ganz and colleagues[30] and others[32] observed unusually rapid evolution of electrocardiographic changes after successful reperfusion, as illustrated in Figure 2. Similarly, rapid evolution of creatine phosphokinase curves, with peaking at 9 to 13 hours rather than the usual 22 hours for conventionally treated patients, is also seen.[30,32] Reperfusion arrhythmias are also commonly noted immediately after reopening of the obstructed vessel.[30,32] Typically, these arrhythmias consist of frequent premature ventricular beats, but episodes of ventricular tachycardia and fibrillation sometimes occur, requiring prompt pharmacologic or electrical cardioversion. Malacoff and coworkers[34] have described inducible ventricular tachycardia in 6 of 12 patients who received streptokinase and had electrophysiologic studies 7 to 25 days later. No correlation between occurrence of reperfusion arrhythmias and inducibility of ventricular tachycardia was found. The clinical significance of this finding is unknown.

Lee[35] and Smalling[36] and their colleagues have shown that reperfusion is more likely to be achieved when streptokinase infusion is begun as early as possible after the onset of infarction symptoms. Following reperfusion, a high-grade residual fixed stenosis, presumably atherosclerotic, usually persists at the site of former occlusion. Less frequently, the residual stenosis is relatively insignificant (Fig. 3). Spherical, teardrop-shaped, or sausage-like intraluminal

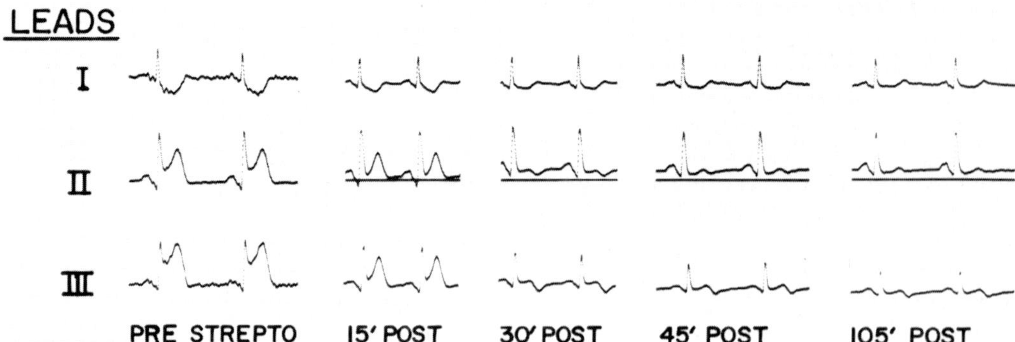

Figure 2. This ECG shows the rapid evolution of electrocardiographic changes of an acute inferior myocardial infarction in a patient whose right coronary artery was reperfused after 10 minutes of intracoronary streptokinase. In this patient, elevated ST segments returned rapidly to baseline, and new Q waves did not develop.

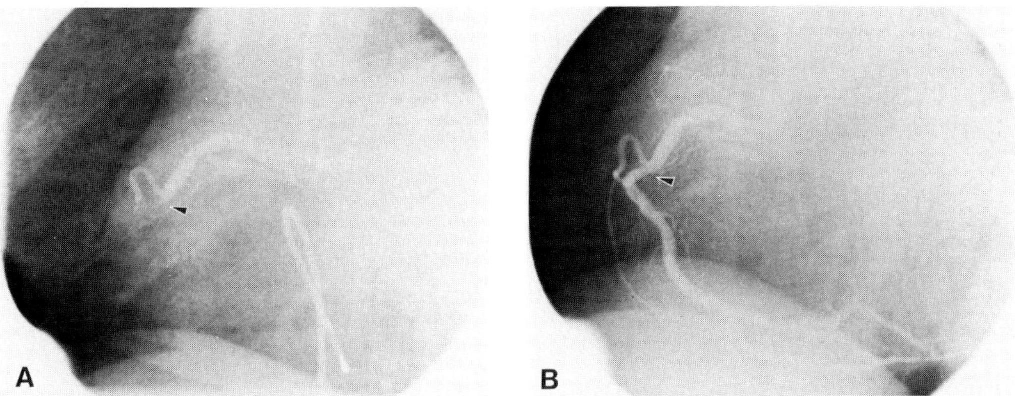

Figure 3. *A,* Shown here is the total occlusion of the main right coronary artery *(arrow)* in a patient receiving intravenous streptokinase for an acute inferior myocardial infarction. Note that the residual stenosis after reperfusion (*B*) is less than 50 percent *(arrow)*. This patient was treated medically and anticoagulated for 4 months. She had no recurrent symptoms.

lucencies or filling defects representing residual thrombotic material are often seen attached to the stenotic site immediately following reperfusion (Fig. 4). Typically, these thrombi shrink or disappear during streptokinase infusion or on subsequent repeat angiography. Occasionally, they can be seen embolizing distally, as in Figure 5. Reclosure of the infarct-related vessel is occasionally seen during the streptokinase infusion.[37] The mechanism is unknown.

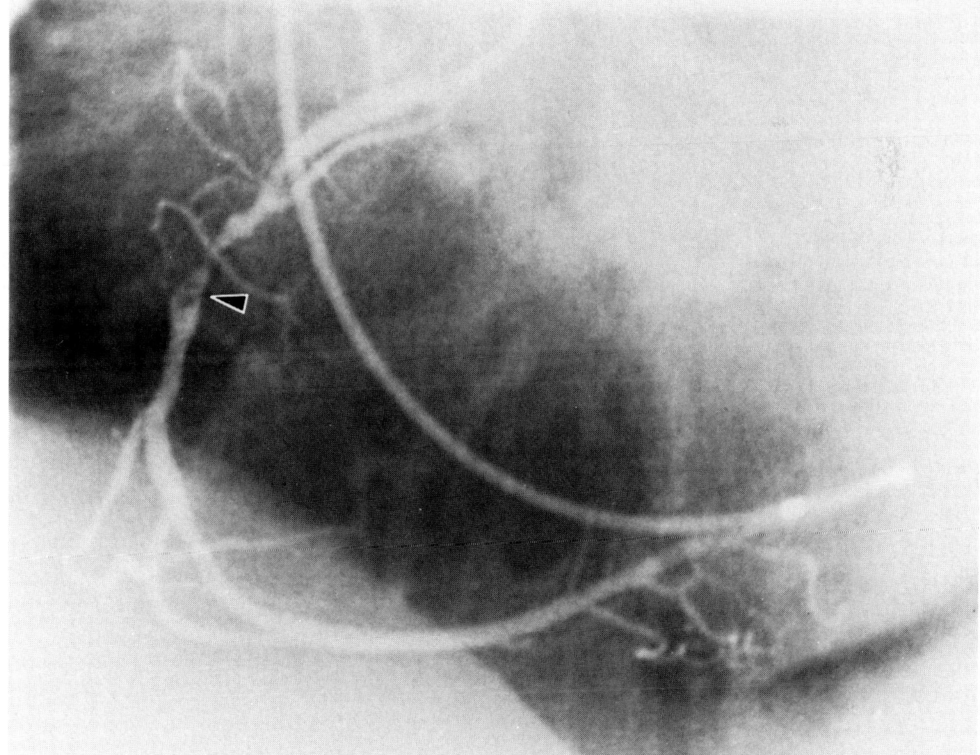

Figure 4. Spherical intraluminal thrombus *(arrow)* shown attached to a severe right coronary artery stenosis.

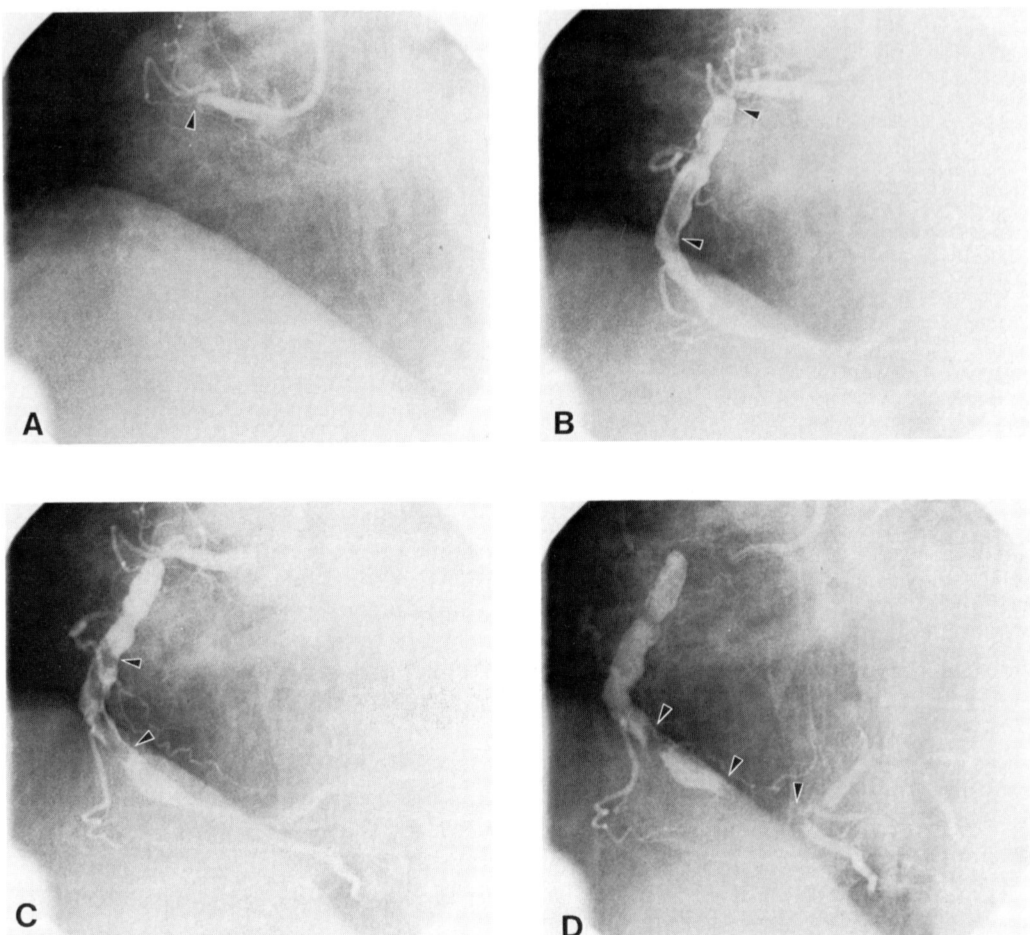

Figure 5. Distal embolization of an intracoronary thrombus during intracoronary streptokinase infusion. *A,* The right coronary artery is totally occluded *(arrow). B,* The vessel is seen reopened, with a sausage-shaped thrombus (*between arrows*) attached to a tight stenosis at the site of former occlusion. *C,* The thrombus has become detached and is seen moving distally *(between arrows). D,* It has broken up and become impacted in the distal vessel *(arrows).*

Reclosure also may occur during subsequent days or weeks. Timmis and associates reported an 18 percent incidence of reclosure within 2 weeks.[38] There is widespread opinion among experienced investigators that careful maintenance of full anticoagulation—initially with heparin and subsequently with warfarin—is effective in reducing the incidence of reclosure, but this has not been rigorously documented.

There is no general agreement on what other steps may be necessary to prevent reinfarction in patients who have had successful reperfusion. Options include continuing medical therapy with anticoagulation for 3 to 6 months, early percutaneous transluminal coronary angioplasty, or early coronary bypass surgery. We have adopted a policy of individualizing therapy, based upon several factors. We have elected to continue medical management, including anticoagulation, in patients in whom the residual stenosis appears not to be significant or when there are electrocardiographic, enzyme, and angiographic evidences that most of the myocardium at risk has undergone necrosis. However, it is important to delay assessment of residual ventricular function until about 3 weeks after reperfusion. Reperfused myocardium may initially

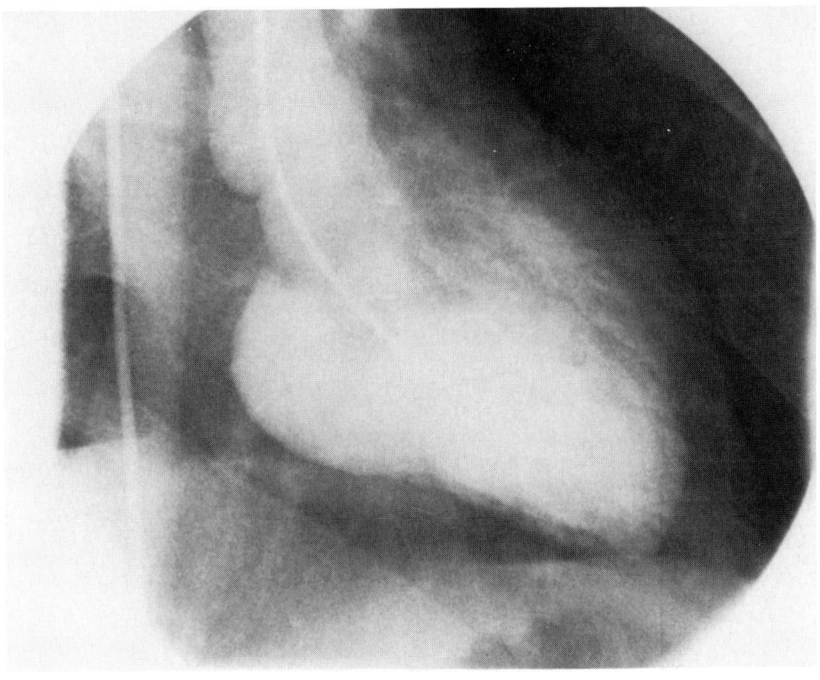

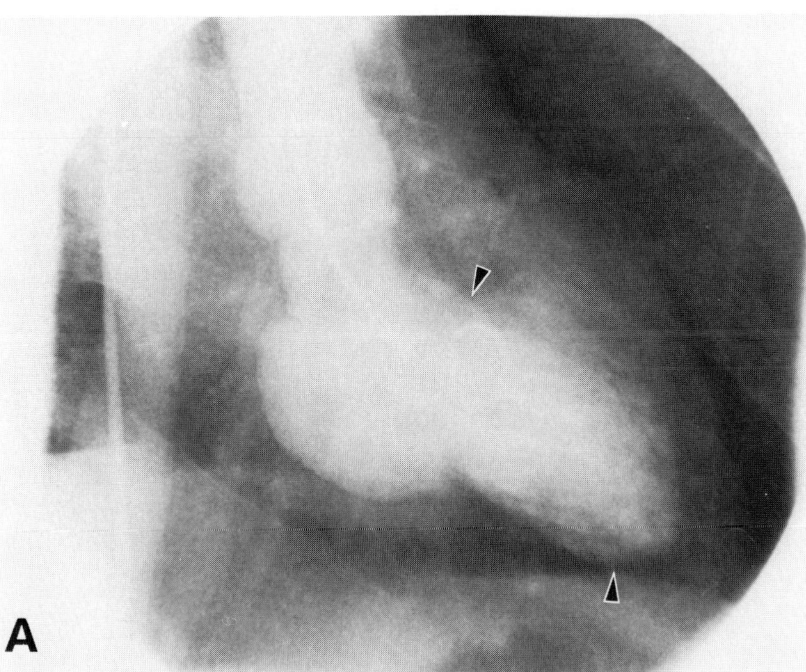

Figure 6. Delayed return of ventricular function following coronary reperfusion. All panels show end-diastole at the top and end-systole at the bottom. *A*, Anterior and apical akinesis *(between arrows)* appear prior to streptokinase infusion.

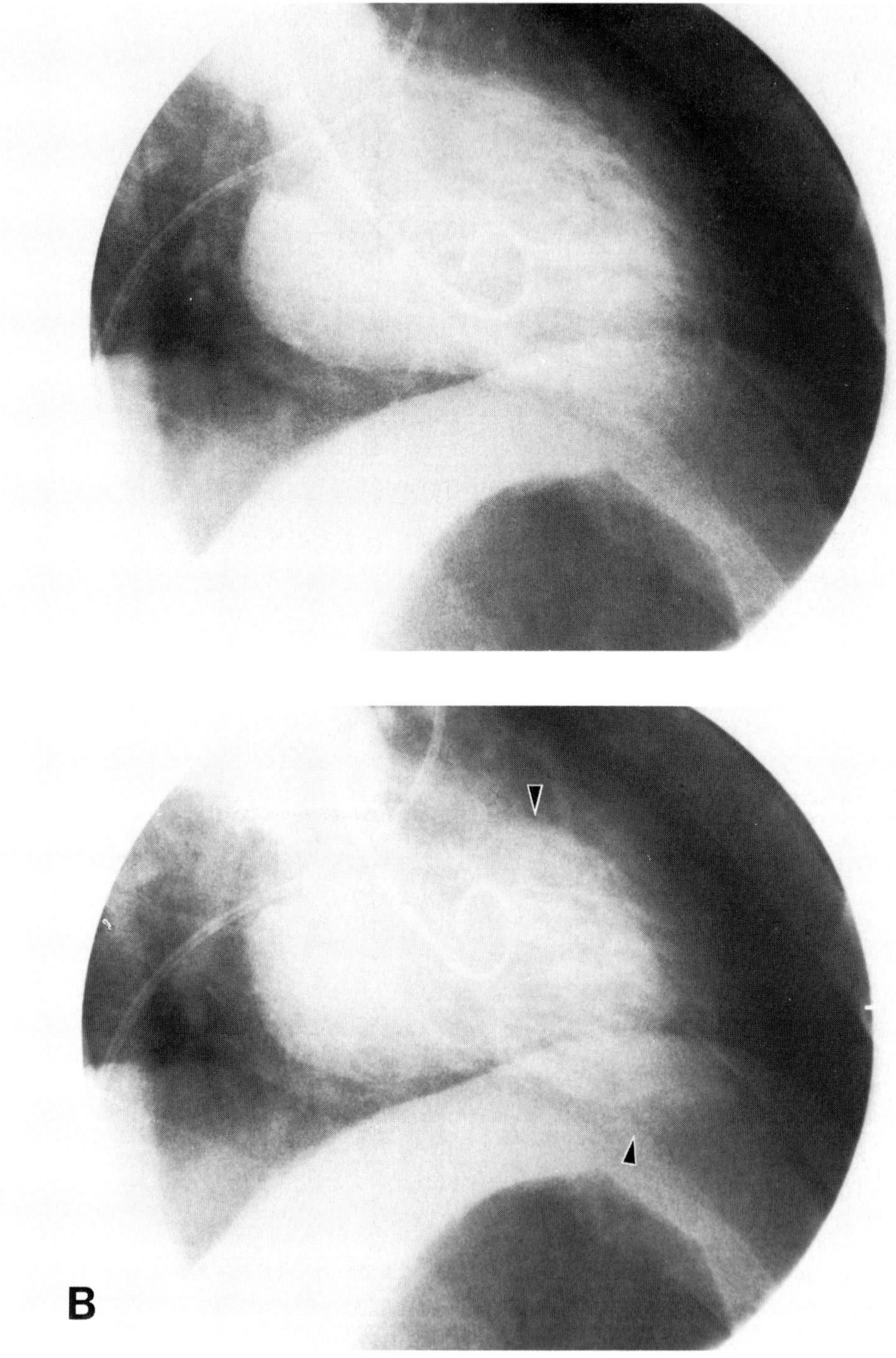

Figure 6. *Continued. B,* There is a slight worsening of anterior wall motion immediately after successful left anterior descending artery reperfusion *(between arrows).*

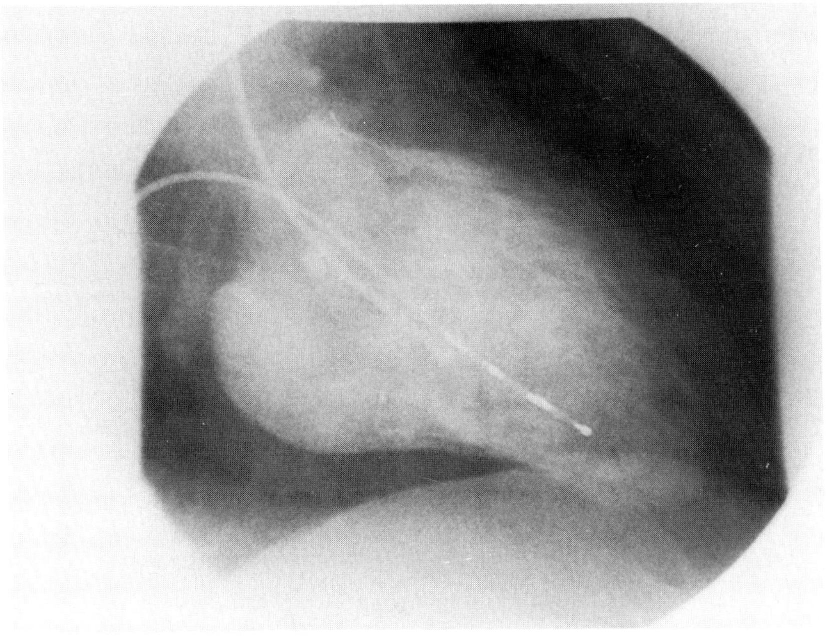

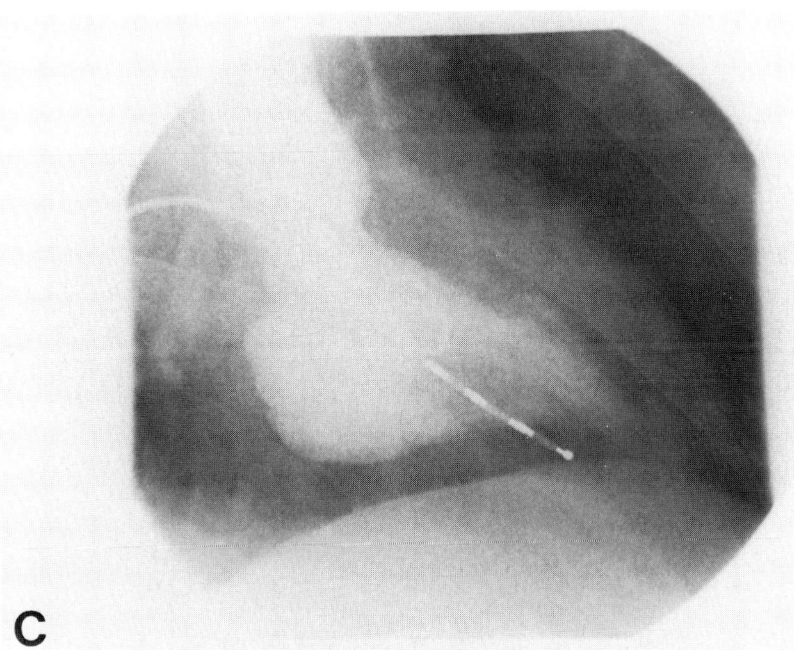

Figure 6. *Continued. C,* Substantial recovery of anterior wall motion is evident 21 days after reperfusion.

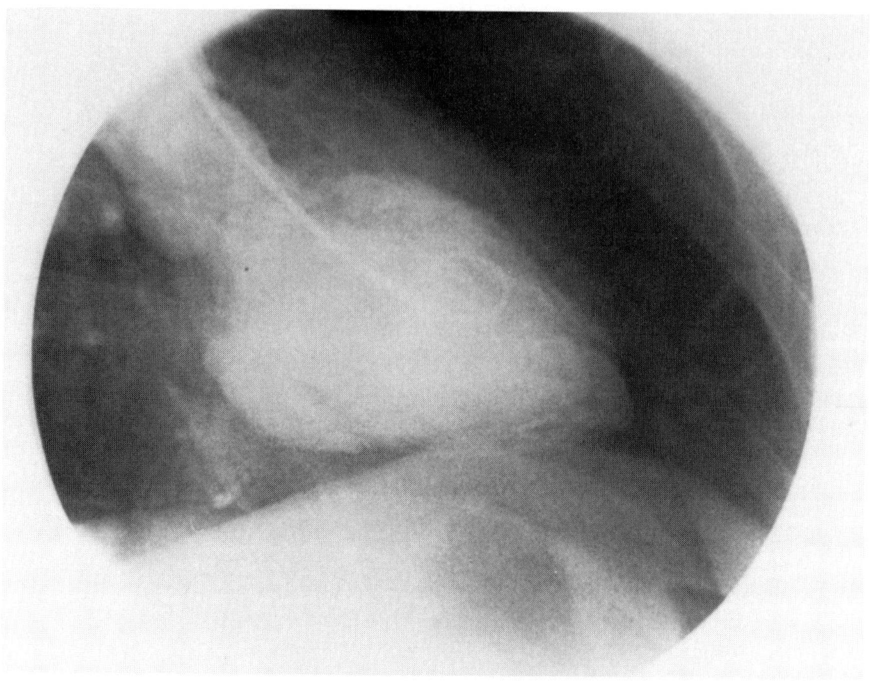

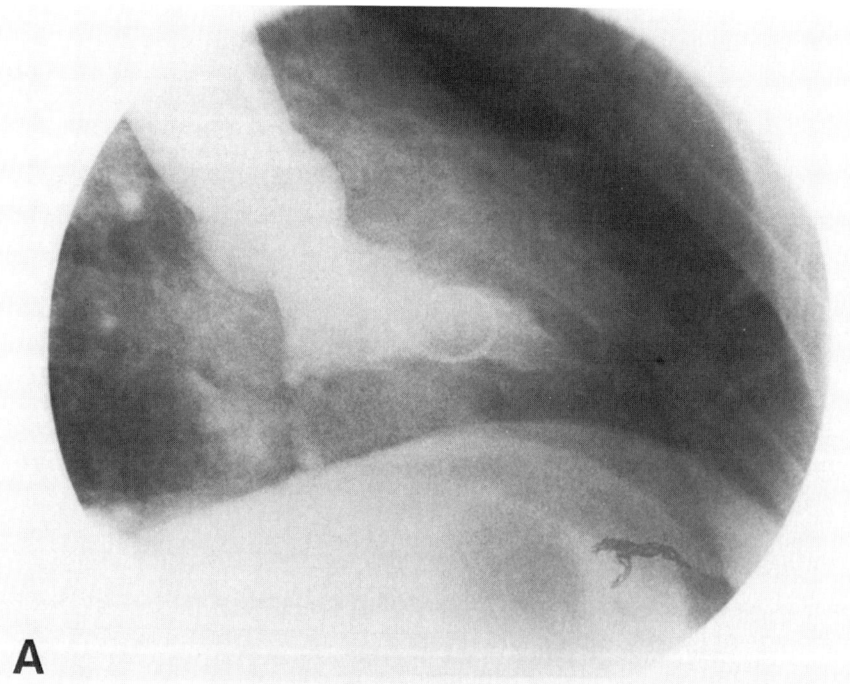

A

Figure 7. *A*, Shown is the normal left ventricular wall motion in a patient with unstable angina. Three days later the patient had an acute anteroseptal MI while in the hospital. The patient received intracoronary streptokinase with reopening of the occluded left anterior descending artery 75 minutes after onset of the MI.

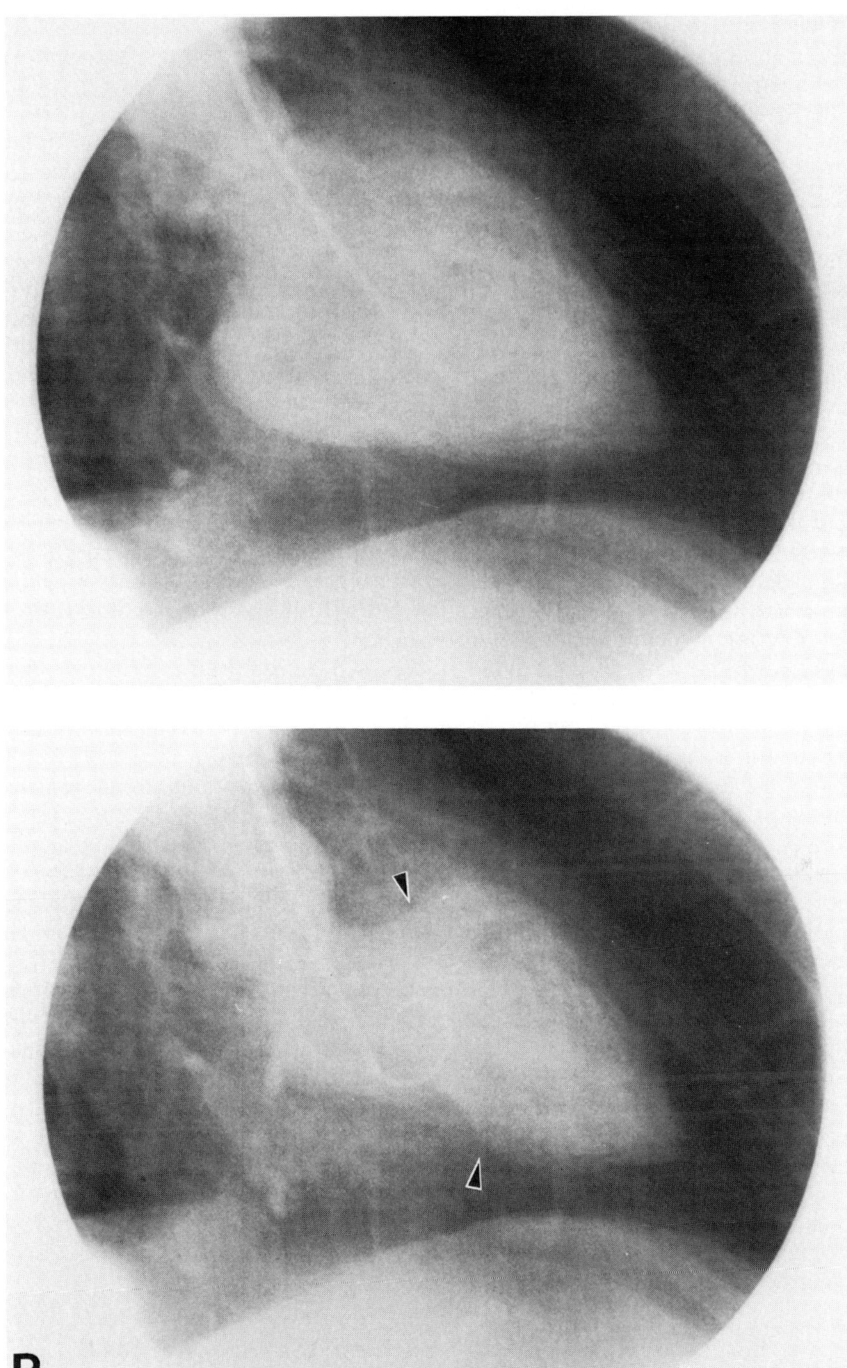

Figure 7. *Continued. B,* Extensive anterior and apical akinesis *(between arrows)* appear just after reperfusion. Repeat angiography 20 days later showed no improvement. Compare with Figure 6, in which most anterior wall function returned following 6 hours of left anterior descending artery occlusion.

appear to have been destroyed yet subsequently show remarkable return of function (Fig. 6). We employ percutaneous transluminal coronary angioplasty or coronary bypass surgery in patients in whom the residual stenosis is severe and when there is evidence that considerable function has been preserved in the myocardial zone at risk.

Rentrop,[31] Mathey,[32] and Reduto[33] and their associates have all demonstrated modest improvement in left ventricular ejection fractions in patients who have had successful thrombolysis. Reduto has also emphasized that ventricular function may not return for 2 or 3 weeks. There is support for this concept from animal studies, in which wall motion and certain myocardial metabolic processes take weeks to recover fully following periods of total coronary occlusion too brief to cause extensive necrosis.[39,40] Factors believed to influence the extent of myocardial salvage in man include time from onset of infarction to reperfusion, size and extent of the vessel involved, presence or absence of preformed collateral circulation, completeness of occlusion of the infarct-related vessel, and hemodynamic determinants of myocardial oxygen demand, such as heart rate, blood pressure, and metabolic state. However, some remarkable inconsistencies in response to thrombolytic therapy and reperfusion are sometimes seen. Figure 7 shows a ventriculogram with systolic and end-diastolic frames from before and 3 weeks after anterior infarction and left anterior descending artery thrombolysis in a patient who infarcted while in the hospital. Reperfusion was achieved in just 75 minutes from the onset of chest pain and ST segment elevation, and yet, no measurable salvage of myocardium occurred. This case should be contrasted to the results in the patient in Figure 6 in whom reperfusion was not achieved until 6 hours from onset of symptoms. Probably not all factors affecting myocardial salvage are known.

Obviously, large randomized controlled studies will be required to critically evaluate the overall usefulness of intracoronary thrombolysis in salvaging myocardium and in preventing death, congestive heart failure, and other complications of acute myocardial infarction. This evaluation should be substantially easier to accomplish now than in the past, given the availability of reliable techniques for invasive and noninvasive determination of ventricular wall motion. Some preliminary reports are available at this time. Walton and coworkers[41] with 34 randomized patients and Leiboff and associates[42] with 27 patients reported no significant differences in left ventricular wall motion or mortality between streptokinase-treated patients and controls. Conversely, Anderson and coworkers[43] with 41 patients, Serruys and associates[44] with 51 patients, and Veroni and coworkers[45] with 25 patients, reported improved ventricular wall motion in their randomized studies. Obviously, all these studies involve far too few patients to permit reliable conclusions, and it is not surprising that divergent results have been reported. Kennedy and colleagues[46] and the other investigators in the Western Washington Intracoronary Streptokinase in Acute Myocardial Infarction Trial have performed the only large-scale study to date. In this multicenter study of 250 patients, a 3.7 percent 30-day mortality in streptokinase-treated patients contrasted with 11.2 percent in controls ($p < 0.02$). However, these results represent a total of only 18 deaths to date. Thus, some caution in interpretation of these preliminary data is indicated. Further study in larger numbers of patients over a longer interval is needed.

At present, intracoronary thrombolysis represents a promising new approach to salvage of myocardium in patients with acute infarction. However, its efficacy has not been firmly established at this time, and it must still be considered experimental therapy.

RECENT INTRAVENOUS STREPTOKINASE STUDIES

Intracoronary administration of streptokinase or urokinase is an unwieldy form of therapy. Acutely ill, frightened patients must give their permission for an invasive procedure without time to consider or to consult with family members. Catheterization facilities are not available in all institutions or may already be in use. Delay may result while catheterization personnel are in transit. Although it was originally hoped that the relatively low total doses of throm-

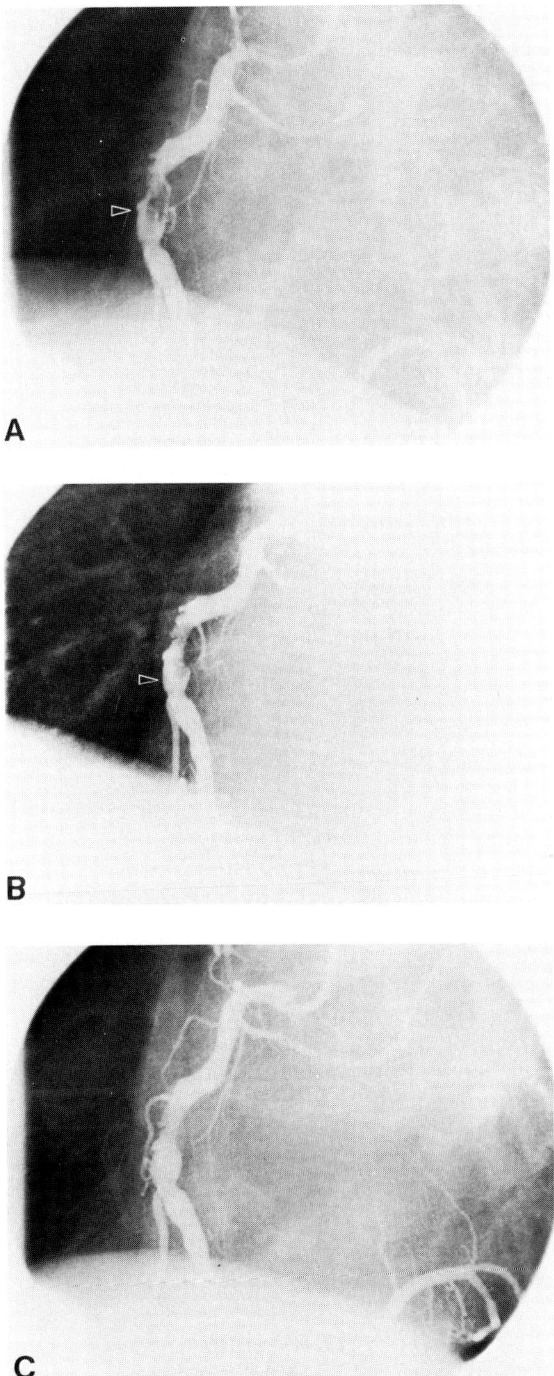

Figure 8. *A*, This is the right coronary artery of a patient with unstable angina. There is a severe stenosis and a large intracoronary filling defect *(arrow)*. *B*, Immediately after intracoronary streptokinase infusion the filling defect is smaller and the stenosis is less severe. *C*, The same artery is shown 1 week later. The filling defect is gone, and the stenosis is even less severe. This patient was managed medically and anticoagulated for 3 months. Symptoms did not return.

bolytic agents used with intracoronary thrombolysis would preclude development of a systemic bleeding tendency ("lytic state"), this disorder occurs in the majority of patients treated.[47] Significant bleeding is particularly likely to occur when arterial catheters are withdrawn following treatment.

Intravenous infusion of thrombolytic agents, if efficacious, would preclude many of these logistical difficulties as well as some bleeding problems. To date, only preliminary studies angiographically documenting the effects of high-dose, brief-duration, intravenous streptokinase administration have been done.[48–50] These studies have shown a somewhat lower (45 to 67 percent) incidence of rapid reperfusion than that seen with the intracoronary route. Blunda and coworkers[49] also showed that the average time from beginning of the infusion to reperfusion was about twice that for intracoronary streptokinase, that is, 54 minutes for intravenous versus 26 minutes for intracoronary streptokinase. Nevertheless, the rapidity with which intravenous streptokinase can be instituted might compensate for the longer reperfusion time needed.

NEWER PLASMINOGEN ACTIVATORS

Perhaps the most exciting development on the horizon is the potential availability of newer clot-selective plasminogen activators. Bergman and associates[51] have used human extrinsic plasminogen activator in a canine model to lyse intracoronary thrombi within 10 minutes with either intracoronary or intravenous administration. If this activator or similar preparations prove safe and similarly effective in man, their potential for myocardial salvage seems exciting indeed.

THROMBOLYSIS IN ISCHEMIC SYNDROMES OTHER THAN ACUTE TRANSMURAL MYOCARDIAL INFARCTION

The rediscovery of intracoronary thrombi as an etiologic factor in acute transmural myocardial infarction has raised the question of their involvement in unstable angina pectoris and nontransmural myocardial infarction. Holmes[52] and Vetrovec[53] and their coworkers recently described intracoronary filling defects similar to those seen during reopening of infarct vessels in patients catheterized for unstable angina or nontransmural infarction. Wolf and colleagues[54] have documented dissolution of such defects and improvement, in some instances, of stenotic lumen diameters when intracoronary streptokinase was administered to patients with these syndromes (Fig. 8). Furthermore, Lawrence and coworkers[55] in a small controlled study showed clinical improvement in patients with unstable angina who received intravenous streptokinase. Much further study is needed to determine the relative incidence and importance of intracoronary thrombi in these syndromes. However, it is possible that thrombolysis or, more likely, anticoagulation or antiplatelet drugs may come to play a role in their management.

Another possible area of application has recently been suggested by Shapiro and associates.[56] These authors administered intracoronary streptokinase to patients with persistent post-infarction angina. Recanalization was accomplished in 6 of 8 patients some 5 to 13 days post-infarction, with substantial relief of symptoms.

CONCLUSIONS

It is clear that intracoronary streptokinase during acute myocardial infarction results in rapid reopening of occluded coronary arteries. It remains to be seen whether this therapy results in worthwhile salvage of myocardium and reduction of mortality and morbidity in patients. Intravenous administration of streptokinase appears to be less consistently effective and slower acting than the intracoronary approach. However, further study of this more convenient and widely applicable form of therapy is needed. Wider application of thrombolysis to patients with post-infarction angina and unstable angina pectoris has been proposed. Pending results of currently ongoing and future studies, thrombolysis remains an experimental therapy for ischemic heart disease.

REFERENCES

1. Peter, T, Norris, RM, Ming, KH, et al: *Reduction of creatine kinase after acute myocardial infarction by propranolol.* Circulation 55, 56(Suppl III):239, 1977.
2. Hockings, BEF, Cope, GD, Clarke, GM, et al: *Randomized controlled trial of vasodilator therapy after myocardial infarction.* Am J Cardiol 48:345, 1981.
3. Leinbach, RC, Gold, HK, Harper, RW, et al: *Early intra-aortic balloon pumping for anterior myocardial infarction without shock.* Circulation 58:204, 1978.
4. DeWood, MA, Spores, J, Notske, R, et al: *Prevalence of total coronary occlusion during the early hours of transmural myocardial infarction.* N Engl J Med 303:897, 1980.
5. Roberts, WC, and Buja, LM: *The frequency and significance of coronary arterial thrombi and other observations in fatal acute myocardial infarction.* Am J Med 52:425, 1972.
6. Spain, DM and Bradess, VA: *The relationship of coronary thrombosis to coronary atherosclerosis and ischemic heart disease.* Am J Med Sci 240:701, 1960.
7. Erlich, JC and Shinohara, Y: *Low incidence of coronary thrombosis in myocardial infarction.* Arch Pathol 78:432, 1964.
8. Buja, LM and Willerson, JT: *Clinicopathologic correlates of acute ischemic heart disease syndromes.* Am J Cardiol 47:343, 1981.
9. Ridolfi, RL and Hutchins, GM: *The relationship between coronary artery lesions in myocardial infarction: Ulceration of atherosclerotic plaques precipitating coronary thrombosis.* Am Heart J 93:468, 1977.
10. Sharma, GVRK, Alla, G, Parisi, AF, et al: *Thrombolytic therapy.* N Engl J Med 306:1268, 1982.
11. Sherry, S: *Personal reflections on the development of thrombolytic therapy and its application to acute coronary thrombosis.* Am Heart J 102:1134, 1982.
12. Meister, SG, Untereker, WJ, Singh, S, et al: *Failure of streptokinase to lyse thrombi on second attempts.* Clin Res 29:656A, 1981.
13. Richter, IH, Musachio, FE, Clifton, EE, et al: *Experiences with clot-lysing agents in coronary thrombosis.* Am J Cardiol 6:534, 1960.
14. Boucek, RJ and Murphy, WP Jr: *Segmental perfusion of the coronary arteries with fibrinolysin in man following a myocardial infarction.* Am J Cardiol 6:525, 1960.
15. Dewar, HA, Stephenson, P, Horter, AR, et al: *Fibrinolytic therapy of coronary thrombosis.* Br Med J 1:195, 1963.
16. Arnery, A, Roeber, G, Vermeulen, HJ, et al: *Single-blind randomized multicenter trial comparing heparin and streptokinase treatment in recent myocardial infarction.* Acta Med Scand 505(Suppl):5, 1969.
17. European Working Party: *Streptokinase in recent myocardial infarction: A controlled multicentre trial.* Br Med J 3:325, 1971.
18. Heikinheimer, R, Ahrenburg, P, Honkapohja, H, et al: *Fibrinolytic treatment in acute myocardial infarction.* Acta Med Scand 189:7, 1971.
19. *European Cooperative Study Group for streptokinase treatment in acute myocardial infarction.* N Engl J Med 301:797, 1979.
20. Dioguardi, N, Mannucci, PM, Lotto, A, et al: *Controlled trial of streptokinase and heparin in acute myocardial infarction.* Lancet 2:891, 1971.
21. Breddin, K, Ehrly, AM, Fechler, L, et al: *Die kurzzhutfebrinolyse biem akuten myokardinfarct.* Dtsch Med Wochenschr 98:861, 1973.
22. Bett, JNN, Biggs, JC, Castaldi, PA, et al: *Australian multicentre trial of streptokinase in acute myocardial infarction.* Lancet 1:57, 1973.
23. Aber, CP, Bass, NM, Berry, CL, et al: *Streptokinase in acute myocardial infarction: A controlled multicentre study in the United Kingdom.* Br Med J 2:1100, 1976.
24. Fratantoni, JC, Ness, P, and Simon, TC: *Thrombolytic therapy.* N Engl J Med 293:1073, 1975.
25. Reisner, KA, Lowe, JE, Rasmussen, MM, et al: *The wavefront phenomenon of ischemic cell death; myocardial infarction size vs duration of coronary occlusion in dogs.* Circulation 56:785, 1977.

26. Muera, M, Thomas, R, Ganz, W, et al: *The effect of delay of propranolol administration on reduction of myocardial infarct size after experimental coronary artery occlusion in dogs.* Circulation 59:1148, 1979.

27. Stampfer, MJ, Goldhaber, SZ, Yseref, S, et al: *Effect of intravenous streptokinase on acute myocardial infarction.* N Engl J Med 307:1180 1982.

28. Dotter, CT, Rösch, J, and Seaman, AJ: *Selective clot lysis with low-dose streptokinase.* Radiology 111:31, 1974.

29. Rentrop, P, Blanke, H, Köstering, K, et al: *Acute myocardial infarction: Intracoronary application of nitroglycerin and streptokinase in combination with transluminal recanalization.* Clin Cardiol 5:354, 1979.

30. Ganz, W, Buchbinder, N, Marcus, H, et al: *Intracoronary thrombus in evolving myocardial infarction.* Am Heart J 101:4, 1981.

31. Rentrop, P, Blanke, H, Karsch, KR, et al: *Selective intracoronary thrombolysis in acute myocardial infarction and unstable angina pectoris.* Circulation 63:307, 1981.

32. Mathey, DG, Kuck, KH, Tilsner, V, et al: *Nonsurgical coronary artery recanalization in acute myocardial infarction.* Circulation 63:489, 1981.

33. Reduto, LA, Smalling, RW, Freund, GC, et al: *Intracoronary infusion of streptokinase in patients with acute myocardial infarction: Effects of reperfusion on left ventricular performance.* Am J Cardiol 48:403, 1981.

34. Malacoff, R, McGovern, B, Ruskin, J, et al: *Ventricular electrical instability in patients treated with streptokinase during acute myocardial infarction.* J Am Coll Cardiol 1 (Part 2):604, 1983.

35. Lee, G, Amsterdam, E, Low, R, et al: *Efficacy of percutaneous transluminal recanalization utilizing streptokinase thrombolysis. Patients with acute myocardial infarction.* Am Heart J 102:1159, 1981.

36. Smalling, RW, Fuentes, F, Freund, GC, et al: *Beneficial effects of intracoronary thrombolysis up to eighteen hours after onset of pain in evolving myoardial infarction.* Am Heart J 104:912, 1982.

37. Feldman, RJ, Crick, LVF, Conti, CR, et al: *Quantitative coronary angiography during intracoronary streptokinase in acute myocardial infarction: How long to continue thrombolytic therapy?* Catheterization & Cardiovasc Diag 9:9, 1983.

38. Timmis, CG, Gangodharan, V, Hauser, AM, et al: *Intracoronary streptokinase in clinical practice.* Am Heart J 104:925, 1982.

39. Heyndricken, GR, Millard, RW, McRitchie, RJ, et al: *Regional myocardial functional and electrophysiologic alterations after brief coronary occlusion in conscious dogs.* J Clin Invest 56:978, 1975.

40. Theroux, P, Ross, JR, Franklin, D, et al: *Coronary arterial reperfusion III. Early and late effects on regional myocardial function and dimensions in conscious dogs.* Am J Cardiol 38:599, 1976.

41. Walton, J Jr, O'Neill, W, Colfer, H, et al: *Failure of intravenous thrombolysis to preserve ventricular function: Report of a randomized clinical trial.* Circulation 66(Suppl II):1336, 1982.

42. Leiboff, RN, Katz, RJ, Wasserman, AG, et al: *A randomized controlled trial of intracoronary streptokinase in acute MI: Preliminary (cautionary) observations.* Circulation 66(Suppl II):1337, 1982.

43. Anderson, JL, Marshall, HW, Bray, BE, et al: *A randomized trial of intracoronary streptokinase in acute myocardial infarction.* Circulation 66(Suppl II):1338, 1982.

44. Serruys, PW, Ribiero, V, Bos, RJ, et al: *Preserved left ventricular function following intracoronary thrombolysis: Report of a randomized trial.* J Am Coll Cardiol 1:591, 1983.

45. Veroni, MS, Tortoledo, FA, Van Reet, RE, et al: *Intracoronary thrombolysis in acute myocardial infarction: Effects on function of myocardium at risk. Preliminary report of a randomized trial.* J Am Coll Cardiol 1:592, 1983.

46. Kennedy, JW, Ritchie, TL, Davis, KB, et al: *The Western Washington Intracoronary Streptokinase in Acute Myocardial Infarction Trial: Analysis of early mortality.* N Engl J Med (in press).

47. Mandelkorn, J, Wolf, NM, Singh, S, et al: *Systemic thrombolytic effect of intracoronary streptokinase.* Circulation 64(Suppl IV):720, 1981.

48. Shröder, R, Biamino, G, Von Leitner, E, et al: *Intravenous short term thrombolysis in acute myocardial infarction.* Circulation 64(Suppl IV):5, 1981.

49. Blunda, M, Wolf, NM, Singh, S, et al: *Intravenous vs intracoronary streptokinase to re-open occluded coronary arteries—preliminary results.* Circulation 66(Suppl II):735, 1982.

50. Spann, S, Sherry, S, Carabello, B, et al: *Rapid coronary reperfusion by high dose, brief intravenous streptokinase in myocardial infarction.* J Am Coll Cardiol 1:629, 1983.

51. Bergman, SR, Keith, AA, Fox, MB, et al: *Coronary thrombolysis achieved with human extrensic plasminogen activator, a clot selective activator, administered intravenously.* J Am Coll Cardiol 1:615, 1983.

52. Holmes, DR Jr, Hartzler, GO, Smith, HC, et al: *Coronary artery thrombosis in patients with unstable angina.* Br Heart J 45:411, 1981.

53. Vetrovec, GW, Cowly, MJ, Overton, H, et al: *Intracoronary thrombus in syndromes of unstable myocardial ischemia.* Am Heart J 102:1202, 1981.

54. Wolf, NM, Mandelkorn, J, LaPorte, S, et al: *Evidence for thrombosis in acute ischemic syndromes other than acute transmural myocardial infarction.* Circulation 64(Suppl IV):744, 1981.

55. Lawrence, JR, Shepherd, JT, Bone, I, et al: *Fibrinolytic therapy in unstable angina pectoris: A controlled clinical trial.* Thromb Res 17:767, 1980.

56. Shapiro, EP, Brinker, JA, Guzman, PA, et al: *Late thrombolysis with intracoronary streptokinase: Therapy for post infarction angina.* J Am Coll Cardiol 1:604, 1983.

Evaluation of Myocardial Function by Invasive Methods

Richard O. Cannon, III, M.D., and
Douglas R. Rosing, M.D.

The cardiac catheterization laboratory offers a unique setting for direct evaluation of cardiac performance. Although angiographic studies of anatomy and intracardiac pressure measurements at rest provide important information describing cardiac function, measurements obtained in the resting state often underestimate the severity of cardiac disease. In fact, because of myocardial adaptation and compensation, the presence of myocardial dysfunction may be missed entirely. This chapter will initially provide a discussion of the determinants of cardiac performance. An overview of invasive measurements of ventricular volume and performance will follow, detailing the contributions of loading conditions and myocardial contractility. Intervention testing, which often allows subtle cardiac abnormalities to be detected, will then be discussed.

CARDIAC PERFORMANCE—PRINCIPLES

Although right ventricular function cannot be ignored, particularly in congenital heart disease, left ventricular function is usually the primary determinant of cardiac performance. An understanding of the factors that influence left ventricular pump function is necessary before hemodynamic adaptations in cardiac disease states can be appreciated. The most easily measured index of cardiac performance, the resting cardiac output, by itself offers little insight relative to cardiac reserve and may be normal in the face of severe cardiac dysfunction. Overall cardiac performance involves four fundamental components: heart rate, preload, afterload, and myocardial contractility. It is the complex interaction among these components that produces the cardiac response to strenuous exercise by the healthy heart and allows some preservation of cardiac performance in a variety of disease states that compromise cardiac function.

Preload refers to sarcomere stretch or myocardial fiber length at the end of diastole. Studies utilizing the isolated muscle preparation[1] demonstrated a relationship between preload and the force generated during contraction (Fig. 1*A*). Within physiologic limits, the greater the muscle is stretched prior to stimulation, the greater the tension that is developed during contraction. Experiments using a heart-lung preparation[2] demonstrated this length-tension relationship between preload, as measured by end-diastolic volume or pressure, and the overall work of the heart, as measured by stroke work or stroke volume (Fig. 1*B*). This classic Frank-Starling relationship demonstrated that, up to certain limits, increases in ventricular filling resulted in improved ventricular performance because of the ability of the stretched cardiac muscle to contract with increased force. Conversely, a decline in preload would result in decreased cardiac performance (reduced stroke volume). Studies also demonstrated that

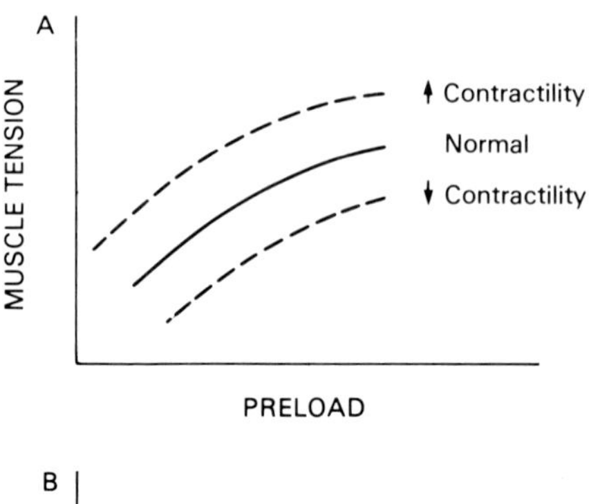

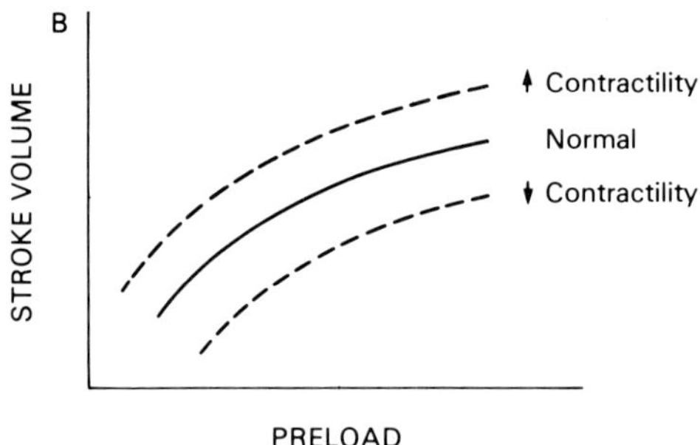

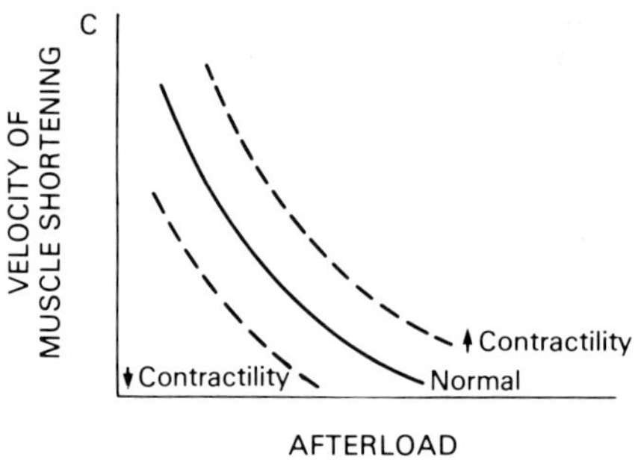

Figure 1. Determinants of left ventricular performance. *A,* This length-tension curve relates the initial stretch of the muscle (preload) to tension developed by stimulated isolated muscle preparation. *B,* This is the Frank-Starling relation—the dependence of overall ventricular performance on filling of the heart. Note that along each curve the relationships are independent of myocardial contractility: Changes in myocardial contractility result in shifts in placement but not in shape of the curves. *C,* The force-velocity curve relates the velocity of muscle shortening of the stimulated muscle to the resistance to contraction encountered by the muscle (afterload).

changes in the contractile state of the myocardium produced a different curve relating preload to stroke volume: Augmented or depressed contractility resulted in increased or reduced work of the heart for any given preload. Thus, a family of ventricular function curves can be constructed for any heart, depending upon the contractile state of the myocardium.[3]

Afterload refers to the resistance against which the myocardium must eject blood during systole and is a function of ventricular systolic pressure, chamber size, shape, and wall thickness (wall stress),* as well as the impedance characteristics of the arterial bed. Isolated muscle preparations demonstrated that increases in afterload, produced by placing weights on a muscle with a fixed preload, reduced the velocity of shortening of muscle (Fig. 1*C*), and that, if afterload became great enough, an isometric contraction resulted. Significant increases in afterload can result in a decline in ventricular performance (Fig. 2), although the healthy heart tolerates a wide range of afterloads with uncompromised performance. However, in the presence of depressed myocardial contractility, mild alterations in afterload can exert a pro-

*According to the Laplace relation: $\sigma = \frac{PR}{2h}$ where σ = wall stress (force/cross-sectional area), P = intraventricular pressure, R = radius of curvature of the wall, and h = wall thickness.

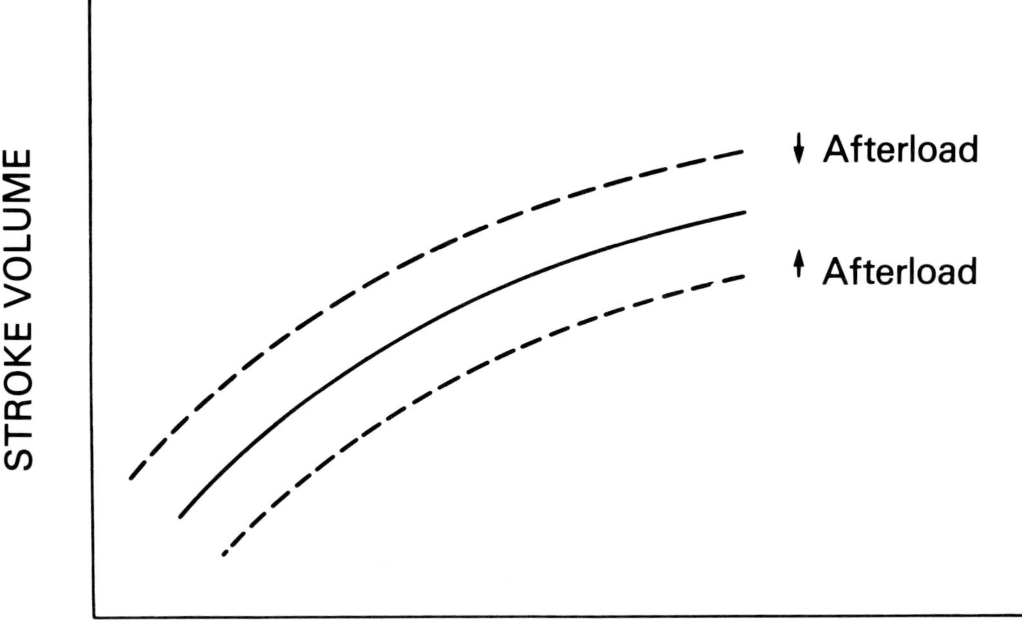

Figure 2. Alteration in ventricular function caused by changes in afterload is particularly important in the setting of depressed contractility, in which even normal afterloads can impair stroke volume. Conversely, decreased afterload (for example, by vasodilator therapy, treatment of hypertension, replacement of a stenotic aortic valve) might result in an upward and leftward shift in the ventricular function curve, with increased stroke volume at any given preload.

found effect on ventricular performance. This observation has served as the impetus for vasodilator therapy to improve cardiac performance in the setting of decreased myocardial contractility.[4]

Heart rate also plays an important role in cardiac performance, as cardiac output is the product of heart rate and stroke volume. With exercise, the normal increase in cardiac output is primarily due to an increase in heart rate, though with strenuous activity the stroke volume increases owing to increased myocardial contractility from sympathetic stimulation and circulating catecholamines. An increase in heart rate alone, as during cardiac pacing, results in a mild increase in myocardial contractility, although this increase does not result in a significant shift in the ventricular function curve.[5,6] At very high heart rates approaching 200 beats per minute, either pacing-induced or as a result of spontaneous supraventricular tachyarrhythmias, the portion of the cardiac cycle devoted to diastole becomes shortened so that ventricular filling is compromised and cardiac output falls.

Numerous attempts have been made to examine myocardial contractility as an independent factor and to quantitate its effect on overall pump performance. However, almost all indices of contractility, such as the maximal rate of change of left ventricular pressure (dp/dt) during isovolumic contraction, ejection fraction, velocity of internal diameter shortening corrected for the end-diastolic diameter (Vcf), and fractional shortening of the ventricular end-diastolic diameter, are influenced by changes in afterload.

More recently, a linear relationship between end-systolic volume and end-systolic pressure (Fig. 3) has been determined in animals as well as in humans by pressure-volume measurements at different afterloads.[7–10] This relationship describes the state of myocardial contrac-

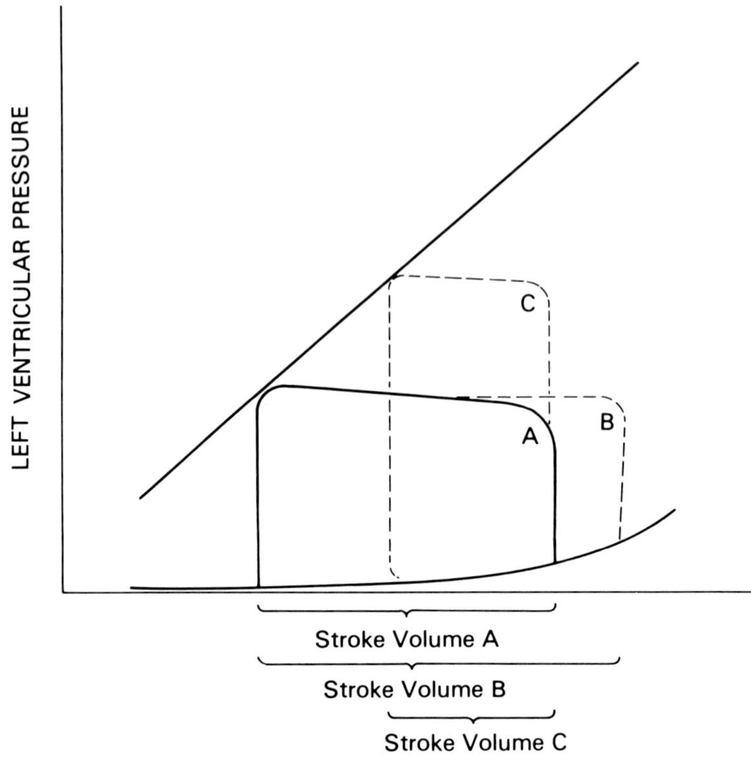

Figure 3. This graph represents pressure-volume relationships in the normal ventricle. The diagonal line represents the end-systolic pressure-volume relationship, and the lower curvilinear line, the relationship for ventricular filling. See Figure 6 for a description of the construction of the pressure-volume curve. Note that the increased preload of beat B relative to A results in a larger stroke volume despite unchanged contractility. Conversely, increased afterload results in reduced stroke volume during beat C relative to beat A.

tility, independent of preload, while incorporating afterload into the analysis. This line defines the limit of ventricular ejection volume, regardless of the initial preload and afterload encountered during systole. In a heart with normal contractility, increases in preload result in increases in stroke volume (Fig. 3B). On the other hand, increases in afterload can result in a reduction of stroke volume (Fig. 3C). Increased myocardial contractility results in an increased stroke volume, and depressed contractility results in a reduction of stroke volume at the same preload, because of shifts in the end-systolic pressure-volume relationship (Fig. 4).

In the previous discussion of ventricular function curves, we indicated that preload could be described as either left ventricular end-diastolic volume or end-diastolic pressure. However, the relationship between end-diastolic pressure and volume is curvilinear (Fig. 5). At low left ventricular end-diastolic pressures, the slope is reduced, and changes in end-diastolic volume are associated with small changes in pressure. At larger end-diastolic volumes, the curve becomes steeper, and small increments in volume are associated with large changes in pressure. Thus, ventricular compliance (dV/dP) declines (that is, the ventricle stiffens) with increased filling, such as volume loading, and increases with volume depletion, such as after nitroglycerin or diuretic administration.[11,12] The end-diastolic pressure–volume relationship is shifted leftward by conditions producing thickening or stiffening of the myocardium (for example, hypertrophy, fibrous scar, amyloid infiltration, or myocardial ischemia). In this set-

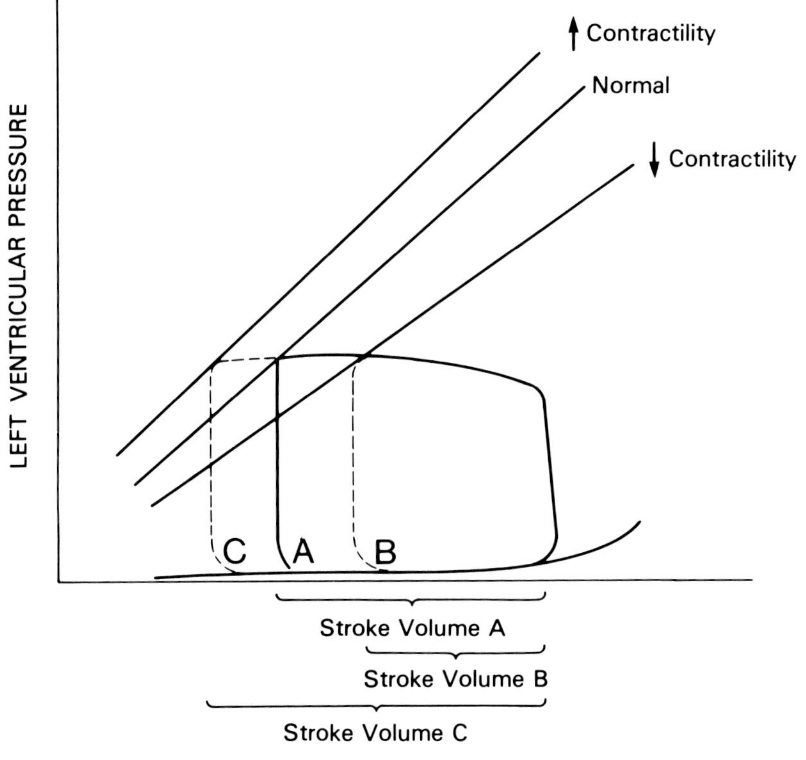

Figure 4. This graph represents changes in the pressure-volume relationship owing to alterations in contractility. Depressed contractility results in a downward and rightward shift of the end-systolic pressure-volume relation and reduced stroke volume of beat B relative to beat A. Conversely, increased contractility results in an upward, leftward shift of the end-systolic pressure-volume relation, and beat C accomplishes a greater stroke volume than beat A. In both beats preload and afterload are unchanged.

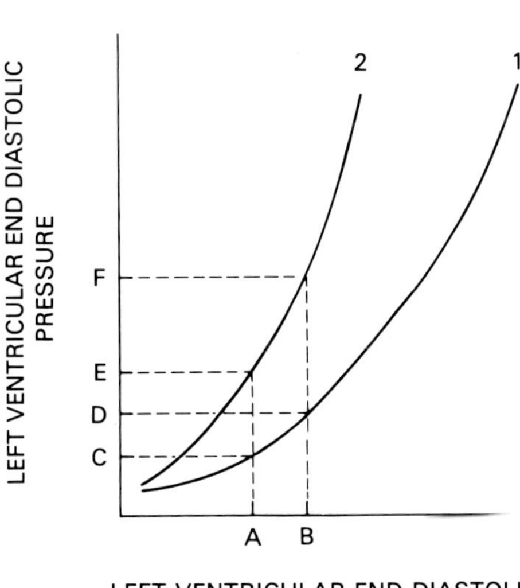

Figure 5. This graph represents ventricular end-diastolic pressure-volume relationship. Curve 1 represents the normal relationship, with increasing steepness of the curve at higher volumes reflecting decreasing compliance (dV/dP). Curve 2 represents a leftward shift in the relationship owing to ventricular stiffening (ischemia, fibrosis, hypertrophy, infiltration). Volume changes (A,B) that ordinarily would result in a minimal pressure elevation (C,D) now result in much greater pressure elevation (E,F).

ting, decreased compliance will be detectable at lower end-diastolic volumes compared with the curve generated by normal hearts. In recent years, increased attention has been focused on the diastolic properties of the ventricle at the initiation of diastole,[13] from closure of the aortic valve to opening of the mitral valve (isovolumic relaxation), and during early diastolic filling of the ventricle.[14]

MEASUREMENT OF VENTRICULAR VOLUME AND EJECTION FRACTION

A detailed derivation and discussion of angiographic methods for measuring ventricular volume and ejection fraction is beyond the scope of this review, and the interested reader is referred to several excellent discussions on the subject.[15–17] Only broad principles and methods will be discussed in this section. Because of the observation that the heart approximates an ellipsoid, Dodge[15] derived a formula for calculating ventricular volumes utilizing measurements from contrast ventriculography. Essentially, the opacified ventricular chamber is traced at end-diastole and end-systole. By measuring the width and length of the tracing, especially in two projections, the volume of the left ventricle in systole and diastole can be calculated. Corrections must be made for x-ray magnification and distortion of the angiographic image. Additionally, a regression equation must be utilized to correct for the small discrepancy between calculated volumes and volumes measured from casts of human left ventricles at autopsy. Stroke volume is determined by subtracting the end-systolic volume from the end-diastolic volume, and ejection fraction is the stroke volume divided by the end-diastolic volume.

Computation of ventricular volumes at multiple points in the cardiac cycle can be plotted against time divisions of the cardiac cycle, which allows construction of volume curves. These volume measurements can also be combined with simultaneously measured left ventricular pressures to construct pressure-volume curves.[18,19] As illustrated (Fig. 6), the pressure-volume curve demonstrates mechanical performance of the ventricle during the cardiac cycle, including isovolumic contraction, systolic ejection, isovolumic relaxation, and diastolic filling. Computer techniques allow rapid determination of angiographic ventricular volumes, although radionuclide techniques are becoming more popular for such measurements,[20,21] because of the ease of data acquisition and the lack of need for the administration of contrast medium, which can alter myocardial contractility as well as loading conditions.

The measurement of left ventricular volumes can also be used to quantitate the amount of valvular regurgitation in patients with aortic or mitral regurgitation. Normally, in the presence of competent valves, the forward stroke volume measured by Fick or indocyanine green dye indicator dilution methods equals the stroke volume determined by angiographic measurement. In patients with valvular regurgitation, however, the total stroke volume as mea-

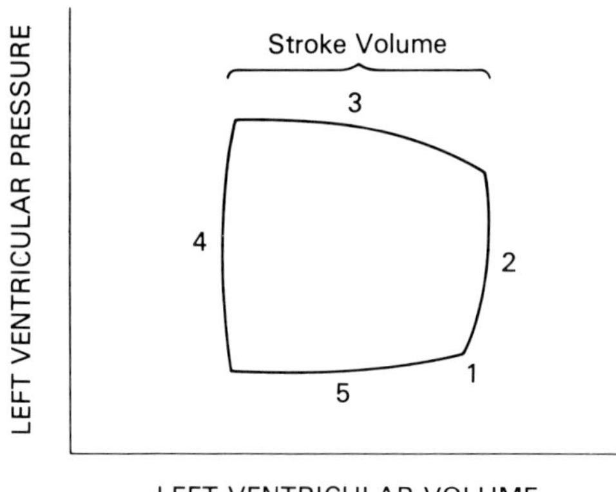

Figure 6. Simultaneous measurements of left ventricular pressure and volume allow construction of a pressure-volume diagram. The cardiac cycle begins at end-diastole (1), continuing through ventricular isovolumic contraction (2), opening of the aortic valve and systolic ejection (3), isovolumic relaxation (4), and diastolic filling of the ventricle (5) for relationship of loop to cardiac cycle.

sured by angiography equals the forward stroke volume, measured by Fick or dilution-techniques, plus the regurgitant volume. Subtraction of the forward stroke volume from the angiographic stroke volume equals the regurgitant stroke volume. The regurgitant stroke volume divided by the angiographic stroke volume gives the regurgitant fraction. In chronic aortic regurgitation, the ventricle dilates as a consequence of the volume overload, and the total ventricular stroke volume may be four to five times normal (up to 300 ml), resulting in flows across the aortic valve of up to 30 liters per minute at rest. Although the end-diastolic volume is increased proportionally to the regurgitant volume, the end-systolic volume is also increased so that the rest ejection fraction may remain normal. In mitral regurgitation the left ventricle also enlarges to accommodate the large diastolic volume, and the left atrium dilates to accommodate the large regurgitant volume.

Left ventricular mass can be estimated angiographically[22] by determining the average wall thickness between the contrast-filled chamber and the cardiac silhouette, adding this measurement to the end-diastolic dimension, and calculating a total cardiac volume. Subtraction of the chamber volume yields an estimate of myocardial volume, which relates to the myocardial mass when multiplied by the specific gravity of muscle. Although this method has been validated by comparison with postmortem studies, errors occur when hypertrophy is eccentric or nonuniform, or when pericardial disease is present.

MEASUREMENTS OF CARDIAC PERFORMANCE

Accurate measurements of left ventricular pressure using high-fidelity micromanometer-tipped catheters and of left ventricular volume using angiographic or radionuclide techniques have resulted in insights as to how myocardial contractility relates to ventricular pump performance and how changes in loading conditions (preload and afterload) affect both. In spite of the intuitive assumption that myocardial muscle and pump function parallel one another, disparities frequently occur owing to the influence of loading conditions.[23] For example, sudden mechanical overload, as may occur with the volume overload produced by acute aortic or mitral regurgitation or the pressure overload of severe hypertension, can result in markedly reduced pump performance without significant impairment of myocardial contractility. Valve replacement or treatment of the hypertension would be expected to result in the restoration of normal myocardial function. Conversely, severe impairment of myocardial contractility can be masked in chronic mitral regurgitation because of left ventricular systolic emptying into a low impedance left atrium. Thus, when mitral valve replacement removes the relatively low pressure vent, myocardial dysfunction becomes evident.

Keeping in mind these considerations and the concepts reviewed previously, altered cardiac function in a variety of disease states can be better evaluated. Ross[24] has introduced the term "afterload mismatch with limited preload reserve" to explain how the sudden imposition of increased afterload, such as the development of acute aortic or mitral valvular regurgitation, can result in pump failure despite normal myocardial contractility. Even at high end-diastolic pressures, there appears to be a limit to the amount of sarcomere lengthening that can occur (approximately 2.3 microns), and thus further increases in preload are limited.[25,26] Any further loading of the heart by volume or pressure results in increased wall stress and reduced wall shortening during systole, and thus a decline in stroke volume—even with normal myocardial contractility. As a result, increased loading results in an apparent "descending limb" of the Frank-Starling ventricular function curve, not because of sarcomere "overstretch" but because of excessive afterload.[23,27] As mentioned previously, valve replacement would usually result in a restoration of normal cardiac performance if the abnormal loading has been short-lived. Chronic mechanical overload caused by valvular heart disease or left-to-right shunting produces adaptations such as chamber dilatation with an increase in preload and thus augmented stroke volume, as well as wall hypertrophy to normalize the increased wall stress and to reduce afterload. Cardiac performance in the basal state may thus remain normal. As myocardial contractility deteriorates with time, even normal afterloads are matched with reduced stroke volume. In chronic aortic regurgitation, valve replacement generally results in more favorable loading conditions with improvement in pump performance, especially during exercise.[28] In chronic mitral regurgitation, however, systolic emptying into a relatively low pressure left atrium results in a favorable afterload situation, allowing a large stroke volume despite depressed contractility. Replacement of the mitral valve results in an increase in afterload and reduction in pump performance,[29] although at lower filling pressures with less likelihood of pulmonary congestion.

"Afterload mismatch" can occur with normal afterload in patients with myocardial failure caused by ischemic heart disease, long-standing valvular heart disease, or dilated cardiomyopathy. In the presence of depressed contractility, stroke volume is highly sensitive to changes in afterload (Fig. 7). It is in the situation of such an "afterload mismatch" that vasodilator therapy results in an improvement in cardiac pump function via a reduction of afterload, despite unaltered myocardial contractility.

Up to this point, attention has been directed primarily toward the influence of afterload and contractility on cardiac performance at the upper limits of preload. However, reduction of preload owing to impaired cardiac filling can reduce cardiac performance as well. Chronic constrictive pericarditis, acute cardiac tamponade, and restrictive cardiomyopathies limit preload and result in a reduced stroke volume despite producing an elevation of filling pressures.

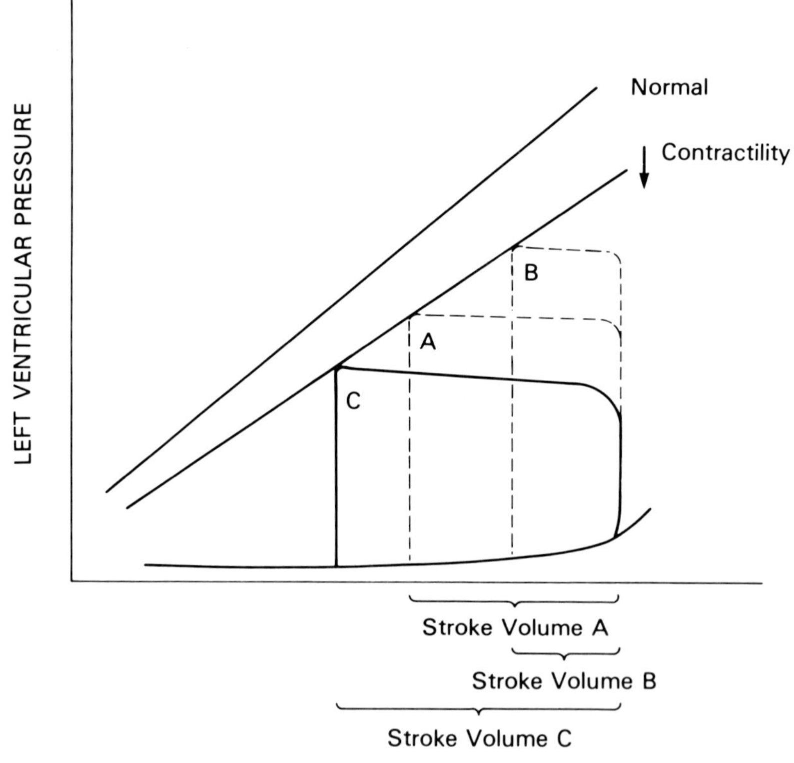

Figure 7. Pressure-volume relationships in myocardial failure are represented in this graph. Even small increases in afterload result in a decrease in stroke volume (beat B relative to beat A), as preload is nearly maximal and further cardiac dilatation impossible. Conversely, a diminished afterload (for example, vasodilator therapy) results in an increase in stroke volume (beat C relative to beat A).

Such a situation occurs even in the face of normal myocardial contractility. Mitral stenosis has a similar effect on cardiac performance in the absence of elevated left ventricular filling pressures. In addition, if preload is reduced by vigorous diuresis or excessive use of vasodilator agents that results in venous pooling of blood, stroke volume may be compromised by reducing end-diastolic volume.

EXERCISE DURING CARDIAC CATHETERIZATION

From the preceding discussion, it is apparent that many patients with significant cardiac disease may have normal resting cardiac performance because of favorable loading conditions despite depressed myocardial contractility. Although complicated analyses of information obtained with the use of micromanometer-tipped catheters and angiographic or radionuclide techniques may identify such situations, the evaluation of cardiac performance in response to stress is a more practical way for most laboratories to detect abnormalities of cardiac function.[30]

During dynamic exercise the increased oxygen demands of working skeletal muscle are met by an increase in cardiac output, primarily owing to an increase in heart rate, and an increase in oxygen extraction from arterial blood. Arterial pressure increases despite a decrease in peripheral vascular resistance, owing to the increase in cardiac output. In individuals with normal or nearly normal pulmonary function and no right-to-left shunting, arterial oxygen saturation remains constant during exercise. Measurement of mixed venous oxygen saturation in the pulmonary artery shows a decline, reflecting an increased arteriovenous oxygen difference owing to increased oxygen consumption. Increased sympathetic nervous system activity, circulating catecholamines, and, to a lesser degree, tachycardia per se result in enhanced myocardial contractility. Preload, as measured by left ventricular end-diastolic volume or pressure, ordinarily remains unchanged or actually declines during vigorous exercise, because of enhanced myocardial contractility and increased stroke volume.

Hemodynamic testing during exercise can be useful in detecting abnormal cardiac performance in patients with heart disease who exhibit normal rest hemodynamics. Epstein and coworkers[31] used upright treadmill exercise in normal volunteers and a group of patients with a variety of cardiac diseases to evaluate cardiac performance. Measurements of total body oxygen consumption, arteriovenous oxygen difference by measurement of mixed venous oxygen saturation in the pulmonary artery and arterial blood oxygen saturation, and cardiac output were made at rest and during strenuous activity. At levels of activity associated with a fall in pulmonary artery oxygen saturation to less than 30 percent (that is, strenuous exercise with significantly increased oxygen consumption), all normal subjects were capable of achieving a cardiac index greater than 7.0 liters per minute per m^2, whereas no patient with cardiac disease achieved a cardiac index of greater than 4.8 liters per minute per m^2 at the same pulmonary artery oxygen saturation. Exercise that was terminated with a pulmonary arterial oxygen saturation greater than 30 percent generally represented noncardiac limitation to exercise (for example, poor conditioning, lack of motivation, "tack in the shoe"). Thus, cardiac performance during exercise can be evaluated and used in assessing the severity of cardiac disease, timing of surgery, and response to therapy.

Measurements of left ventricular end-diastolic pressure and cardiac output during dynamic exercise can also provide an estimate of cardiac performance by allowing construction of ventricular function curves[32] (Fig. 8). The normal response to exercise, as mentioned previously, is an increase in cardiac output with a slight decline in left ventricular end-diastolic pressure (see Fig. 8*A–B*). Patients with limited cardiac reserve rely on the Frank-Starling relation, and thus require an augmented preload to increase cardiac output (A–C). In patients with more advanced heart disease, even an increase in preload cannot augment stroke volume, and cardiac output remains unchanged or actually falls, reflecting depressed myocardial contractility (A–D).

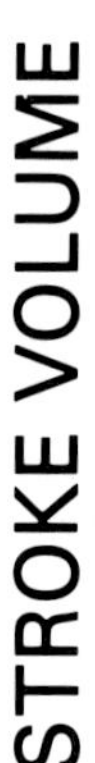

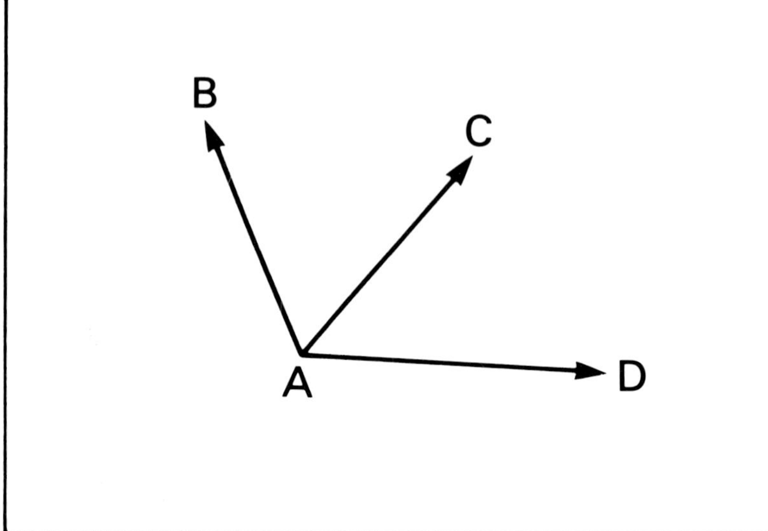

Figure 8. This graph represents a modified ventricular function relationship obtained by measurement of stroke volume and left ventricular end-diastolic pressure (LVEDP) at rest (A) and during exercise. Normally, exercise results in increased stroke volume at a lower preload because of enhanced myocardial contractility (B). With mild myocardial impairment and limited contractile reserve, exercise may necessitate an increase in preload to augment ventricular performance (Frank-Starling relation—C). With myocardial failure, not even increases in preload can augment ventricular performance (D) and may result in an actual decline in stroke volume.

Because dynamic exercise during cardiac catheterization may be impractical, isometric exercise has been utilized employing a handgrip dynamometer. Normally, 3 to 4 minutes of sustained handgrip of approximately one-third maximum grip capacity results in increases in arterial pressure, heart rate, and cardiac output, albeit to lesser degrees than dynamic exercise. Left ventricular function can be evaluated with the measurement of left ventricular end-diastolic pressure and cardiac output, as previously described for dynamic exercise. Care must be taken that the patient does not perform a Valsalva maneuver during handgrip, for this can result in a decrease in preload owing to impaired venous return and can cause a decline in cardiac output even in normal subjects.

ATRIAL PACING DURING CARDIAC CATHETERIZATION

The application of atrial pacing to stress the heart has also been used to study left ventricular function in patients with coronary artery disease.[33] Although increasing heart rate by pacing does increase myocardial oxygen consumption, the increase in myocardial oxygen demand is not as great as with identical heart rates achieved during exercise. However, the evaluation of cardiac performance during pacing allows examination of function without concomitant changes occurring in cardiac output, afterload, and circulating catecholamines. Pacing can be performed with a unipolar or bipolar pacing electrode, with the right atrial appendage or coronary sinus being stable locations. At paced heart rates of approximately 130 to 150 bpm, many cardiac patients as well as normal subjects will develop atrioventricular conduction delays, usually Wenckebach phenomenon, with increasing incidence of heart block at higher heart rates. Similar heart rates during exercise are generally not associated with

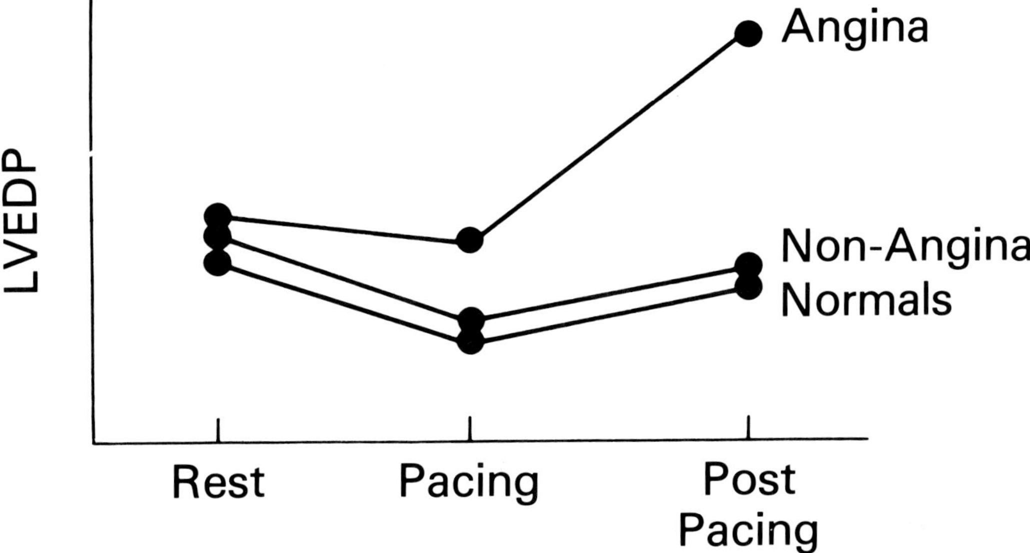

Figure 9. In normal subjects and patients with coronary artery disease not experiencing angina with pacing, the left ventricular end-diastolic pressure (LVEDP) falls during pacing and immediately returns to rest levels post-pacing. In contrast, patients with coronary artery disease experiencing angina during pacing have a higher post-pacing LVEDP.

Wenckebach block because of facilitation of atrioventricular conduction by circulating catecholamines.

Total body oxygen consumption, cardiac output, and blood pressure remain unchanged during pacing. The increase in heart rate causes relative reduction of the diastolic portion of the cardiac cycle and thus decreases diastolic time. As a result, the preload falls and stroke volume declines while the ejection fraction remains essentially unchanged in normal subjects. During pacing at heart rates of greater than 120 to 130 bpm, assessment of preload changes by measuring left ventricular end-diastolic pressure is difficult because of catheter artifact in diastole. Immediately post-pacing, however, left ventricular end-diastolic pressure returns to normal in normal subjects. In patients with coronary artery disease who are paced to angina, the left ventricular end-diastolic pressure (LVEDP) does not fall. Immediately after termi-

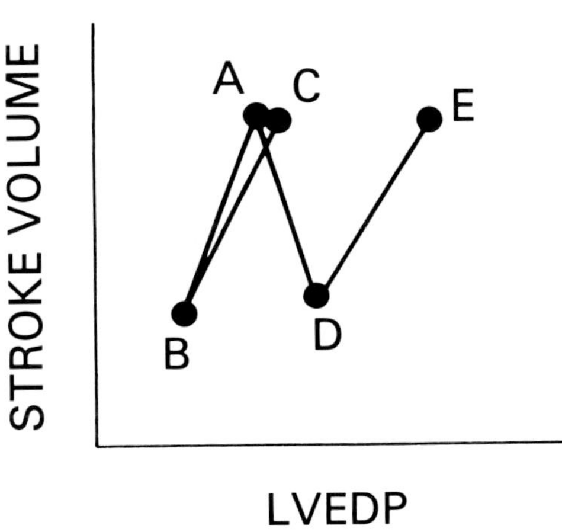

Figure 10. This graph represents the modified ventricular function curve during atrial pacing. In normal, healthy subjects and in patients with coronary artery disease not experiencing chest pain, atrial pacing results in a fall in stroke volume and preload (B), with return to rest values (A) immediately post-pacing (C). Conversely, patients with coronary artery disease experiencing chest pain during atrial pacing demonstrate no decrease in preload as stroke volume drops (D) and post-pacing returns to a higher preload (E), indicating a downward, rightward shift in ventricular function owing to myocardial ischemia.

nation of pacing, the end-diastolic pressure is still elevated above baseline leads, reflecting decreased compliance of the ischemic myocardium with a higher pressure for a given filling volume (Fig. 9). An increase in LVEDP of ≥5 mm Hg from rest to post-pacing or an absolute value ≥17 mm Hg after pacing is suggestive of ischemia, provided the blood pressure and heart rate are similar during the two periods.[33] These changes in preload and stroke volume allow construction of ventricular function curves, analogous to those obtained with exercise, relating left ventricular stroke volume to end-diastolic pressure[34] (Fig. 10).

PHARMACOLOGIC INTERVENTION FOR ASSESSMENT OF VENTRICULAR FUNCTION

As discussed earlier, depressed myocardial contractility, even if not apparent clinically, can be brought out by changes in afterload. Infusion of a pressor agent such as angiotensin will have little effect on performance of the normal heart—stroke volume generally remains unchanged. In the presence of contractile dysfunction, the increased afterload will result in a fall in stroke volume.[35] Cardiac performance can also be assessed during reduction of afterload by nitroprusside, hydralazine, and other agents which, in the presence of depressed contractile function,[4] should increase stroke volume and cardiac output, generally without an increase in heart rate. Diuresis may have a variable effect; a decline in preload may result in decreased cardiac size and thus a decreased wall stress. On the other hand, a drop in preload may result in a fall in stroke volume if the heart is operating on a steep portion of the ventricular function curve (see Fig. 1*B*). A modest fall in filling pressures may be necessary to relieve pulmonary congestion, however, resulting in improved systemic and cardiac oxygen delivery.

SUMMARY

The evaluation of myocardial performance requires an understanding of the contributions of loading conditions (preload and afterload), heart rate, and contractility. Although the measurement of these parameters often requires specialized techniques, more easily performed invasive evaluation can take place applying the principles derived from an understanding of the factors affecting cardiac performance. The construction of ventricular function curves permits the evaluation of the influence of preload on the work of the heart. Changes in afterload and/or myocardial contractility can produce a series of such function curves. Construction of pressure-volume loops and the examination of end-systolic pressure-volume relationships offer insights into the status of myocardial contractility apart from loading conditions, as well as into the response of the heart to acute and chronic alteration in loading conditions. Ventricular function curves can be obtained during exercise, pacing, and pharmacologic intervention in order to detect subtle cardiac dysfunction, to assess the severity of dysfunction, and to gauge the response to therapy.

REFERENCES

1. Abbott, BC and Mommaerts, WFHM: *A study of inotropic mechanisms in the papillary muscle preparation.* J Gen Physiol 42:533, 1959.
2. Frank, O: *On the dynamics of cardiac muscle.* Am Heart J 58:282, 467, 1959.
3. Sarnoff, SJ: *Myocardial contractility as described by ventricular function curves; observations on Starling's law of the heart.* Physiol Rev 35:107, 1955.
4. Chatterjee, K and Parmley, WW: *The role of vasodilator therapy in heart failure.* Prog Cardiovasc Dis 19:301, 1977.

5. MITCHELL, JH, WALLACE, AG, AND SKINNER, NS: *Intrinsic effect of heart rate on left ventricular performance.* Am J Physiol 205:41, 1963.
6. HIGGINS, CB, VATNER, SF, FRANKLIN, D, ET AL: *Extent of regulation of the heart's contractile state in the conscious dog by alteration in the frequency of contraction.* J Clin Invest 52:1187, 1973.
7. SUGA, H, SAGAWA, K, AND SHOUKAS, AA: *Load independence of the instantaneous pressure-volume ratio of the canine left ventricle and effects of epinephrine and heart rate on the ratio.* Circ Res 32:314, 1973.
8. MAHLER, F, COVELL, JW, AND ROSS, J: *Systolic pressure-diameter relations in the normal conscious dog.* Cardiovasc Res 9:447, 1975.
9. GROSSMAN, W, BRAUNWALD, E, MANN, T, ET AL: *Contractile state of the left ventricle in man as evaluated from end-systolic pressure-volume relationships.* Circulation 56:845, 1977.
10. MEHMEL, HE, STOCKINS, B, RUFFMANN, K, ET AL: *The linearity of the end-systolic pressure-volume relationship in man and its sensitivity for assessment of left ventricular function.* Circulation 63:1216, 1981.
11. GROSSMAN, W AND MCLAURIN, LP: *Diastolic properties of the left ventricle.* Ann Intern Med 84:316, 1976.
12. GAASCH, WH, LEVINE, HJ, QUINONES, MA, ET AL: *Left ventricular compliance: Mechanisms and clinical implications.* Am J Cardiol 38:645, 1976.
13. WEISS, JL, FREDERICKSEN, JW, AND WEISFELDT, ML: *Hemodynamic determinants of the time-course of fall in canine left ventricular pressure.* J Clin Invest 58:751, 1976.
14. BONOW, RO, BACHARACH, SL, GREEN, MV, ET AL: *Impaired left ventricular diastolic filling in patients with coronary artery disease.* Circulation 64:315, 1981.
15. DODGE, HT, SANDLER, H, BALLEW, DW, ET AL: *The use of biplane angiocardiography for the measurement of left ventricular volume in man.* Am Heart J 60:762, 1960.
16. RACKLEY, CE, HOOD, WP, AND GROSSMAN, W: *Measurement of ventricular volume, mass and ejection fraction.* In GROSSMAN, W (ED): *Cardiac Catheterization and Angiography.* Lea and Febiger, Philadelphia, 1980, p 232.
17. DODGE, HT AND SHEEHAN, FH: *Quantitative contrast angiography for assessment of ventricular performance in heart disease.* J Am Coll Cardiol 1:73, 1983.
18. BUNNELL, IL, GRANT, C, AND GREENE, DC: *Left ventricular function derived from the pressure-volume diagrams.* Am J Med 39:881, 1965.
19. DODGE, HT, SANDLER, H, BARTLEY, WA, ET AL: *Usefulness and limitation of radiographic methods for determining left ventricular volume.* Am J Cardiol 18:10, 1956.
20. DEHMER, GJ, LEWIS, SE, HILLIS, LD, ET AL: *Exercise-induced alterations in left ventricular volumes and pressure-volume relationship: A sensitive indicator of left ventricular dysfunction in patients with coronary artery disease.* Circulation 63:1008, 1981.
21. MAGORIEN, DJ, SHAFFER, P, BUSH, CA, ET AL: *Assessment of left ventricular pressure-volume relations using gated radionuclide angiography, echocardiography, and micromanometer pressure recordings.* Circulation 67:844, 1983.
22. RACKLEY, CE, DODGE, HT, COBE, TD, ET AL: *A method for determining left ventricular mass in man.* Circulation 29:266, 1964.
23. ROSS, J *Cardiac function and myocardial contractility: A perspective.* J Am Coll Cardiol 1:52, 1983.
24. ROSS, J: *Afterload mismatch and preload reserve: A conceptual framework for the analysis of ventricular function.* Prog Cardiovasc Dis 18:255, 1976.
25. MONROE, RG, GAMBLE, WJ, LAFARGE, CG, ET AL: *Left ventricular performance at high end-diastolic pressures in isolated, perfused dog hearts.* Circ Res 26:85, 1970.
26. ROSS, J, SONNENBLICK, EH, TAYLOR, RR, ET AL: *Diastolic geometry and sarcomere lengths in the chronically dilated canine left ventricle.* Circ Res 28:49, 1971.
27. MACGREGOR, DC, COVELL, JW, MAHLER, F, ET AL: *Relations between afterload, stroke volume, and descending limb of Starling's curve.* Am J Physiol 227:884, 1974.
28. BONOW, RO, ROSING, DR, KENT, KM, ET AL: *Timing of operation for chronic aortic regurgitation.* Am J Cardiol 50:325, 1982.
29. SCHULER, G, PETERSON, K, JOHNSON, A, ET AL: *Temporal response of left ventricular performance to mitral valve surgery.* Circulation 59:1218, 1979.
30. GROSSMAN, W AND MCLAURIN, LP: *Dynamic and isometric exercise during cardiac catheterization.* In GROSSMAN, W (ED): *Cardiac Catheterization and Angiography.* Lea and Febiger, Philadelphia, 1980, p 215.
31. EPSTEIN, SE, BEISER, GD, STAMPFER, M, ET AL: *Characterization of the circulatory response to maximal upright exercise in normal subjects and patients with heart disease.* Circulation 35:1049, 1967.
32. ROSS, J, GAULT, JH, MASON, DT, ET AL: *Left ventricular performance during muscular exercise in patients with and without cardiac dysfunction.* Circulation 34:597, 1966.

33. PARKER, JO: *Atrial pacing: Pacing ventricular function curves.* In GROSSMAN, W (ED): *Cardiac Catheterization and Angiography.* Lea and Febiger, Philadelphia, 1980, p 223.

34. PARKER, JO, KHAJA, F, AND CASE, RB: *Analysis of left ventricular function by atrial pacing.* Circulation 43:241, 1971.

35. ROSS, J AND BRAUNWALD, E: *The study of left ventricular function in man by increasing resistance to ventricular ejection fraction with angiotensin.* Circulation 29:739, 1964.

Endomyocardial Biopsy

Jeffrey A. Laser, M.D., Robert E. Fowles, M.D., and Jay W. Mason, M.D.

Since its introduction in the early 1960s the technique of transvascular endomyocardial biopsy has become a safe diagnostic tool commonly used throughout the world. Percutaneous needle biopsy and open thoracotomy to obtain heart tissue have been largely abandoned owing to high complication rates and the risks and inconvenience associated with surgery. Presently endomyocardial biopsy is useful in the evaluation of a number of problems, including cardiac allograft rejection, myocarditis, anthracycline-induced cardiotoxicity, and infiltrative cardiomyopathies. In addition, this procedure is used as a research tool to elucidate myocyte-drug interactions and biochemical, enzymatic, and immunologic abnormalities associated with numerous cardiac diseases.

The purpose of this chapter is to review the history and to describe the techniques of endomyocardial biopsy and to discuss how it is used in cardiology nowadays.

HISTORY

Microscopic examination of solid organ biopsy specimens has been clinically possible since Silverman first described his biopsy needle technique in 1938.[1] Percutaneous biopsy of the heart was performed in dogs in 1953 by Casten.[2] Human heart biopsies were initially obtained by Sutton in 1956 through a limited thoracotomy using a Vim-Silverman biopsy needle.[3] A number of percutaneous needle biopsy techniques were described during the 1960s and 1970s, all of which failed to gain widespread popularity because of unacceptably high incidences of pneumothorax and cardiac tamponade.[4–8]

The major breakthrough in endomyocardial biopsy technology came in 1962 when Sakakibara and Konno[9] described their transvascular approach using a biopsy catheter called a bioptome. In 1972, Caves and associates[10] modified this bioptome in order to optimize its use for percutaneous, transvenous approach to the right ventricular septum through the internal jugular vein. Richardson[11] and Brooksby and his associates[12,13] in 1974 reported the use of the King's College bioptome, which is a modified Olympus bronchoscope biopsy forceps capable of right and left ventricular biopsies. Mason and associates[14,15] have further modified the bioptome developed by Caves for improved and broadened use in biventricular endomyocardial biopsies. Kawai and Kitaura[16] have designed a biopsy catheter with a steerable tip to facilitate entry into the left ventricle and to direct it at specific biopsy sites. Children have been safely biopsied using a smaller bioptome.[17] Nowadays the bioptome developed at Stanford University is most frequently used in North America, whereas the King's College bioptome is used primarily in the United Kingdom and Europe and the Konno bioptome in Europe, Japan, and elsewhere.

ENDOMYOCARDIAL BIOPSY TECHNIQUES

Konno Method

The Konno bioptome, first described in 1962,[9] is usually inserted by cutdown technique in the basilic or saphenous veins or brachial artery. Percutaneous insertion through a sheath is difficult because of the large width of the biopsy head.[11,18] The bioptome jaws consist of two cups that open via a double-swivel mechanism. A drive wire operated by a thumb ring in the handle pushes the jaws open and pulls them closed. The catheter shaft consists of stainless steel covered with Teflon. The bioptome is 100 cm in length, with two available sizes for the outer jaw diameter (2.5 and 3.5 mm). Biopsy specimens are often 3 to 4 mm in diameter. There are some limitations found by investigators using the Konno bioptome. The catheter shaft is rigid, with limited intravascular maneuverability which can prevent successful entry into the ventricles. Some investigators have reported difficulties properly operating the drive wire mechanism.[11,14,15,18]

King's Method

The King's bioptome, which is similar to the Konno instrument, was first described by Richardson in 1974.[11] The bioptome can be inserted percutaneously through an 8 French, long sheath into veins and arteries. The instrument is a modified Olympus fiberoptic bronchoscope biopsy forceps made of stainless steel. An inner drive wire connects a ring in the handle to the jaws. A spring maintains tension, holding the jaws closed until the ring is pushed in, which opens the jaws in a scissor action. The shaft is 105 cm long with a diameter of 2 mm and is made of a flexible, coiled stainless steel covered with Teflon.

The diameter of the jaws is 1.8 mm, which yields the smallest biopsy specimens. The increased shaft flexibility and length has led to a higher rate of successful biopsies than the Konno bioptome. The smaller catheter tip has made vessel insertion easier. The King's bioptome is also subject to breakdown of the drive wire mechanism.

Stanford Method

The Stanford bioptome, which is a modification of the Konno bioptome, was first described by Caves and associates[10] in 1973. It has undergone subsequent modification by Scholten (Mason and associates[14,15,18]) (Fig. 1).

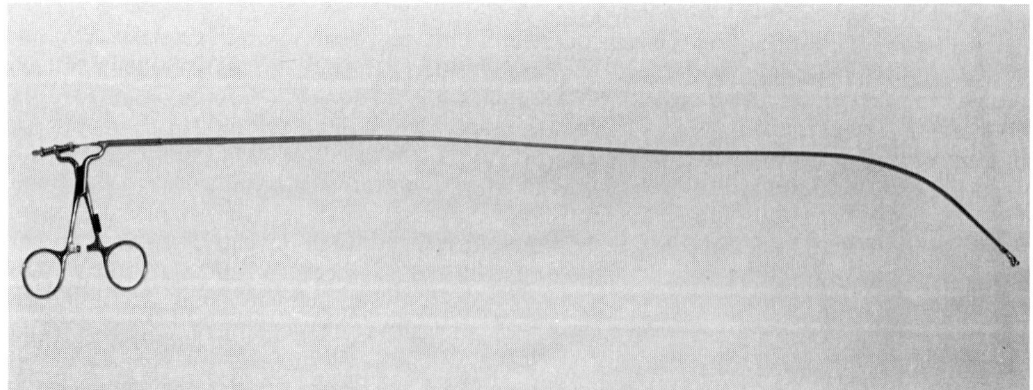

Figure 1. This is the bioptome presently used at Stanford for right ventricular biopsies.

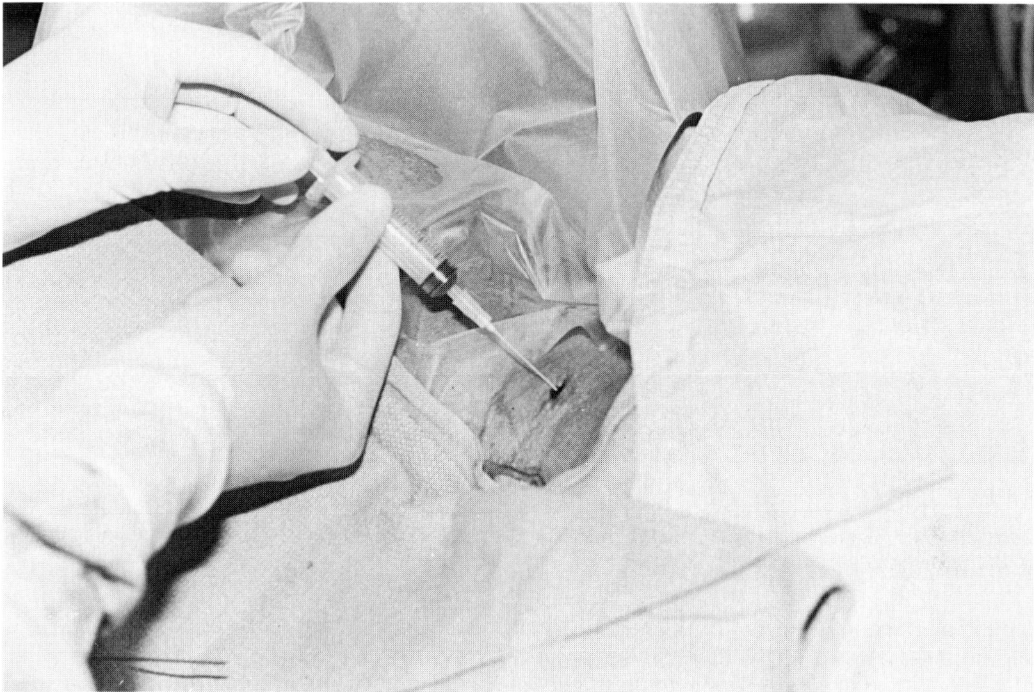

Figure 2. This is the 22-gauge seeker needle being placed in the right internal jugular vein. The patient's head is behind the plastic drape to the left of the picture. The seeker needle is pointed toward the right breast, angled posteriorly.

The bioptome, designed specifically for right ventricular septal biopsy, is inserted through a 9 French sheath via percutaneous puncture into the right internal jugular vein. The following procedure is used in cannulation of the right internal jugular vein: The patient's head is turned to the left as far as possible. The sternal (medial) and clavicular (lateral) bellies of the sternocleidomastoid muscle are identified by having the patient tense this muscle by lifting the head. The insertion site is located between these two muscle bellies 3 to 4 cm above the superior border of the clavicle. A small amount of local anesthetic is injected into the skin and subcutaneous tissue followed by a 1 cm horizontal incision with a no. 11 blade. The skin is then bluntly separated with a small hemostat. The vein is first entered using a 1.5 inch, 22 gauge "seeker" needle attached to a 5 ml syringe. The needle is angled 60° posteriorly from the horizontal plane and 30° laterally toward the right breast (Fig. 2). The needle is slowly advanced while continuously aspirating from the syringe. The vein is usually found 1 to 3 cm deep to the skin. The seeker needle is left in the vein to act as a guide for a 3 inch, 18 gauge, thin wall needle that is advanced in the same manner alongside the 22 gauge needle. If the vein is not located with the 22 gauge seeker needle, it should be redirected first laterally and then medially. If the carotid artery is entered, pressure should be applied to the area for a few minutes before continuing. Maneuvers that dilate the internal jugular vein often facilitate its cannulation. The patient can be put in the Trendelenburg position and can be asked to perform a Valsalva maneuver during insertion of the needles. Figure 3 demonstrates how the Valsalva maneuver can dilate the internal jugular vein. Once the 18 gauge needle is in the vein with blood easily aspirated into the syringe, a 0.035 inch, 40 cm guide wire is inserted through the needle into the right atrium and both needles are removed. A 9 French sheath and dilator are advanced over the wire into the vein, the dilator is removed, and a catheter

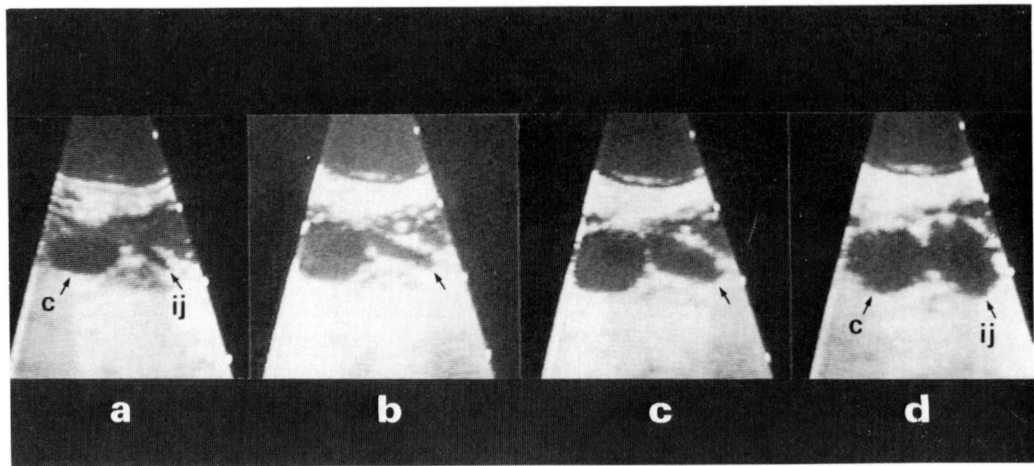

Figure 3. *a,* This is an ultrasound sector scan of the right carotid artery (c) and the internal jugular vein (ij) taken 3 cm above the clavicle in a reclining patient at rest. *b,* Patient begins to perform a Valsalva maneuver. Note the internal jugular vein beginning to dilate. *c,* Three seconds after the Valsalva maneuver began. *d,* Maximum dilation of the internal jugular vein (ij) 6 seconds after the Valsalva maneuver.

plug is inserted into the end of the sheath when it is not being used (Fig. 4). In order to avoid aspiration of air into the vein, a rubber diaphragm is attached to the end of the sheath. This diaphragm is made by cutting off two fingers of a sterile glove and placing them over the end of the sheath, one on top of the other. The fingers are secured to the hub of the sheath with chromic suture, and a hole is made in the diaphragm with an 18 gauge needle.

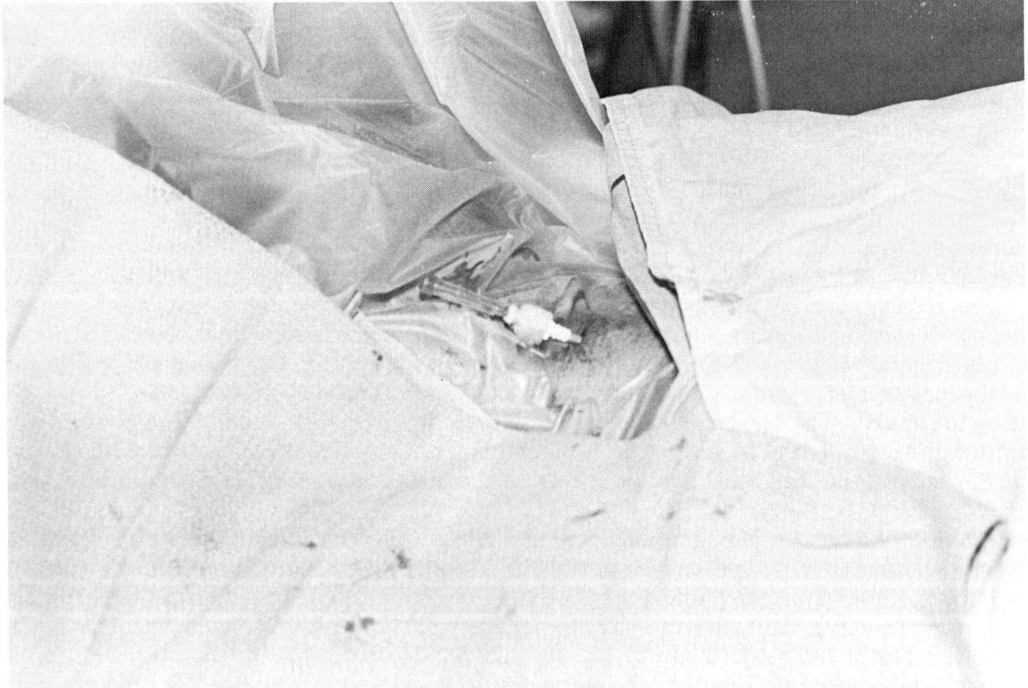

Figure 4. Shown is a 9 French sheath with rubber diaphragm in place in the internal jugular vein.

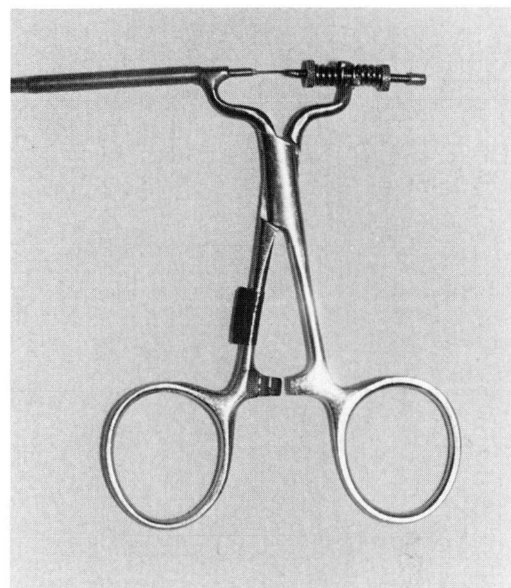

Figure 5. The handle of the Stanford bioptome is a modified mosquito hemostat.

The shaft of the bioptome is made of relatively stiff coiled stainless steel covered with non-thrombogenic plastic and has a 45° bend near the tip. This curve in the shaft is in the same plane as the handle, so that the orientation of the jaws is always known. The handle is a modified mosquito hemostat connected to the jaws by a drive wire running through the core of the shaft (Fig. 5). The shaft is 50 cm long and has a diameter slightly less than 9 French. The jaws consist of two hollow cups joined with a single hinge, so one cup is fixed while the other opens (Fig. 6). The jaws have an internal diameter of 2.5 mm and obtain an average sample size of 2.5 by 3 mm. The cutting force of the jaws can be varied through an adjustable spring mechanism at the handle (Fig. 7). The spring-buffered, variable force applied to the cutting jaws has increased the longevity of this bioptome. The feature of a relatively stiff, short shaft with an adjustable bend in conjunction with the nearly direct entry into the right ventricle from the jugular vein has greatly increased the efficiency and safety of this technique. The catheter tip can be easily and accurately positioned against the right ventricular

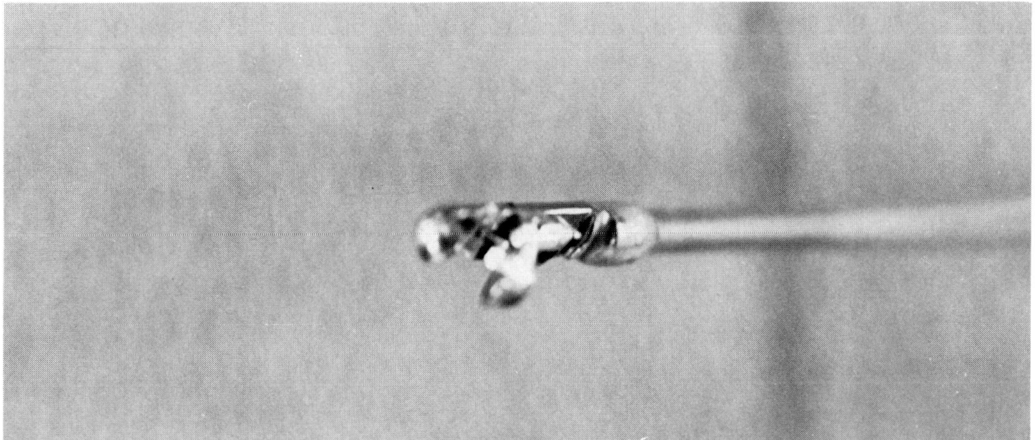

Figure 6. These are the single-hinged jaws of the Stanford bioptome.

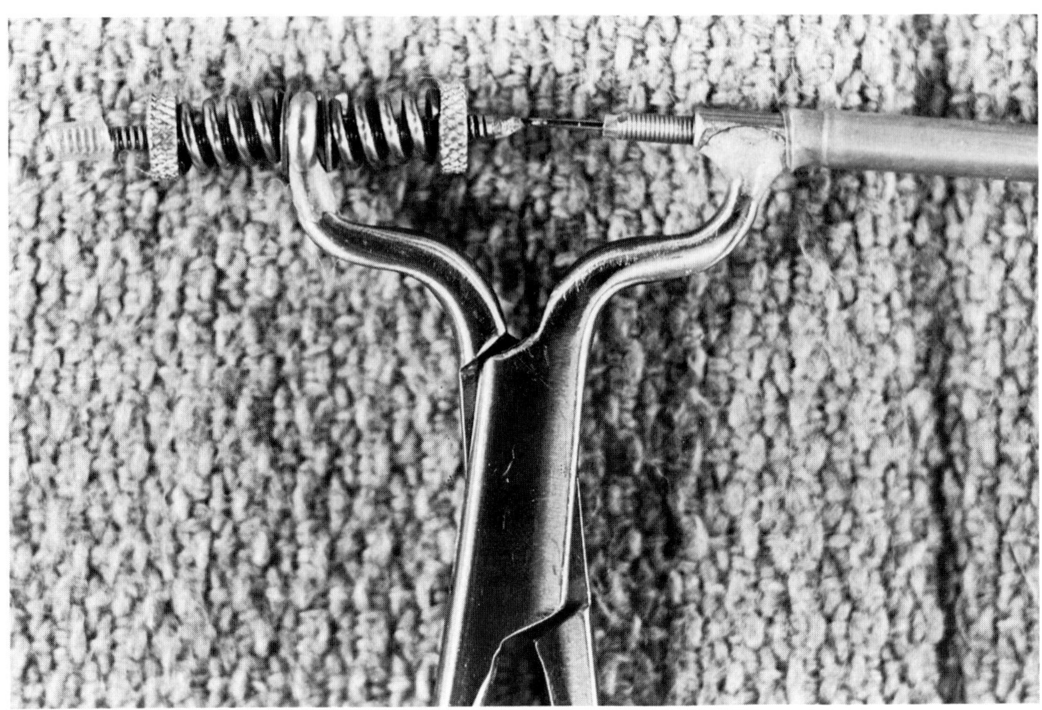

Figure 7. This is a close-up of the spring-buffered mechanism in the handle.

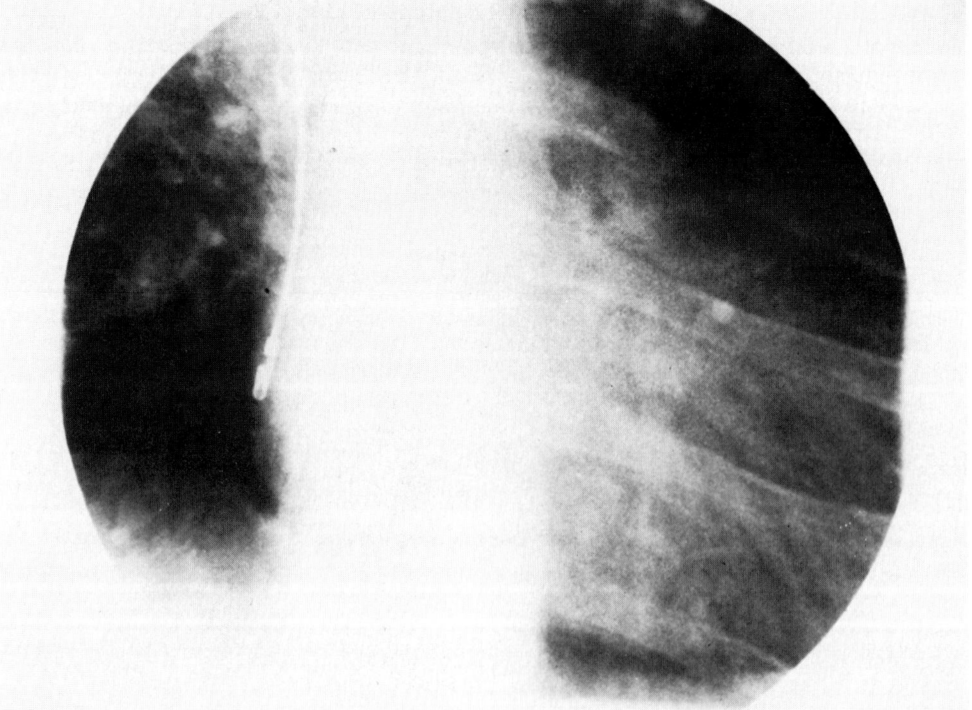

Figure 8. This is a fluoroscopy of the heart showing the Stanford bioptome in the right atrium with the tip of the catheter pointing laterally.

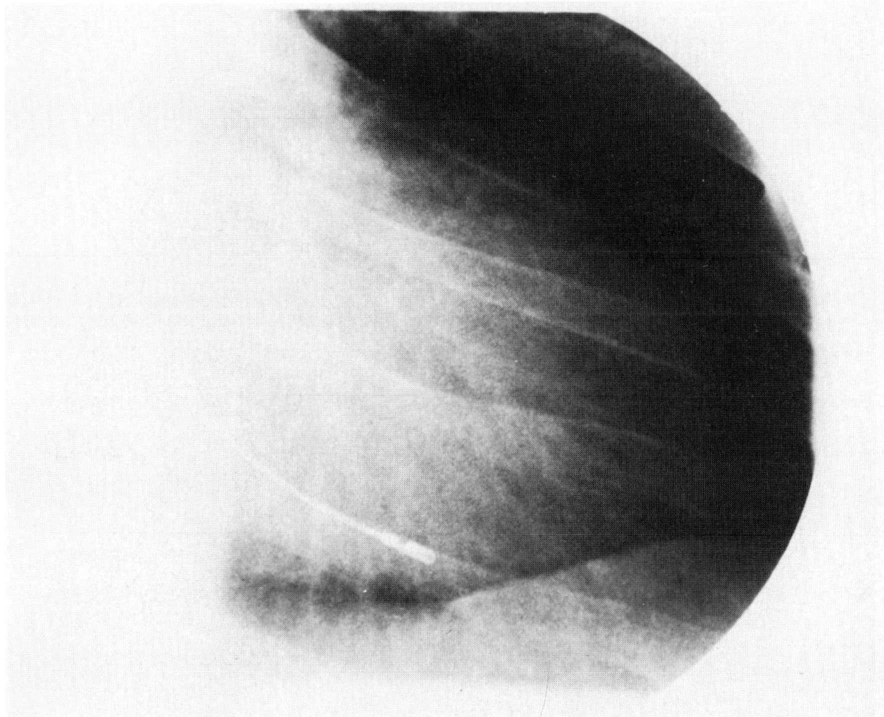

Figure 9. The bioptome tip is in the right ventricle pointing toward the interventricular septum.

septum where biopsies are safely obtained. The bioptome is advanced through the sheath and superior vena cava into the right atrium, with the handle and catheter tip pointing laterally, as shown in Figure 8. The handle is rotated medially when the catheter tip is in the lower third of the right atrium, which facilitates passage through the tricuspid valve into the right ventricle (Fig. 9). Once the catheter tip is in the right ventricle, the bioptome handle is rotated posteriorly so that it is pointing leftward and inferiorly. This maneuver directs the jaws toward the intraventricular septum. Correct positioning of the bioptome is confirmed by seeing the tip well past the left border of the vertebral column and below the shadow of the left diaphragmatic dome. The contraction of the heart will usually be transmitted to the bioptome handle and PVCs are encountered when the catheter tip makes contact with the septum. The bioptome is then withdrawn 1 cm and the jaws opened, as seen in Figure 10. The bioptome is readvanced until contact is made, immediately closed, and withdrawn from the ventricle. A small tug is often felt as the bioptome is withdrawn, and the patient may feel momentary discomfort. Rarely a moderately forceful tug will not free the specimen from the ventricular wall, in which case the jaws should be reopened and a repeat attempt at the biopsy should be performed. Three to five specimens are obtained for analysis by light and electron microscopy (Fig. 11). Adequate biopsy specimens are obtained 98 percent of the time with this technique.[14] When the right internal jugular vein cannot be successfully cannulated, the femoral or subclavian vein can be used. These two approaches, however, require negotiating curvatures in the vascular system, and ideal right ventricular septal placement is often difficult or impossible. Additionally, the femoral vein approach usually requires a longer bioptome. An acceptable alternative is to perform a left ventricular biopsy via the percutaneous femoral artery approach. The left ventricular bioptome used at Stanford is a modification of the right ventricular instrument. It is 100 cm in length and has a 6 French diameter. A 90 cm radiopaque Teflon sheath is advanced into the left ventricle over a 100 cm 6.7 French pigtail catheter. Once the sheath is located in the left ventricle, it is connected to a continuous

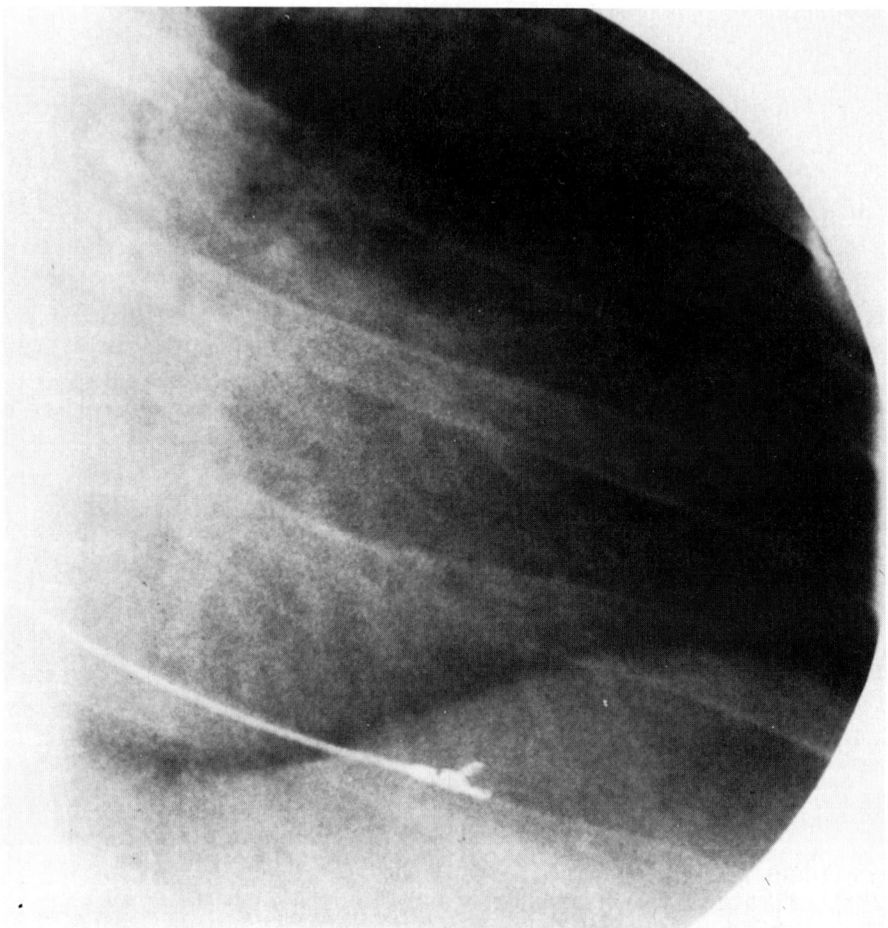

Figure 10. The bioptome jaws are opened. The tip of the catheter is well past the left border of the vertebral column and below the shadow of the left hemidiaphragm.

drip via a side-arm tubing. The bioptome can then be safely advanced through the sheath to the left ventricular apex where the thicker left ventricular myocardium greatly reduces the risk of free wall perforation.

LEFT VENTRICULAR VS RIGHT VENTRICULAR BIOPSY

Most pathologic processes that can be diagnosed by examination of endomyocardial biopsy specimens will affect both ventricles, making the need for left ventricular biopsy infrequent.[18,19] There are, however, certain instances in which left ventricular biopsy is specifically indicated: study of myocardial changes owing to aortic and mitral valve disease, hypertrophic cardiomyopathy, certain forms of endomyocardial fibrosis, scleroderma heart disease involving only the left ventricle, left ventricular irradiation, and when right ventricular biopsy cannot be successfully performed. At Stanford the safety record for left ventricular biopsy is similar to that of right ventricular biopsy.[14,18]

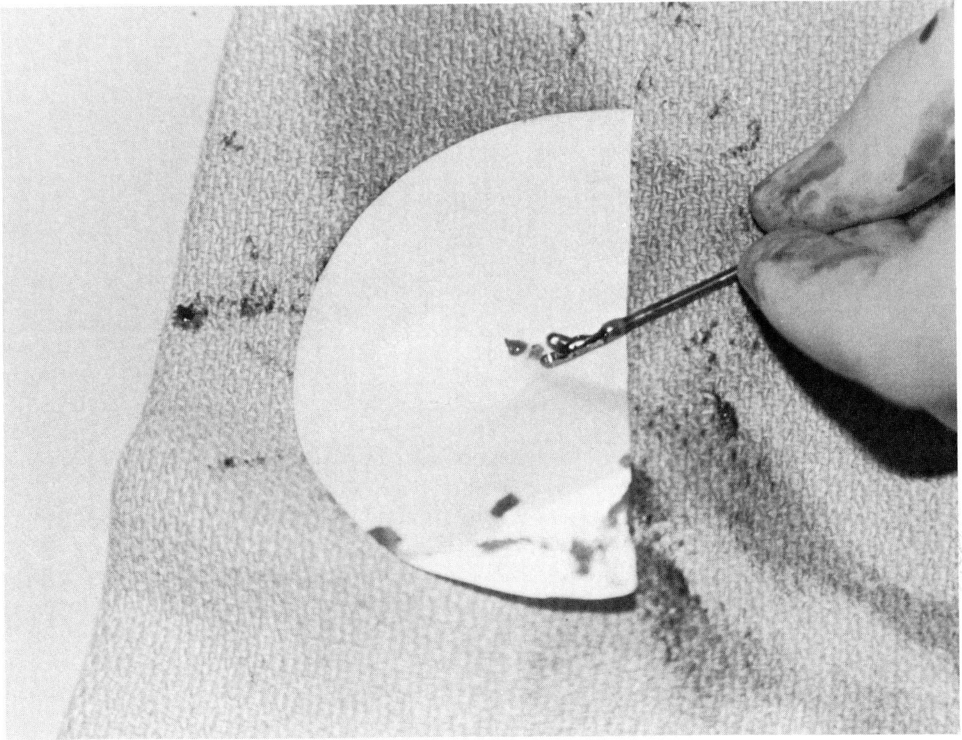

Figure 11. This is a photograph of a typical biopsy specimen obtained with the Stanford right ventricular bioptome.

SAFETY OF ENDOMYOCARDIAL BIOPSY

The low incidence of complications associated with transvascular endomyocardial biopsy has been one of the major reasons for its world-wide popularity as an invasive diagnostic tool in cardiology. Konno and coworkers[20] reported no major complications in their initial series of 450 patients. In contrast, there has been a significant complication rate associated with transthoracic needle biopsy techniques. Shirey and associates[5] found an 8 percent incidence of cardiac tamponade, with half these patients requiring thoracotomy. There was a total major complication rate of 10 percent.

Table 1 lists the complications that have been associated with transvascular endomyocardial biopsy. Hemopericardium with cardiac tamponade owing to free wall perforation is the most significant major complication.

A world-wide biopsy survey conducted by Sekiguchi and Take[21] has found an overall major complication rate of 1.17 percent in 6739 patients. Twenty-eight patients (0.42 percent) suffered cardiac perforation, and two (0.03 percent) of them died.

Experience in the United Kingdom, where both the Konno and King's bioptomes are used,[22,23] has shown a 1.1 percent incidence of major complications, with death occurring very rarely. At Stanford, over 4000 biopsies have been performed since 1973, with only 6 patients (0.15 percent) developing cardiac tamponade. All six patients were successfully treated with pericardiocentesis. There have been no deaths at Stanford associated with endomyocardial biopsies. Our incidence of other complications such as atrial fibrillation, ventricular tachyarrhythmias, pneumothorax, uncomplicated air embolism, transient paresis of the recurrent laryngeal nerve and phrenic nerve, and Horner's syndrome has been 0.5 percent.

Table 1. Complications of endomyocardial biopsy

Complication	Association
Cardiac perforation Cardiac tamponade Ventricular arrhythmia Atrial fibrillation Pericardial inflammation	Associated with both RV and LV biopsy procedures
Cerebral embolism	Associated with LV biopsy
Right pneumothorax Air embolism Temporary recurrent laryngeal nerve paresis Phrenic nerve paresis Horner's syndrome	Associated with right internal jugular vein cannulation

Our patients undergoing left ventricular biopsy are heparinized, and we have had no cases of arterial embolization in over 200 procedures.

The biopsing of tissue from the right ventricular septum or from the left ventricle does not seem to significantly impair cardiac performance.

The safety of endomyocardial biopsy compares favorably to other solid organ biopsy procedures, such as liver biopsy. Bleeding, the most common serious complication of liver biopsy, has an incidence ranging from 0.4 to 1 percent.[24-29] Mahal and associates[30] at Stanford found 22 of 3080 patients (0.7 percent) had significant bleeding after liver biopsy. Seventeen patients were given blood transfusions, and 6 required laparotomies to control their bleeding.

DISORDERS THAT ARE SPECIFICALLY DIAGNOSED BY BIOPSY

The disorders that can be specifically diagnosed by endomyocardial biopsy are listed in Table 2.

Cardiac Allograft Rejection

The bioptome developed by Caves and Schultz was first introduced into the clinical heart transplant program at Stanford University in August 1972. The routine use of right ventricular biopsy during the post-transplant followup has made a major impact on the early diagnosis and management of allograft rejection.[31] The method of monitoring objective morpho-

Table 2. Disorders which can be specifically diagnosed by biopsy

Anthracycline cardiotoxicity
Carcinoid heart disease
Cardiac allograft rejection
Cardiac amyloidosis
Cardiac hemochromatosis
Cardiac sarcoidosis
Cardiac tumors
Endocardial fibroelastosis
Endocardial fibrosis
Fabry's disease of the heart
Glycogen storage diseases
Irradiation fibrosis of the heart
Myocarditis

Table 3. Grading of endomyocardial biopsies in acute human cardiac rejection

Mild rejection	Minimal endocardial and perivascular lymphocytic infiltrate. Lymphocytes are pyroninophilic. Endocardial and interstitial edema. Reversible.
Moderate rejection	Endocardial, perivascular, and interstitial lymphocytic infiltrate of a moderate degree; focal areas of myocyte lysis. Reversible.
Severe rejection	Heavy lymphocytic and neutrophilic infiltrate throughout the tissue. Interstitial hemorrhage with vessel and myocyte necrosis. Reversible with difficulty.
Resolving rejection	Nonpyroninophilic lymphocytes with active fibrosis. Lipochrome pigment is seen.

logic findings on heart biopsies, rather than clinical signs of rejection, has greatly improved the success rate of cardiac transplantation. In addition, since the use of cyclosporine (cyclosporin A) as an immunosuppressant, the "common" clinical signs of rejection—such as the development of heart failure, an S_3 gallop, arrhythmias, and loss of ECG voltage—occur very late in the rejection episode, if at all. During the initial post-transplant course, patients are biopsied weekly or more often if any clinical or histologic signs suggest an acute rejection episode. The repeated biopsy procedures, which are usually performed on an outpatient basis, are tolerated quite well by our transplant recipients (many of whom have had over 20 biopsy procedures performed).[31] Transplant patients are given prophylactic antibiotics 1 hour before

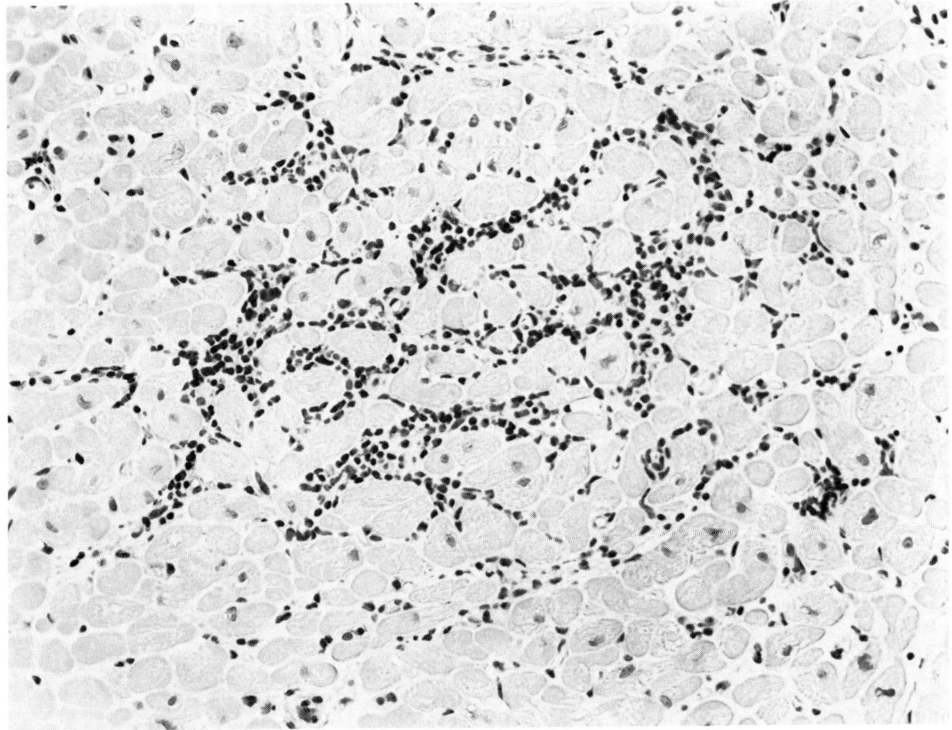

Figure 12. Mild acute rejection (H&E, ×192). Mild interstitial and perivascular lymphocytic infiltrate without myocyte necrosis.

the procedure. Local anesthesia is used for the placement of the sheath in the internal jugular vein. Each biopsy procedure entails the removal of three to five pieces from the right ventricular septal wall.

Multiple specimens significantly increase the accuracy of biopsy interpretation, resulting in good histologic correlation between biopsy pieces and autopsy specimens.[19,31] These specimens are stained with hematoxylin and eosin, Masson's Trichrome, and methyl-green pyronin stains. The severity of acute rejection is determined as shown in Table 3.

MILD REJECTION. Mild rejection shows early or minimal lymphocytic infiltration of the perivascular and endocardial tissues. These lymphocytes are of T cell origin and avidly take up pyronin stain owing to their high RNA turnover rate. In addition there is often endocardial and interstitial edema. These alterations are easily reversible (Fig. 12).

MODERATE REJECTION. In this stage of rejection the infiltrate is heavier and has extended into the interstitial tissue. In areas with clumps of lymphocytes there is evidence of early myocyte death. These findings are usually reversible (Fig. 13).

SEVERE REJECTION. Severe rejection is characterized by the same histopathology encountered in moderate rejection, with the addition of polymorphonuclear leukocytes and interstitial hemorrhage caused by vascular damage. There is also more evident and diffuse myocyte necrosis. This is often irreversible (Fig. 14).

RESOLVING REJECTION. After rejection has been successfully treated, the inflammatory infiltrate quickly clears, leaving only scant mononuclear leukocytes that take up pyronin stain poorly. Within 3 days active fibrosis occurs and leads to scar tissue by 1 week. Lipochrome pigment signifying old myocyte death can also be seen.

The use of cyclosporine for cardiac allograft recipients has caused some additional changes seen on endomyocardial biopsies. Soon after transplant a sparse, poorly staining, mononuclear

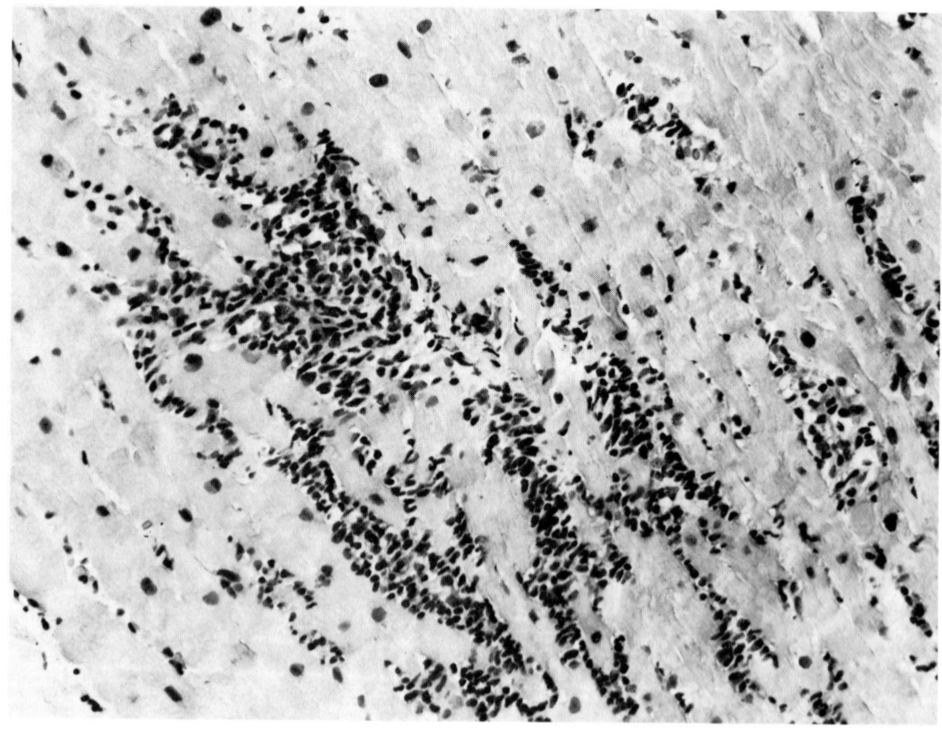

Figure 13. Moderate acute rejection (H&E, ×192). Moderate interstitial lymphocytic infiltrate with focal myocyte necrosis.

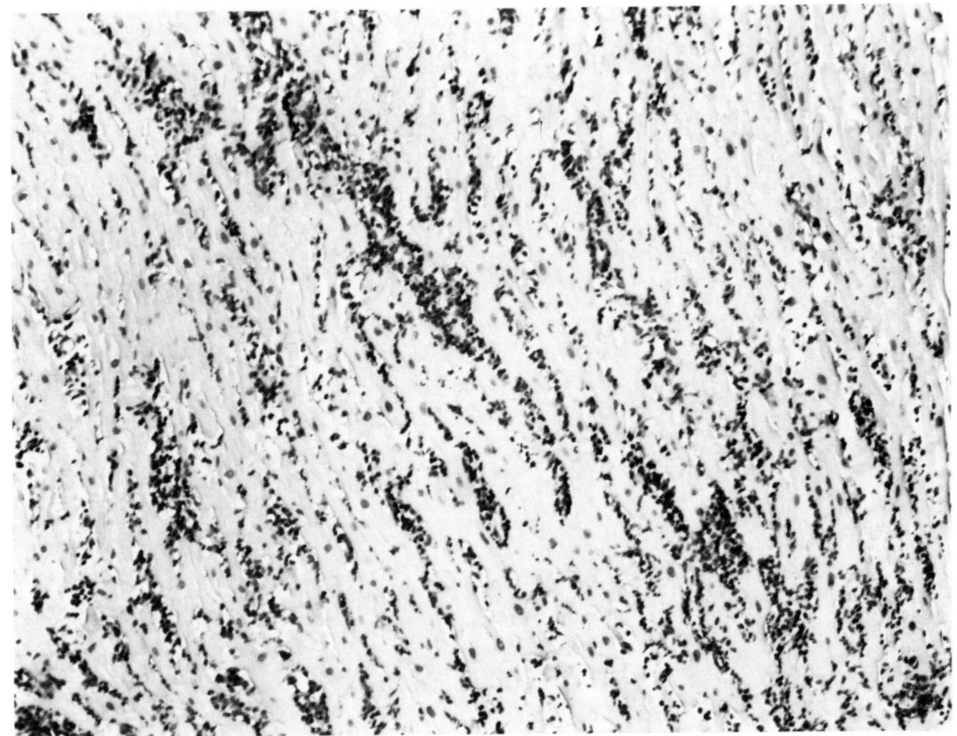

Figure 14. Severe acute rejection (H&E, ×120). Dense, widely distributed lymphocytic infiltrate with occasional neutrophils and small hemorrhages. Myocyte necrosis is more extensive.

interstitial infiltrate is often present, which probably does not represent acute rejection. In addition, all patients receiving cyclosporine also have a fine, diffuse interstitial fibrosis that is unrelated to previous acute rejection episodes.[31]

Myocarditis

According to currently available information, the definitive diagnosis of myocarditis can be made only by examination of myocardial tissue.[19,32] Endomyocardial biopsy provides a safe method for diagnosing myocarditis. The clinical diagnosis of myocarditis has previously been made in patients who present with sudden onset of congestive heart failure often preceded by a viral upper respiratory illness. Patients are usually younger than 40 years, have nonspecific electrocardiographic abnormalities, and are found to have cardiomegaly, biventricular failure, and absence of valvular and coronary artery disease. At most, only 25 percent of these patients, however, are found to have inflammatory cellular infiltrates on biopsy.[32,33] An example of biopsy-proven acute myocarditis, with a dense infiltrate composed of lymphocytes, neutrophils, and eosinophils, is shown in Figure 15. The low incidence of these findings on biopsy in this group of patients may account for the initial clinical impression that corticosteroid therapy fails to improve myocarditis.

We have found that immunosuppressive therapy with prednisone and azathioprine in patients with biopsy-proven myocarditis is usully associated with improvement or stabilization of myocardial function.[34] Early withdrawal of immunosuppressive therapy can result in clinical and biopsy-proven relapse. Recently, Fenoglio and associates[35] have suggested that myocarditis can be divided into clinically meaningful histologic subsets of patients with predictive

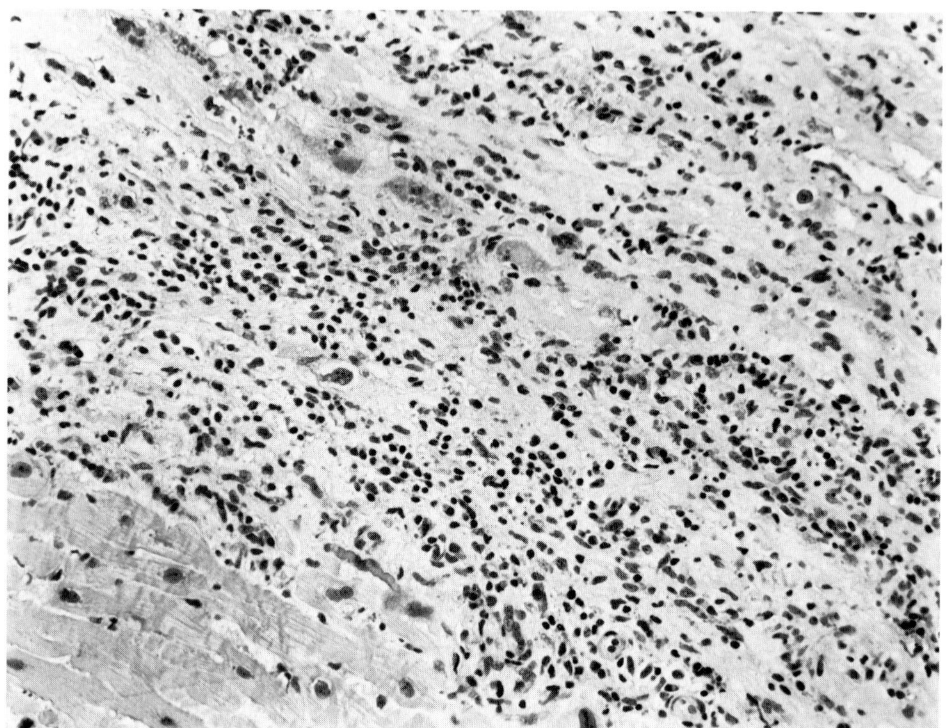

Figure 15. Severe myocarditis (H&E, ×192). Dense infiltrate composed of lymphocytes, neutrophils, and eosinophils. Occasional multinucleated giant cells are found. Myocyte necrosis is extensive with fibrosis; myocytes at the periphery are unremarkable.

therapeutic response and prognosis. Their classification, however, is derived from relatively small patient groups and may be confounded by vague histologic criteria used to distinguish true myocarditis from cardiomyopathy.

Opinions differ between pathologists regarding the diagnosis of myocarditis. Some require the presence of extensive, diffuse mononuclear infiltration with evidence of myocyte damage; others have more liberal criteria, accepting focal patches of mononuclear cells as sufficient evidence. There is a need for a quantitative histologic grading system acceptable to most pathologists to help clarify the diagnosis of myocarditis.[36] A multicenter cooperative trial is presently underway to test the efficacy of immunosuppressive therapy in myocarditis. It is hoped that this study will also serve to define better the relationship between histologic appearance and clinical manifestations of myocarditis and to identify which patients will best respond to immunosuppressive therapy. It should be re-emphasized that endomyocardial biopsy is an essential tool in the evaluation of patients with suspected myocarditis and that immunosuppressive drugs, with their serious side effects, should not be given to anyone without histologically proven myocarditis.

Anthracycline Cardiotoxicity

Anthracycline antibiotics, particularly doxorubicin hydrochloride, are potent wide-spectrum antitumor agents.[37–39] The major drawback to the use of doxorubicin is its dose-related cardiotoxicity, which can lead to a rapidly deteriorating cardiomyopathy. Initial observation of this toxicity has led to the policy of administering to a patient a total maximum dose of 500 to 550 mg per m^2.[37,39] Unfortunately, some patients develop fatal heart failure despite this dose limitation, and others, who could tolerate higher doses, are denied further needed antitumor therapy because they have reached the "maximum" dose. Alexander and associates[40] have used a drop in the radionuclide ejection fraction as a harbinger of the development of clinically significant cardiomyopathy. One group of observers has recently reported a lack of correlation between clinical heart failure and anthracycline cardiotoxicity seen on autopsy specimens of myocardium.[41] Their findings are at variance with previously reported observations,[37,38,42–44] and we believe their conclusions are incorrect for the following reasons: (1) They misidentified normal postmortem changes and normal central myocyte paleness as anthracycline toxicity; (2) specimens were only examined under light microscopy, which can miss early findings, and not under the more sensitive electron microscope; and (3) the clinical diagnosis of heart disease was made from review of medical records, which makes the diagnosis questionable in some of their patients. In contrast, we have found that the use of histopathologic grading of endomyocardial biopsies in conjunction with right heart catheterization findings during rest and exercise has allowed us to accurately predict the risk of developing cardiomyopathy with further doxorubicin therapy.[37] At Stanford, since 1978 we have monitored over 100 patients using endomyocardial biopsy and right heart catheterization and have had only 2 cases of anthracycline-induced cardiomyopathy while giving an average cumulative dose of 600 mg per m^2. After receiving 400 to 450 mg per m^2, patients are biopsied before every additional 150 to 200 mg per m^2 dosage. Some patients have received total cumulative dosages greater than 1100 mg per m^2 without developing heart failure.

There are two typical features of anthracycline-induced damage seen on nearly all endomyocardial biopsies from treated patients.[45] The first type is partial or total myofibrillar loss

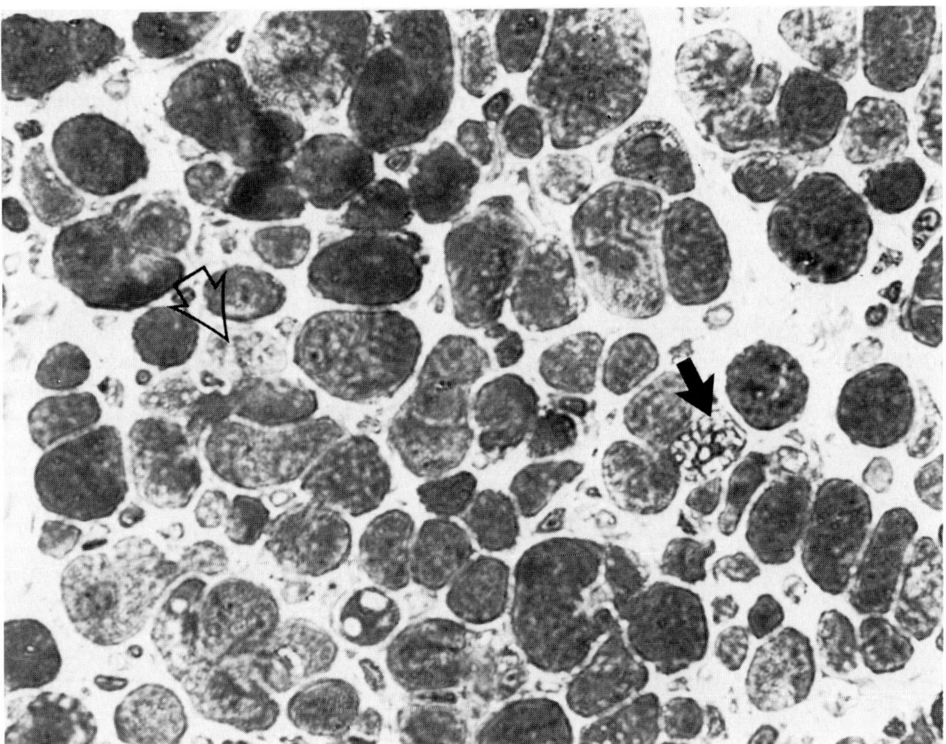

Figure 16. Adriamycin cardiotoxicity (Toluidine Blue, ×480). One micron plastic embedded sections with myocytes showing myofibrillar loss *(open arrow)* and cytoplasmic vacuolization *(closed arrow)*.

Table 4. Grading of endomyocardial biopsies of anthracycline cardiotoxicity

Grade 0	Normal myocardium
Grade 1	Partial myofibrillar loss and/or distended sarcotubular system in isolated myocytes with normal neighboring myocytes
Grade 1.5	Features between Grades 1 and 2
Grade 2	More extensive myofibrillar loss and/or cytoplasmic vacuolization in groups or clusters of myocytes
Grade 2.5	Features between Grades 2 and 3
Grade 3	Severe myofibrillar loss and cytoplasmic vacuolization diffusely present with myocyte necrosis seen

from myocytes. The nucleus and mitochondria are intact but only Z-band remnants remain. The second finding is sarcoplasmic reticulum dilation and coalescence leading to cytoplasmic vacuolization. These two features can be found separately or in the same myocyte and are easily seen on electron microscopic examination (Fig. 16). The extent to which these two abnormalities are found on a biopsy specimen determines the grade of damage, as shown in Table 4. With grades 0 to 1.5 an additional 100 to 200 mg of anthracycline can be given with less than 10 percent risk of heart failure. With grades 2.0 to 2.5 additional anthracycline dosages carry a moderate risk (10 to 25 percent) of heart failure, and the need for continued therapy must be individually weighed against the risk. With grade 3.0 additional anthracycline therapy carries a greater than 25 percent risk of heart failure and should not be given.[37] Interstitial fibrosis is a common finding in cardiotoxicity but is too nonspecific, and it is not used in grading the severity of damage. Postmortem examinations in humans have shown that anthracycline-induced damage involves both ventricles symmetrically and occurs first in the endomyocardium.

Cardiac Hemochromatosis

It is quite unusual for the diagnosis of systemic hemochromatosis to be made initially by endomyocardial biopsy. By the time that the heart has accumulated significant amounts of iron, many other organs—especially the liver and pancreas—have been sufficiently damaged to cause clinical signs. On occasion, however, the cardiac manifestations, such as heart failure and arrhythmias, may be so severe that a patient will first present to a cardiologist. At that time a biopsy will make the definitive diagnosis of hemochromatosis. Figure 17 demonstrates the dense deposits of iron seen in the myocyte cytoplasm of a patient with primary hemochromatosis.

Once the diagnosis is made and therapy to remove iron is begun, serial endomyocardial biopsies can be used to monitor organ iron depletion.[46] Cases have been reported in which patients developed hypoferremia and iron-deficiency anemia while still retaining significant myocardial iron.[46] Continued treatment will eventually remove this iron, and cardiotoxicity can be improved. Additionally, endomyocardial biopsy may be used to monitor and to prevent iatrogenic cardiac hemosiderosis in patients who require numerous blood transfusions to treat diseases such as thalassemia. However, some investigators believe that biopsies are too insensitive for monitoring patients, because of variations in the extent of iron deposition in the epicardium and endocardium and in different myocardial regions.[47]

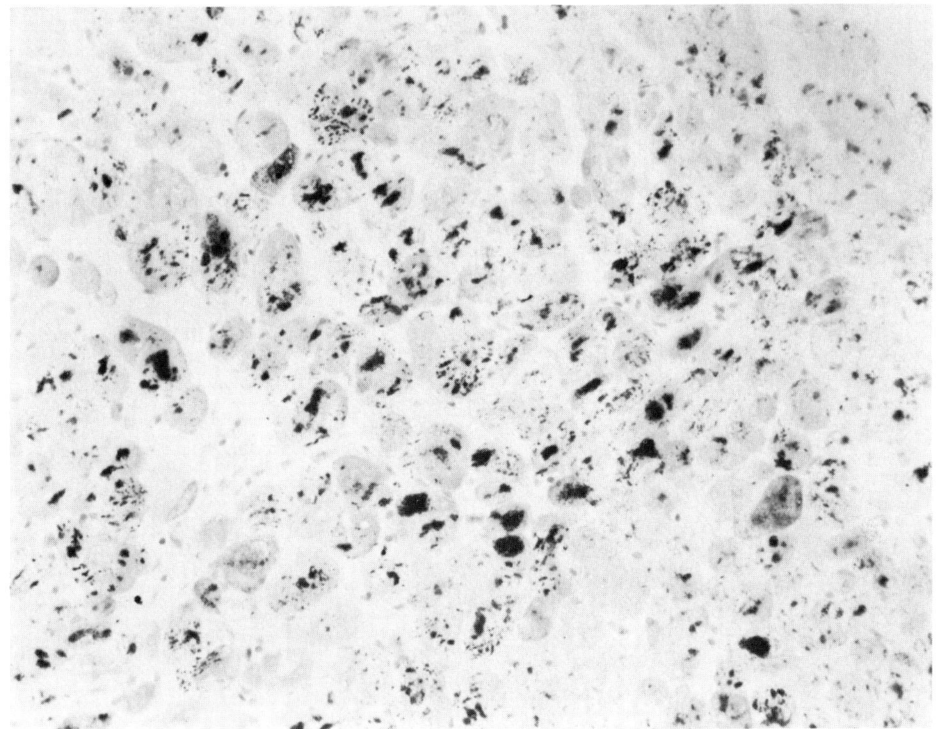

Figure 17. Hemochromatosis (Prussian Blue, ×192). Myocytes show dense cytoplasmic iron deposits, especially in the perinuclear regions. Interstitial fibrosis is mildly increased.

Cardiac Amyloidosis

The diagnosis of cardiac amyloidosis can be made easily using heart biopsies. Figure 18 shows the typical homogenous eosinophilic amyloid deposits surrounding myocytes and blood vessels in an advanced case of cardiac amyloidosis. The myocytes show hypertrophy with degenerative changes. Special staining techniques, such as congo red and thioflavin-T, as well as electron microscopy may be needed to detect early myocardial amyloid deposits.[48] In addition, endomyocardial biopsy may help differentiate amyloidosis from other disease processes that present with similar hemodynamic and clinical pictures, such as pericardial constriction.

Cardiac Sarcoidosis

Inasmuch as steroidal therapy can be life-saving in cases of cardiac sarcoidosis, the diagnosis should be aggressively pursued when clinically suspected.[49] Heart failure and arrhythmias may be the initial signs of the disease. Because sarcoid granulomata occur focally, with normal areas in between lesions, the possibility of a false-negative biopsy is large. On obtaining multiple specimens, however, it is possible to see the typical noncaseating granulomata that are found in greatest density in the interventricular septum (which is the area biopsied with the right ventricular biopsy procedure).

Endocardial Fibrosis

Although a certain amount of fibrosis can be found in the endocardium of many types of cardiomyopathy, the term endocardial fibrosis refers specifically to Loeffler's endocarditis

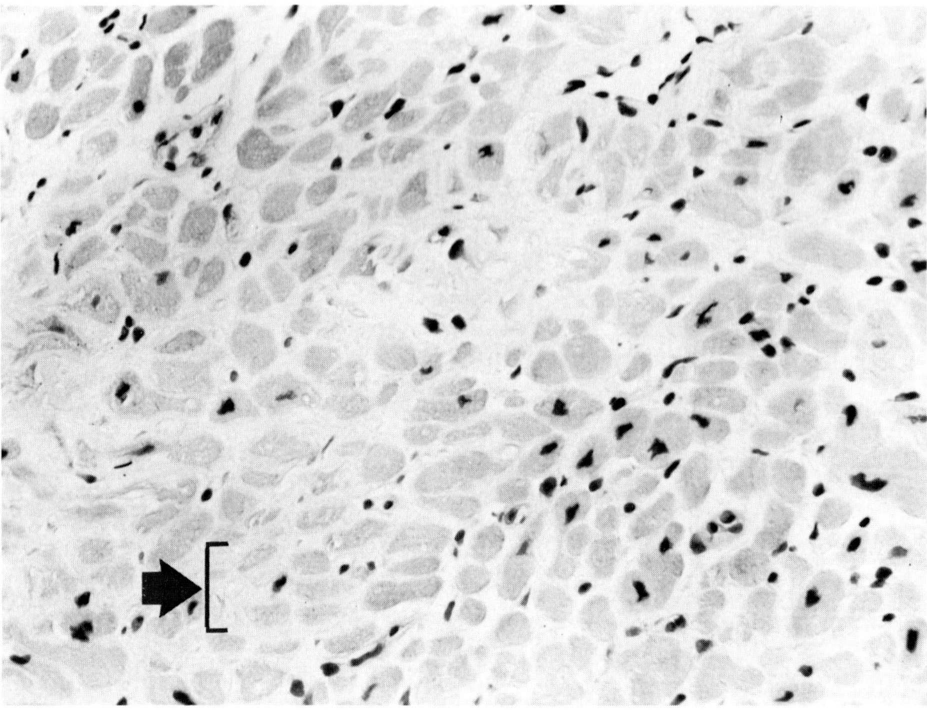

Figure 18. Amyloidosis (H&E, ×300). Homogenous eosinophilic amyloid protein is present around myocytes and blood vessels *(bracket)*. Myocytes show hypertrophy and degenerative changes.

with eosinophilia and to Davies' tropical endomyocardial fibrosis. These two disorders are characterized by marked fibrosis of the endocardium, with minimal or no myocardial or epicardial involvement.[50] Typically, patients present with a clinical picture of restrictive disease. The most common sites of endocardial involvement are the apex and body of the right ventricle and the inferior inflow region of the left ventricle. Endomyocardial biopsy can be useful in establishing the diagnosis and in localizing the extent of involvement, which would help direct the surgical therapy of this disorder.

Fabry's Disease of the Heart

Fabry's disease, a disorder characterized by abnormal accumulation of neutral glycolipids in various tissues, can involve the heart, leading to congestive heart failure. Specific findings such as perinuclear vacuolization, cytoplasmic inclusion bodies containing glycolipid, and lacework appearance of myocardial fibers have been found on endomyocardial biopsy specimens.[51] The diagnosis of Fabry's disease may be made by biopsy in patients who do not clinically exhibit the other signs of the disease.

Myocardial diseases such as carcinoid heart disease, cardiac tumors, and glycogen storage diseases are occasionally diagnosed first by endomyocardial biopsy, though this is not the method of choice.

DIFFERENTIATION BETWEEN MYOCARDIAL RESTRICTION AND PERICARDIAL CONSTRICTION

Separating myocardial restriction from pericardial constriction on clinical grounds is often difficult. Calcification on chest x-ray or abnormal pericardium on echocardiography is not

Table 5. Indications for endomyocardial biopsy

Suspected cardiac allograft rejection
Monitoring cardiac allograft recipients
Suspected myocarditis
Suspected anthracycline cardiotoxicity
Monitoring anthracycline cardiotoxicity
Suspected diagnosis of secondary cardiomyopathies (hemochromatosis, amyloidosis, sarcoidosis, and so forth)
Differentiation between restrictive and constrictive cardiac disease

always present in constrictive disease. Furthermore, hemodynamic abnormalities seen on cardiac catheterization may fail to identify correctly the disease process. Endomyocardial biopsy can be helpful in differentiating pericardial constriction from myocardial restriction. Biopsy should be performed in patients undergoing pericardectomies unless this differentiation is clearly evident preoperatively.

INDICATIONS FOR ENDOMYOCARDIAL BIOPSY

The indications presently believed to be appropriate for endomyocardial biopsy are listed in Table 5. It is now widely accepted that cardiac allograft transplantation programs cannot successfully function without monitoring patients for rejection using biopsies.[31] Signs of clinical rejection occur late and unreliably in patients treated with cyclosporine.[34] Biopsies should be performed on patients who present clinically with myocarditis. The incidence of histologically confirmed myocarditis in this group of patients is low, and therefore immunosuppressive therapy should not be given without biopsy evidence of the disease. Because cancer patients receiving anthracycline antibiotics often have cardiac dysfunction related to mediastinal radiation, valvular or coronary heart disease, it may be difficult clinically to diagnose drug-induced cardiotoxicity. Electron microscopic examination of endomyocardial biopsies is a highly specific and sensitive method of diagnosing and monitoring anthracycline-induced cardiotoxicity.[37] Therefore, ideally, biopsies should be used when following these patients. This approach allows the patient to receive the maximum safe dose of this widely useful antitumor medication. In cases of suspected secondary cardiomyopathy, endomyocardial biopsy should be performed.[45] Because successful therapeutic options are available for many of these diseases, such as hemochromatosis, sarcoidosis, and hepatolenticular degeneration, attempts to confirm these diagnoses should be made. When the differentiation between restrictive and constrictive heart disease is not clear and surgical intervention is being considered, endomyocardial biopsy is indicated.

Biopsy is not indicated in most obvious cases of hypertrophic or congestive cardiomyopathy. There are no pathognomonic findings in these two conditions, and the biopsy results will not affect patient management or predict outcome more accurately than other means.[19]

There are two major contraindications to performing endomyocardial biopsies. The first is the presence of a bleeding disorder such as thrombocytopenia or abnormal coagulation. These disorders put the patient at an increased risk of hemorrhage and tamponade if cardiac perforation should occur. The second contraindication is a left ventricular thrombus. Left ventricular biopsy in patients with left ventricular mural thrombus may lead to systemic embolization. Biopsy in the presence of a right ventricular thrombus has not led to clinically significant pulmonary embolization in our experience, but adequate tissue may not be obtainable if the endocardium is thoroughly covered by organized thrombi.

RESEARCH APPLICATIONS AND SPECIAL INVESTIGATIONS

There are various research methods that currently employ endomyocardial biopsy tissue. Major areas of active investigation include biochemical and structural analysis, pharmacology, membrane receptor enzymology, and immunology.

Biochemical Studies

Cellular enzyme concentrations are presently being measured on biopsy specimens of heart tissue. Concentrations of cyclic adenosine monophosphate (c-AMP), cyclic guanosine monophosphate (c-GMP), adenosine triphosphate (ATP), adenosine triphosphatase (ATPase), lactate dehydrogenase (LDH) and creatine phosphokinase (CK) have been measured in various disease states. Intraoperative transmural biopsies have been done on patients with coronary artery disease undergoing bypass surgery.[52] Such studies have shown higher levels of ATP and CK in the subendocardium compared with the subepicardium of myocardium supplied by normal arteries. Biopsies taken from ischemic areas supplied by diseased coronary arteries showed a reverse gradient with higher levels of ATP and CK in the subepicardial tissue.[52] A few investigators have found increased levels of LDH and decreased levels of ATP in biopsy specimens taken from patients with cardiomyopathies.[53–55] In contrast, one investigator found decreased LDH activity in myopathic ventricles.[56] Torp and associates studied tissue lipid concentrations in patients with cardiomyopathies.[57,58] Though there is some sampling error as well as technical difficulty in obtaining adequate specimens for assays, accurate and reproducible enzyme measurements can be performed on endomyocardial biopsies.[59]

Myocardial cell structure and tissue fibrosis have been studied using biopsy specimens in an attempt to clarify the pathophysiology of various cardiac diseases. Ultrastructural morphometry has revealed, for example, differences between volume-loaded ventricles in mitral insufficiency and normal tissue and distinctions between volume-loaded and pressure-loaded ventricles.[60] Myocardial stiffness as measured by hemodynamic monitoring correlates with the degree of fibrosis seen on biopsy from patients with congestive cardiomyopathies and aortic valve disease.[61] In ischemic heart disease, morphometry on operative biopsy samples has disclosed quantitatively less myocardial fibrosis in regions supplied by collateral vessels than in those without collaterals.[62] Other morphometric studies have shown a correlation between ventricular wall segment contractile function and the extent of fibrosis.[63]

Pharmacologic Studies

Myocardial tissue concentrations of cardioactive drugs probably represent a more meaningful value than serum levels for examining the effects of a given drug on the heart. Myocardial digitoxin concentrations have been shown to be higher than serum levels.[64] Kates and Jaillon[65] have compared plasma and tissue concentrations of various drugs and found clinically useful information about pharmacokinetics. Endomyocardial biopsies have also been used to study the action of glucagon on the heart.[58]

Receptor Enzymology and Immunology

Bristow and associates[66] have shown a significant decrease in beta-adrenergic receptor density in severely myopathic hearts of cardiac transplant recipients. We are presently measuring beta-adrenergic receptors in endomyocardial biopsy tissue from patients with varying degrees of cardiomyopathy. There seems to be a correlation between the degree of heart failure and the amount of receptor density reduction.[67] Immunologic abnormalities have been reported in patients with idiopathic congestive cardiomyopathy. Peripheral blood lymphocytes have decreased suppressor function[68] as well as some cytotoxic effects against endomyocardial biopsy tissue.[19,69]

SUMMARY

Endomyocardial biopsy is an accepted, useful invasive tool for the analysis of human endomyocardium at the cellular and subcellular levels. It is applicable in the evaluation of specific diseases including cardiac allograft rejection, myocarditis, anthracycline cardiotoxicity, and infiltrative cardiomyopathies. The procedure can be performed in a cardiac catheterization room on an outpatient basis. The technique is quite safe when performed by trained cardiologists. Left ventricular biopsies are also safe but require systemic heparinization to prevent thromboembolization.

The clinical indications for performing an endomyocardial biopsy include routine followup and suspected rejection of cardiac allograft, suspected myocarditis, monitoring or diagnosis of suspected anthracycline cardiotoxicity, and suspected secondary cardiomyopathies. Left ventricular endomyocardial biopsy is indicated for diseases that predominately involve the left side of the heart, including left heart irradiation, cardiac fibroelastosis in infants, endomyocardial fibrosis, and scleroderma heart disease, and when right ventricular biopsy is unsuccessful. Endomyocardial biopsy is increasingly being used for research in the areas of tissue biochemistry, primary and valvular cardiomyopathies, immunology, beta receptor enzymology, drug interactions, and myocardial fibrosis.

Endomyocardial biopsy has not been shown to be clinically useful in the evaluation of primary, dilated, hypertrophic, or alcoholic cardiomyopathies. These disease processes all lack pathognomomic microscopic abnormalities, and subclassification has neither been successful nor therapeutically useful. In addition, this technique is limited in diagnosing any cardiac abnormality that is not diffuse, inasmuch as only a few samples of the endomyocardial layer are obtained for evaluation. Therefore, a negative biopsy result is not 100 percent specific in excluding certain diseases. A further limitation of this technique is the need for an experienced cardiac pathologist who is well versed in interpretation of biopsy specimens. Finally, there should be a sufficiently large case load to train and to maintain skilled practitioners so that the procedure can be performed with little risk.

The role of endomyocardial biopsy will continue to expand as research continues to find more uses for the technique and as more clinicians become skilled in its use.

REFERENCES

1. Silverman, I: *A new biopsy needle.* Am J Surg 40:671, 1938.
2. Casten, AL and March, JB: *Metabolic studies on cardiac tissue obtained by needle biopsy of the intact anesthetized dog.* Circ Res 1:226, 1953.
3. Sutton, DC, Sutton, GC, and Kent, G: *Needle biopsy of the human ventricular myocardium.* Q Bull Northwestern Univ Med School 30:213, 1956.
4. Timmis, GC, Gordon, S, Baron, RH, et al: *Percutaneous myocardial biopsy.* Am Heart J 70:499, 1965.
5. Shirey, EK, Hawk, WA, Mukerji, D, et al: *Percutaneous myocardial biopsy of the left ventricle. Experience in 198 patients.* Circulation 46:112, 1972.
6. Bercu, B, Heinz, J, Choudhry, A, et al: *Myocardial biopsy. A new technic utilizing the ventricular septum.* Am J Cardiol 14:675, 1964.
7. Shugoll, GI: *Percutaneous myocardial and pericardial biopsy with the Menghini needle.* Am Heart J 85:35, 1973.
8. Shugoll, GI: *Percutaneous myocardial and pericardial biopsy with the Menghini needle.* Am Heart J 85:35, 1973.
9. Sakakibara, S and Konno, S: *Endomyocardial biopsy.* Jpn Heart J 3:537, 1962.
10. Caves, PS, Stinson, EB, Graham, AF, et al: *Percutaneous transvenous endomyocardial biopsy.* JAMA 225:288, 1973.
11. Richardson, PJ: *King's endomyocardial bioptome.* Lancet 1:660, 1974.
12. Brooksby, IAB, Swanton, RH, Jenkins, BS, et al: *Long sheath technique for introduction of catheter tip manometer or endomyocardial bioptome into left or right heart.* Br Heart J 36:908, 1974.
13. Brooksby, IAB, Jenkins, BS, Coltart, DJ, et al: *Left-ventricular endomyocardial biopsy.* Lancet 2:1222, 1974.
14. Mason, JW: *Techniques for right and left ventricular endomyocardial biopsy.* Am J Cardiol 41:887, 1978.
15. Mason, JW, Billingham, ME, and Ricci, DR: *Treatment of acute inflammatory myocarditis assisted by endomyocardial biopsy.* Am J Cardiol 45:1037, 1980.

16. Kawai, C and Kitaura, Y: *New endomyocardial biopsy catheter for the left ventricle.* Am J Cardiol 40:63, 1977.

17. Lurie, PR, Fujita, M, and Neustein, HB: *Transvascular endomyocardial biopsy in infants and small children: Description of a new technique.* Am J Cardiol 42:453, 1978.

18. Mason, JW and Billingham, ME: *Myocardial biopsy.* In Yu, PN and Goodwin, JF (eds): *Progress in Cardiology,* Lea and Febiger, Philadelphia, 1980.

19. Fowles, RE and Mason, JW: *Endomyocardial biopsy.* Ann Intern Med 97:885, 1982.

20. Konno, S, Sekiguchi, M, and Sakakibara, S: *Catheter biopsy of the heart.* Radiol Clin No Am 9:491, 1971.

21. Sekiguchi, M and Take, M: *World survey of catheter biopsy of the heart.* In Sekiguchi, M and Olsen, EGJ (eds): *Cardiomyopathy. Clinical, Pathological, and Theoretical Aspects.* University Park Press, Baltimore, 1980.

22. Olsen, EGJ: *Endomyocardial biopsy.* Br Heart J 40:95, 1978.

23. Brooksby, IA, Jenkins, BS, Davies, MJ, et al: *Left ventricular endomyocardial biopsy. 1: Description and evaluation of the technique.* Cathet Cardiovasc Diagn 3:115, 1977.

24. Edmondson, HA and Schiff, L: *Needle biopsy of the liver.* In Edmondson, HA and Schiff, L (eds): *Diseases of the Liver.* JB Lippincott Company, Philadelphia, 1975.

25. Zamcheck, N and Klausenstock, O: *Liver biopsy (concluded) II. The risk of needle biopsy.* N Engl J Med 249:1062, 1953.

26. Linder, H: *Grenzen und gefahren der Perkutanen Leberbiopsie mit der Menghini-Nadel: Erfahrungen bei 80,000 Leberbiopsien.* Deutsch Med Wschr 92:1751, 1967.

27. Ovlisen, B and Baden, H: *Liver biopsy by the method of Menghini.* Nord Med 83:297, 1970.

28. Parets, A: *Detection of intrahepatic metastases by blind needle liver biopsy.* Am J Med Sci 237:335, 1959.

29. Perrault, J, McGill, DB, Ott, BJ, et al: *Liver biopsy: Complications in 1000 inpatients and outpatients.* Gastroenterology 74:103, 1978.

30. Mahal, AS, Knauer, M, and Gregory, PB: *Bleeding after liver biopsy.* West J Med 134:11, 1981.

31. Billingham, ME: *Diagnosis of cardiac rejection by endomyocardial biopsy.* Heart Transplantation 1:25, 1982.

32. Mason, JW and Billingham, ME: *Acute inflammatory myocarditis.* In Fenoglio, JJ Jr (ed): *Endomyocardial Biopsy: Techniques and Applications.* CRC Press, Inc., Boca Raton, Florida, 1982.

33. Kuhn, H, Breithardt, G, Knieriem, H, et al: *Die bedeutung der endomyotcardialen katheterbiopsie fur die diagnostitc und die beurteilund der prognose der congestiven cardiomyopathie.* Dtsch Med Wochenschr 100:717, 1975.

34. Mason, JW, Billingham, ME, and Ricci, DR: *Treatment of acute inflammatory myocarditis assisted by endomyocardial biopsy.* Am J Cardiol 45:1037, 1980.

35. Fenoglio, JJ Jr, Ursell, PC, et al: *Diagnosis and classification of myocarditis by endomyocardial biopsy.* N Engl J Med 308:12, 1983.

36. Edwards, WD, Holmes, DR Jr, and Reeder, GS: *Diagnosis of active lymphocytic myocarditis by endomyocardial biopsy.* Mayo Clin Proc 57:419, 1982.

37. Bristow, MR, Lopez, MB, Mason, JW, et al: *Efficacy and cost of cardiac monitoring in patients receiving doxorubicin.* Cancer 50:32, 1982.

38. Legha, SS, Benjamin, RS, Mackay, B, et al: *Reduction of doxorubicin cardiotoxicity by prolonged continuous intravenous infusion.* Ann Intern Med 96:133, 1982.

39. Blum, RH and Carter, SK: *Adriamycin, a new anticancer drug with significant clinical activity.* Ann Intern Med 80:249, 1974.

40. Alexander, J, Dainak, N, Berger, HJ, et al: *Serial assessment of doxorubicin cardiotoxicity with quantitative radionuclide angiocardiography.* N Engl J Med 300:278, 1979.

41. Isner, JM, Ferrans, VJ, Cohen, SR, et al: *Clinical and morphologic cardiac findings after anthracycline chemotherapy. Analysis of 64 patients studied at necropsy.* Am J Cardiol 51:1167, 1983.

42. Mason, JW, Bristow, MR, Billingham, ME, et al: *Invasive and noninvasive methods of assessing adriamycin cardiotoxic effects in man: Superiority of histopathologic assessment using endomyocardial biopsy.* Cancer Treat Rep 62:857, 1978.

43. Bristow, MR, Mason, JW, Billingham, ME, et al: *Dose-effect and structure-function relationships in doxorubicin cardiomyopathy.* Am Heart J 102:709, 1981.

44. Friedman, MA, Bozdech, MJ, Billingham, ME, et al: *Doxorubicin cardiotoxicity. Serial endomyocardial biopsies and systolic time intervals.* JAMA 240:1603, 1978.

45. Billingham, ME: *The role of endomyocardial biopsy in the diagnosis and treatment of heart disease.* In Silver, MD (ed): *Cardiovascular Pathology* (Volume 2). Churchill Livingstone, New York, 1983.

46. Short, EM, Winkle, RA, and Billingham, ME: *Myocardial involvement in idiopathic hemochromatosis. Morphologic and clinical improvement following venesection.* Am J Med 70:1275, 1981.

47. Fitchett, DH, Coltart, DJ, Littler, WA, et al: *Cardiac involvement in secondary hemochromatosis: A catheter biopsy study and analysis of myocardium.* Cardiovasc Res 14:19, 1980.

48. Schroeder, JS, Billingham, ME, and Rider, AK: *Cardiac amyloidosis: Diagnosis by transvenous endomyocardial biopsy.* Am J Med 59:269, 1975.

49. Lorell, B, Alderman, EL, and Mason, JW: *Cardiac sarcoidosis: Diagnosis with endomyocardial biopsy and treatment with corticosteriods.* Am J Cardiol 42:143, 1978.

50. Chew, CYC, Ziady, GM, Raphael, JM, et al: *Primary restrictive cardiomyopathy: Non-tropical endomyocardial fibrosis and hypereosinophilic heart disease.* Br Heart J 39:399, 1981.

51. Matsui, S, Murakami, E, Takekoshi, N, et al: *Cardiac manifestations of Fabry's disease: Report of a case with pulmonary regurgitation diagnosed on the basis of endomyocardial biopsy findings.* Jpn Circ J 41:1023, 1977.

52. Jones, RN, Peyton, RB, Sabina, RL, et al: *Transmural gradient in high-energy phosphate content in patients with coronary artery disease.* Ann Thorac Surg 32:546, 1981.

53. Schultheiss, HP, Bolte, HD, and Cyran, J: *Lactic dehydrogenase isoenzyme pattern in myocardial biopsies of patients with congestive cardiomyopathy and with alcoholic cardiomyopathy—clinical and experimental results.* In Bolte, HD (ed): *Myocardial Biopsy. Diagnostic Significance.* Springer-Verlag, Berlin, 1980.

54. Peters, TJ, Brooksby, IAB, Webb-Peploe, MM, et al: *Enzymic analysis of cardiac biopsy material from patients with valvular heart disease.* Lancet 1:269, 1976.

55. Peters, TJ, Wells, G, Oakley, CM, et al: *Enzymic analysis of endomyocardial biopsy specimens from patients with cardiomyopathies.* Br Heart J 39:1333, 1977.

56. Barrie, SE, Saad, EA, Ubatuba, S, et al: *Myocardial enzyme activities in congestive cardiomyopathy.* Res Commun Chem Pathol Pharmacol 23:375, 1979.

57. Belfrange, P, Johanson, BW, Torp, A, et al: *Micromethods for analysis of lipids in endomyocardial biopsy specimens.* Acta Med Scand 205:283, 1979.

58. Torp, A: *Special investigations in COCM (congestive cardiomyopathy): Biochemical analysis of cardiac biopsies.* Postgrad Med J 54:494, 1978.

59. Unverferth, DV, Fertel, RH, Altschuld, R, et al: *Biochemical measurements of endomyocardial biopsies.* Cathet Cardiovasc Diagn 7:55, 1981.

60. Fleischer, M, Wippo, W, Themann, H, et al: *Ultrastructural morphometric analysis of human myocardial left ventricles with mitral insufficiency. A comparison with normally loaded and hypertrophied human left ventricles.* Virchows Arch (Pathol Anat) 389:205, 1980.

61. Hess, OM, Scheider, J, Koch, R, et al: *Diastolic function and myocardial structure in patients with myocardial hypertrophy: Special reference to normalized viscoelastic data.* Circulation 63:360, 1981.

62. Schwarz, F, Schaper, J, Becker, V, et al: *Coronary collateral vessels: Their significance for left ventricular histologic structure.* Am J Cardiol 49:291, 1982.

63. Stinson, EB and Billingham, ME: *Correlative study of regional left ventricular histology and contractile function.* Am J Cardiol 39:378, 1977.

64. Storstein, L: *Studies on digitalis: X. Digitoxin metabolites in human myocardium and relationship between myocardial and serum concentrations of digitoxin in patients on maintenance treatment.* Clin Pharmacol Ther 21:395, 1976.

65. Kates, RE and Jaillon, P: *A model to describe myocardial drug disposition in the dog.* J Pharm Exp Ther 214:31, 1980.

66. Bristow, MR, Ginsburg, R, Minobe, W, et al: *Decreased catecholamine sensitivity and beta-adrenergic-receptor density in failing human hearts.* N Engl J Med 307:205, 1980.

67. Laser, JA and Bristow, MR: Unpublished data, 1983.

68. Fowles, RE, Bieber, CP, and Stinson, EB: *Defective in vitro suppressor cell function in idiopathic congestive cardiomyopathy.* Circulation 59:483, 1979.

69. Jacobs, B, Matsude, Y, Deodhar, S, et al: *Cell-mediated cytotoxicity to cardiac cells of lymphocytes from patients with primary myocardial disease.* Am J Clin Pathol 72:1, 1979.

Evaluation of Valvular Heart Disease by Invasive Methods

Mary E. Fontana, M.D., and Richard P. Lewis, M.D.

Invasive evaluation is indispensable in the management of patients with valvular heart disease. St. John Sutton attempted to justify that catheterization studies were not necessary before performing valvular surgery,[1] but the vast majority of cardiologists share Roberts's view that hemodynamic-angiographic evaluation is essential for optimum management of patients with valvular heart disease.[2] Catheterization studies (1) allow accurate diagnosis of all valvular lesions and their severity; (2) identify coexisting types of heart disease, such as coronary artery disease, myocardial or pericardial disease, and congenital heart disease; (3) avoid unexpected findings at surgery; (4) provide baseline data for comparison with postoperative data; (5) help decide what surgical approach or procedure is best; (6) give prognostic information to help better define the natural (or rather, unnatural, since the advent of surgery) history of valvular heart lesions.

The extent of an invasive procedure is determined by careful clinical evaluation of each patient and can range from flow-directed balloon-tipped catheterization of the right heart with thermodilution outputs[3,4] to multiple approach right and left heart catheterization with fluid-filled and micromanometer catheters, with shunt detection, cardiac output determinations, intracardiac sound recordings, multiple angiography, myocardial biopsy, drug administration, and even therapeutic procedures such as balloon valvuloplasty, which has recently been reported.[5] Electrophysiologic evaluation also may be needed if tachydysrhythmias or bradydysrhythmias complicate the clinical picture and might require additional surgical procedures, such as bypass tract division or pacemaker insertion. The use of noninvasive evaluation by electrocardiogram (ECG), chest x-ray, echocardiography, systolic time intervals, Holter monitoring, and radionuclide angiography is important for the design and proper timing of the catheterization procedure, but these tests do not replace carefully done hemodynamic studies. Most patients with valvular heart disease will require baseline measurements of right and left heart pressures, cardiac output determinations, valvular gradient measurements, and cineangiography for definition of valve anatomy and dysfunction and analysis of ventricular function and mass. Because long-term followup of patients with valvular heart disease implicates ventricular function as a major determinant of survival and functional improvement,[6–18] analysis of ventricular function by quantitative volume, ejection fraction, and mass determinations is of prime importance. The use of 30° right anterior oblique (RAO), biplane posteroanterior and lateral, or biplane right and left anterior oblique (LAO) projections, with or without cranial-caudal angulation, for ventricular analysis are all accepted techniques.[19–26] The area-length method for determining volumes from RAO cineangiograms is used most commonly. Quantitation of right ventricular function by angiographic techniques has been far less precise, primarily because the right ventricle does not resemble any geometric figure for which a volume formula is available. Radionuclide angiography appears to be the most useful technique for assessing right ventricular function. Computer analysis allows easy calculation of many parameters of ventricular function; so further advances in this area will surely be forthcoming.

Cardiac output measurements may be performed by indicator dilution, thermodilution, Fick, or angiographic methods. Indicator curves (generally with indocyanine green) are easily performed and calculated (by hand or by computer) and are satisfactory in most cases. However, the presence of significant left heart valvular regurgitation, a huge left atrium, very low cardiac output, or coexisting shunt may interfere with accurate measurements owing to curve distortion. Thermodilution outputs are not useful in the presence of right heart valvular regurgitation and do not reflect left heart output if a left-to-right shunt is present. The Fick method is generally most accurate if collections are made properly, especially in low output situations, but requires more time and equipment to perform and is difficult to do in patients with resting dyspnea. Angiographic outputs should be calculated from several beats and are not valid in the presence of an irregular rhythm, for example, atrial dysrhythmia or ventricular ectopy.

We routinely use hydrogen inhalation for shunt detection in all patients having right heart catheterization in our laboratories and have found unsuspected left-to-right shunts in 1 percent of patients.[27] Over one half of these patients have valvular heart disease, especially mitral valve disease. Although most of the shunts are small, their presence occasionally has surgical implications.

Clinical symptoms may not match the baseline hemodynamic measurements in patients with valvular heart disease, especially in patients with mitral valve disease, in elderly patients, and in patients who have been excessively diuresed or who have had prolonged hospitalizations prior to catheterization studies. Interventions during catheterization then become essential to assess the true hemodynamic significance of the patient's problem. Exercise testing, cardiac pacing, drug administration, and post-angiographic or volume infusion pressure measurements will greatly enhance the value of a catheterization study. To not use these techniques can be a great disservice to a patient, particularly if a surgical decision is involved.

Intracardiac sound recordings are considered a luxury by many, because of the expense of the catheters, the extra time added to the procedure, and the lesser influence on decision-making compared with other standard catheterization techniques. We find intracardiac sound studies extremely useful in the evaluation of right-sided regurgitant lesions, as well as unexplained murmurs.[28,29]

The inclusion of coronary arteriography in the evaluation of patients with valvular heart disease depends on the patient's symptoms, age, and ventricular function. Most patients over age 40 should have coronary arteriography even in the absence of symptoms. Patients with chest pain and patients with abnormalities of ventricular function should have their coronary arteries investigated routinely.

The following discussions concern considerations in the evaluation of individual valvular lesions.

MITRAL STENOSIS

The cornerstone in the evaluation of mitral stenosis (MS) is the measurement of the gradient across the mitral valve, generally by simultaneously recording pulmonary capillary wedge or left atrial pressure and left ventricular pressure. Cardiac output measurements must also be done as closely as possible to and under the same conditions as the gradient measurement, so that the severity of MS can be assessed. The Gorlin formula is usually used to calculate mitral valve area.[30,31] Valve area of 1.5 cm^2 or less generally dictates surgery.

Inasmuch as patients with mitral stenosis usually have exertional dyspnea, reflecting left atrial pressure elevation with stress, resting hemodynamic measurements may not accurately assess the functional severity.[32,33] Interventions therefore are necessary during catheterization studies in patients with symptoms who have small gradients and normal or modestly elevated

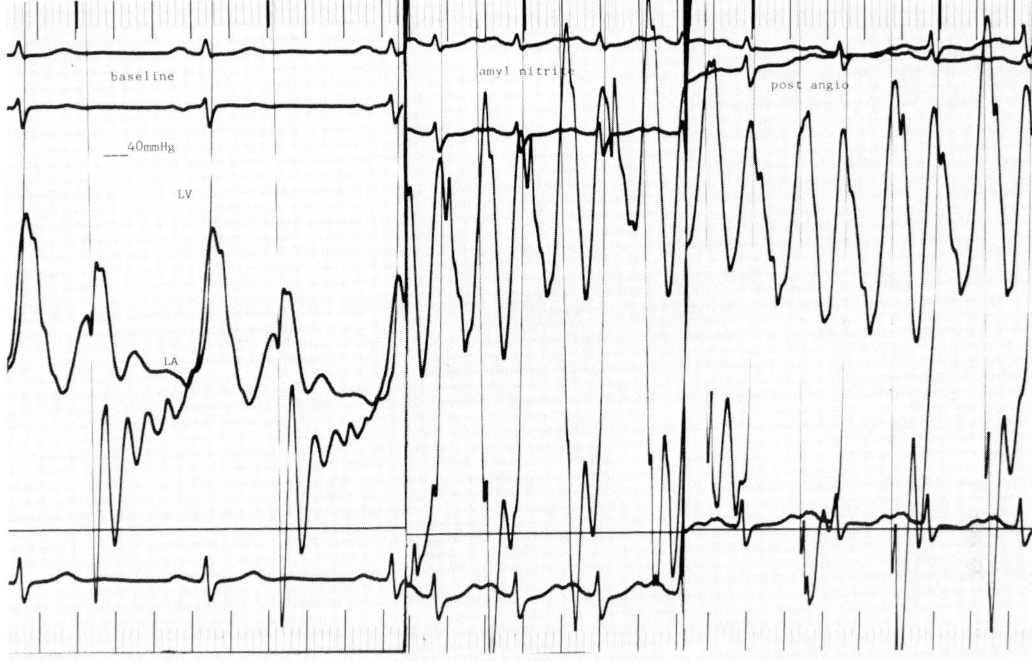

Figure 1. The left panel demonstrates the baseline mitral valve gradient in a patient with mitral stenosis (LA = 18, LVEDP = 14, HR = 61). In the center panel, the gradient is markedly accentuated after inhalation of amyl nitrite (LA = 37, LVEDP = 8, HR = 136). On the right, contrast injection produces a similar response to amyl nitrite, but at a slower heart rate, owing to plasma volume expansion (LA = 36, LVEDP = 8, HR = 120). LA = left atrium, LV = left ventricle.

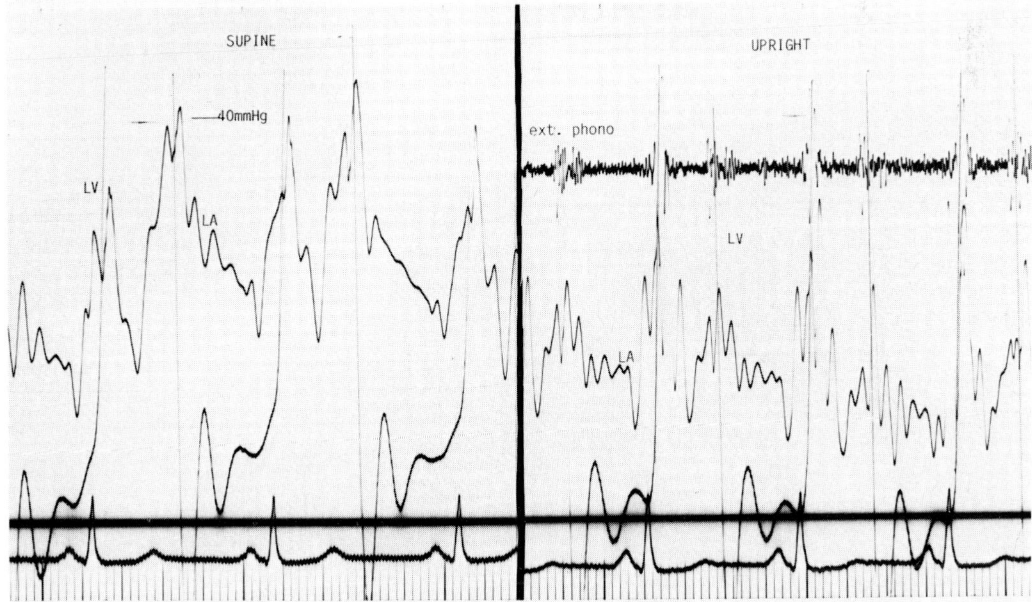

Figure 2. The left panel shows a large mitral gradient with a markedly elevated left atrial pressure in the supine position (LA = 25, LVEDP = 12). The right panel shows a significant drop in left atrial and left ventricular diastolic pressures and mitral gradient in the same patient tilted upright (LA = 16, LV = 2), even though the heart rate is faster, owing to reduction in central blood volume.

pressures at rest. Supine bicycle exercise with gradient and output measurements will produce striking pressure elevations with or without subnormal output responses in many of these patients, confirming the need for surgery. Atrial pacing can increase the gradient by reducing diastolic filling time. Inhalation of amyl nitrite produces a reflex tachycardia and will exaggerate the mitral valve gradient in patients with significant mitral stenosis, whereas left atrial and left ventricular end-diastolic pressures will both go down in mild disease. We routinely measure the mitral valve gradient after left ventricular cineangiography (Fig. 1). The plasma volume expansion and tachycardia that result from contrast administration can produce considerable elevation in left atrial pressure with little effect on the left ventricular end-diastolic pressure, resulting in a large mitral gradient.

Some patients will have exaggerated wedge pressure responses during supine bicycle exercise that are greater than would be expected from their symptoms. Upright exercise tolerance may be more relevant than supine exercise in patients with mitral stenosis, owing to lower left atrial pressure when upright (peripheral pooling, smaller central blood volume) (Fig. 2). This fact requires consideration in those patients with more modest degrees of stenosis (mitral valve area 1.5 to 2.0 cm^2). Echocardiography can be used to follow patients with nonsurgical disease to assess valve mobility and thickening and to approximate valve area.

Cineangiography demonstrates the thickness of the leaflets, their mobility, presence or absence of calcification, thickened chordae, distortion of ventricular anatomy, and the narrowing of the front of nonopacified blood entering the left ventricle (Fig. 3).[34] Although the 30° RAO left ventricular cineangiogram shows many of these features well, a left ventricular injection in the 60° LAO projection is very useful in assessing the mobility of the anterior leaflet of the mitral valve and in actually visualizing the orifice of the mitral valve (Fig. 4).

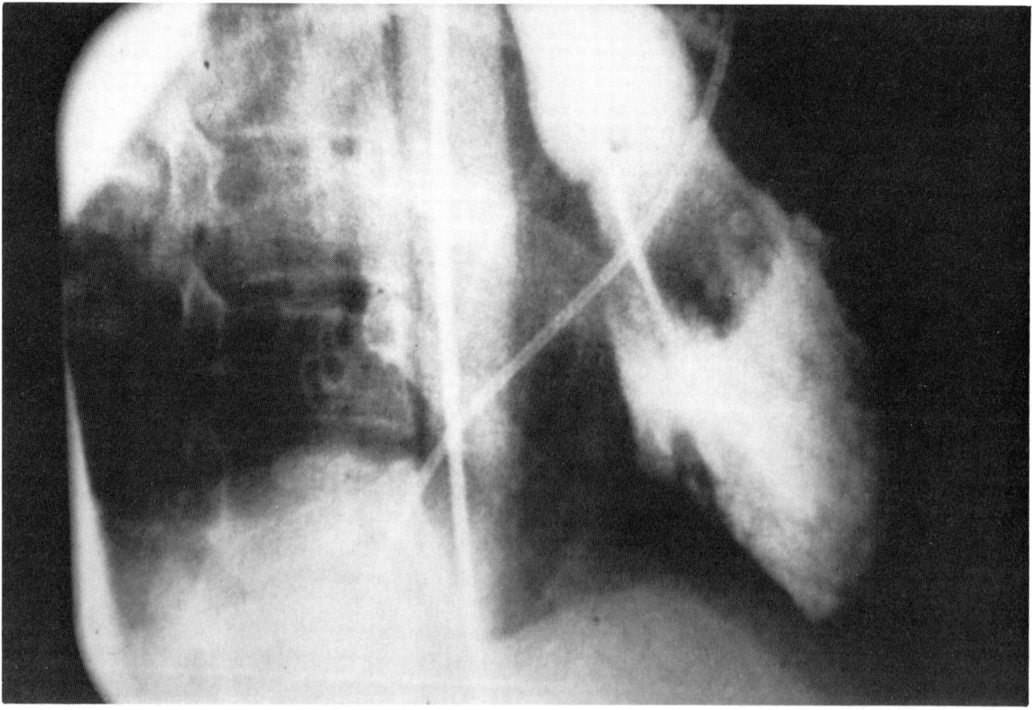

Figure 3. Thirty degree RAO left ventricular cineangiogram in a patient with mitral stenosis. The thickened, mobile, mitral leaflet complex descends into the ventricle in diastole. The posteromedial papillary muscle is pulled into the left ventricular cavity by thick, shortened chordae tendineae. No distinct filling wave from the left atrium is seen, suggesting severe stenosis.

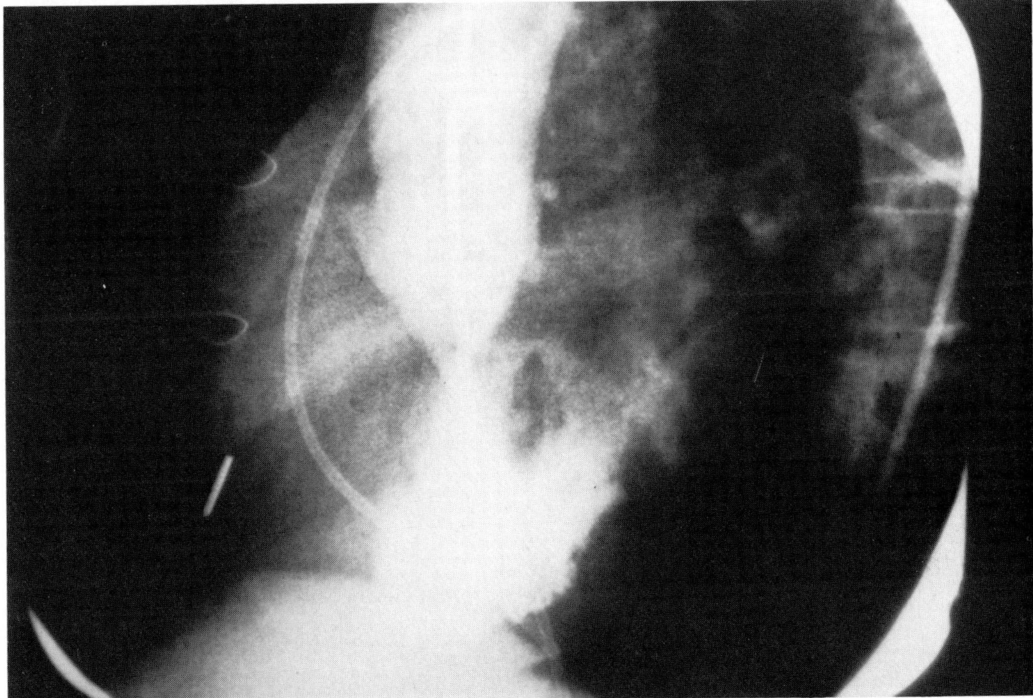

Figure 4. Diastolic frame from a 60° LAO left ventricular injection in a patient with mitral stenosis. The curved interface protruding into the LV outflow tract is formed by the mobile anterior mitral leaflet. The "fishmouth" orifice of the stenotic valve is clearly seen.

This technique is particularly important when coexisting lesions that cause elevation of left ventricular end-diastolic pressure—such as aortic valve disease, myocardial disease, or pericardial disease—are present, inasmuch as the mitral gradient will be minimized under such a condition. A serious underestimation of the severity of the stenosis could result if only hemodynamic measurements were made without cineangiography.

MITRAL REGURGITATION

The findings at catheterization in mitral regurgitation depend upon the duration of the lesion, the size of the left atrium and ventricle, the left ventricular function, and the volume status of the patient when studied. Again, careful pressure and output measurements with angiographic evaluation are all necessary. The left atrial pressure will show prominent V waves in severe mitral regurgitation when the left atrium is mild to moderately enlarged, as is usually the case in patients with acute mitral valve disruption. These patients are often very dyspneic and may require emergency studies if they cannot be stabilized. Balloon-tipped catheterization is often done at the bedside. Finding large V waves in the left atrial pressure pulse is not specific for mitral regurgitation, inasmuch as any situation where left atrial compliance is reduced or excessive volume overload of the left atrium occurs (for example, ventricular septal defect, pulmonary edema) can produce large V waves.[35] The converse is also important—the V waves will be unimpressive even with severe mitral regurgitation if the left atrium is large, as in chronic mitral regurgitation. Also, the V wave will be small in volume depletion, which is often present in elderly patients and in patients who have been diuresed excessively (often not clinically recognized). We find it very valuable to measure wedge pres-

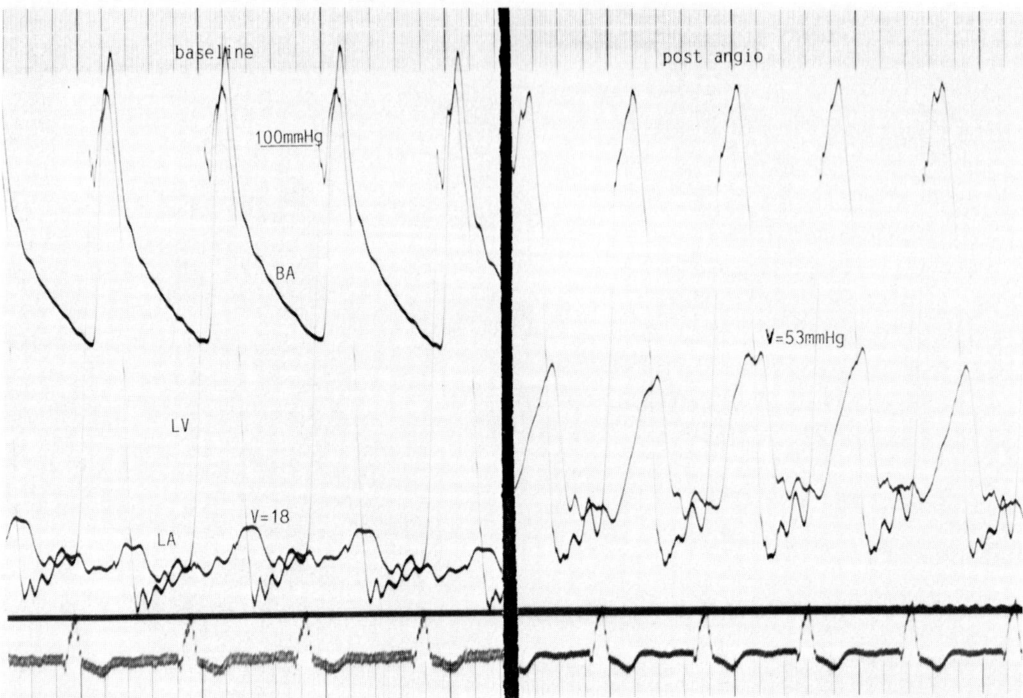

Figure 5. The left panel shows the left heart pressures in an elderly lady who was vigorously diuresed before catheterization studies. The left atrial pressure is low with a normal V wave. After LV cineangiography, large V waves characteristic of severe mitral regurgitation are clearly seen. The cineangiogram showed severe mitral regurgitation.

sure after left ventricular cineangiography in these patients, looking for the large V wave and elevated left atrial pressure that can confirm hemodynamically significant mitral regurgitation (Fig. 5).

Indicator dilution cardiac outputs may be so distorted by regurgitation and a large left atrium that accurate output measurements cannot be made by this technique. Right-sided thermodilution outputs or Fick outputs are more desirable in this setting.

Left ventricular cineangiography demonstrates the severity of the regurgitation, graded primarily according to the relative concentration of contrast in the left atrium and left ventricle (Table 1)(Fig. 6).[36–39] The degree of regurgitation can be underestimated if the left ventricle is large and/or poorly functioning, and/or the left atrium is very large, due to dilution of the contrast media.[40] Measurement of a regurgitant fraction by comparing actual left ventricular stroke volume from quantitative cineangiographic volume measurements with peripheral cardiac output measurements (Fick, indicator, thermodilution) is useful in assessing severity;[38] regurgitant fractions in excess of 50 percent denote severe regurgitation. All outputs must be determined under the same conditions, and the rhythm must be regular during angiography to make regurgitant fraction calculations useful. A variety of techniques using indicators are also available for quantitating regurgitation, but all have limitations, just as angiographic regurgitant fraction does.[41] Obtaining good data on the amount of regurgitation is essential; further technical developments are needed. Determination of left ventricular volumes and ejection fraction is necessary, inasmuch as it has been shown that surgical mortality and long-term survival are closely related to left ventricular function.[6–8] Thirty degree RAO and 60° LAO or left lateral left ventricular cineangiography with or without angulation are used to assess ventricular size and function and to define the anatomy of the

Table 1. Angiographic quantitation of valvular regurgitation

Mitral Regurgitation	*Aortic Regurgitation*
+ mild LA opacification; clears rapidly, often jet-like	+ small regurgitant jet only; LV ejects contrast each systole
++ moderate LA opacification, less than LV	++ regurgitant jet faintly opacifies LV cavity; not cleared each systole
+++ diffuse contrast regurgitation; LA opacification = LV; LA significantly enlarged*	+++ persistent LV opacification = aortic root density; LV enlargement*
++++ LA opacification > LV, persistent; systolic pulmonary vein opacification may occur; often marked LA enlargement*	++++ persistent LV opacification > aortic root concentration; often marked LV enlargement*

*chronic regurgitation
LA = left atrium
LV = left ventricle

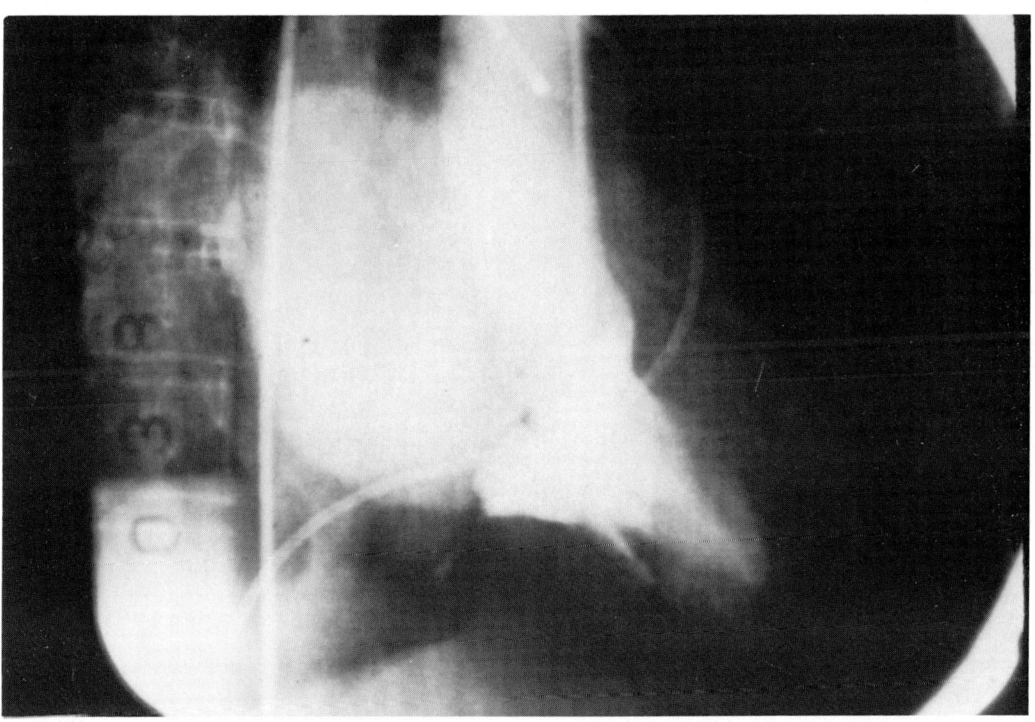

Figure 6. A left ventricular cineangiogram in the 30° RAO projection demonstrating the thickened, prolapsing posterior mitral leaflet and marked left atrial enlargement. The contrast density is equal in left atrium and left ventricle, denoting 3+ mitral regurgitation.

mitral valve, particularly mitral valve prolapse, which is now clearly the most common cause of mitral regurgitation in patients requiring valve replacement (see Figure 6).[26,42] In patients with significant mitral regurgitation (3 or 4+) and reduced left ventricular function (ejection fraction <40 percent), it can be very difficult to decide if the regurgitation is the cause of or the result of the poor left ventricular function. Ventricles of greater than twice normal end-diastolic volume are likely the cause of mitral regurgitation. Drug interventions with afterload reducing agents can be useful in evaluating this group of patients to aid in therapeutic decisions.

AORTIC STENOSIS

Every patient with cardiac symptoms who has findings on clinical examination to suggest aortic stenosis should have catheterization studies performed. Noninvasive tests such as systolic time intervals and echocardiography can effectively exclude aortic stenosis but are less reliable in assessing severity. Invasive evaluation of aortic stenosis requires measurement of the valve gradient and cardiac output along with cineangiographic assessment of left ventricular function, mass and valve anatomy. The gradient should be measured from simultaneous left ventricular and aortic or peripheral artery (brachial or femoral) pressures using planimetry (Fig. 7). A gradient determined from a pullback from left ventricle to aorta can be

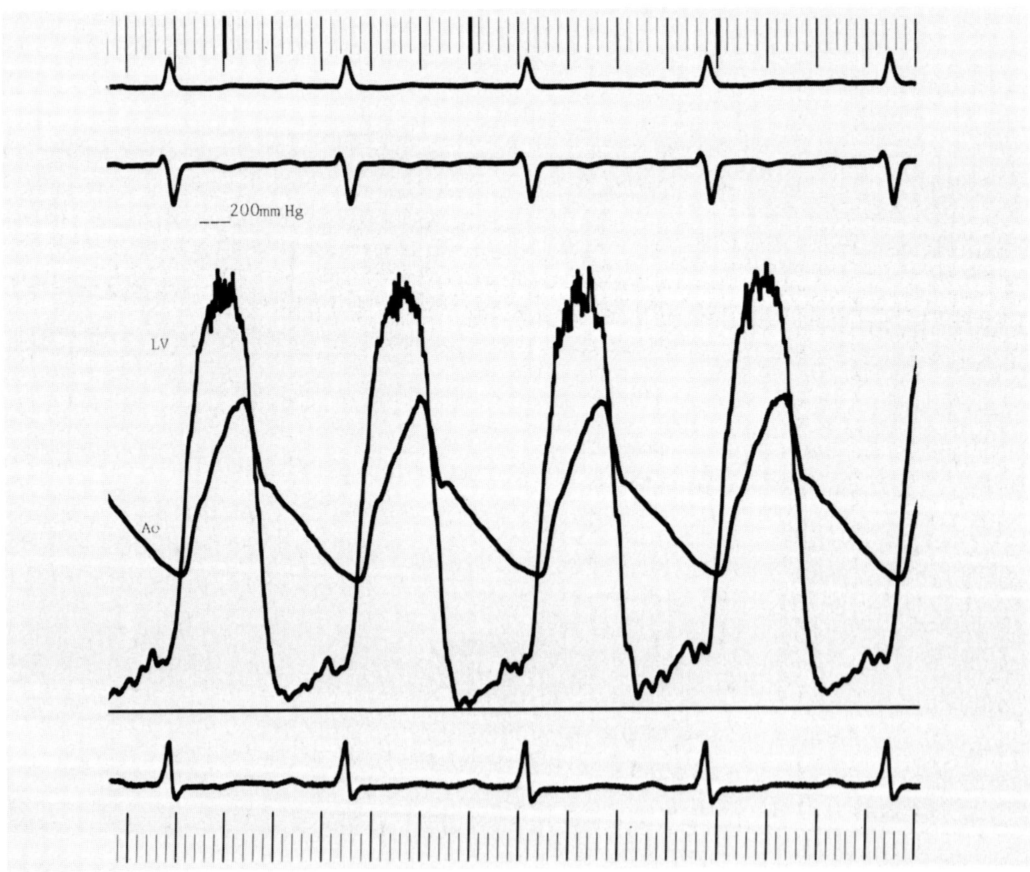

Figure 7. Simultaneous left ventricular (LV) and aortic (Ao) pressure pulses in a patient with calcific aortic stenosis. The aortic pressure pulse shows the slow upstroke; the gradient is planimetered and equals 54 mm Hg. The LV pressure pulse is distorted by catheter vibration from the high velocity jet crossing the stenotic valve.

used, but it is not simultaneous and is invalid in the presence of an irregular rhythm or atrio-ventricular dissociation (for example, ventricular pacing). Cardiac output measurements must be made as close to and under identical conditions as the gradient measurement. The aortic valve area is calculated using the Gorlin formula.[30] A valve area of 0.75 cm^2 or less is accepted as an indication for surgery. Patients with left ventricular dysfunction or volume depletion may have small gradients owing to a depressed cardiac output but will still have severe stenosis by valve area calculation. Therefore, valve gradients should always be interpreted in light of the flow across the valve. Elderly patients with atherosclerotic peripheral vessels with or without hypertension may have wide arterial pulse pressures with high systolic pressures. The severity of the stenosis can be underestimated in this situation. Cineangiography in conjunction with clinical and noninvasive evaluation is necessary to evaluate adequately such patients.

The status of the left ventricle is less critical to decision making in aortic stenosis, because the surgical result is often good even with low ejection fractions.[42–44] Selective coronary arteriography is necessary in most patients with aortic stenosis, inasmuch as most adults with symptomatic aortic stenosis are over 40 years of age and chest pain is a common symptom. In markedly symptomatic patients, coronary arteriography should be done before left ventricular or aortic cineangiography, because large contrast loads may precipitate symptoms that may make completion of studies difficult. Inasmuch as these patients will usually have clinical and noninvasive evidence of significant aortic stenosis, completing the evaluation for coronary disease is the most important part of their evaluation, because bypass surgery for

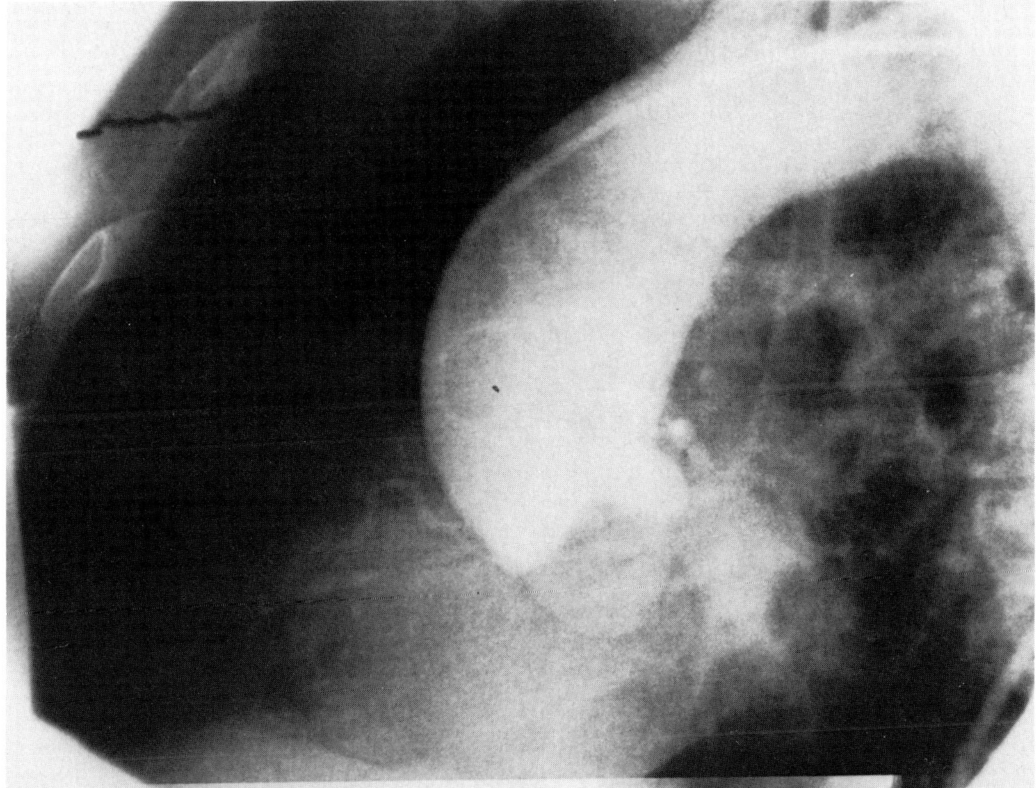

Figure 8. Sixty degree LAO aortic root cineangiogram in a young man with a stenotic bicuspid aortic valve. In this systolic frame, the leaflets "dome" into the aorta, little nonopacified blood enters the aorta, and poststenotic dilatation of the aortic root is seen.

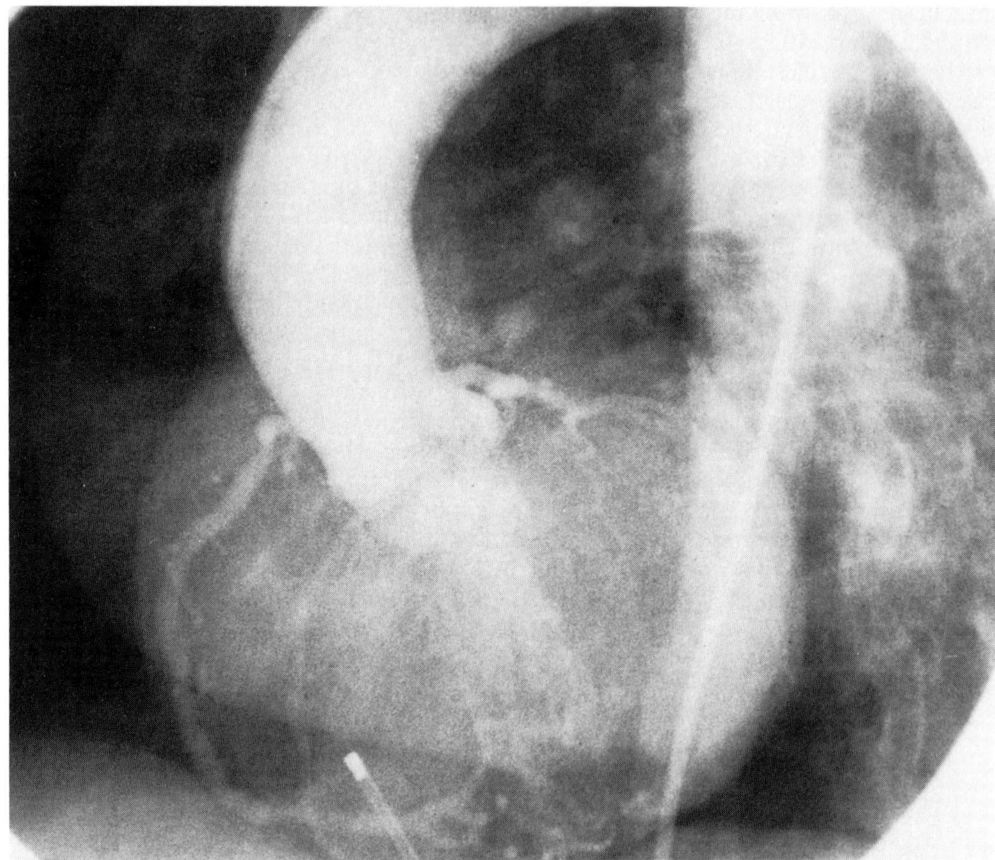

Figure 9. Sixty degree LAO aortic root cineangiogram in a 72-year-old woman with severe degenerative aortic stenosis. The aortic sinuses are symmetrical, the leaflets immobile, thickened, and calcified. The jet entering the aortic root is centrally located, and poststenotic dilatation is absent.

critical lesions should be done at the time of aortic valve replacement.[37] Supravalvular aortic cineangiography performed in the 45° to 60° LAO projection demonstrates the reduced cusp mobility, calcification, and narrow jet entering the aortic root that characterize aortic stenosis. Important information on etiology of the stenosis is also obtained. Cusp assymmetry, "doming" of fused leaflets, varying amounts of commissural calcifications, and poststenotic dilatation of the aortic root characterize congenital aortic stenosis (Fig. 8), whereas rigid cusps with sinus and leaflet calcifications, central orifice, and lack of poststenotic dilatation characterize the degenerative aortic stenosis of the elderly (Fig. 9).[34] Angulated views can be used to enhance the definition of valve anatomy as well.[45]

AORTIC REGURGITATION

The timing of the invasive evaluation of aortic regurgitation is different from many of the other valvular lesions, in that waiting for symptoms may be too late as far as a good surgical result is concerned.[9–15] Any patient with an acute onset of aortic regurgitation or evidence of progressive cardiac enlargement with previously diagnosed aortic regurgitation, even without symptoms, should have careful invasive evaluation to determine the severity of the lesion and the etiology, so that therapeutic decisions can be accurately made.

The invasive evaluation of aortic regurgitation includes baseline pressure measurements, cardiac outputs, and cineangiographic evaluation of left ventricular size and function, aortic valve and aortic root morphology. Coronary arteriography is necessary for patients over 40 years, those with chest pain, or those in whom there is a concern about the integrity of the ostia of the vessels, for example, in syphlitic aortitis or aortic aneurysms.

In chronic, severe aortic regurgitation, elevated systolic pressures in the left ventricle and aorta with a wide aortic pulse pressure, related also to a low diastolic pressure, and absence of the dicrotic notch are generally found. The left ventricular end-diastolic pressure may be normal or elevated. Indicator dilution cardiac output curves can be distorted in severe aortic regurgitation, so the Fick or thermodilution method may be more appropriate. In acute aortic regurgitation, usually in the setting of infective endocarditis or aortic dissection, the hemodynamic picture reflects acute left ventricular volume overload with failure and a high end-diastolic pressure that may nearly equal the aortic diastolic pressure. The aortic pulse pressure will often be normal. The angiocardiographic evaluation is most crucial. A 30° right anterior oblique left ventricular angiogram free of ectopic beats is necessary for the determination of volumes and mass, ejection fraction, and regurgitant fraction.[38] A left lateral or LAO left ventricular cineangiogram may give additional information about left ventricular function. Supravalvular cineangiography in the 45° to 60° LAO position is essential to determine aortic valve and aortic root morphology and to assess the severity of regurgitation. If aortic dissection is suspected, then biplane large film angiography is necessary to define best

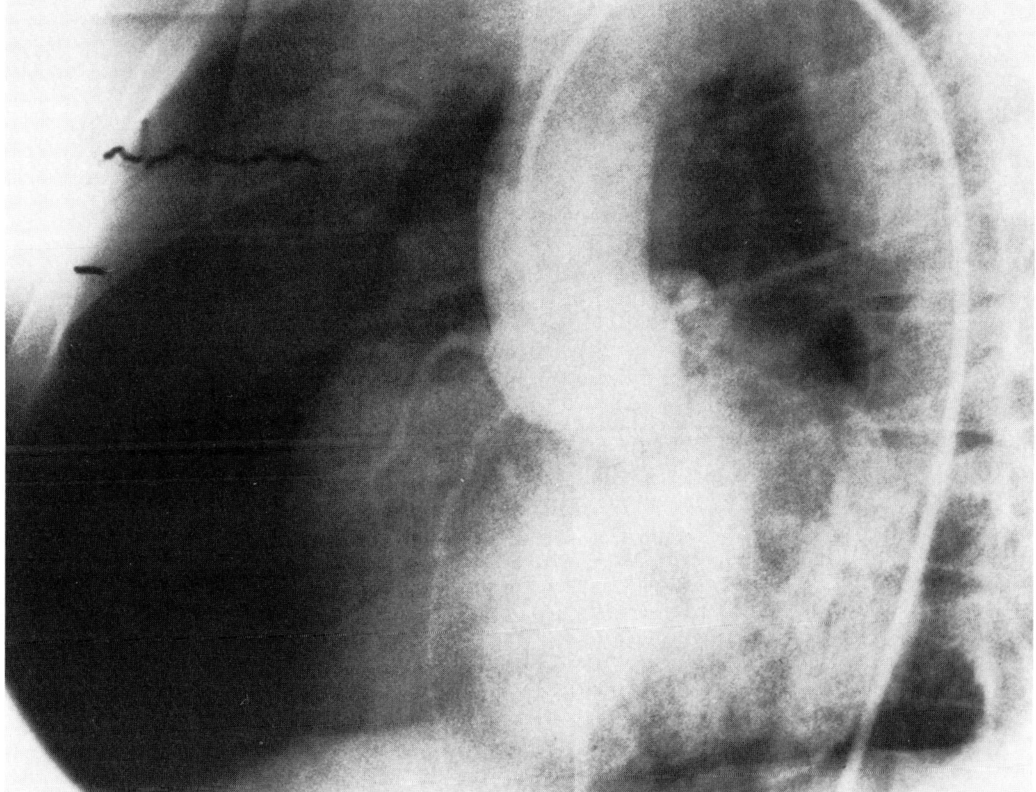

Figure 10. Supravalvular cineangiogram in the 60° LAO projection in a patient with chronic aortic regurgitation demonstrating reflux of contrast into the left ventricle through a trisinus aortic valve. The left ventricular cavity is enlarged. Aortic and left ventricular contrast densities are equal, consistent with 3+ regurgitation.

the extent of the dissection and the compromise of aortic branches. Cineangiography may show the intimal flap of a dissection, but the field is often too restricted to define the total involvement. In infective endocarditis, the left ventricle may be adequately evaluated by an aortic root injection in the 30° RAO projection if the valve is known to have vegetations by echocardiography. There is, however, no significant increase in risk for catheterization studies in endocarditis, and unsuspected pathology important to management is often found.[47]

The severity of regurgitation is determined by relative density of contrast in the aorta and left ventricle (see Table 1) (Fig. 10).[37,38,48] Mild regurgitation is also characterized by the ventricle ejecting the regurgitated volume during the subsequent systole. This applies only if left ventricular function is normal or nearly normal. Because even severe aortic regurgitation can be tolerated for years without symptoms, the determination of left ventricular function and reserve often determines future management—surgical versus medical.[9–15] Evidence of abnormal left ventricular systolic performance dictates the need for surgery. Inasmuch as the optimum time for surgery is likely before resting left ventricular dysfunction occurs, hemodynamic or angiographic measurements during exercise or isometrics may be useful when baseline measurements are normal. Exercise reduces regurgitant flow owing to the induced tachycardia shortening diastole, but systolic pressure elevations are often dramatic, resulting in increased oxygen demand. Elevation of diastolic pressure reflects decreased left ventricular reserve. Systolic left ventricular performance during stress is best evaluated by nuclear techniques. Stress nuclear angiography, along with echocardiography, is becoming more useful in

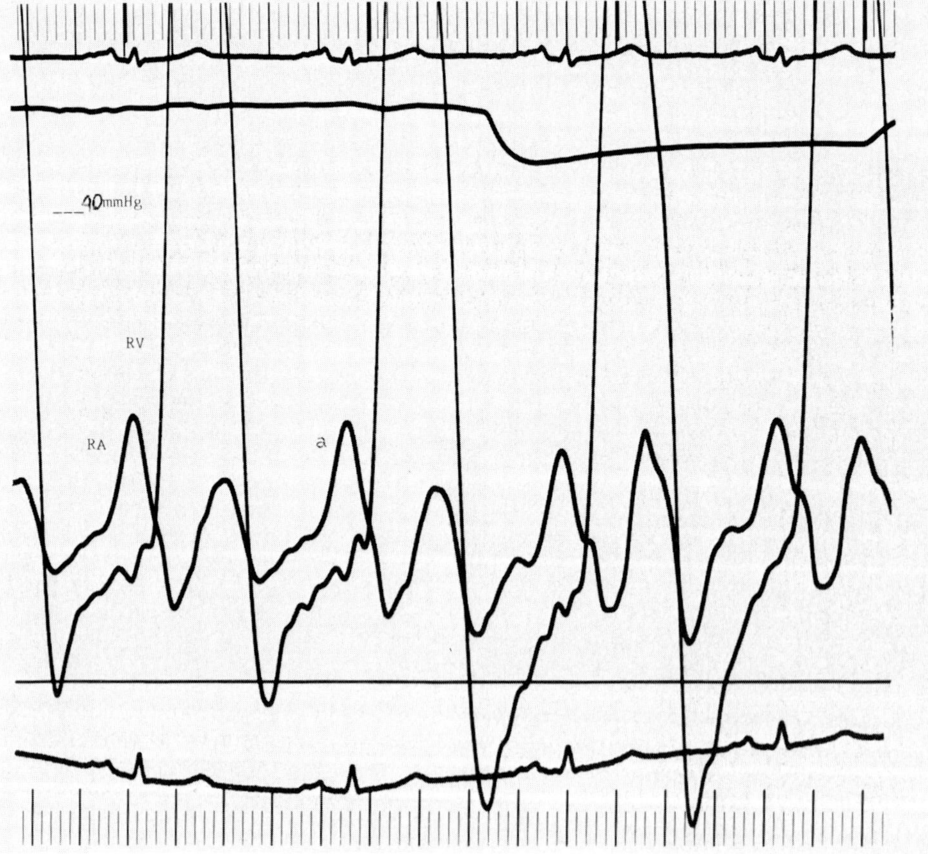

Figure 11. Simultaneous right atrial (RA) and right ventricular (RV) pressure pulses recorded with equisensitive catheters in a patient with tricuspid stenosis, demonstrating a diastolic pressure gradient, particularly prominent during the large "a" wave of the RA pressure pulse.

determining the timing of catheterization studies and surgical intervention in patients with chronic aortic regurgitation. Myocardial biopsy also may be useful in assessing the status of the left ventricle.[49]

TRICUSPID STENOSIS

Tricuspid stenosis (TS) is relatively uncommon compared with aortic and mitral valvular stenosis and is also easy to miss on clinical examination or during catheterization.[50,51] The valve gradient is only a few millimeters, even in severe stenosis, so measurement of the gradient requires simultaneous right atrial and right ventricular pressure measurements using two similar catheters or a double lumen catheter (Fig. 11). A gradient measured by pullback may be detectable in sinus rhythm when the tall spiky "a" wave of TS is easily seen and not transmitted to the ventricle, but it is useless in atrial fibrillation when no "a" wave is present and beat-to-beat variations in pressure occur owing to the irregular R-R intervals. Cardiac output is determined under similar conditions, and valve area is calculated using the Gorlin formula, which has had little pathologic validation in tricuspid stenosis. Valve areas less than 2 cm^2 are significant.

Right atrial cineangiography in the 20° RAO projection demonstrates the thickened, mobile, fused leaflet complex funnelling into the right ventricle in diastole, with a narrowed front of contrast entering the ventricle.[34] We have found that calculating percent tricuspid stenosis from a right atrial cineangiogram accurately reflects the severity of TS determined from pathologic analysis of excised tricuspid valves (Fig. 12).[52] The width of the contrast front entering the right ventricle is used as the height of an equilateral triangle, and the annular sized is used as the diameter of a circle. Annular area − orifice area/annular area yields percent stenosis. Clinically detectable tricuspid stenosis occurs at >75 percent stenosis of the

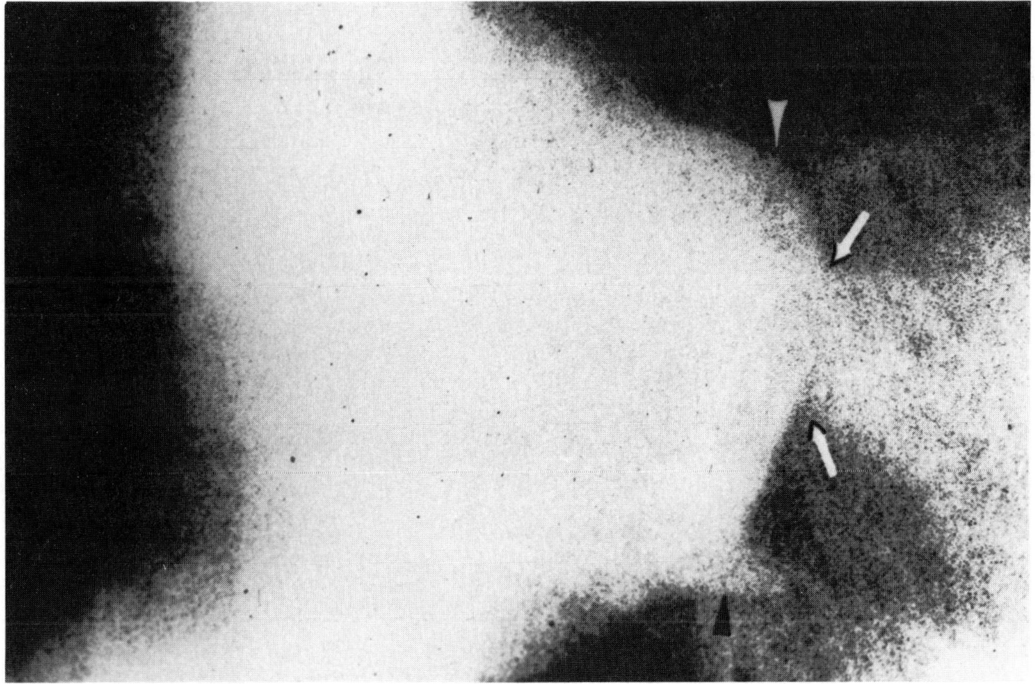

Figure 12. Right atrial cineangiogram in the 20° projection in a patient with severe tricuspid stenosis. The central pair of arrows defines the narrow dye front entering the ventricle. The outer pair of arrows defines the tricuspid annulus. Percent stenosis can be calculated as described in the text.

valve. Right ventricular cineangiography demonstrates the same anatomy as right atrial cineangiography plus the invariable presence of tricuspid regurgitation if the stenosis is severe.[53]

TRICUSPID REGURGITATION

Tricuspid regurgitation can be difficult to document and to quantitate owing to technical factors and the connection of the right atrium to the large, capacitant caval-venous system.[54,55] Measurement of right atrial pressure will demonstrate elevated mean right atrial pressure with prominent C-V waves that increase on inspiration in moderate or severe tricuspid regurgitation. The larger the right atrium, the less impressive the pressure pulse abnormalities. Mild tricuspid regurgitation may produce no pressure pulse abnormalities, even with little right atrial enlargement. Right ventricular pressure measurement is important, in that if it is severely elevated (>60 mm Hg), the regurgitation may be secondary to right ventricular dilatation, whereas if it is low, a structural valve abnormality is more likely.

Indicator injection into the right ventricle with sampling from the right atrium can demonstrate the early appearance of contrast in the right atrium, confirming tricuspid regurgitation; and methods of quantitation using indicator techniques have been developed.[55–57]

Right ventricular cineangiography is essential to demonstrate tricuspid regurgitation but is complicated by the need to have a catheter across the valve. This plus induction of ectopy during contrast injection makes interpretation difficult, especially in mild regurgitation. Using specially preformed catheters, and/or careful attention to positioning the catheter low in the right ventricular inflow tract, and using slow injection rates can avoid these problems.[58] The

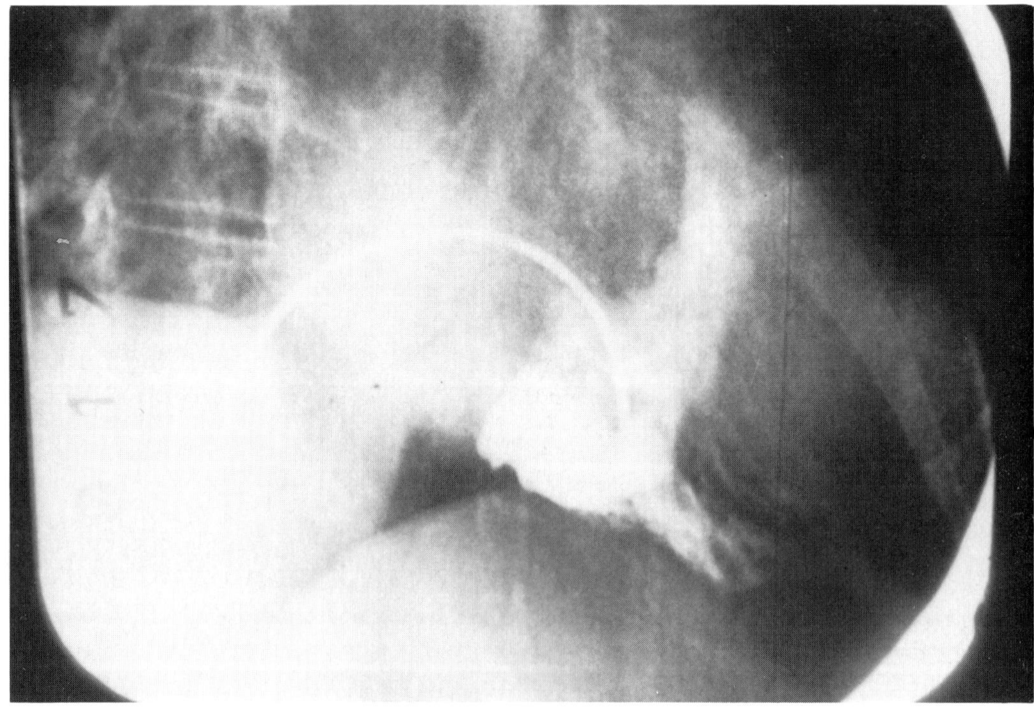

Figure 13. Right ventricular cineangiogram in the 20° RAO projection in a patient with tricuspid valve prolapse with regurgitation. The regurgitant jet enters the atrium inferiorly, below the position of the catheter, eliminating catheter interference as the cause. The right atrium is nearly fully opacified, but the concentration is less than in the right ventricle, constituting mild or 2+ regurgitation.

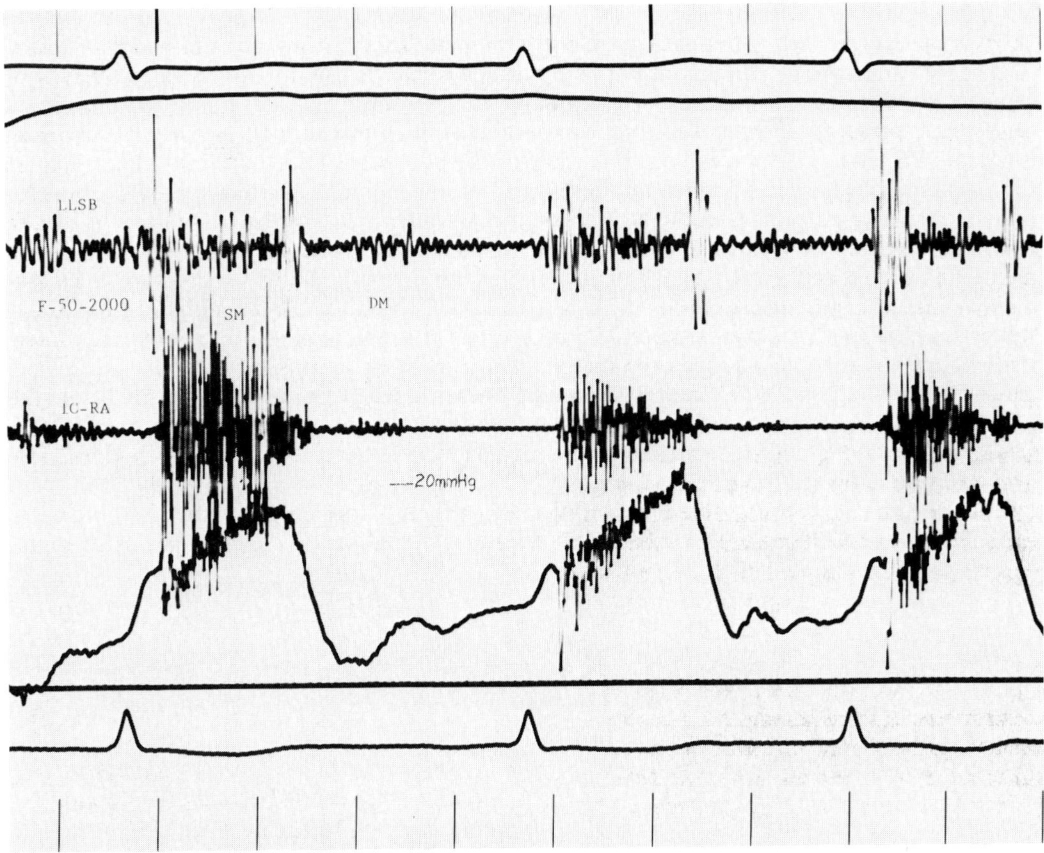

Figure 14. Intracardiac sound and pressure recording from near the tricuspid valve using micromanometer catheter in a patient with severe tricuspid regurgitation. The "ventricularized" right atrial pressure pulse with a large CV wave is seen. The upper sound recording shows the pansystolic murmur of tricuspid regurgitation and diastolic flow rumble recorded externally at the lower left sternal border (LLSB). The intense pansystolic murmur is recorded in the right atrium as well as a soft diastolic flow rumble (2nd line = intracardiac sound).

20° to 30° RAO position is best as it moves the tricuspid valve off the spine, making the valve plane more perpendicular to the imaging plane, thus allowing definition of the valve (for example, prolapsing, thickened). The severity of tricuspid regurgitation angiographically is determined similarly as in mitral regurgitation with the same reservations (Fig. 13). Systolic reflux into the vena cavae denotes severe regurgitation. Echocardiography combined with microbubble injection or Doppler studies can be very helpful in documenting tricuspid regurgitation. Intracardiac sound recordings are particularly useful in tricuspid regurgitation inasmuch as the murmur can be recorded without crossing or interfering with the valve (Fig. 14). The technique is particularly helpful in mild lesions, when angiography is not technically satisfactory, and in demonstrating a diastolic filling rumble in the right ventricle, confirming severe regurgitation.[28,29]

PULMONARY STENOSIS

Valvular pulmonary stenosis (PS) can present as a spectrum ranging from a surgical emergency in a neonate to an asymptomatic murmur in older children and adults. Catheterization studies are necessary to assess the severity of obstruction and the presence of coexisting lesions. Right heart catheterization with measurement of the pressure gradient across the valve is necessary, with a pullback gradient commonly used. In infants and small children, formal measurement of cardiac output as described earlier is usually not done, so severity of stenosis is judged by the degree of right ventricular pressure elevation, absolute and related to systemic pressure. In mild PS, right ventricular systolic pressure is less than 50 mm Hg; moderate PS, 50 to 100 mm Hg or up to systemic levels; severe PS, >100 mm Hg or greater than systemic.[59] This classification implies normal or low pulmonary artery pressures. In older patients, cardiac output is routinely measured and valve area can be calculated using the Gorlin formula.[30] A valve area of ≤ 1 cm^2 corresponds to the moderate or severe classification mentioned above and generally dictates the need for surgery. Pullback pressure measurements across the pulmonary outflow tract must be done carefully to determine if infundibular stenosis is also present. Intracardiac ECG recordings at the time of pullback may help define the level of obstruction: a more prominent R wave or R′ appearing as the valve is crossed, and greater voltage with a dominant S wave appearing when the catheter drops below the infundibulum. Exercise testing during catheterization is of value in borderline cases of PS. Marked elevation of right ventricular pressures and/or a subnormal cardiac output response with exercise indicates the need for surgery.[60–62]

Routine shunt detection should be performed (oximetry, foreign gas inhalation, indicator curves) because of the possible coexistence of a shunt (atrial septal defect, ventricular septal defect, patent foramen ovale).

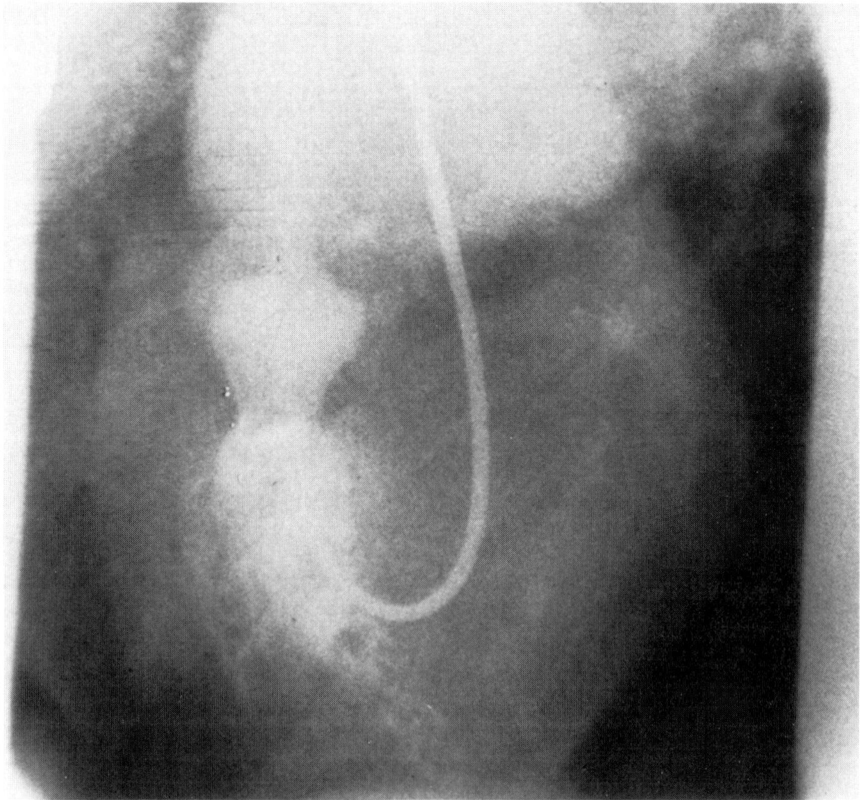

Figure 15. A left lateral cineangiogram in a patient with valvular pulmonary stenosis demonstrating the thickened leaflets "doming" toward the pulmonary artery in systole and the narrow jet of contrast crossing the valve, opacifying a dilated main pulmonary artery.

Right ventricular cineangiography in the posteroanterior and lateral projections will demonstrate the anatomy of the valve, infundibulum, and proximal pulmonary arteries (Fig. 15).[34] The systolic "doming" of the thickened, fused leaflets, the narrowed jet entering the pulmonary artery, and the poststenotic dilatation of the main and proximal left pulmonary artery all characterize typical congenital valvular pulmonary stenosis.

PULMONARY REGURGITATION

The evaluation of pulmonary regurgitation requires right heart catheterization with measurement of pressures and cineangiography. In low pressure pulmonary regurgitation from an abnormal valve, absent valve, or dilated valve ring, both pulmonary artery and right ventricular systolic pressures will be low, and pulmonary artery and right ventricular diastolic pressures will tend to equilibrate. In severe pulmonary hypertension, no pressure pulse abnormalities may be present to distinguish the presence or absence of pulmonary regurgitation. Cardiac outputs by thermodilution and indicator dilution with pulmonary artery injection will be distorted by the regurgitation; Fick outputs or indicator injection at a more distal site are preferred. Indicator techniques can be used for detection of pulmonary regurgitation as in

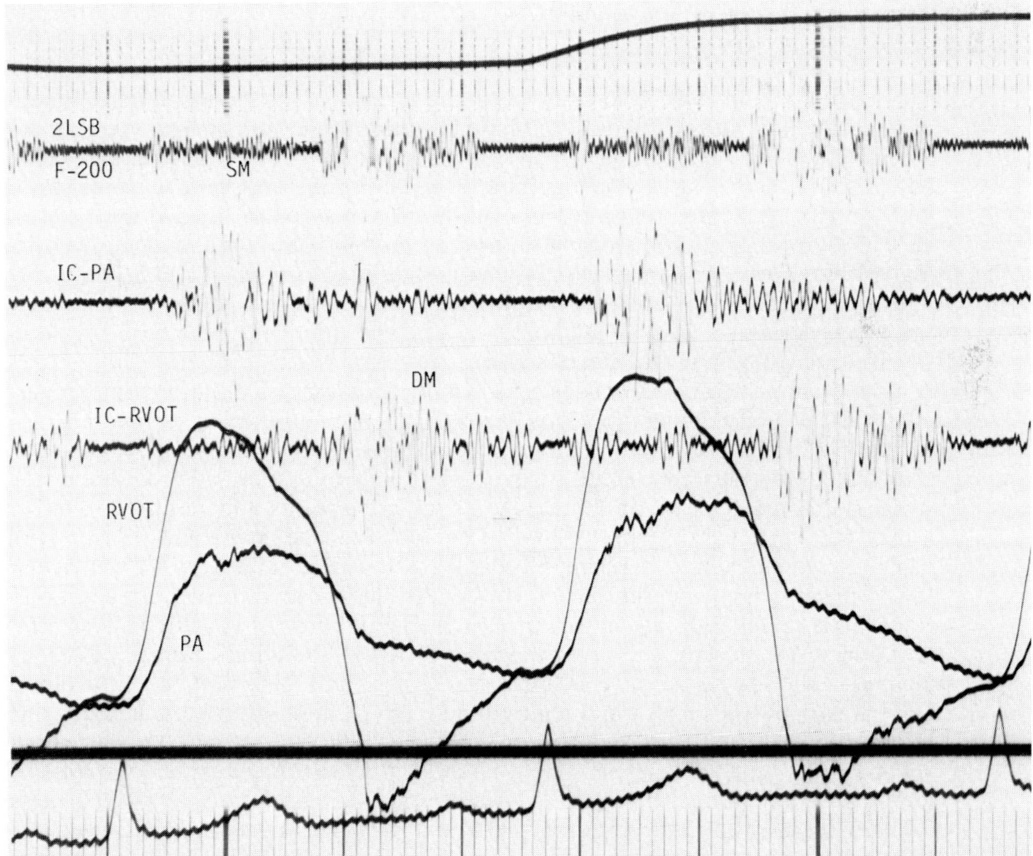

Figure 16. Congenital pulmonary regurgitation in a young man. From top to bottom: External phonocardiogram from the 2nd intercostal space, left sternal border (2LSB) showing a soft systolic murmur and crescendo-decrescendo diastolic mumur; intracardiac (IC) phono from pulmonary artery (PA) with ejection murmur; IC phono from right ventricular outflow tract (RVOT) showing diastolic murmur (DM) of pulmonary regurgitation; micromanometer pressures from the RVOT and PA showing equilibration in diastole. A small (~10 mm Hg) pressure gradient is present across the pulmonary valve.

other regurgitant lesions.[57] Technically good cineangiography is difficult in pulmonary regurgitation owing to the catheter being across the valve, rapid systolic emptying of pulmonary artery, and potential for catheter recoil with the high flow rates of injection usually necessary for good opacification.[63] Intracardiac sound and pressure studies are valuable, demonstrating the crescendo-decrescendo diastolic murmur in the right ventricular outflow tract or just below it in low pressure pulmonary regurgitation (Fig. 16), or the high-pitched decrescendo diastolic murmur of high pressure pulmonary regurgitation.[28,29,64] Doppler echocardiography may be useful in the noninvasive detection of pulmonary regurgitation.

COMBINED VALVULAR DISEASE

The symptomatic patient with multivalvular disease requires more complete catheterization studies with right and left heart pressure measurements, cardiac output measurements, and cineangiography as described for the individual lesions. Even carefully done studies with measurement of appropriate gradients, flows, and angiography may not accurately assess the severity of the individual valve lesions. A high index of suspicion, in addition to objective data, in the evaluation of each patient is necessary, because if planned surgery does not correct all significant lesions, the result will be unsatisfactory. In some cases, direct inspection of the valve at surgery will be necessary to ascertain need for repair or replacement. Important considerations in the invasive evaluation of multivalvular disease include the following:

(1) The most proximal valve lesion may mask the severity of more distal lesions. Examples include: (a) Mitral stenosis may limit cardiac output, diminishing the gradient across a stenotic aortic valve. Valve area calculation may indicate significant obstruction nonetheless. Aortic regurgitation may be underestimated in similar fashion. (b) The gradient across a stenotic aortic valve may be minimized by the presence of mitral regurgitation, owing to the regurgitated volume reducing left ventricular output. The same applies to pulmonary stenosis with tricuspid regurgitation. (c) Tricuspid stenosis will "protect" the pulmonary circuit in coexisting mitral stenosis (invariably present), so that pulmonary artery and pulmonary capillary pressures will be lower than in mitral stenosis alone.

(2) A distal stenotic lesion will enhance the hemodynamic severity of a proximal regurgitant lesion. For example, in aortic stenosis, mitral regurgitation can be manifest by high left atrial pressure with large V waves and be angiographically significant, even though the valve is structurally intact. The increased afterload produced by the stenosis, combined with left ventricular dilatation, which could result from either lesion, produces these findings. Surgical decisions can be very difficult, even with complete hemodynamic-angiographic data, inasmuch as influences on ventricular function and hemodynamics of each valve individually cannot be determined.

(3) Valve area calculations are inaccurate when combinations of stenotic and regurgitant lesions are present, because calculation of actual flow across a given valve may be impossible. The aortic valve area in aortic stenosis and regurgitation, or the mitral valve area in mitral stenosis and regurgitation, can be approximated if angiographic left ventricular output can be determined.[65] Not to take into account the regurgitant volume will result in underestimation of the valve area. Right heart combination lesions are more difficult to evaluate owing to the lack of firmly established criteria for normal right ventricular volumes and function, such as exist for the left ventricle.

(4) Elevation of diastolic pressure in the ventricle as a result of distal semilunar valve disease, diastolic dysfunction of the ventricle, or pericardial disease can lead to serious underestimation of atrioventricular valve stenosis by minimizing the measured gradient. Angiographic assessment of the valve is crucial in this setting.

(5) When two regurgitant lesions are present (for example, aortic and mitral regurgitation), quantitation of regurgitant fraction will represent the total regurgitation for

both valves. Assessing the severity of each lesion individually is difficult. Again, analysis of all invasive and noninvasive data is necessary in reaching conclusions.

(6) Combined aortic stenosis and regurgitation is worse than either lesion alone, owing to the presence of both pressure and volume loads on the left ventricle. The quantitation of each lesion may well be less than the usual surgical criteria for each lesion, but the ventricle will usually show considerable enlargement, markedly increased mass, and/or reduced systolic function as a result of the combined workload. Parameters of left ventricular function are therefore important in therapeutic decision-making.

(7) The presence of coronary artery disease in patients with aortic stenosis and/or regurgitation with markedly increased left ventricular mass will produce symptoms earlier than in any condition without increased left ventricular mass. The coronary arteries are often very large and carry high flows in these patients. A 50 percent lesion may have enough influence on flow to cause symptoms, but the cross-sectional area at the point of stenosis may be similar to that of a normal artery. Therefore, correction of the valve lesion with resultant regression of hypertrophy and coronary size will render the lesion insignificant. Lesions with $\geq$75 percent obstruction generally require bypass. In contrast to the situation with increased mass, severe coronary obstruction ($\geq$75 percent) may produce no symptoms in patients with valvular disease with decreased left ventricular work, for example, mitral stenosis. Angina may appear when left ventricular preload is increased by mitral valve surgery, if bypasses are not performed at the same time.

SUMMARY

The need for and the design of invasive procedures in patients with valvular heart disease should be based on the careful evaluation of the patient with history, physical examination, and appropriate noninvasive testing. The number of parameters measured, angiograms performed, and interventions performed during catheterization is determined by the suspected pathology and the clinical status of the patient. The ability to amend the planned sequence and number of measurements as the study progresses must be preserved, so that the most useful data to be used in patient management can be obtained. Knowledge of the limitations as well as the advantages of each technique is necessary to obtain the most accurate data and to interpret the results obtained. It must be recognized that invasive procedures will not always answer all the questions and, in fact, may raise new ones. They are, however, an indispensible part of the evaluation of patients with valvular heart disease, as most surgical and many medical decisions cannot be made without them.

REFERENCES

1. St John Sutton, MG, St John Sutton, M, Oldershaw, P, et al: *Valve replacement without preoperative cardiac catheterization.* N Engl J Med 305:1233, 1981.
2. Roberts, WC: *No cardiac catheterization before cardiac valve replacement—a mistake.* Am Heart J 103:930, 1982.
3. Swan, HJC, Ganz, W, Forrester, J, et al: *Catheterization of the heart in man with use of flow-directed balloon tipped catheter.* N Engl J Med 283:447, 1970.
4. Ganz, W and Swan, HJC: *Measurement of blood flow by thermodilution.* Am J Cardiol 29:241, 1972.
5. Kan, JS, White RI, Mitchell, SE, et al: *Transluminal balloon valvuloplasty for the treatment of congenital pulmonary valve stenosis.* J Am Coll Cardiol 1(Part 2):588, 1983.
6. Tyrell, MJ, Ellison, RC, Hugenholtz, PG, et al: *Correlation of degree of left ventricular volume overload with clinical course in aortic and mitral regurgitation.* Br Heart J 32:683, 1970.
7. Phillips, HR, Levine, FH, Carter, JE, et al: *Mitral valve replacement for isolated mitral regurgitation: Analysis of clinical course and late postoperative left ventricular ejection fraction.* Am J Cardiol 48:647, 1981.
8. Schuller, G, Peterson, KL, Johnson, A, et al: *Temporal response of left ventricular performance to mitral valve surgery.* Circulation 59:1218, 1979.

9. CLARK, DG, MCANULTY, JH, AND RAHIMTOOLA, SH: *Valve replacement in aortic regurgitation with left ventricular dysfunction.* Circulation 61:411, 1980.
10. HENRY, WL, BONOW, RO, BORER, JS, ET AL: *Observations on the optimum time for operative intervention of aortic regurgitation.* Circulation 61:471, 1980.
11. GREVES J, RAHIMTOOLA, SH, MCANULTY, JH, ET AL: *Preoperative criteria predictive of late survival following valve replacement for severe aortic regurgitation.* Am Heart J 101:300, 1981.
12. BONOW, RO, ROSING, DR, KENT, KM, ET AL: *Timing of operation for chronic aortic regurgitation.* Am J Cardiol 50:325, 1982.
13. DONALDSON, RM, FLORIO, R, RICKARDS, AF, ET AL: *Irreversible morphologic changes contributing to depressed cardiac function after surgery for chronic aortic regurgitation.* Br Heart J 48:589, 1982.
14. KENNEDY, JW, DOCES, J, AND STEWART, DK: *Left ventricular function before and following aortic valve replacement.* Circulation 56:944, 1977.
15. KRAYENBUEHL, JP, TURINA, M, HESS, OM, ET AL: *Preoperative and postoperative left ventricular contractile function in patients with aortic valve disease.* Br Heart J 41:204, 1979.
16. HOSSACK, KF, NEUTZE, JM, LOWE, JB, ET AL: *Congenital valvar aortic stenosis: Natural history and assessment for operation.* Br Heart J 43:561, 1980.
17. GRAHAM, TP, JR: *Ventricular performance in adults after operation for congenital heart disease.* Am J Cardiol 50:612, 1982.
18. RAHIMTOOLA, SH: *Valvular heart disease: A perspective.* J Am Coll Cardiol 1:199, 1983.
19. RACKLEY, CE: *Quantitative evaluation of left ventricular function by radiographic techniques.* Circulation 54:862, 1976.
20. KASSER, IS, AND KENNEDY, JW: *Measurement of left ventricular volumes in man by single-plane cineangiocardiography.* Invest Radiol 4:83, 1969.
21. KENNEDY, JW, TRENHOLM, SE, KASSER, KS: *Left ventricular volumes and mass from single plane cineangiocardiogram: A comparison of anteroposterior and right anterior oblique methods.* Am Heart J 80:343, 1970.
22. DODGE, HT, SANDLER, H, BALLEW, DW, ET AL: *The use of biplane angiocardiography for the measurement of left ventricular volume in man.* Am Heart J 60:762, 1960.
23. WYNNE, J, GREEN, LH, MANN, T, ET AL: *Estimation of left ventricular volumes in man from biplane cineangiograms filmed in oblique projections.* Am J Cardiol 41:726, 1978.
24. KENNEDY, JW, REICHENBACH, DD, BAXLEY, WA, ET AT: *Left ventricular mass. A comparison of angiocardiographic measurements with autopsy weight.* Am J Cardiol 19:221, 1967.
25. RACKLEY, CE, DODGE, HT, COBLE, YD, JR, ET AL: *A method for determining left ventricular mass in man.* Circulation 29:666, 1964.
26. ROGERS, WJ, SMITH, LR, BREAM, PR, ET AL: *Quantitative axial oblique contrast left ventriculography: Validation of the method by demonstrating improved visualization of regional wall motion and mitral valve function with accurate volume determinations.* Am Heart J 103:185, 1982.
27. WILSON, MR, FONTANA, ME, AND WOOLEY, CF: *Routine use of the hydrogen platinum electrode system in shunt detection.* Cath Cardiovasc Diag 1:207, 1975.
28. WOOLEY, CF, AND FONTANA, ME: *Intracardiac sound and pressure: Right heart events. Toward an ultimate classification of auscultatory events.* In FOWLER, NO (ED): *Diagnostic Methods in Cardiology.* FA Davis, Philadelphia, 1975.
29. WOOLEY, CF: *Intracardiac phonocardiography: Intracardiac sound and pressure in man.* In *Reviews of Contemporary Laboratory Methods.* American Heart Association Monograph #66, 1980, p 111.
30. GORLIN, R AND GORLIN, SG: *Hydraulic formula for calculation of the area of stenotic mitral valve, other cardiac valves, and central circulatory shunts.* Am Heart J 41:1, 1951.
31. COHEN, MV AND GORLIN, R: *Modified orifice equation for the calculation of mitral valve area.* Am Heart J 84:839, 1972.
32. HAKKI, AH, ISKANDRIAN, AS, BEMIS, CE, ET AL: *A simplified valve formula for the calculation of stenotic cardiac valve areas.* Circulation 63:1050, 1981.
33. LIBANOFF, AJ AND RODBARD, S: *Atrioventricular pressure half-time. Measure of mitral valve orifice area.* Circulation 38:144, 1968.
34. BARON, MG: *The angiographic diagnosis of valvular stenosis.* Circulation 44:143, 1971.
35. PICHARD, AD, KAY, R, SMITH, H, ET AL: *Large V waves in the pulmonary wedge pressure tracing in the absence of mitral regurgitation.* Am J Cardiol 50:1044, 1982.
36. SANDLER, J, DODGE, HT, HAY, RE, ET AL: *Quantitation of valvular insufficiency in man by angiocardiography.* Am Heart J 65:501, 1963.
37. SELLERS, RD, LEVY, MJ, AMPLATZ, K, ET AL: *Left retrograde cardioangiography in acquired cardiac disease. Technique, indications, and interpretations in 700 cases.* Am J Cardiol. 14:437, 1964.

38. HUNT, D, BAXLEY, WA, KENNEDY, JW, ET AL: *Quantitative evaluation of cineaortography in the assessment of aortic regurgitation.* Am J Cardiol 31:696, 1973.

39. BJORK, VO, LODIN, H, AND MALERS, E: *The evaluation of the degree of mitral insufficiency by selective left ventricular angiocardiography.* Am Heart J 60:691, 1960.

40. BOLDEN, JL AND ALDERMAN, EL: *Ventriculographic and hemodynamic features of mitral regurgitation of cardiomyopathic, rheumatic, and nonrheumatic etiology.* Am J Cardiol 39:177, 1977.

41. YANG, SS, BENTIVOGLIO, LG, MARANHAO, V, ET AL: *Assessment of valvular regurgitation.* In *From Cardiac Catheterization Data to Hemodynamic Parameters.* FA Davis, Philadelphia, 1978.

42. WALLER, BF, MORROW, AG, MARON, BJ, ET AL: *Etiology of clinically isolated, severe, chronic, pure mitral regurgitation: Analysis of 97 patients over 30 years of age having mitral valve replacement.* Am Heart J 104:276, 1982.

43. SMITH, N, MCANULTY, JH, AND RAHIMTOOLA, SH: *Severe aortic stenosis with impaired left ventricular function and clinical heart failure: Results of valve replacement.* Circulation 58:255, 1978.

44. CARABELLO, BA, GREEN, LH, GROSSMAN, W, ET AL: *Hemodynamic determinants of prognosis of aortic valve replacement in critical aortic stenosis and advanced congestive heart failure.* Circulation 62:42, 1980.

45. FOLGER, GM, JR, SABBAH, HN, AND STEIN, PD: *Evaluation of the anatomy of congenitally malformed aortic valves by orifice-view aortography.* Am Heart J 100:152, 1980.

46. HAKKI, AH, KIMBIRIS, D, ISKANDRIAN, AS, ET AL: *Angina pectoris and coronary artery disease in patients with severe aortic valvular disease.* Am Heart J 100:441, 1980.

47. WELTON, DE, YOUNG, JB, RAIZNER, AE, ET AL: *Value and safety of cardiac catheterization during active infective endocarditis.* Am J Cardiol 44:1306, 1979.

48. LEHMAN, JS, BOYLE, JJ, AND DEBBAS, JN: *Quantitation of aortic valvular insufficiency by catheter thoracic aortography.* Radiology 79:361, 1962.

49. DONALDSON, RM, FLORIO, R, RICKARDS, AF, ET AL: *Irreversible morphologic changes contributing to depressed cardiac function after surgery for chronic aortic regurgitation.* Br Heart J 48:589, 1982.

50. KILLIP, T AND LUKAS, DS: *Tricuspid stenosis. Physiologic criteria for diagnosis and hemodynamic abnormalities.* Circulation 16:3, 1957.

51. KITCHIN, A AND TURNER, R: *Diagnosis and treatment of tricuspid stenosis.* Br Heart J 26:354, 1964.

52. FONTANA, ME, BABA, N, KILMAN, JW, ET AL: *Tricuspid stenosis—a superior method for evaluating the severity of obstruction.* Circulation 62 (Part II):III-217, 1980.

53. HADJIGEORGE, C, PAPADOPOULOS, A, GIALAFOS, J, ET AL: *The contribution of right ventricular angiocardiography to the diagnosis of tricuspid valvular stenosis.* Acta Cardiol 31:210, 1976.

54. CAIRNS, KB, KLOSTER, FE, BRISTOW, JD, ET AL: *Problems in the hemodynamic diagnosis of tricuspid insufficiency.* Am Heart J 75:173, 1968.

55. HANSING, CE AND ROWE, GG: *Tricuspid insufficiency: A study of hemodynamics and pathogenesis.* Circulation 45:793, 1972.

56. BAJEC, DF, BIRKHEAD, NC, CARTER, SA, ET AL: *Localization and estimation of severity of regurgitant flow at the pulmonary and tricuspid valves.* Mayo Clin Proc 33:569, 1958.

57. COLLINS, NP, BRAUNWALD, E, AND MORROW, AG: *Detection of pulmonic and tricuspid valvular regurgitation by means of indicator solutions.* Circulation 20:561, 1959.

58. LINGAMNENI, R, CHA, SD, MARANHAO, V, ET AL: *Tricuspid regurgitation: Clinical and angiographic assessment.* Cath Cardiovasc Diag 5:7, 1979.

59. EMMANOUILIDES, GC: *Obstructive lesions of the right ventricle and the pulmonary arterial tree.* In MOSS, AJ, ADAMS, FH, AND EMMANOUILIDES, GC (EDS): *Heart Disease in Infants, Children, and Adolescents.* Williams & Wilkins, Baltimore, 1977.

60. LEWIS, JM, MONTERO, AC, KINARD, SA, ET AL: *Hemodynamic response to exercise in isolated pulmonic stenosis.* Circulation 29:854, 1964.

61. IKKOS, D, JOHNSON, B, AND LINDERHOLM, H: *Effect of exercise in pulmonary stenosis with intact ventricular septum.* Br Heart J 28:316, 1966.

62. MOLLER, JH, RAO, S, AND LUCAS, RV: *Exercise hemodynamics of pulmonary valvular stenosis: Study of 64 children.* Circulation 46:1018, 1972.

63. COLLINS, NP, BRAUNWALD, E, AND MORROW, AG: *Isolated congenital pulmonic valvular regurgitation: Diagnosis by cardiac catheterization and angiocardiography.* Am J Med 18:159, 1960.

64. LEVIN, HS, RUNCO, V, WOOLEY, CF, ET AL: *Pulmonic regurgitation following staphylococcal endocarditis: An intracardiac phonocardiographic study.* Circulation 30:411, 1964.

65. ASKENAZI, J, CARLSON, CJ, ALPERT, JS, ET AL: *Mitral valve area in combined mitral stenosis and regurgitation.* Circulation 54:480, 1976.

Electrophysiologic Study in Supraventricular Arrhythmias

David L. Ross, M.B., B.S., F.R.A.C.P., A. Robert Denniss, M.B., B.S., B.Sc. (Med), M.Sc., F.R.A.C.P., and John B. Uther, B.Sc. (Med), M.D., B.S., F.R.A.C.P.

Investigation of supraventricular arrhythmias by clinical electrophysiologic studies began in the late 1960s.[1–5] These and subsequent studies resulted in a vastly improved understanding of supraventricular tachycardias (SVT) and have opened up new areas of treatment such as specific antitachycardia surgery guided by electrophysiologic mapping,[6–27] use of implanted antitachycardia pacemakers,[28–31] and catheter ablation of the His bundle.[32] In addition, a more rational approach to antiarrhythmic drug therapy is facilitated. Electrophysiologic studies in patients with supraventricular arrhythmias have therefore been transformed from largely research tests to routine clinical investigations with frequent direct benefits to patient management.

A significant proportion of the electrophysiologic laboratory caseload is devoted to investigation of SVT. For example, in the last three years (1980 to 1982, inclusive) we studied 1402 patients in our electrophysiologic laboratory; 258 patients (18 percent) had inducible SVT. The breakdown into the various types of SVT is shown in Table 1. Although recent electrophysiologic advances have been mainly in the field of ventricular arrhythmias and postinfarct research, electrophysiologic investigation of supraventricular tachycardia continues to be important because of its direct benefits in patient management. In general, the study of SVT in the electrophysiologic laboratory is more complex than ventricular tachycardia, and the investigator requires specialized electrophysiologic training and experience.

The indications, methods, complications, and benefits of electrophysiologic studies for SVT are covered in the following discussions. Attention has been confined to SVT, and supraventricular bradyarrhythmias have not been considered.

Table 1. Types of supraventricular tachycardias induced at electrophysiologic study*

Tachycardias utilizing an atrioventricular accessory pathway	114	(44%)
AV junctional re-entry tachycardias	107	(41%)
Atrial tachycardias	18	(7%)
Re-entrant tachycardias using a nodo-ventricular fiber	5	(2%)
Miscellaneous	14	(5%)
Total	258	

*These figures are based on consecutive cases over a 3-year period (1980 to 1982, inclusive). The miscellaneous group mainly comprised patients with atrial fibrillation or flutter as their sole clinical arrhythmia.

CLINICAL INDICATIONS FOR ELECTROPHYSIOLOGIC STUDY IN SUPRAVENTRICULAR TACHYCARDIA

Electrophysiologic study is indicated for:

(1) *Establishing the presence of arrhythmia*
This indication applies to patients with recurrent palpitations suggestive of paroxysmal tachycardia but which have never been documented on an electrocardiogram or to patients with undiagnosed syncope suggestive of a cardiac origin. Ambulatory electrocardiographic monitoring is rarely useful in these patients unless the frequency of arrhythmia episodes is high. Electrophysiologic study, on the other hand, frequently provides a definitive diagnosis.

(2) *Clarifying the diagnosis*
Diagnostic problems arise with broad complex tachycardias that may or may not be ventricular tachycardia, or multiple types of tachycardia within an individual patient. These problems can usually be resolved at electrophysiologic study.

(3) *Determination of therapeutic options*
The range of treatment available depends greatly on the type of supraventricular tachycardia. Electrophysiologic study permits the making of a definitive diagnosis and facilitates the drawing up of a treatment plan that caters to the medical needs and personal wishes of the patient. This method usually achieves more effective treatment more quickly and is usually more acceptable to patients.

(4) *Guiding therapy*
Patients with arrhythmias refractory to standard antiarrhythmic drugs require electrophysiologic study to determine suitability for other methods of treatment, such as antitachycardia pacing, antiarrhythmia surgery, or catheter His bundle ablation.

(5) *Identification of patients at risk for sudden death*
This group includes patients with a rapid ventricular response during atrial fibrillation owing to antegrade conduction over an atrioventricular accessory pathway, or patients in whom the antegrade effective refractory period of an atrioventricular accessory pathway is suspected to be short on the basis of an ajmaline or procainamide test.[33,34] Patients with asymptomatic Wolff-Parkinson-White syndrome who are airline pilots, train drivers, and so on also fall within this group. A reasonably strong case can be made for investigating *all* patients with Wolff-Parkinson-White syndrome to determine the antegrade effective refractory period of the bypass tract (excluding patients with second-degree antegrade block over the accessory pathway in sinus rhythm).

(6) *Patients with supraventricular tachycardia who are undergoing open heart surgery for other reasons*
Tachycardias that are due to a free wall atrioventricular accessory pathway can be cured by accessory pathway section at the same time with little increase in risk.

(7) *Postoperative evaluation*
Patients who have undergone a cardiac surgical attempt at cure or modification of tachycardia require further electrophysiologic investigation to determine whether surgery has been successful.

METHODS OF ELECTROPHYSIOLOGIC STUDIES FOR SUPRAVENTRICULAR TACHYCARDIA

The general method for these studies as performed in our laboratory will be described first and specific modifications will be discussed separately for each type of SVT.

Precatheterization Procedures

Standard pre-cardiac catheterization checks regarding pregnancy, allergies, bleeding tendencies, and so on are performed. It is important that all antiarrhythmic medications (including digoxin) be stopped well before the study, if at all possible. We stop antiarrhythmic medications 1 week prior to the test because some medications (for example, beta blockers) can have prolonged effects despite the absence of significant blood levels. Recurrence of sustained arrhythmia during this week is uncommon. Patients with life-threatening arrhythmias should have their antiarrhythmic drugs stopped while in the hospital; the remaining patients can stop their medications prior to hospital admission.

Each patient is provided with a detailed information booklet that explains the general reasons for electrophysiologic study, the techniques by which the test is done, the types of arrhythmias which may develop and how they will be handled, the sensations the patient will feel during the test, the complications which may occur, the possible need for cardioversion, the likelihood of needing further electrophysiologic studies, and the difference between an electrophysiologic study and hemodynamic and angiographic catheterizations. This total disclosure method has worked well for most patients. Excessively anxious patients tend to skip sections that cause them undue concern. In general, better patient education prior to the test has reduced anxiety.

Premedication

Diazepam, 10 mg p.o. 1 hour prior to the study, is used for premedication. The same dose should be used in children older than 5 years. The dose should be reduced to 5 mg for elderly or sick patients. Premedications with morphine or its analogs, antihistamines, and major tranquilizers should be avoided because these drugs have anticholinergic actions that frequently impair induction of tachycardias, such as atrioventricular nodal reentry. Diazepam produces no significant electrophysiologic effects.[35]

Local Anesthesia

Lidocaine 1 percent is used for local anesthesia. The usual dose is 5 to 10 ml.

Catheter Insertion and Placement

Standard catheter insertion sites in our laboratory are the right femoral vein and a left antecubital vein. Three (and on occasions, four) catheters are inserted via the right femoral vein. All catheters are 6 French and are introduced using the Seldinger needle, guide wire, and sheath technique. The sheath is withdrawn back to the base of the catheter when the catheter has been passed to the inferior vena cava. Some electrophysiologic laboratories recommend upper limits of a total of 14 French of catheters in any one femoral vein. We have had minimal problems using a total of 18 French of catheters in one vein as a routine. The same technique may also be used in children older than 5 years of age.

Coronary sinus catheterization is usually best done with an approach via the superior vena cava. We favor percutaneous catheterization of a medially running left antecubital vein. If no medial vein is present, a laterally running vein will permit coronary sinus catheterization in approximately 70 percent of cases. In the remainder, the catheter will not negotiate the shoulder. In these cases and in those in which no superficial antecubital vein can be catheterized, alternative approaches such as an antecubital cutdown, use of a right antecubital vein, or subclavian or internal jugular vein approach should be used. The coronary sinus also may be catheterized from below in most cases.[36] This latter approach is less satisfactory for mapping along the coronary sinus. Patients tolerate an antecubital approach better than a subclavian or internal jugular approach, and the percutaneous method permits re-use at subsequent studies.

Using fluoroscopy, the coronary sinus catheter is inserted first and positioned as distal in the coronary sinus as possible. A quadripolar catheter is placed in the right atrial appendage for recording the high right atrial electrogram and for atrial pacing.

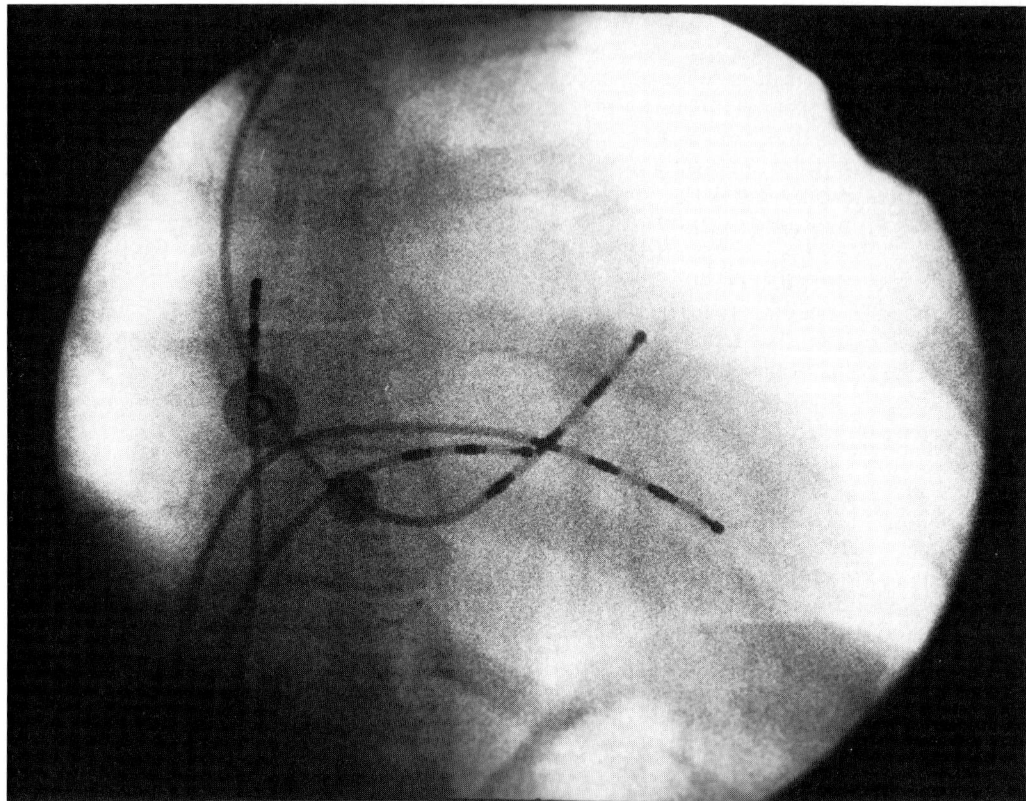

Figure 1. Catheter positions during electrophysiologic study for supraventricular tachycardia.

A tripolar catheter is placed in the His bundle region to record a proximal His bundle electrogram. However, almost any catheter may be used for this purpose, including quadripolar or other multipolar catheters (most with interelectrode distances of 1 cm) or bipolar catheters of various sizes with interelectrode distances of 5 to 10 mm. When a catheter position producing a good His bundle electrogram has been obtained, those same electrodes are used for pacing. If this causes atrial or His bundle pacing (the latter popularized by Narula[37,38]), this is termed a proximal site.

If the QRS morphology shows mainly a normal morphology, with a minor initial deflection owing to direct ventricular septal stimulation, this is termed an intermediate site. If the QRS morphology is wide, reflecting mainly ventricular pacing, this recording site is termed distal. Using this technique, the catheter is positioned at a proximal or, if this is not possible, an intermediate site.

If a stable His bundle recording site cannot be obtained, recording from a proximal electrode pair rather than a distal pair using a tripolar or quadripolar catheter may be helpful. Occasionally, a more stable recording may be obtained with a small floppy catheter (4 French bipolar pacing catheter).

A further quadripolar catheter is positioned at the right ventricular apex for pacing and recording the right ventricular electrogram. Final catheter positions are shown in Figure 1.

X-ray Facilities

If the electrophysiology laboratory is self-sufficient (that is, not using the angiographic laboratory facilities), a relatively cheap and satisfactory system can be assembled with a radiolucent trolley (which can also be used for patient transport) and a small mobile C-arm image intensifier of the type used for setting fractures.

Heparin

We do not give routine heparin during electrophysiologic studies unless the left heart or arterial circulation is to be entered. Several laboratories do heparinize routinely for electrophysiologic studies. However, we do not believe that the benefits of routine heparinization outweigh its risks during electrophysiologic studies on the right heart.

Recording of Electrograms

At least three surface electrocardiographic leads should be recorded, preferably orthogonal leads. We record leads X, Y, and Z of the Frank vectorcardiogram.[39] Leads I, aVF and V_2 of the scalar electrocardiogram may be used. These leads enable recognition of changes in QRS morphology, such as aberrancy and pre-excitation, and they permit accurate measurements of the HV interval.[38] These leads should be recorded simultaneously with multiple intracardiac electrograms. We routinely record simultaneous electrograms from the high right atrium, proximal coronary sinus, distal coronary sinus, His bundle region, and right ventricular apex. A band pass filter of 50 to 1000 Hz is used, and amplifier gain is adjusted to give satisfactorily sized electrograms on paper. A direct-writing recorder is mandatory for electrophysiologic studies. By far the best systems currently available are ink jet recorders. These systems give good quality direct recordings on graticuled cheap paper and have an adequate frequency response. This paper does not require frequent changes. Recording systems using photographic paper cause a vast increase in paper costs and markedly increase the cost of each study. Heat stylus and ink pen recorders do not have an adequate frequency response.

The recording system should have a paper speed error of <1 percent and should be capable of speeds of at least 25 mm per second, 100 mm per second (standard electrophysiologic study paper speed), and a faster speed such as 200 or 250 mm per second for very accurate measurements, such as during mapping.

All equipment in the electrophysiology laboratory must be of Class A standard to ensure the electrical safety of patients.

It is essential to achieve good quality, low noise recordings to permit a satisfactory standard of electrophysiologic study to be performed. Adequate earthing of equipment using a common ground bus, shielding of cables, and elimination of noisy equipment is required.

The preceding description applies to an eight-channel system. A larger system permits more surface and intracardiac leads to be recorded simultaneously but in general adds little clinical benefit.

Tape Recording

A high quality FM tape recorder is an advantage but not a necessity. It can be used to capture arrhythmias missed on the paper recorder, and it also permits replay of tracings at various speeds for the preparation of figures for publication and so on.

Programmed Stimulator

A programmed stimulator delivering drive chains of programmable cycle length, plus at least two individually programmable extrastimuli, is necessary. Several satisfactory stimulators are commercially available.

Stimulation Protocol

Recording of Basic Conduction Intervals

This is best done at a paper speed of 200 to 250 mm per second. A 100 mm per second paper speed is satisfactory for most other parts of the electrophysiologic study except where indicated. Standard definitions for interval measurements and refractory periods are used.[40]

Antegrade Conduction Study

We use an atrial driving cycle length as close as possible to 600 msec. A current intensity of twice diastolic threshold is used. An atrial extrastimulus is delivered after every eight drive beats. The prematurity of the extrastimulus is decreased by 50 msec decrements to 400 msec and by 20 msec decrements thereafter. Refractory periods of the atrium and conduction system are determined to an accuracy of 10 msec.

Retrograde Conduction Study

An identical protocol to that used for an antegrade study is used with ventricular instead of atrial pacing.

Atrioventricular (AV) Wenckebach Threshold

Beginning at rates just in excess of sinus, the atrium is paced at gradually increasing rates until second-degree AV block occurs. It is important to ensure that atrial capture has not been lost intermittently. This procedure should be repeated with pacing from the coronary sinus.

Ventriculoatrial (VA) Wenckebach Threshold

An identical protocol to that for AV Wenckebach threshold is used with ventricular pacing until second-degree VA block occurs.

Sinus Node Recovery Times

These measurements are worthwhile if sinus node disease is a possibility.[41] Occasionally the prolonged pacing at fast rates will facilitate induction of supraventricular tachycardia. Note: If atrial fibrillation has occurred previously, it is wise to perform all ventricular stimulation before atrial stimulation is commenced.

Induction of Tachycardia

If tachycardia has not been induced by this stage, atrial or ventricular burst pacing at about the AV or VA Wenckebach threshold is usually the most productive maneuver. If this method fails, use of double atrial or ventricular stimuli may be successful. Different atrial sites should be stimulated. If these maneuvers fail, pharmacologic stimulation is tried next (atropine 0.5 to 1.5 mg intravenously (IV) or isoprenaline infusion 4 to 12 μg per minute IV). Isoprenaline infusion is quickly reversible, whereas atropine lasts several hours. However, atropine is effective and easy to administer in most cases. If no arrhythmia is induced (and a documented, definitely supraventricular tachycardia is being chased), atrial pacing at rates up to 300 to 400 beats per minute is used.

If the arrhythmia remains noninducible, we perform a ventricular stimulation protocol designed to elicit ventricular tachycardias, especially if the clinical rhythm has been poorly documented and may be ventricular tachycardia.

Catheter Mapping

Mapping is performed for precise localization of an arrhythmia "focus" or components of a re-entry circuit. Clinically it is useful in localizing an atrioventricular accessory pathway or the origin of a true atrial tachycardia (that is, a tachycardia that does not include AV junctional tissues in its mechanism). All recordings are made at 250 m per second.

CORONARY SINUS MAPPING. Coronary sinus mapping is used for suspected or possible left free wall or septal atrioventricular accessory pathways. Two anatomical markers are identified: (1) the mouth of the coronary sinus (identified by advancing the catheter and making it buckle at the orifice of the coronary sinus), and (2) the point at which the coronary sinus rounds the obtuse margin of the heart. Up to five coronary sinus catheter positions can then be determined (Fig. 2). At each position, both the proximal and distal pairs of each electrode are recorded or stimulated. It is rather uncommon to be able to place the coronary sinus catheter in a very distal position. However, a distal or midcoronary sinus position can be reached in almost all cases.

An *antegrade* map is performed by pacing from the proximal and distal pairs of electrodes in turn at each catheter position. Stimulus to delta intervals are measured. The catheter position and electrode pair with the shortest interval indicate the atrial location of the accessory pathway used for antegrade conduction. A *retrograde* map is performed during supraventricular tachycardias using the AV node—His Purkinje system for antegrade conduction and an atrioventricular accessory pathway for retrograde conduction. Identical catheter positions to those used for an antegrade map are used. Coronary sinus electrograms are recorded from each electrode pair at each site. The shortest onset of QRS to atrial electrogram interval indicates the atrial site closest to the accessory pathway used for retrograde conduction (note: this is not necessarily the same as that used for antegrade conduction).

It is important not to include part of the P wave as the onset of the delta wave in an antegrade map; and the same lead with the best onset of delta should be used for measurements at each site. During antegrade mapping, direct stimulation of the left ventricle may occur (often with a similar QRS morphology to pre-excited beats), especially with distal coronary sinus positions. This is obvious when ventricular activity is simultaneous with or precedes the atrial electrogram at that catheter position. Current intensity should be adjusted to the lowest giving stable atrial pacing at that site (this may be in the 5 to 10 mA range for some coronary sinus positions).

RIGHT AND LEFT ATRIAL MAPPING. If the accessory pathway is right sided or septal, mapping of the atrium adjoining the tricuspid ring should be performed. A 7 French bipolar catheter with a stilette (similar to a Brockenbrough needle), designed by Gallagher and associates,[42] is suitable for this purpose. The proximal end of the stilette indicates the direction of the catheter tip. During tachycardia, atrial electrograms from this catheter are recorded from the low right atrium (just above the tricuspid valve) from each of the medial, anteromedial, anterior, anterolateral, lateral, posterolateral, posterior, and posteromedial positions (the latter position is close to the His bundle area). The close bipolar electrodes (2 mm interelectrode distance) are not suitable for pacing and cannot usually be used to perform an antegrade map (that is, analysis of stimulus to delta intervals in the presence of antegrade pre-excitation). The accuracy of the tricuspid ring map is reasonable but not very precise because of the difficulties involved in staying close to the tricuspid ring. Endocardial mapping at surgery is always required to confirm catheter findings prior to any attempt at surgical interruption of an accessory pathway.

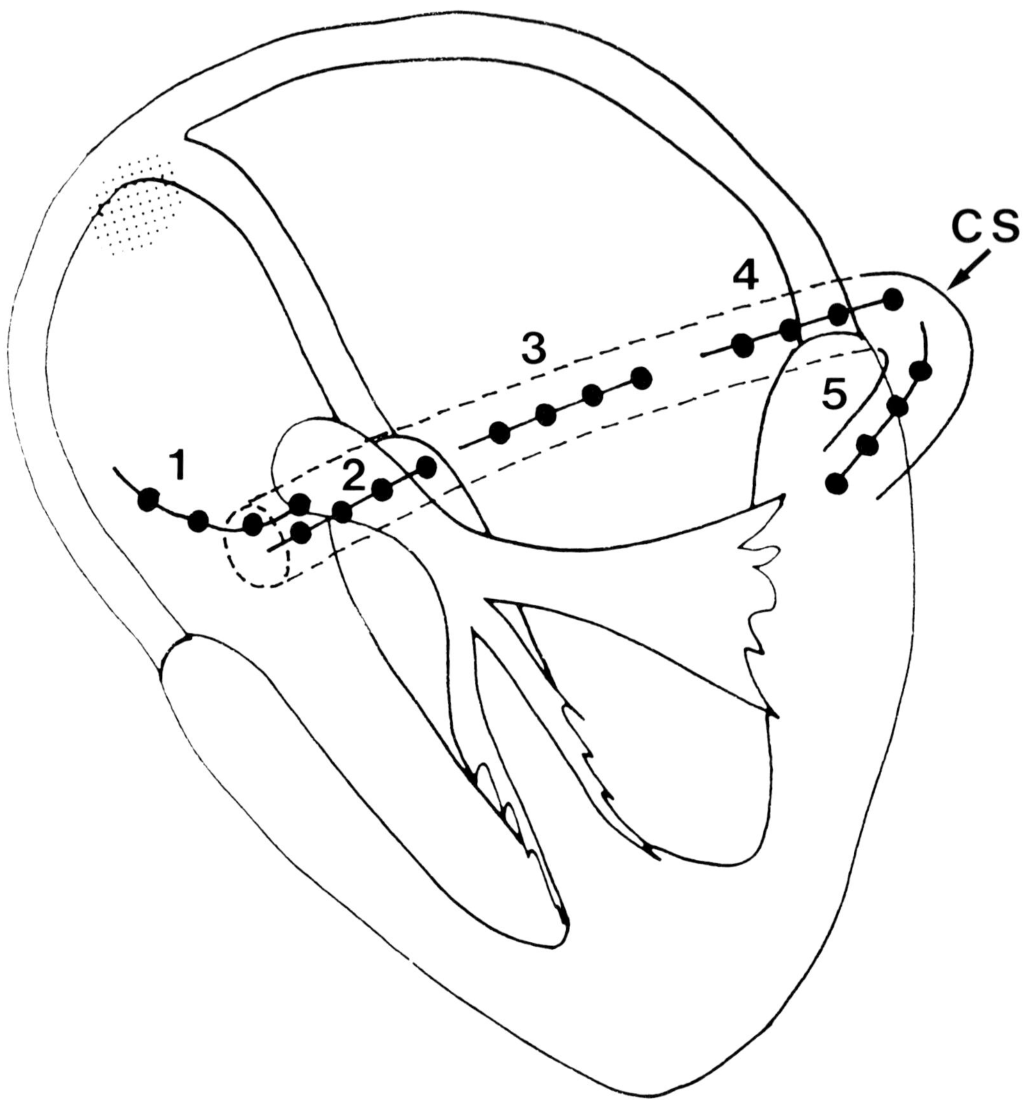

Figure 2. Coronary sinus (CS) catheter positions for coronary sinus mapping. The five sites are (1) very proximal CS; (2) proximal CS; (3) mid CS; (4) distal CS; (5) very distal CS.

Mapping of the remainder of the right atrium is useful for right atrial tachycardias. The Gallagher catheter is used in the aforementioned way at three atrial levels: low, mid, and high. More limited information is usually obtained with catheter left atrial maps. The posterior and lateral mitral ring activation is mapped with the coronary sinus catheter. A probe-patent foramen ovale may permit direct access to the left atrium. A catheter positioned in the main pulmonary artery records anterior left atrial activity, and a catheter in the right pulmonary artery records activity from the roof of the left atrium. In practice, left atrial tachycardias are much less common than right atrial tachycardias.

Analysis of the Cardiac Tissues Involved in the Tachycardia Mechanism

Conduction intervals and sequences of activation during tachycardia are recorded at paper speeds of 200 to 250 mm per second. In general terms, introduction of programmed atrial

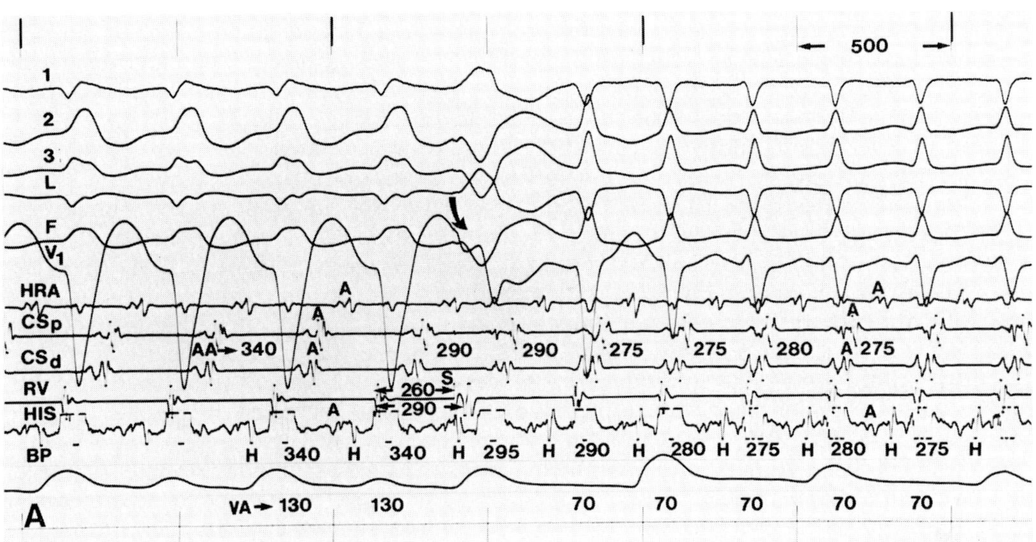

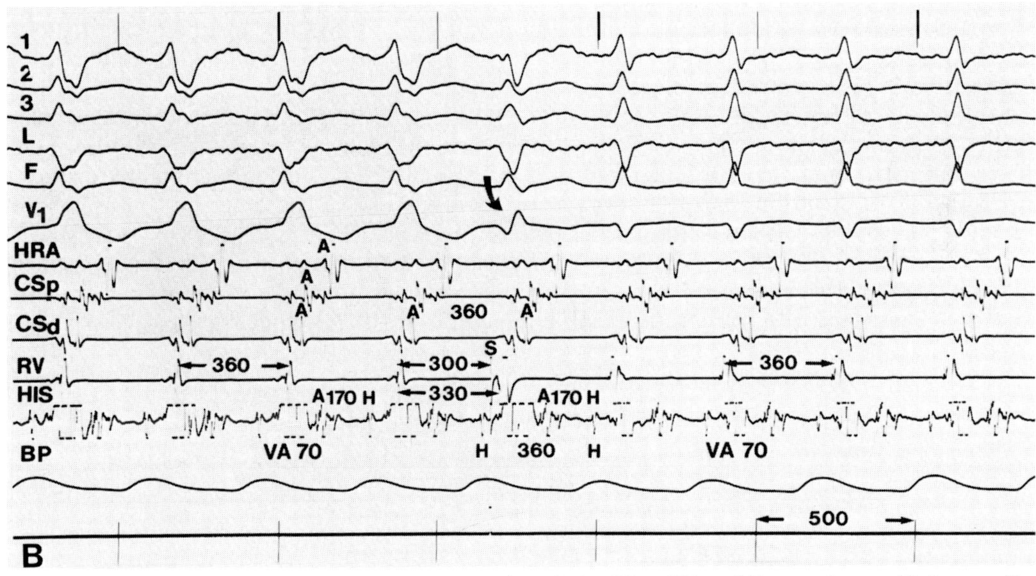

Figure 3. Simultaneous recording of surface ECG leads 1, 2, 3, aVL, aVF, and V_1, are shown with intracardiac leads from the high right atrium (HRA), proximal (p) and distal (d) coronary sinus (CS), right ventricular apex (RV), and His bundle region (HIS). Simultaneous intra-arterial blood pressure (BP) recordings are also shown. A represents atrial activation, H represents the His bundle electrogram, and V represents ventricular activation. S represents programmed stimuli. These same abbreviations are used in subsequent figures. Frank vectorcardiographic orthogonal leads X, Y, Z are used in place of standard ECG leads in most of these illustrations. *A, B,* Orthodromic supraventricular tachycardia (SVT) using a left free wall atrioventricular accessory pathway is shown. Note the typical sequence and timing of atrial activation. *A,* LBBB aberrancy is converted to normal conduction following a critically timed, introduced ventricular premature beat *(arrow)*. Note that tachycardia cycle length and VA interval are longer during LBBB (that is, bundle branch block *ipsilateral* to the accessory pathway). *B,* The same patient with SVT with RBBB aberrancy is converted to normal conduction by a critically timed ventricular stimulus. VA interval does not change, and tachycardia cycle length is unaltered (that is, bundle branch block contralateral to the accessory pathway has no effect).

and ventricular extrastimuli during tachycardia and the effects of bundle branch block or atrioventricular block during tachycardia identify the tissues involved. The major diagnostic maneuvers that should be performed for the major types of supraventricular tachycardia are summarized in the discussions that follow. This is an extensive subject, and the reader is referred to several authoritative papers and reviews in the literature for more detail.[40,43–59] Cardiologists performing electrophysiologic studies for supraventricular tachycardia should be well versed in this subject because prompt recognition of the probable arrhythmia type and performance of the required diagnostic maneuvers during the study are essential.

Supraventricular Tachycardia Utilizing an Atrioventricular Accessory Pathway. The atrial activation sequence during orthodromic tachycardia identifies left and right free wall pathways. Ipsilateral bundle branch block prolongs the VA interval in tachycardias using free wall accessory pathways (Fig. 3). Atrioventricular block terminates the tachycardia. Programmed atrial and ventricular stimulation are able to advance the subsequent tachycardia cycle. The major diagnostic problem is identification of concealed (retrograde function only) septal accessory pathways. These are distinguished from AV junctional re-entry by programmed ventricular stimulation during tachycardia at a time when the His bundle is refractory owing to the antegradely conducted tachycardia impulse. Advancement of subsequent atrial activation by the ventricular extrastimulus confirms the presence of a ventriculoatrial accessory pathway (Fig. 4). In addition, the ventriculo-earliest-atrial-activation interval is usually less than 50 msec in AV junctional re-entry, whereas in tachycardias using a ventriculoatrial accessory pathway this interval is usually greater than 60 msec.[60]

Antidromic tachycardia is recognized by a similar QRS morphology to maximally pre-excited beats seen during the antegrade study, absence of a preceding His spike, the ability of programmed atrial stimulation to alter timing but not morphology of subsequent ventricular activation without producing an antegrade His bundle electrogram, and termination of tachycardia by atrioventricular block.

Multiple accessory pathways are recognized by different sets of atrial activation sequences during tachycardia; discordance of earliest activation sites during antegrade and retrograde maps; and more than one morphology of fully pre-excited beats during an antegrade study, atrial pacing, or atrial flutter/fibrillation. Bundle branch block should not be confused with a second morphology of pre-excitation in this latter instance (Fig. 5).

AV Junctional Re-entry. Atrial activation mapping during tachycardia reveals earliest activation in the His bundle lead or in the proximal coronary sinus adjacent to its orifice. This pattern is consistent with retrograde atrial activation over the AV node[42] or very close to it.

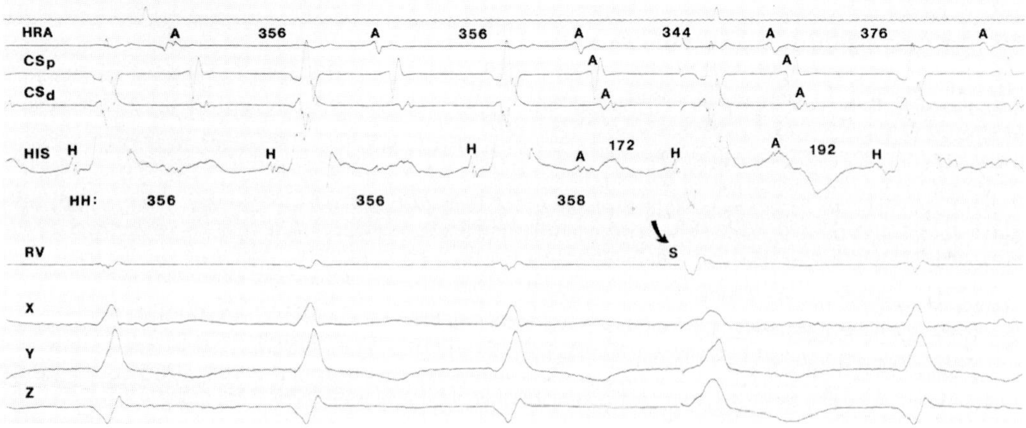

Figure 4. Supraventricular tachycardia using a septal ventriculoatrial accessory pathway is present. A programmed, induced ventricular premature beat that follows antegrade tachycardia His bundle depolarization is able to advance subsequent atrial activation by 12 ms, confirming the presence of a second pathway for VA conduction.

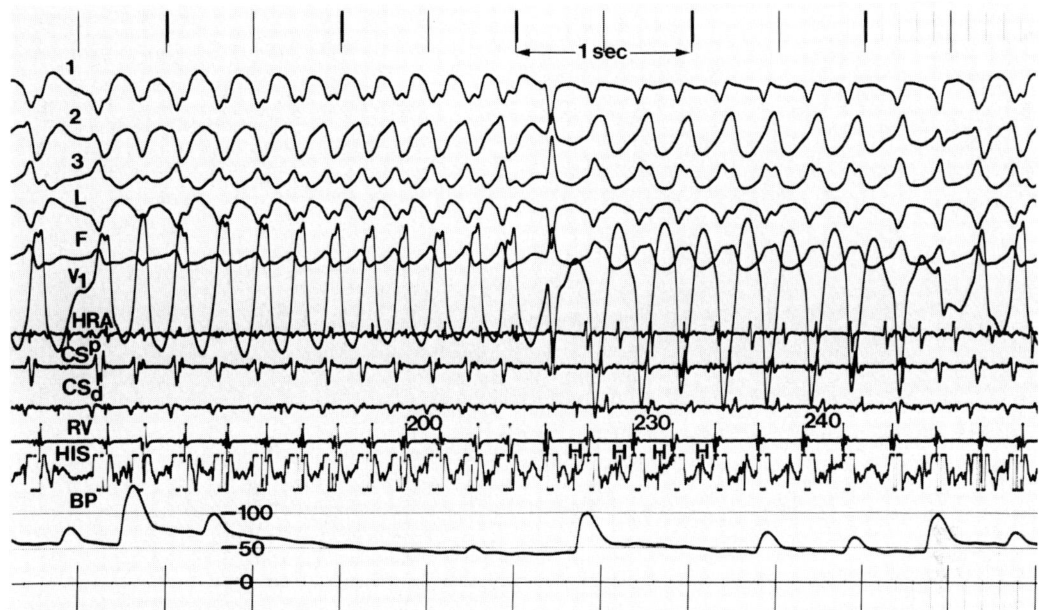

Figure 5. Atrial flutter/fibrillation in a patient with a left free wall accessory atrioventricular connection is shown. Note the very rapid ventricular response (approximately 300 beats per minute) and its effect on blood pressure. A run of maximally pre-excited beats is shown on the left-hand side of the trace. A second morphology of broad complex QRS is shown on the right-hand portion following an intermediate normally conducted beat. This second morphology is preceded by a His spike and represents LBBB aberrancy caused by rapid conduction over the AV node-His Purkinje system. Note that the rate is only slightly slower. This is due to the presence of enhanced AV nodal function.

In the most common antegrade slow pathway, retrograde fast pathway form, the H-to-earliest-atrial-activation interval is short in the majority of AV junctional re-entrant tachycardias, and atrial activation is often visible at the end of the HV interval prior to the onset of ventricular activation (Fig. 6). This finding, and continuation of tachycardia in the presence of second-degree AV block (either proximal or distal to the bundle of His[61]), indicates that the ventricles are not part of the re-entry circuit. Rarely, second-degree block of retrograde activation to the atria during tachycardia indicates that the atria are not part of the re-entry circuit.[61] AV junctional re-entry is distinguished from low septal atrial tachycardias by (1) the rare phenomenon above, (2) achievement of a critical AH interval before tachycardia can be induced, (3) need for block in an antegrade fast pathway with subsequent conduction over an antegrade slow pathway before tachycardia can be induced with atrial extrastimuli (this rule applies to most but not all AV junctional tachycardias), and (4) the ability of maneuvers causing changes in antegrade AV nodal conduction times during tachycardia to produce very similar changes in tachycardia cycle lengths while maintaining constant (or very nearly so) HA intervals, thus implying that the AV node is part of the circuit. The last three of these criteria are suggestive but not absolutely diagnostic for AV junctional re-entry.

AV junctional re-entry is distinguished from a concealed septal ventriculoatrial accessory pathway re-entrant tachycardia by (1) continuation of tachycardia in the face of antegrade AV block, usually distal to the His bundle (this phenomenon occurs in 5 to 10 percent of cases with AV junctional re-entry); (2) inability to pre-excite the atria by a ventricular extrastimulus delivered during tachycardia when the His bundle is refractory; (3) VA interval less than 60 msec; and (4) atrial activity preceding onset of ventricular activation (that is, HA interval shorter than HV). AV junctional re-entry tachycardias *may* be advanced by pre-

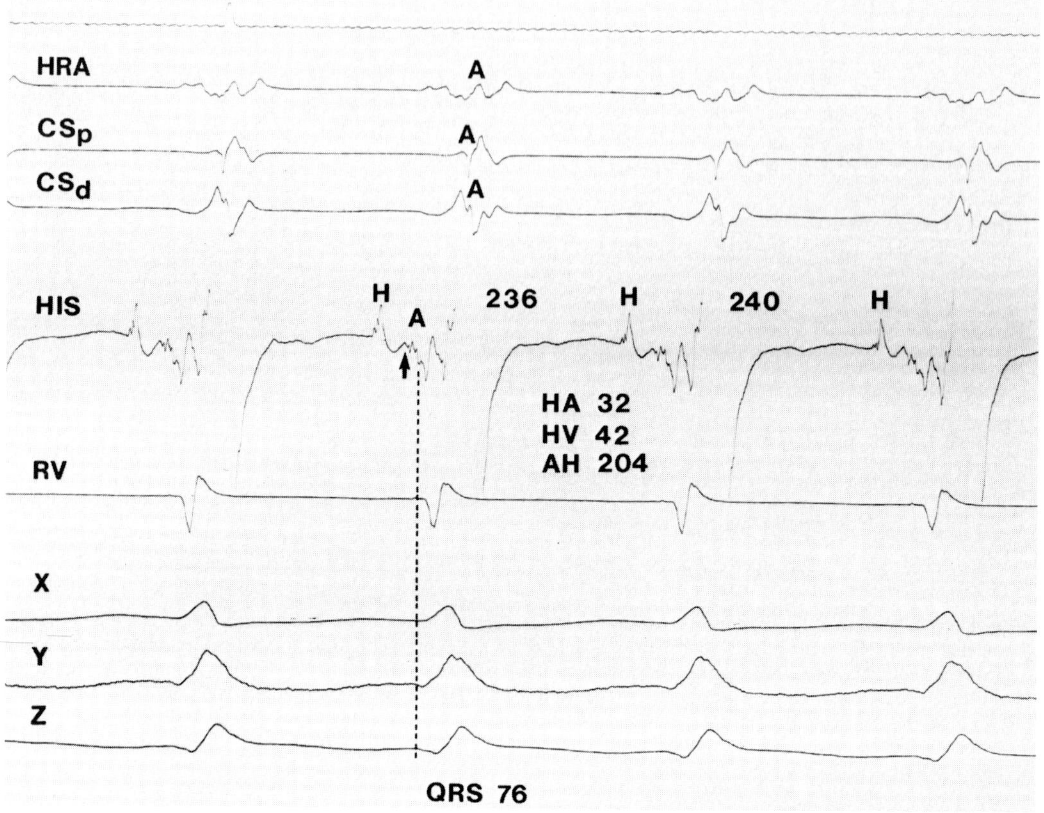

Figure 6. A typical example of AV junctional re-entry tachycardia is shown. Paper speed is 250 mm per second. Note that atrial activation is simultaneous with ventricular activation. Atrial activation is earliest in the His bundle lead and *precedes* onset of ventricular activation by 10 msec. This excludes the ventricles from being part of the re-entry circuit. Note that some AV junctional re-entry tachycardias are capable of rapid rates (250 per minute in this case).

mature ventricular extrastimuli given during tachycardia before antegrade His bundle activation is expected. Stimuli given more than an HV interval before inscription of the antegrade His spike can theoretically advance subsequent atrial activation but almost never do so until the stimulus precedes His bundle activation by more than 80 msec. AV junctional re-entry is most easily initiated by atrial pacing but may also be initiated by ventricular pacing. It is often stated that if retrograde conduction (that is, VA conduction) is absent with ventricular pacing at rates greater than 100 per minute, then AV junctional re-entry is ruled out. However, the retrograde pathway may be dependent on autonomic tone and become capable of rapid conduction at a later time (for example, Fig. 7). The reader is referred to Hariman, Gomes, and El Sherif[62] for further information. It is worth noting that AV junctional re-entry tachycardias are among the most capricious of those inducible in the electrophysiologic laboratory. They may be abolished by anticholinergic premedications, are very dependent on autonomic tone, and commonly require atropine to facilitate conduction.[63] A high index of suspicion for this arrhythmia should be maintained and vigorous efforts made to induce it when other types of arrhythmias have been excluded.

The antegrade fast pathway, retrograde slow pathway type of AV junctional re-entry is a very rare cause of sustained tachycardia.[51]

Atrial Tachycardias. Atrial activation sequence and P wave morphology usually differ from sinus beats (Fig. 8). Atrial mapping during tachycardia usually reveals an earliest site

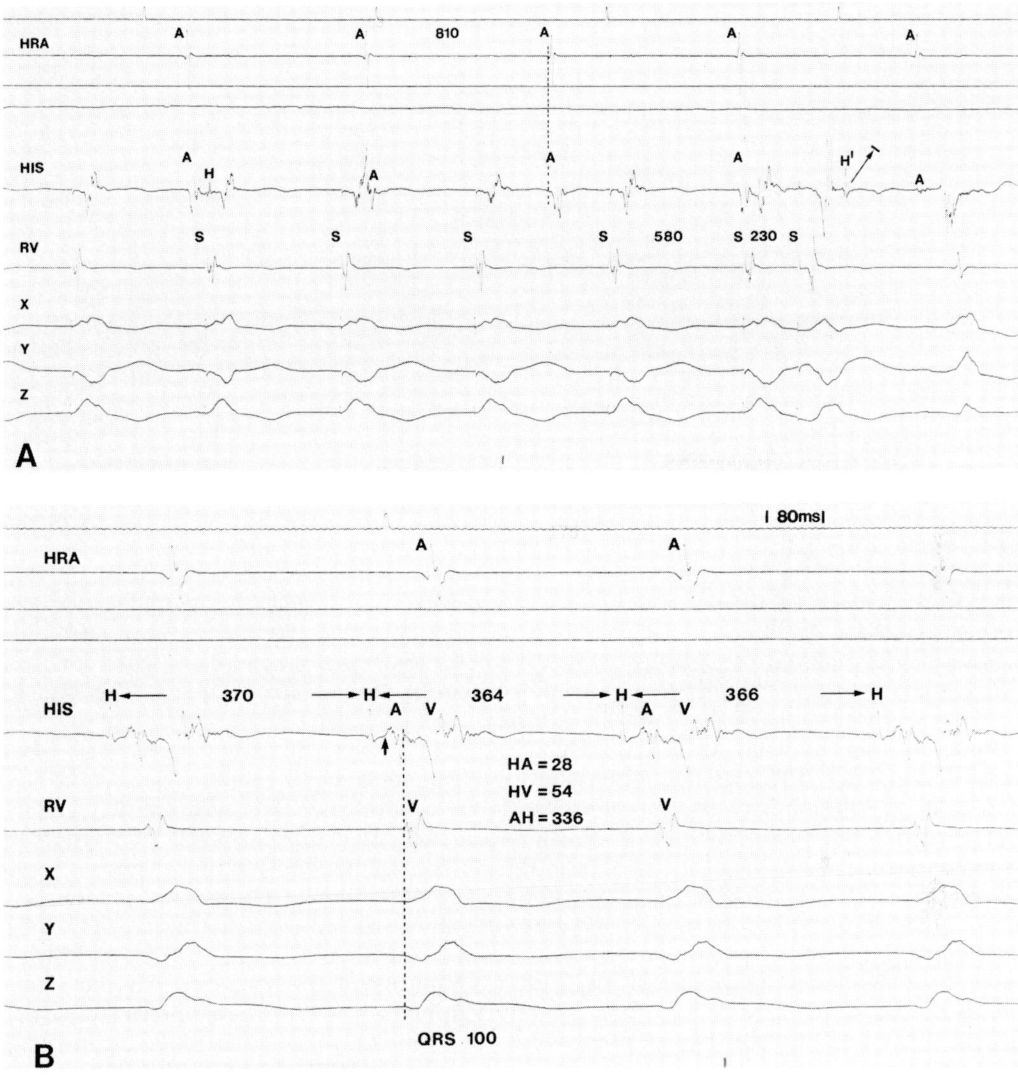

Figure 7. *A,* This ECG shows VA dissociation during ventricular pacing at a cycle length of 580 ms. The appearance of a retrograde His bundle electrogram following the extrastimulus indicates that retrograde block occurred at the level of the AV node. *B,* This ECG shows AV junctional re-entry tachycardia at a cycle length of 360–370 ms in the same patient at the same electrophysiologic study. Note that retrograde atrial activation precedes onset of ventricular activation. No pharmacologic agents were used, and no unusual circumstances occurred to cause this change in capability for retrograde conduction. This change, therefore, presumably represents variable spontaneous autonomic influence on the retrograde fast pathway used in this tachycardia.

which is *not* adjacent to the atrioventricular ring. Measures that alter AV nodal conduction times, such as ventricular stimulation with concealed penetration of the AV node, fail to alter atrial tachycardia cycle length. Ventricular premature stimulation during tachycardia does not advance atrial activation with the same atrial activation sequence as the tachycardia beats. Tachycardia continues unaltered in the presence of AV nodal and more distal atrioventricular block. Carotid sinus massage may slow and terminate atrial tachycardias.[53] Re-entrant atrial tachycardias may be initiated and terminated by atrial pacing or by ventricular pacing if VA conduction is intact.

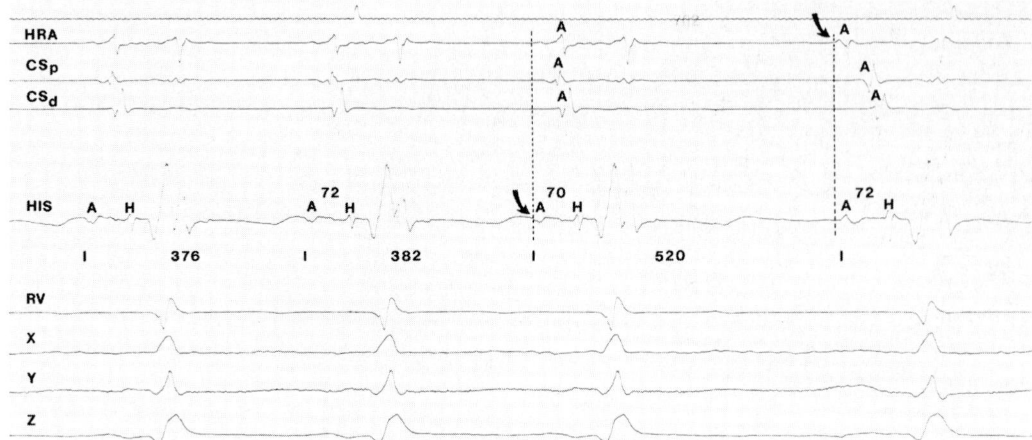

Figure 8. The last two cycles of a true atrial tachycardia are shown prior to spontaneous termination and resumption of sinus rhythm. Note that earliest atrial activation in tachycardia arises in the low right atrium. In sinus rhythm, earliest atrial activation is in the high right atrium. The two P wave morphologies are clearly different. Spontaneous termination is quite frequent in inducible atrial tachycardias.

NODO-VENTRICULAR FIBERS. The pattern of pre-excitation during an antegrade study has a typical LBBB configuration and not the usual type of broad bizarre complex seen with atrioventricular accessory connections. The A-to-delta interval is much longer than that seen with conventional pre-excitation and is independent of site of atrial pacing. The typical appearance during tachycardia is shown in Figure 9.

Maneuvers that prolong AV nodal conduction prolong the tachycardia cycle. Atrial premature stimulation advances tachycardia without changing QRS morphology. Atrial and ventricular *association* is present in more than 50 percent of cases. Tachycardia may be terminated with atrial or ventricular stimuli. In some cases, the nodo-ventricular fiber seems to be an entirely separate AV connection from the normal conduction system.[64]

INCESSANT AV RE-ENTRANT TACHYCARDIAS. This term should be reserved for unusual tachycardias using a posterior septal concealed ventriculoatrial accessory pathway with a long conduction time (two to three times that of conventional atrioventricular accessory pathways) and with conduction properties consistent with incorporation of AV nodal tissue in the accessory pathway.[56–58] Tachycardia is present nearly continuously and is often initiated following a single sinus beat (Fig. 10). The rate may vary over a wide range, and because of the inverted P waves this tachycardia is often mislabelled as a "coronary sinus rhythm." The RP interval is longer than the PR interval, a characteristic similar to atrial tachycardias. A typical example is shown in Figure 10. This type of tachycardia is distinguished from slow-fast AV junctional re-entry by the ability to advance tachycardia when the His bundle is refractory.

Electrophysiologic Laboratory Staff

For economic reasons we use the minimum number of staff necessary for the performance of good quality, safe, and technically satisfactory studies. Each study requires a cardiologist, electrophysiologic technician, and a registered nurse.

Fluoroscopy Times, Study Durations and Costs

Fluoroscopy times for 59 consecutive patients undergoing electrophysiologic study at Westmead Centre for supraventricular tachycardia are shown in Table 2. The protocol used in these studies (described earlier) was designed to induce the arrhythmia(s), to make an accu-

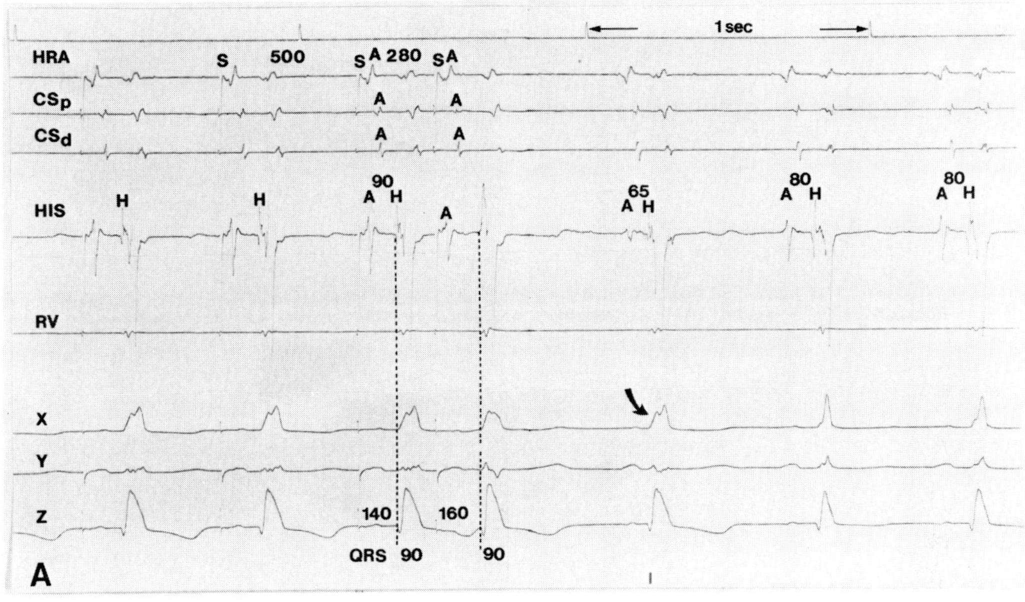

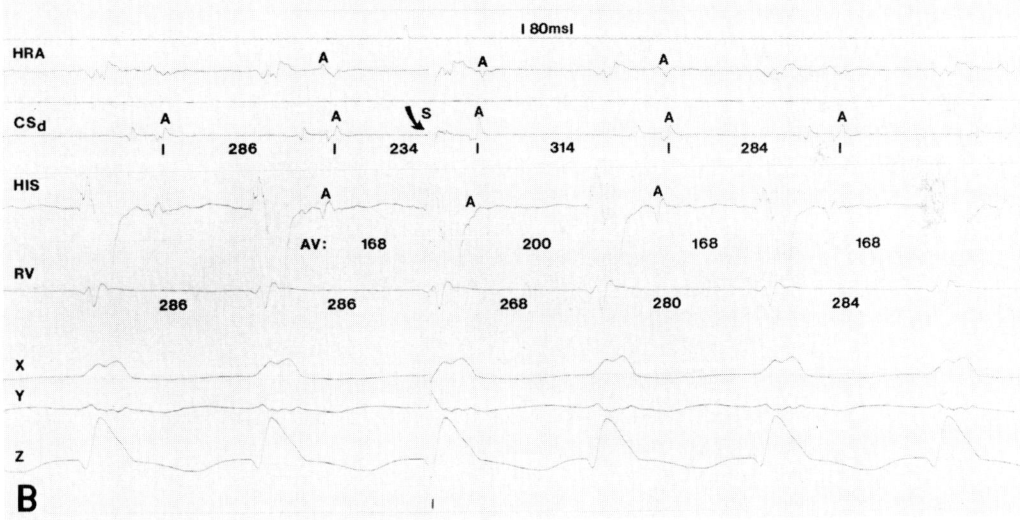

Figure 9. These tracings are typical of a nodo-ventricular fiber. *A*, This ECG shows atrial pacing at cycle length 500 ms. Note the short HV and the typical LBBB pattern of QRS morphology. Following an extrastimulus at 280 ms, the His bundle electrogram is lost in ventricular activation consistent with ventricular pre-excitation. There is some prolongation of stimulus-to-V interval. The first beat following the premature beat is probably a junctional ectopic beat inasmuch as the AH interval was shorter than any sinus AH interval. Note that more pre-excitation is present with the junctional ectopic beat than in subsequent sinus beats. Several beats of this kind were recorded during this study. *B*, This ECG shows supraventricular tachycardia using the nodo-ventricular fiber for antegrade conduction and presumably the normal conduction system for retrograde conduction. Antegrade His bundle activation is not visible. An atrial premature beat *(arrow)* delivered during tachycardia advances subsequent ventricular activation despite a prolonged A to V time. QRS morphology is identical to other tachycardia beats. The A to V times during tachycardia are much longer than those found with antidromic tachycardias using an atrioventricular accessory pathway of the conventional type. The findings here (*B*) exclude ventricular tachycardia.

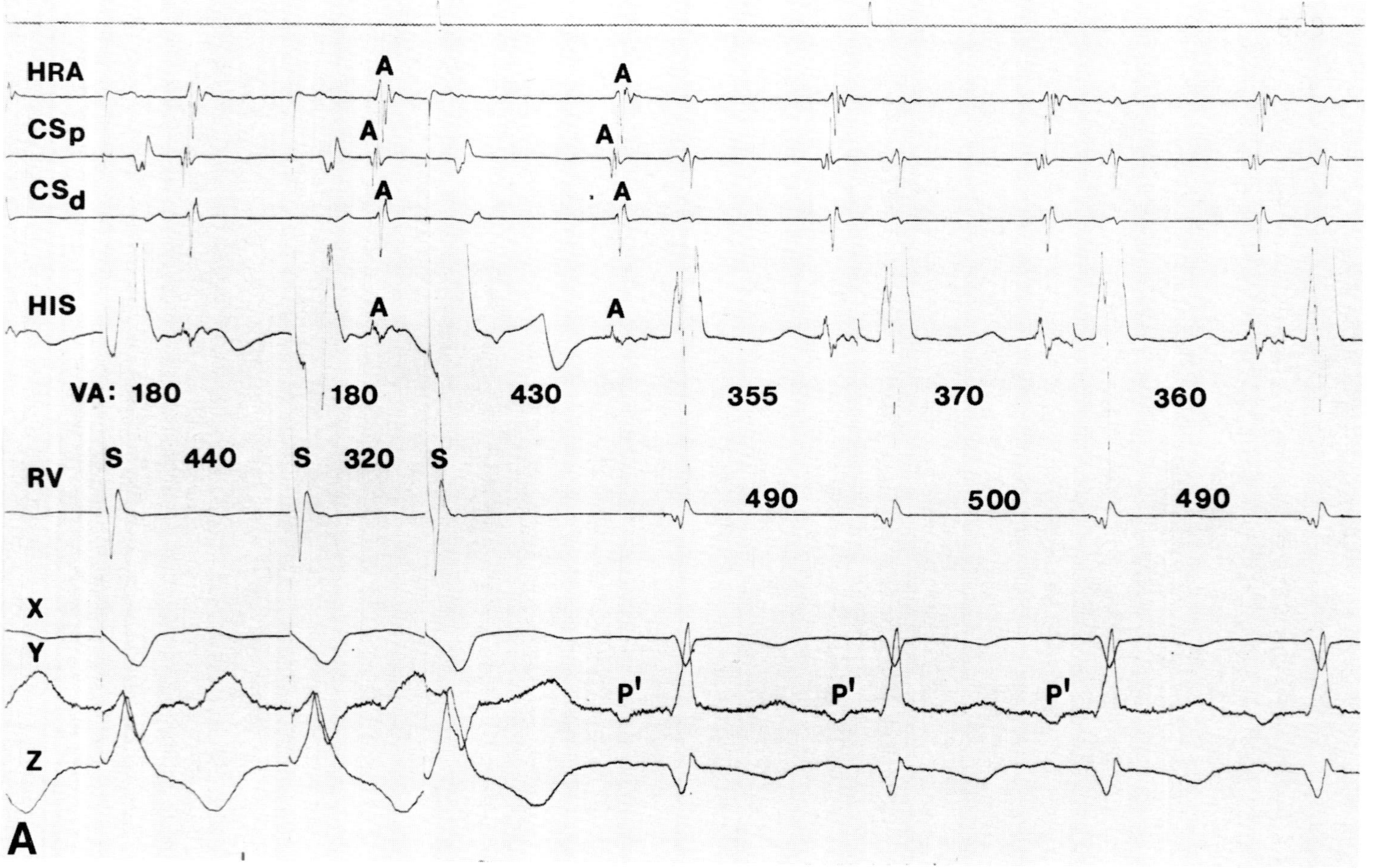

Figure 10. Salient observations during an incessant tachycardia using a posterior septal ventriculoatrial accessory pathway with a long conduction time are illustrated. *A*, Ventricular pacing with delivery of a single extrastimulus is shown. VA conduction during drive beats is consistent with retrograde conduction over the AV node. Following the extrastimulus, VA time is markedly prolonged (with only minimal changes in atrial activation sequence), and tachycardia is initiated. This is due to retrograde block in the normal pathway and retrograde conduction over the accessory pathway with a long conduction time. Note the typical inverted P waves in lead Y during tachycardia. The PR interval is much less than the RP interval.

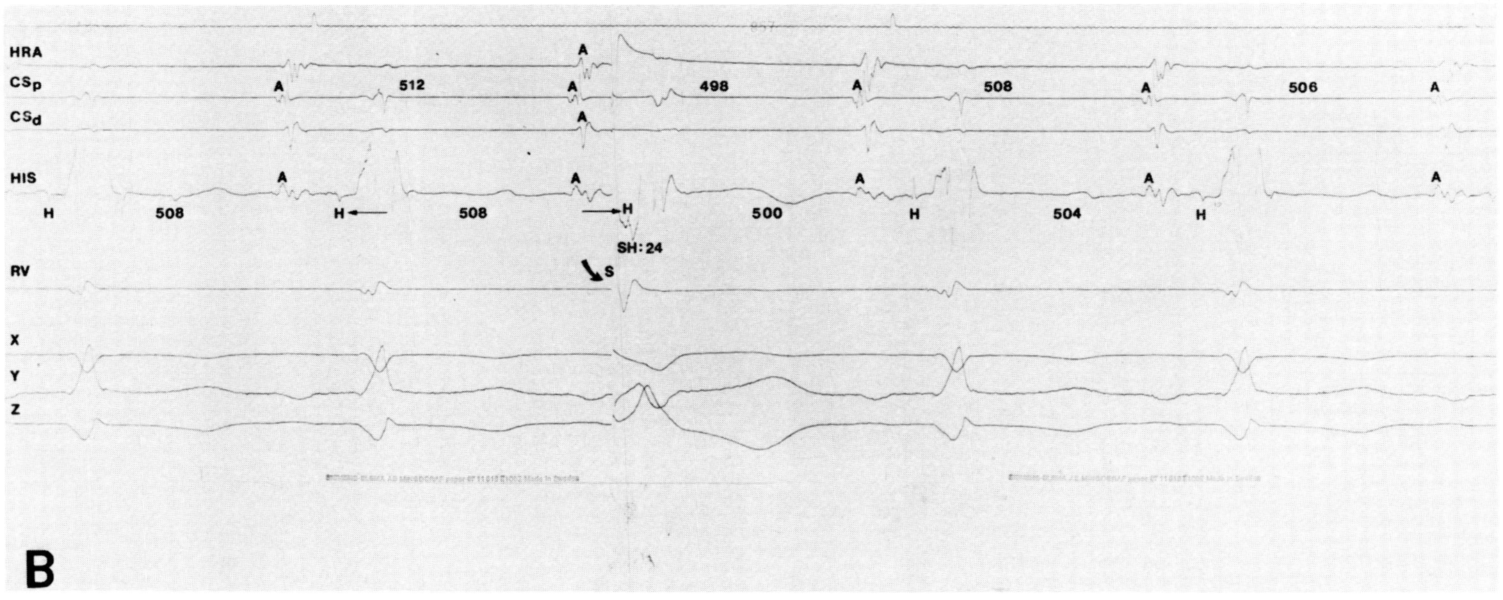

Figure 10. *Continued. B,* A ventricular extrastimulus is delivered during tachycardia. Antegrade His bundle activity falls on time, yet subsequent retrograde atrial activation is advanced, confirming the presence of a ventriculoatrial accessory pathway.

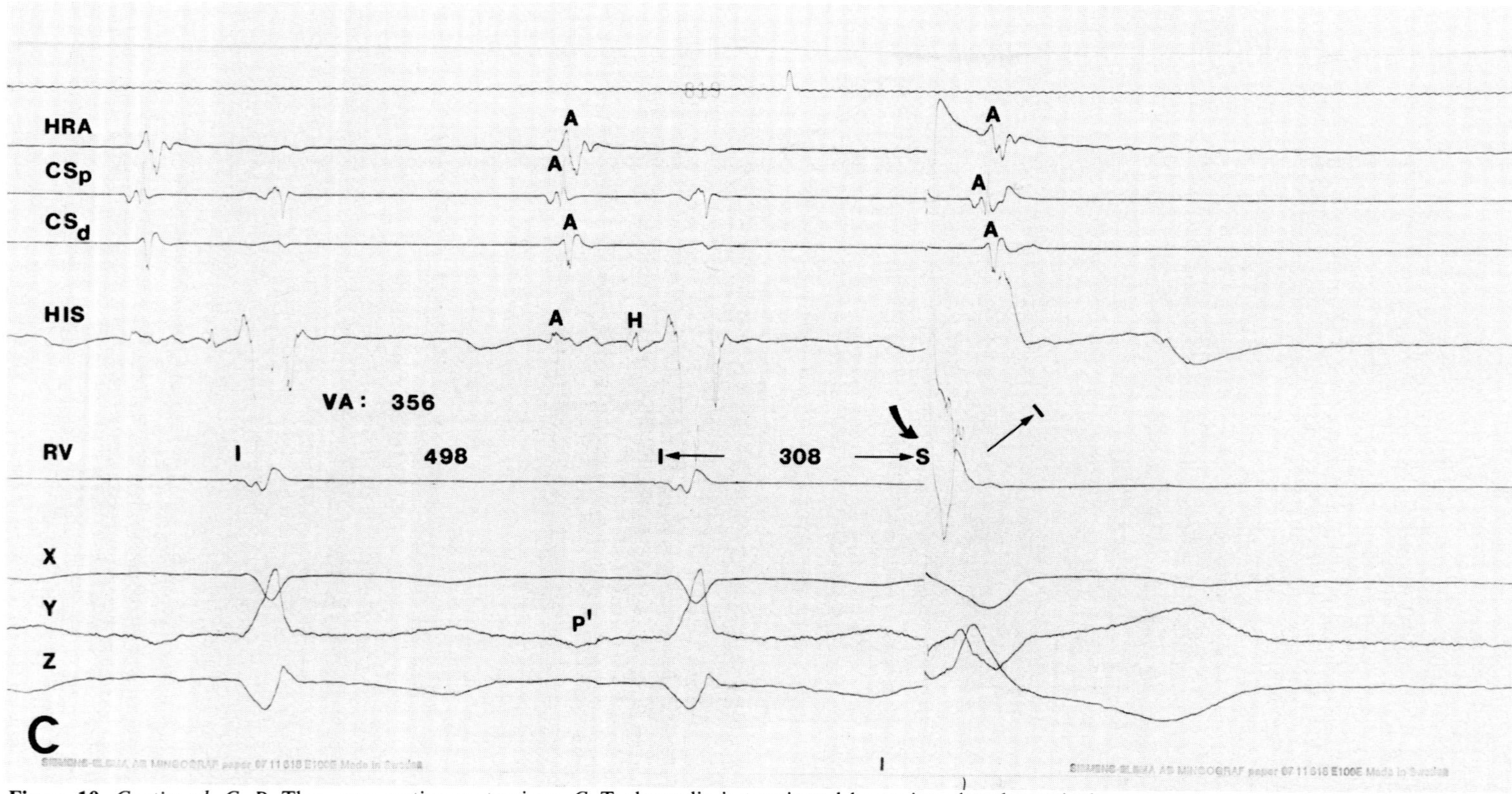

Figure 10. *Continued. C, D,* These are continuous tracings. *C,* Tachycardia is terminated by an introduced ventricular premature beat that fails to be conducted retrogradely to the atria.

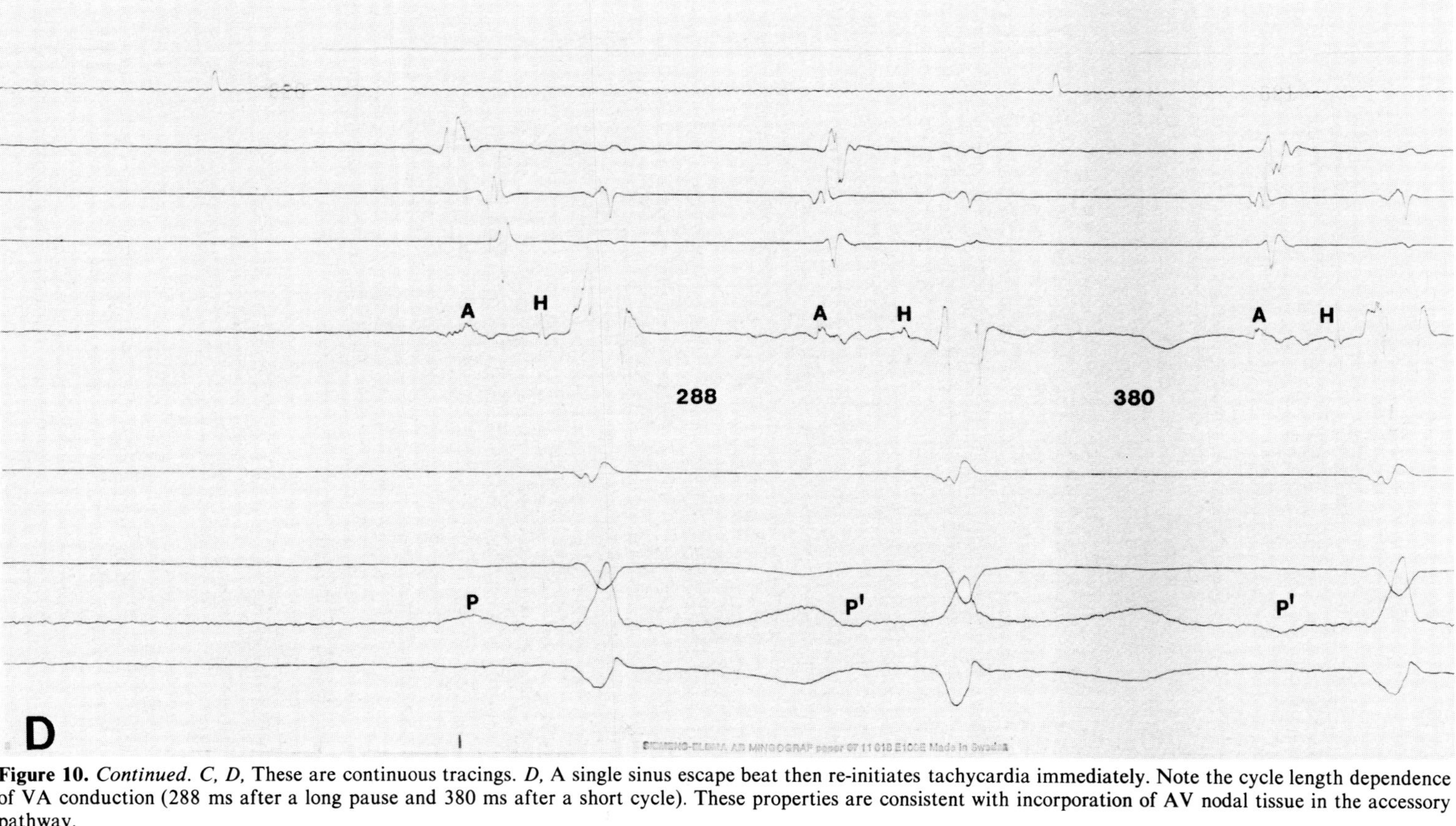

Figure 10. *Continued. C, D,* These are continuous tracings. *D,* A single sinus escape beat then re-initiates tachycardia immediately. Note the cycle length dependence of VA conduction (288 ms after a long pause and 380 ms after a short cycle). These properties are consistent with incorporation of AV nodal tissue in the accessory pathway.

Table 2. Fluoroscopy and duration of study times in electrophysiologic studies for supraventricular tachycardia

	n	*Median*	*Mean* ± *S.D.*	*Range*
Fluoroscopy time	59	10 min	11.8 ± 8.3 min	3–47 min
Duration of study*	59	110 min	121.0 ± 35.0 min	55–220 min

*Duration of study was measured from the time the patient was placed on the table to the time of removal of the patient from the laboratory (this time includes skin electrode preparation and placement and scrub up and draping times).

rate diagnosis of the tissues involved in the tachycardia circuit (or to localize the focus in non-re-entrant rhythms), and to study methods of pace termination of the arrhythmia. Acute antiarrhythmic drug testing was not performed. Thus, the information obtained was clinically relevant and did not include research procedures. This approach reduces the duration of the electrophysiologic study by greater than 30 minutes (25 percent of the total study time) when compared with previously published data.[36] In our laboratory the costs of all consumables plus the salary of an electrophysiology technician for the full financial year 1982 cost 120 dollars Australian per case. Electrode catheters are very expensive and are sterilized and re-used until nonfunctional to achieve this rather low cost. The additional costs of patient bed costs, equipment purchase and maintenance, nurse and cardiologist, sterilization, laboratory space, cleaning, electricity, and so on are not included.

COMPLICATIONS

Complications are rare. Over the last three years (1980 to 1982 inclusive), the only serious complication in our series was a deep vein thrombosis in one patient (an incidence of 0.4 percent). This complication occurred in an elderly diabetic man with a thrombotic tendency. Eleven cases (4.3 percent) developed sustained atrial fibrillation that required cardioversion under general anesthetic so that the study could continue or for hemodynamic reasons in patients with a rapidly conducting accessory atrioventricular connection. An additional 11 patients (4.3 percent) developed sustained atrial fibrillation near the end of the study after all relevant information had been obtained. None suffered hemodynamic impairment, and all reverted spontaneously to sinus rhythm within 24 hours of the conclusion of the study without any specific treatment.

This low rate of complications is due to the inherent low risk of these types of studies and the fact that most patients with supraventricular tachycardia are otherwise free of heart disease and are in good general health. Josephson and Seides also noted a low incidence of complications related to electrophysiologic study.[40]

BENEFITS DERIVED FROM ELECTROPHYSIOLOGIC STUDY

Definitive Diagnosis

As with most diseases, a definitive diagnosis enables a clearer and more effective plan of management to be drawn up that is more satisfying to both patient and physician. "Tachycardia" or "SVT" is no more a diagnosis than is "heart failure" or "systolic murmur." Furthermore, paroxysmal tachycardias are often difficult to capture on ECG because of spontaneous termination or a low frequency of arrhythmia episodes. Many of these patients are therefore diagnosed as suffering from anxiety, nervous disorders, and so on. Induction of sustained supraventricular tachycardia at electrophysiologic study frequently provides the diagnosis in these cases, confirming to the patient that he or she has not become neurotic but indeed suffers from an organic disorder.

Electrophysiologic studies also enable erroneous provisional diagnoses to be corrected. The most common errors are ventricular tachycardia previously labelled as supraventricular tachycardia with aberrant conduction, supraventricular tachycardia with aberration diagnosed as ventricular tachycardia, confusion of intraventricular conduction defects with Wolff-Parkinson-White syndrome and vice versa, and antidromic tachycardias using an atrioventricular accessory pathway or tachycardias utilizing a nodo-ventricular fiber wrongly diagnosed as ventricular tachycardia.

In addition, on the basis of a surface ECG, AV junctional re-entry is often hard to distinguish from supraventricular tachycardias using an atrioventricular accessory pathway.

Another group in which electrophysiologic study clarifies diagnosis are those patients with two different types of tachycardia, for example, two different types of supraventricular tachycardia, or both supraventricular tachycardia and ventricular tachycardia (Fig. 11), or multiple accessory pathway tachycardias.

Choice of Therapy

Four different types of treatment are currently available for supraventricular tachycardia: antiarrhythmic drugs, antitachycardia pacemakers, antiarrhythmic surgery, and, recently, catheter His bundle and/or AV node ablation.

AV nodal blocking drugs (for example, digoxin, beta blockers, verapamil) are the first line of treatment for AV junctional tachycardias. Quinidine and like drugs are the first line of treatment for most circus-movement tachycardias utilizing an AV accessory pathway. Digoxin, or verapamil, or quinidine-like drugs are the first-line treatment for atrial tachycardias. AV nodal blocking drugs and/or quinidine-like drugs are useful for nodo-ventricular fiber tachycardias. Incessant tachycardias are slowed by AV nodal blocking drugs, but the tachycardia is not usually abolished. A few of the newer antiarrhythmic drugs such as amiodarone, oral encainide, and sotalol may be effective in all types of supraventricular tachycardias.

Antitachycardia pacemakers are most useful for AV junctional re-entry tachycardias (where surgery currently abolishes symptoms at the expense of heart block); incessant tachycardias (by using simultaneous atrial and ventricular pacing);[2] and drug refractory cases of AV accessory pathway tachycardias unsuitable for surgery. Current automatic antitachycardia pacemakers recognize tachycardia and use either programmable bursts or programmable multiple extrastimuli for tachycardia termination.[30,31] These methods must first be shown to be reliable and effective at electrophysiologic study before permanent pacemaker implantation.

Surgical section of an atrioventricular accessory pathway abolishes supraventricular tachycardias incorporating that pathway in the circuit and prevents rapid AV conduction over the accessory pathway. In addition, recurrence of atrial fibrillation is abolished in approximately 75 percent of patients with preoperative atrial fibrillation who are younger than 40 years old and free of myocardial disease (JB Uther, unpublished data). With free wall accessory pathways, failure to section the accessory pathway now occurs in less than 1 percent of cases, and operative mortality is less than 1 percent in uncomplicated cases.[24,27] Success rates are lower for septal accessory pathways, but current success rates are in the 50 to 90 percent range and rising.[24,27] Successful section of the accessory pathway therefore "cures" the patient with an operation of low mortality and morbidity. The most common cause for an unsuccessful result from surgery nowadays is the failure to recognize preoperatively or intraoperatively the presence of an additional accessory pathway or other mechanism of tachycardia. Additional pathways or tachycardias occur in about 5 to 10 percent of cases. It is hoped that failures that

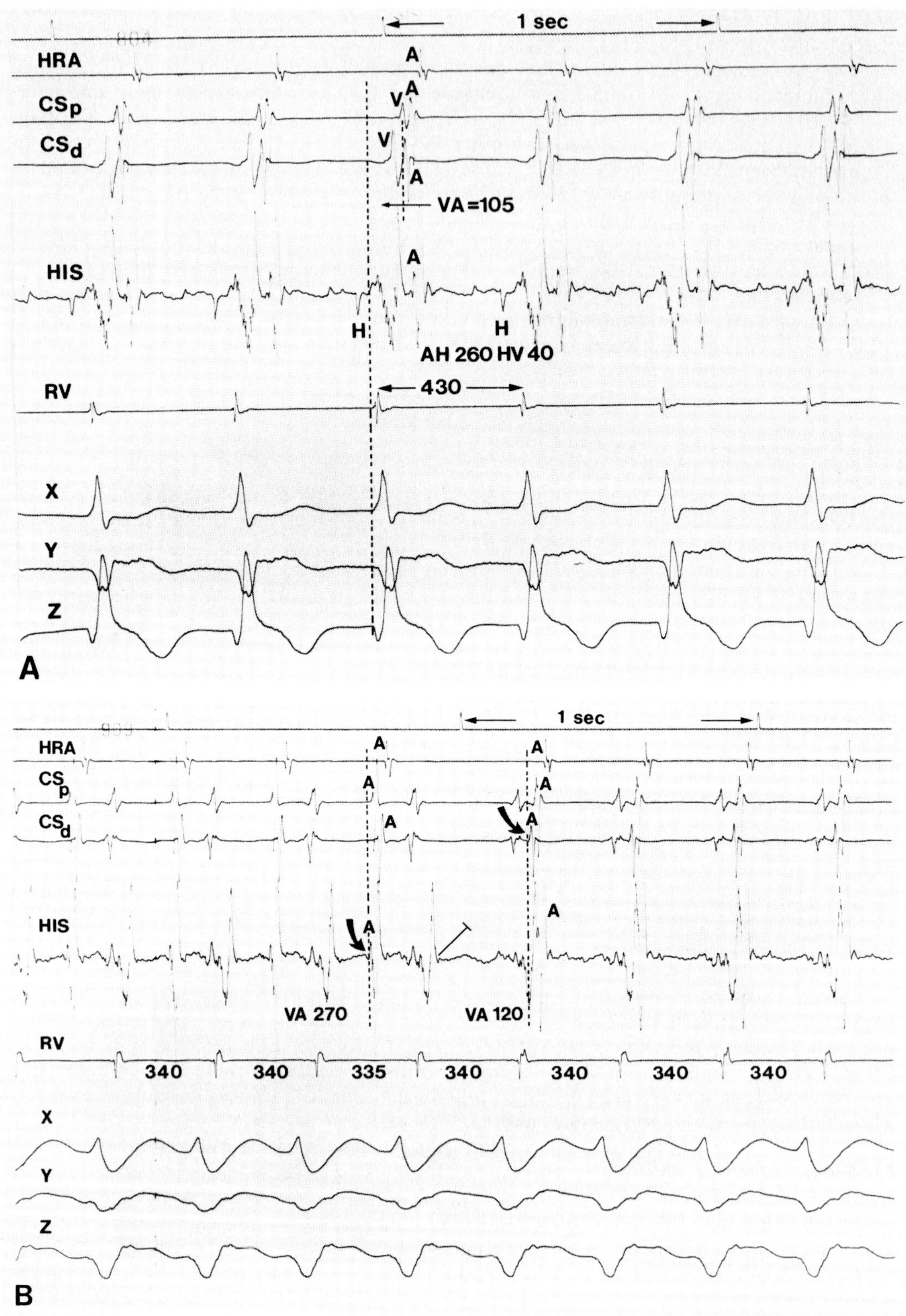
1 sec
HRA
CSp
CSd
A
V
VA=105
HIS
H
AH 260 HV 40
RV
430
X
Y
Z
A
1 sec
HRA
CSp
CSd
HIS
VA 270
VA 120
RV
340
335
X
Y
Z
B

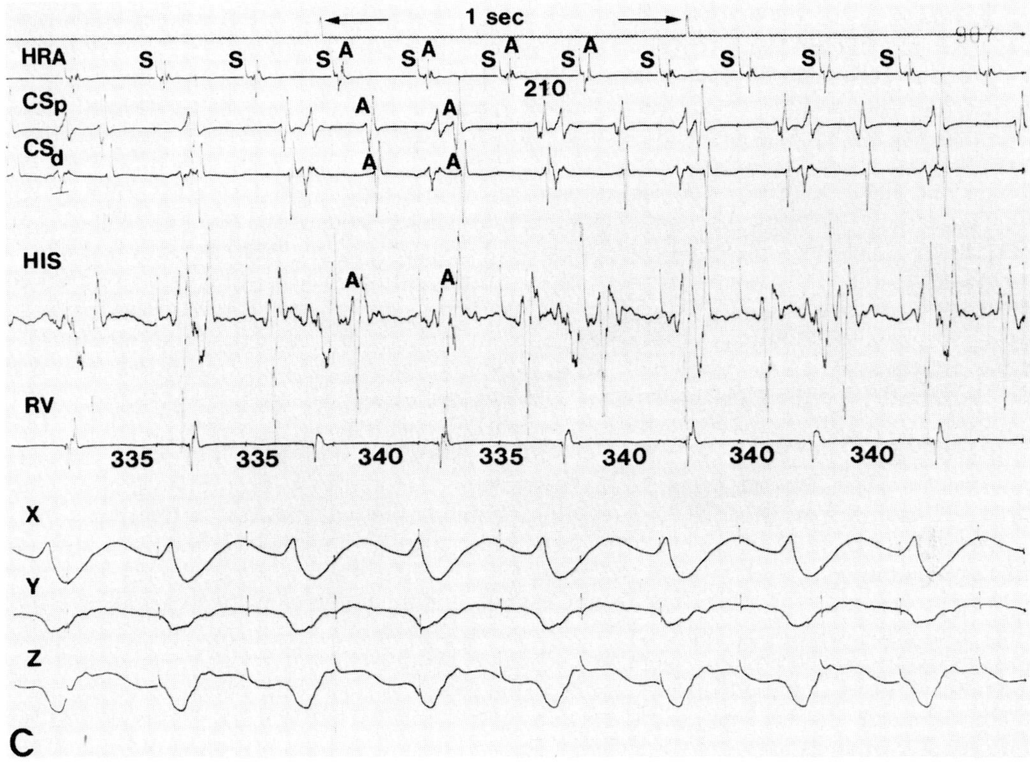

Figure 11. These figures were obtained during investigation of a patient with two different types of paroxysmal tachycardia: one narrow complex QRS and the other wide complex QRS. *A*, This ECG shows typical tracings of a supraventricular tachycardia using a concealed left free wall ventriculoatrial accessory pathway with earliest atrial activation in the distal coronary sinus lead. *B*, This ECG shows a broad complex tachycardia. Anterograde His bundle activation is not present. The left-hand portion is consistent with retrograde conduction over the AV node. VA block occurs following a minor shortening of tachycardia cycle length, and VA conduction then resumes over the left-sided ventriculoatrial accessory pathway. *C*, This ECG shows rapid atrial pacing during the broad complex tachycardia. Note that the broad complex tachycardia continues unchanged despite complete dissociation of atrial and ventricular activation. Thus, both ventricular tachycardia and supraventricular tachycardia using a concealed left free wall ventriculoatrial connection were present in one patient, causing understandable diagnostic problems.

are due to missed pathways will diminish in the future with appropriate vigilance for this problem in the preoperative assessment.

Intractable AV junctional re-entry tachycardia may be symptomatically treated by ablation of the AV node or section of the His bundle, usually with placement of a permanent pacemaker to protect against unstable escape rhythms. This operation does not restore normal anatomy and leaves both patient and doctor with the problem of permanent pacing.

A similar technique may be used for intractable atrial tachycardias, but alternative methods of excision of the atrial re-entrant circuit or automatic "focus" are feasible and successful in approximately 70 percent of cases.[26] Atrial tachycardias that are inducible by programmed stimulation have a higher chance of surgical success than noninducible automatic tachycardias. The increase in left ventricular function in these patients after years of almost constant tachycardia is uniform and sometimes spectacular (for example, increase from a preoperative ejection fraction of 19 percent to 70 percent postoperatively).

We have surgically interrupted re-entry circuits using a nodo-ventricular fiber in two cases, in one by selective section of the nodo-ventricular fiber and in another by His bundle section.

AV conduction over the nodo-ventricular fiber was preserved in the latter case. Both patients have had no recurrence of arrhythmia on long-term followup and have intact AV conduction. Gillette and coworkers have also successfully sectioned nodo-ventricular type fibers.[64]

The accessory pathway used in incessant tachycardias using a septal ventriculoatrial accessory pathway with a long conduction time is located close to the normal AV conduction system, making selective surgical section of the accessory pathway technically different. Gallagher and Sealy have reported successful surgical interruption of this tachycardia by His bundle section.[57] Retrograde conduction over the accessory connection remained intact.

Catheter ablation of the His bundle area has been successfully used for treatment of AV junctional re-entry, atrial tachycardias, atrial fibrillation or flutter with a rapid ventricular response,[32] and one case of an incessant tachycardia using a septal VA accessory pathway with a long conduction time.[65] This type of approach, although nonoperative, suffers from the same defects as operative His bundle section. Normal anatomy is not usually restored, and the tachycardia is often replaced with a permanent pacemaker. This result is an improvement, indeed, but not a total cure as with accessory pathway section.

It is obvious from the aforementioned considerations that rational and effective choice of treatment is dependent on a total electrophysiologic diagnosis. The performance of an electrophysiologic study is therefore the key to determining the best methods of treatment.

Lastly, the choice of treatment depends on balancing the patient's symptoms against the efficacy and morbidity of treatment. Although usually not a life-threatening disease, recurrent supraventricular tachycardia adds an unpleasant, unpredictable element to a patient's life, thus affecting personality, approach to life, participation in sporting and social activities, response to stress, and ability to perform certain occupations. Only the patient can accurately judge the severity of the incapacitation. Physicians can offer accurate advice about the likely success and side effects of proposed treatment, but the balancing of these factors against the severity of symptoms and their wider influence on life-style is best left to the patient. Many patients approached in this way choose an attempt at surgical cure if their tachycardia is a suitable type. Fortunately, almost 50 percent of supraventricular tachycardias are suitable for curative surgery.

CONCLUSIONS

Electrophysiologic studies permit a comprehensive electrophysiologic assessment of a supraventricular tachycardia and thereby define the various options of treatment. Although surgery is only one avenue of treatment, it should be emphasized that surgical cure of tachycardia is possible in almost 50 percent of all patients with supraventricular tachycardia and is currently available at an acceptably low mortality and morbidity. We believe that in addition to patients with life-threatening or refractory tachycardias, appropriate patients with non-life-threatening tachycardias should be offered the option of surgical treatment earlier than is current practice and that each patient should make his or her choice of treatment after full explanation of the pros and cons of the alternative methods available. Performance of an electrophysiologic study is necessary for this type of approach to treatment of supraventricular tachycardia.

ACKNOWLEDGEMENTS

We wish to acknowledge the major contributions of our colleagues David Cody, David Richards, Paul Russell, and Alan Young. David Johnson performed all the cardiac surgery for arrhythmias at Westmead Centre. We are especially grateful to our electrophysiologic technicians and to our research technicians, Kathy Palmer and Judy Waywood.

REFERENCES

1. Durrer, D, Schoo, L, Schuilenburg, RM, et al: *The role of premature beats in the initiation and termination of supraventricular tachycardia in the Wolff-Parkinson-White syndrome.* Circulation 36:644, 1967.
2. Coumel, P, Cabrol, C, Fabiato, A, et al: *Tachycardie permanente par rhythme reciproque (I) Preuves du diagnostic par stimulation auriculaire et ventriculaire (II) Traitement par l'implantation intracorporelle d'un stimulateur cardiaque avec entrainement simultane de l'oreillette et du ventricle.* Arch Mal Coeur 60:1830, 1967.
3. Hunt, NC, Cobb, FR, Waxman, MB, et al: *Conversion of supraventricular tachycardias with atrial stimulation: Evidence for re-entry mechanism.* Circulation 38:1060, 1968.
4. Barold, SS, Linhart, JW, Sarnet, P, et al: *Supraventricular tachycardia initiated and terminated by a single electrical stimulus.* Am J Cardiol 24:37, 1969.
5. Goldreyer, BN and Bigger, JT Jr: *Spontaneous and induced re-entrant tachycardia.* Ann Intern Med 70:87, 1969.
6. Cobb, FR, Blumenschein, SD, Sealy, WC, et al: *Successful surgical interruption of the bundle of Kent in a patient with Wolff-Parkinson-White syndrome.* Circulation 38:1018, 1968.
7. Sealy, WC, Hattler, BC, Blumenschein, SD, et al: *Surgical treatment of the Wolff-Parkinson-White syndrome.* Ann Thorac Surg 8:1, 1969.
8. Iwa, T, Kazui, T, Sugii, S, et al: *Surgical treatment of Wolff-Parkinson-White syndrome.* Kyobu Geka 23:513, 1970.
9. Sealy, WC, Wallace, AG, Ramming, KP, et al: *An improved operation for definitive treatment of the Wolff-Parkinson-White syndrome.* Ann Thorac Surg 17:107, 1974.
10. Wallace, AG, Sealy, WC, Gallagher, JJ, et al: *Surgical correction of anomalous left ventricular preexcitation: Wolff-Parkinson-White syndrome (Type A).* Circulation 49:206, 1974.
11. Coumel, P and Barold, SS: *Mechanisms of supraventricular tachycardia.* In Narula, OS (ed): *His Bundle Electrocardiography and Clinical Electrophysiology.* FA Davis, Philadelphia, 1975.
12. Sealy, WC, Gallagher, JJ, and Wallace, AG: *The surgical treatment of the Wolff-Parkinson-White syndrome: Evolution of the improved methods of identification and interruption of the Kent bundle.* Ann Thorac Surg 22:443, 1976.
13. Iwa, T: *Surgical experiences with the Wolff-Parkinson-White syndrome.* J Cardiovasc Surg 17:549, 1976.
14. Harrison, L, Gallagher, JJ, Kasell, J, et al: *Cryosurgical ablation of the atrioventricular node-His bundle: A new method for producing atrioventricular block.* Circulation 55:463, 1977.
15. Sealy, WC, Gallagher, JJ, and Pritchett, ELC: *The surgical anatomy of Kent bundles based on electrophysiological mapping and surgical exploration.* J Thorac Cardiovasc Surg 76:804, 1978.
16. Baird, DK and Uther, JB: *Surgical management of supraventricular tachycardia.* In Kelly, DT (ed): *Advances in the Management of Arrhythmias.* Telectronics, Sydney, 1978, pp 150–161.
17. Pritchett, ELC, Anderson, RW, Benditt, DG, et al: *Re-entry within the atrioventricular node: Surgical cure with preservation of atrioventricular conduction.* Circulation 60:440, 1979.
18. Sealy, WC and Gallagher, JJ: *The surgical approach to the septal area of the heart based on experiences with 45 patients with Kent bundles.* J Thorac Cardiovasc Surg 79:542, 1980.
19. Iwa, T, Magara, T, Watanabe, Y, et al: *Interruption of multiple accessory conduction pathways in the Wolff-Parkinson-White syndrome.* Ann Thorac Surg 30:313, 1980.
20. Klein, GJ, Sealy, WC, Pritchett, ELC, et al: *Cryosurgical ablation of the atrioventricular node-His bundle: Long-term followup and properties of the junctional pacemaker.* Circulation 61:8, 1980.
21. Camm, J, Ward, DE, Spurrell, RAJ, et al: *Cryothermal mapping and cryoablation of refractory cardiac arrhythmias.* Circulation 62:67, 1980.
22. Wyndham, CRC, Arnsdorf, MF, Levitsky, S, et al: *Successful surgical excision of focal paroxysmal atrial tachycardia. Observations in vivo and in vitro.* Circulation 62:1365, 1980.
23. Sealy, WC and Gallagher, JJ: *Surgical problems with multiple accessory pathways of atrioventricular conduction.* J Thorac Cardiovasc Surg 81:707, 1981.
24. Gallagher, JJ, Sealy, WC, Cox, JL, et al: *Results of surgery for pre-excitation in 200 cases.* Circulation 64 (Suppl IV):146, 1981.
25. Anderson, KP, Stinson, EB, and Mason, JW: *Surgical exclusion of focal paroxysmal atrial tachycardia.* Am J Cardiol 49:869, 1982.
26. Russell, PA, Johnson, DC, Denniss, AR, et al: *Surgical management of right atrial tachycardia.* Am J Cardiol 49:994, 1982.

27. UTHER, JB, JOHNSON, DC, BAIRD, DK, ET AL: *Surgical section of accessory atrioventricular connections in 108 patients.* Am J Cardiol 49:995, 1982.

28. BAROLD, SS: *Therapeutic uses of cardiac pacing in tachyarrhythmias.* In NARULA, OS (ED): *His Bundle Electrocardiography and Clinical Electrophysiology.* FA Davis, Philadelphia, 1975, p 407.

29. WELLENS, HJJ, BAR, FW, GORGELS, AP, ET AL: *Electrical management of arrhythmias with emphasis on the tachycardias.* Am J Cardiol 41:1025, 1978.

30. GRIFFIN, JC, MASON, JW, AND CALFEE, RV: *A programmable tachycardia terminating pacemaker for the treatment of arrhythmias.* In HARRISON, DC (ED): *Cardiac Arrhythmias. A Decade of Progress.* G.K. Hall, Boston, 1981, p 383.

31. SPURRELL, RAJ, NATHAN, AW, BEXTON, RS, ET AL: *Implantable automatic scanning pacemaker for termination of supraventricular tachycardia.* Am J Cardiol 49:753, 1982.

32. GALLAGHER, JJ, SVENSON, RH, KASELL, JH, ET AL: *Catheter technique for closed chest ablation of the atrioventricular conduction system. A therapeutic alternative for treatment of refractory supraventricular tachycardia.* N Engl J Med 306:194, 1982.

33. WELLENS, HJJ, BAR, FW, GORGELS, AP, ET AL: *Use of ajmaline in patients with the Wolff-Parkinson-White syndrome to disclose short refractory period of the accessory pathway.* Am J Cardiol 45:130, 1980.

34. WELLENS, HJJ, BRAAT, S, BRUGADA, P, ET AL: *Use of procainamide in patients with the Wolff-Parkinson-White syndrome to disclose a short refractory period of the accessory pathway.* Am J Cardiol 50:1087, 1982.

35. RUSKIN, JN, CARACTA, AR, BATSFORD, WP, ET AL: *Electrophysiologic effects of diazepam in man.* Clin Res 22:302A, 1974.

36. ROSS, DL, FARRE, J, BAR, FW, ET AL: *Comprehensive clinical electrophysiologic studies in the investigation of documented or suspected tachycardias: Times, staff, problems, costs.* Circulation 61:1010, 1980.

37. NARULA, OS, SCHERLAG, BJ, AND SAMET, P: *Pervenous pacing of the specialized conduction system in man: His bundle and A-V nodal stimulation.* Circulation 41:77, 1970.

38. NARULA, OS: *Validation of His bundle recordings: Limitations of the catheter technique.* In NARULA, OS (ED): *His Bundle Electrocardiography and Clinical Electrophysiology.* FA Davis, Philadelphia, 1975, p 65.

39. FRANK, E: *An accurate clinically practical system for spatial vectorcardiography.* Circulation 13:737, 1956.

40. JOSEPHSON, ME AND SEIDES, SF: *Clinical Cardiac Electrophysiology. Techniques and Interpretations.* Lea & Febiger, Philadelphia, 1979.

41. MANDEL, W, HAYAKAWA, H, DANZIG, R, ET AL: *Evaluation of sino-atrial node function in man by overdrive suppression.* Circulation 44:59, 1971.

42. GALLAGHER, JJ, PRITCHETT, ELC, BENDITT, DG, ET AL: *New catheter techniques for analysis of the sequence of retrograde atrial activation in man.* Eur J Cardiol 6:1, 1977.

43. WELLENS, HJJ AND DURRER, D: *The role of an atrioventricular accessory pathway in reciprocal tachycardia. Observations in patients with and without the Wolff-Parkinson-White syndrome.* Circulation 52:58, 1975.

44. WELLENS, HJJ: *Value and limitations of programmed electrical stimulation of the heart in the study and treatment of tachycardias.* Circulation 57:845, 1978.

45. GALLAGHER, JJ, PRITCHETT, ELC, AND WALLACE, AG: *The pre-excitation syndromes.* Prog Cardiovasc Dis 20:285, 1978.

46. COUMEL, P AND ATTUEL, P: *Reciprocating tachycardia in overt and latent pre-excitation. Influence of functional bundle branch block on the rate of tachycardia.* Eur J Cardiol 1:423, 1974.

47. SPURRELL, RAJ, KRIKLER, DM, AND SOWTON, E: *Concealed bypasses of the atrioventricular node in patients with paroxysmal supraventricular tachycardia revealed by intracardiac stimulation and verapamil.* Am J Cardiol 33:590, 1974.

48. ZIPES, DP, DE JOSEPH, RL, AND ROTHBAUM, DA: *Unusual properties of accessory pathways.* Circulation 49:1200, 1974.

49. NEUSS, H, SCHLEPPER, M, AND THORMANN, J: *Analysis of re-entry mechanisms in three patients with concealed Wolff-Parkinson-White syndrome.* Circulation 51:75, 1975.

50. DENES, P, WU, D, DHINGRA, RC, ET AL: *Demonstration of dual AV nodal pathways in patients with supraventricular tachycardia.* Circulation 48:549, 1973.

51. WU, D, DENES, P, AMAT-Y-LEON, F, ET AL: *An unusual variety of atrioventricular nodal re-entry due to retrograde dual atrioventricular nodal pathways.* Circulation 56:50, 1977.

52. NARULA, OS: *Sinus node re-entry: A mechanism for supraventricular tachycardia.* Circulation 50:1114, 1974.

53. WU, D, AMAT-Y-LEON, F, DENES, P, ET AL: *Demonstration of sustained sinus and atrial re-entry as a mechanism of paroxysmal supraventricular tachycardia.* Circulation 51:234, 1975.

54. CURRY, PVL AND KRICKLER, DM: *Paroxysmal reciprocating sinus tachycardia.* In KULBERTUS, HE (ED): *Reentrant Arrhythmias.* MTP Press, Lancaster, 1977, p 39.

55. Gallagher, JJ, Smith, WM, Kasell, JH, et al: *Role of Mahaim fibers in cardiac arrhythmias in man.* Circulation 64:176, 1981.

56. Coumel, P: *Junctional reciprocating tachycardias. The permanent and paroxysmal forms of AV-nodal reciprocating tachycardia.* J Electrocardiol 8:79, 1975.

57. Gallagher, JJ and Sealy, WC: *The permanent form of junctional reciprocating tachycardia: Further elucidation of the underlying mechanism.* Eur J Cardiol 8:413, 1978.

58. Farre, J, Ross, D, Wiener, I, et al: *Reciprocal tachycardias using accessory pathways with long conduction times.* Am J Cardiol 44:1099, 1979.

59. Narula, OS (ed): *Cardiac Arrhythmias: Electrophysiology, Diagnosis and Management.* Williams & Wilkins, Baltimore, 1979.

60. Uther, JB, Geary, G, Sadick, N, et al: *Electrophysiological investigation of supraventricular tachycardia.* In Kelly, DT (ed): *Advances in the Management of Arrhythmias.* Telectronics, Sydney, 1978.

61. Wellens, HJJ, Wesdorp, JC, Duren, DR, et al: *Second degree block during reciprocal atrioventricular nodal tachycardia.* Circulation 53:595, 1976.

62. Hariman, RJ, Gomes, JAC, and El Sherif, N: *Catecholamine dependent atrioventricular nodal re-entrant tachycardia.* Circulation 67:681, 1983.

63. Wu, D, Denes, P, Bauernfeind, R, et al: *Effects of atropine on induction and maintenance of atrioventricular nodal re-entrant tachycardia.* Circulation 59:779, 1979.

64. Gillette, PC, Garson, A, Cooley, DA, et al: *Prolonged and decremental antegrade conduction properties in right anterior accessory connections: Wide QRS antidromic tachycardia of left bundle branch block pattern without Wolff-Parkinson-White configuration in sinus rhythm.* Am Heart J 103:66, 1982.

65. Critelli, G, Perticone, F, Coltorti, F, et al: *Antegrade slow bypass conduction after closed chest ablation of the His bundle in permanent junctional reciprocating tachycardia.* Circulation 67:687, 1983.

Ventricular Arrhythmia Induction Study

Roger A. Freedman, M.D., and Jay W. Mason, M.D.

Ventricular arrhythmia induction by appropriately timed electrical stimulation of the heart in patients with recurrent, sustained ventricular tachycardia was first described by Wellens and coworkers in 1972.[1] It was subsequently shown that inducibility of arrhythmias after pharmacologic interventions predicted response to long-term therapy.[2–6] Since then, ventricular arrhythmia induction studies have assumed an increasing role in the management of patients with known or suspected ventricular arrhythmias (Table 1). Induction studies are performed not only in patients with recurrent, sustained ventricular tachycardia but also in patients with unsustained ventricular tachycardia, ventricular fibrillation, out-of-hospital cardiac arrest, and syncope of unknown etiology. Most recently, induction studies have been used prospectively to identify patients at high risk for suffering malignant ventricular arrhythmias.[7,8] There is considerable controversy pertaining to the techniques of arrhythmia induction and to the value of induction studies in various patient subgroups.

TECHNIQUES OF VENTRICULAR ARRHYTHMIA INDUCTION STUDY

Patients are studied in the conscious state; light sedation is frequently administered. Several surface electrocardiographic channels are simultaneously monitored. Electrode catheters are positioned at one or more endocardial sites using fluoroscopic guidance. Multipolar catheters are used to allow simultaneous bipolar stimulation and recording of intracardiac electrograms. Electrograms are recorded from ventricular sites, the right atrium, and from the area of the His bundle. Stimuli are rectangular pulses, usually of 1 or 2 msec in duration and twice diastolic threshold in amplitude. Intra-arterial pressure is directly monitored.

Table 1. Proposed indications for ventricular arrhythmia induction study

Sustained ventricular tachycardia*
Unsustained ventricular tachycardia*
Ventricular fibrillation*
Wide-complex tachycardia of uncertain mechanism*
Out-of-hospital cardiac arrest*
Syncope of unknown etiology
Assessment of prognosis in high-risk patients

*not associated with acute myocardial infarction

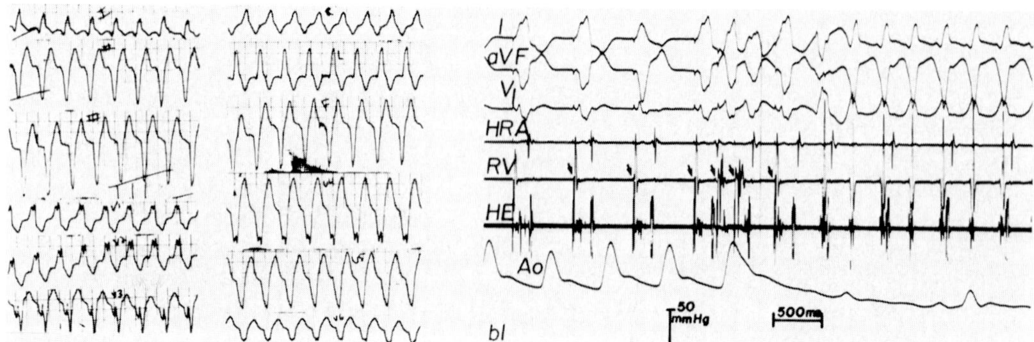

Figure 1. Induction of ventricular tachycardia with morphology similar to spontaneous arrhythmia is illustrated. On the left is a standard surface 12-lead electrocardiogram of spontaneous ventricular tachycardia, with a right bundle branch block, left axis deviation morphology. On the right, ventricular tachycardia of similar morphology is induced with three extrastimuli delivered during ventricular-paced rhythm. Two-to-one ventriculoatrial block is present during tachycardia. His bundle depolarizations are not seen. I, aVF, V_1 = standard surface electrocardiograph leads; HRA = high right atrial electrogram; RV = right ventricular electrogram; HE = His bundle electrogram; Ao = aortic pressure; bl = baseline for blood pressure calibration.

Stimuli are delivered according to a specific protocol or until a predetermined endpoint is reached. Protocol and endpoints vary from one laboratory to the next. In our laboratory, reproduction of the spontaneous arrhythmia is the endpoint in patients with spontaneous ventricular tachycardia or fibrillation. When the spontaneous arrhythmia has not been recorded on a 12-lead electrocardiogram or when it cannot be reproduced, therapy assessment can be based on any sustained, unimorphic, ventricular tachycardia. In patients with out-of-hospital cardiac arrest, the endpoint in our laboratory is a sustained ventricular tachyarrhythmia.

Our stimulation protocol begins with single ventricular stimuli delivered to the right ventricular apex during late diastole during sinus rhythm. The coupling interval of the premature stimulus is decreased until refractoriness is reached. With the first extrastimulus positioned 10 msec after the ventricular refractory period, a second extrastimulus is delivered at decreasing coupling intervals to the first until refractoriness to the second extrastimulus is reached. Up to three extrastimuli are introduced in this manner. Extrastimuli are similarly delivered during ventricular paced rhythm (Fig. 1). Multiple ventricular pacing cycle lengths, ranging from 700 to 400 msec, may be used. Ventricular burst pacing of several seconds duration is delivered at successively shorter cycle lengths until 1:1 capture is no longer obtained. The entire pacing protocol may be repeated at a second right ventricular site, at a left ventricular site, or during isoproterenol infusion.

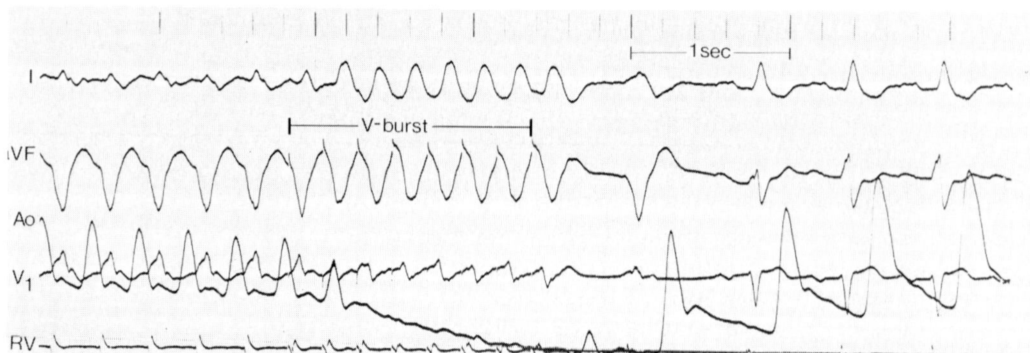

Figure 2. This ECG shows termination of ventricular tachycardia by ventricular burst pacing. Abbreviations as in Figure 1. (From Mason, JW, and Winkle, RA,[4] with permission of the American Heart Association, Inc.)

If a sustained ventricular arrhythmia is induced, the patient's hemodynamic status is assessed. Termination by pacing is attempted during hemodynamically well-tolerated rhythms (Fig. 2); cardioversion is promptly performed when the rhythm is poorly tolerated.

Ventricular arrhythmia induction studies should be performed only by personnel experienced in resuscitating patients from malignant arrhythmias. We strongly recommend that two nurses and two physicians expert in basic cardiopulmonary resuscitation, electrical cardioversion, and the use of emergency cardiac medications be present during the induction of ventricular arrhythmias. Continuous blood pressure monitoring with an arterial catheter facilitates assessment of the patient's hemodynamic status. A posterior defibrillator paddle is positioned with fluoroscopic guidance prior to arrhythmia induction attempts. Two defibrillators, each capable of delivering at least 400 joules, are present. Equipment for airway management and ventilation, including oxygen, endotracheal tubes, and suction, is at hand.

INCIDENCE AND TYPES OF INDUCED ARRHYTHMIAS

Several factors have been identified that influence the incidence and types of induced arrhythmias. The nature of the clinical arrhythmia is an important determinant (Tables 2, 3). Patients with clinically sustained ventricular tachycardia have the highest reported rates of arrhythmia inducibility (71 to 95 percent). Moreover, in most patients with clinically sus-

Table 2. Rates of ventricular arrhythmia inducibility

	Reason for Study	*Author or Institution*	*Inducibility Rate*
Documented VT or VF			
	sustained VT*	Fisher[2]	95%
		Vandepol[70]	95%
		Livelli[10]	71%
		STANFORD[34]	93%
	unsustained VT*	Vandepol[70]	62%
		Livelli[10]	56%
		Schoenfeld[54]	63%
		STANFORD[34]	62%
	VF*	Josephson[52]	60%
		Kehoe[71]	63%
		STANFORD[34]	71%
No documented VT or VF			
	syncope of unknown etiology	DiMarco[55]	36%
		Wellens[56]	7%
		Brandenburg[57]	11%
		Hess[58]	34%
		McAnulty[59]	46%
		Li[60]	0%
		Prystowski[61]	0%
	coronary artery disease	Hamer[7]	28%
		Richards[8]	23%
		Kowey[72]	19%
	SVT, bradyarrhythmias, miscellaneous	Livelli[10]	2%
		Vandepol[70]	0.7%

*not associated with acute myocardial infarction
VT = ventricular tachycardia
VF = ventricular fibrillation
SVT = supraventricular tachycardia

Table 3. Induced tachyarrhythmias at Stanford University Medical Center*

Clinical Arrhythmia	*Induced Arrhythmia*			
	Sustained VT	*Unsustained VT*	*VF*	*None*
Sustained VT (n = 226)	176 (78%)	18 (8%)	15 (6%)	17 (7%)
Unsustained VT (n = 42)	9 (21%)	14 (33%)	3 (7%)	16 (38%)
VF (n = 28)	5 (18%)	5 (18%)	10 (36%)	8 (29%)

VT = ventricular tachycardia
VF = ventricular fibrillation
*Adapted from Mason et al.[34]

tained ventricular tachycardia, the induced arrhythmia is also sustained ventricular tachycardia (see Table 3). By comparison, patients with clinically unsustained ventricular tachycardia or ventricular fibrillation have reported overall arrhythmia inducibility rates ranging from 60 percent to 71 percent. In many of these patients, the induced arrhythmia is different from the clinical arrhythmia (see Table 3).

Patients without documented ventricular tachycardia or fibrillation have lower reported rates of arrhythmia inducibility (see Table 2). Those with syncope of unknown etiology have inducibility rates ranging from 0 percent to 46 percent. Those with no symptoms suggestive of arrhythmias have inducibility rates ranging from less than 1 percent to 28 percent. The higher rates are reported in patients with coronary artery disease or other structural heart disease.

Whether the presence of structural heart disease per se influences rates of ventricular arrhythmia inducibility is controversial. As noted, rates of inducibility reported among patients without documented, spontaneous arrhythmias have been higher in those with structural heart disease. Similarly, among patients with sustained or unsustained ventricular tachycardia, Naccarelli and coworkers[9] found higher inducibility rates in patients with coronary artery disease than in those without. In contrast, Livelli and associates[10] found the presence of structural heart disease to have no effect on the incidence of inducibility in patients with and without known, spontaneous arrhythmias.

The incidence of arrhythmia induction depends on the stimulation protocol used.[11,12] For example, stimulation using up to three extrastimuli at the right ventricular apex results in a greater incidence of arrhythmia induction than when only two extrastimuli are used.[12] Similarly, stimulation at a second right ventricular site,[13,14] in the left ventricle,[15,16] or during isoproterenol infusion[17,18] increases the yield of induced arrhythmias. However, the relative yields and resultant clinical relevance of such techniques are not fully known.

Increasing the complexity of the stimulation protocol increases the yield of induced arrhythmias but results in less specificity. For example, in patients with documented, spontaneous arrhythmias, a more complex stimulation protocol may induce arrhythmias that do not resemble the clinical arrhythmia.[19] Aggressive stimulation protocols may also induce arrhythmias in patients not otherwise thought to be at risk for spontaneous arrhythmias.[20] The optimal stimulation protocol—one that combines high sensitivity with high specificity—remains to be established and may vary among clinical subsets of patients.

THERAPY ASSESSMENT BY INDUCTION STUDY

The widest clinical application of ventricular arrhythmia induction studies is selection and assessment of antiarrhythmic therapy. Induction studies have been used to guide therapy with drugs, surgery, and implantable electric devices.

Antiarrhythmic Drugs

Fisher,[2] Hartzler and Maloney,[3] Mason and Winkle,[4,6] and Horowitz[5] and their coworkers demonstrated that in patients with sustained ventricular tachycardia and inducible arrhythmias the effect of a drug on arrhythmia inducibility predicts clinical outcome during chronic therapy. Since then, there has been widespread use of drug testing during induction studies. The yield and predictive value of invasive drug testing, however, depends on the methodology of testing and the criteria of drug efficacy. Furthermore, there may be some drugs for which the results of testing are not predictive.

INVASIVE DRUG TESTING. A control induction study, before which all antiarrhythmic drugs are discontinued, should be performed first. This is important for several reasons. Arrhythmias induced in the presence of a drug, or failure to induce arrhythmias in the presence of a drug, are best interpreted in relation to a control study. In addition, the nature of arrhythmias induced in the control state and the ease with which they are induced may predict response to acute drug testing[21] and overall prognosis.[22–26]

During the control study, the reproducibility of arrhythmia induction by a specific stimulation method should be confirmed. Afterward, drugs may be administered orally or intravenously and repeat induction studies performed (Fig. 3). With oral dosing, repeat study should be delayed until steady-state concentrations of the drug and its metabolites are reached. Serum drug concentrations should be obtained at the time of testing and used as a guide to chronic therapy.

The results of drug testing during ventricular arrhythmia induction studies at our institution are shown in Tables 4 and 5. It is apparent that the average rate of efficacy for a drug is low (15 percent) and that no single drug appears substantially more effective than the others. Furthermore, the fraction of patients in whom at least one acutely effective drug was found was also low (32 percent). These response rates, and those reported by other investigators, must be interpreted in light of several factors: the methodology of drug testing, the criteria for efficacy, and the clinical characteristics of the patients.

It is generally agreed that to accurately assess efficacy of a drug, stimulation should be performed with at least the same pacing stress and at the same ventricular site at which arrhythmias were induced in the control state. Whether testing with more complex stimulation or at other ventricular sites is also required to establish acute efficacy, and to predict chronic efficacy, is not settled.[16,27,28] We considered a drug acutely effective only if there was prophylaxis against induction by all levels of pacing stress (without pacing at secondary sites). However, we subsequently found[12] that when arrhythmias are induced in the control state with one or two extrastimuli, drug prophylaxis against arrhythmia induction with three extrastimuli is not a more accurate predictor of chronic efficacy than prophylaxis against induction with two extrastimuli. In a small number of patients, DiMarco and colleagues[27] reported that drugs that increased the pacing stress required but did not prevent induction of arrhythmias were chronically effective. More information is needed to determine the extent of pacing stress that should be used to predict drug efficacy. It is clear that an interplay between sensitivity and specificity must be considered.

When sustained arrhythmias were induced in a control study, in the past we arbitrarily considered five induced beats as the maximum consistent with efficacy during drug testing. We recently found[28] that a good prognosis is associated with fifteen or fewer induced beats on therapy and that tachyarrhythmia recurrence rates are independent of the specific number of induced beats as long as these were fifteen or fewer. When only unsustained arrhythmias (less than 15 sec duration) are induced in the control study, choice of the number of induced beats consistent with drug efficacy is less certain; our arbitrary criterion is two or fewer beats.

Clinical factors that predict the likelihood of finding an effective drug during induction studies have recently been examined.[21,29,30] Predictive factors include younger age, female sex,

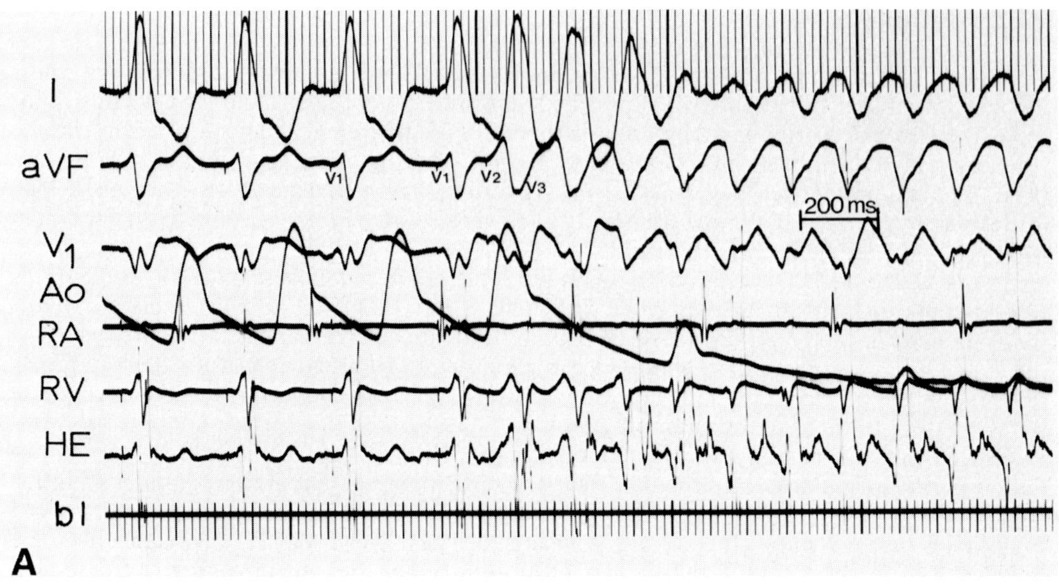

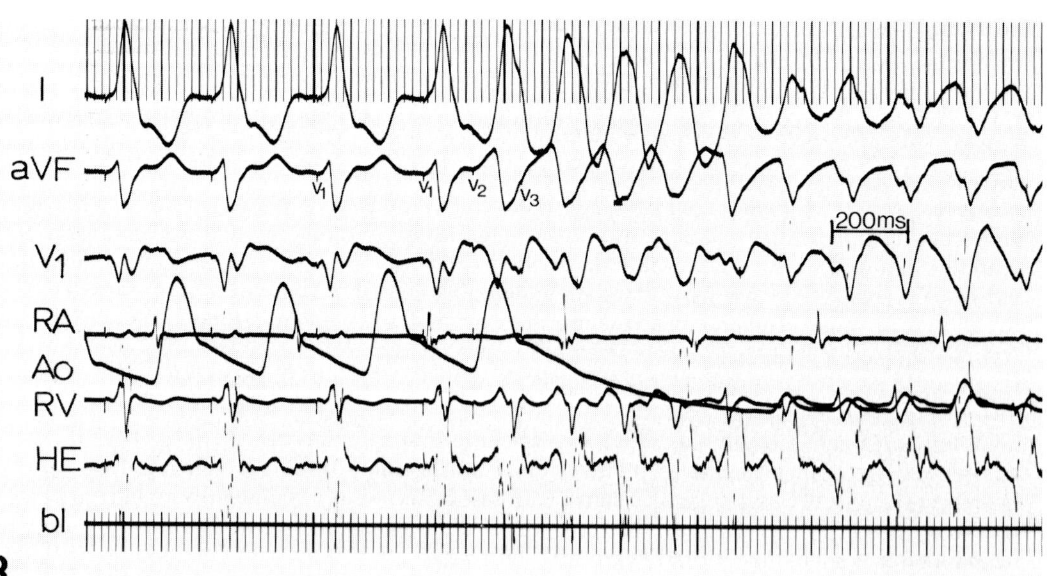

Figure 3. These ECGs show acute drug testing using ventricular arrhythmia induction study. *A,* Control study. Ventricular tachycardia is induced with two extrastimuli delivered during ventricular-paced rhythm. Note atrioventricular dissociation during tachycardia. *B,* After intravenous administration of lidocaine, with serum concentration of 5.2 μg per ml. Ventricular tachycardia with similar morphology and rate is still inducible with two extrastimuli delivered during ventricular-paced rhythm.

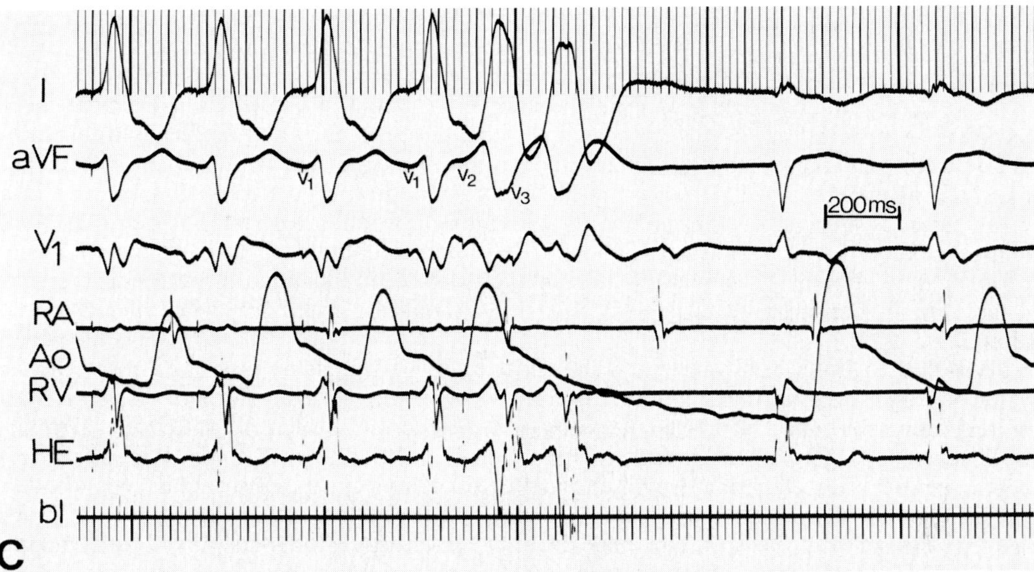

Figure 3. *Continued. C,* After intravenous administration of quinidine, with serum concentration of 8.0 μg per ml. Ventricular tachycardia is not inducible with two extrastimuli delivered during ventricular-paced rhythm. V_1 = paced ventricular drive beats; V_2, V_3 = first and second paced extrastimuli, respectively. Other abbreviations as in Figure 1. (From Mason, JW, and Winkle, RA,[4] with permission of the American Heart Association, Inc.)

Table 4. Efficacy of antiarrhythmic drugs at ventricular arrhythmia induction study*

Drug	*No. of Patients Tested*	*No. of Patients with Effective Trial*	*Efficacy Rate*
Lidocaine	136	18	13%
Quinidine	97	21	22%
Procainamide	66	13	20%
Propranolol	20	5	25%
Disopyramide	12	4	33%
Phenytoin	7	1	14%
Other	203	18	9%
Total	541	80	15%

*Adapted from Mason et al.[34]

Table 5. Efficacy of drug therapy among patients undergoing ventricular arrhythmia induction study*

	Drug-tested Group		*Entire Group*	
Clinical arrhythmia	*N*	*Effective*	*N*	*Effective*
Sustained VT	195	60 (31%)	241	(25%)
Unsustained VT	19	6 (32%)	42	(14%)
VF	15	8 (69%)	28	(29%)
Total	229	74 (32%)	311	(24%)

VT = ventricular tachycardia
VF = ventricular fibrillation
*Adapted from Mason et al.[34]

fewer empiric drug failures, less coronary artery disease, and less left ventricular dysfunction. Given the relatively low yield of effective therapy identified by serial induction studies, such factors should be taken into account in the future selection of appropriate patients for study.

Other recent findings may help limit the number of drug trials to which patients are subjected. Waxman and associates[31] reported that the acute efficacy and inefficacy of procainamide during induction study predicted the response to other conventional antiarrhythmic drugs. Similarly, in our experience the likelihood of finding an acutely effective drug in a given patent is successively diminished after each unsuccessful drug trial. Furthermore, Ross and coworkers[32] showed that combinations of selected antiarrhythmic drugs are very unlikely to be acutely effective at induction study if the drugs used individually were not effective. Thus, combinations of previously ineffective drugs should be tested only when no reasonable alternative exists.

CORRELATION BETWEEN ACUTE AND CHRONIC EFFICACY. Early reports[2–5] of the predictive value of drug testing during induction studies have been augmented with more recent analysis of long-term followup.[6,33,34,73] In our experience,[34] the two-year actuarial incidence of arrhythmia recurrence is 22 percent in patients maintained on an acutely effective drug and 41 percent in patients treated with a drug found ineffective at study. An unresolved issue is whether successful acute drug trials merely identify patients with better prognoses, regardless of subsequent chronic drug therapy. This issue could be definitively addressed only by randomizing patients in whom acutely effective drugs are found to chronic therapy or no therapy—an ethically unacceptable study.

It has now been widely reported[35–37] that in the case of amiodarone, there may be a good clinical response despite the drug's failure to prevent arrhythmia induction. Why amiodarone should be so distinguished from other antiarrhythmic drugs is not known. The value of testing by induction study of each new antiarrhythmic drug should be established.

Surgery for Ventricular Tachycardia

Because of disappointing results of coronary artery bypass surgery and blind aneurysmectomy in the surgical treatment of recurrent ventricular tachycardia,[38] a more recent surgical approach has been myocardial ablation guided by activation-sequence mapping.[38,39] Preoperatively, mapping may be done at multiple right and left ventricular sites with catheter electrodes. Intraoperatively, more detailed epicardial and endocardial mapping is done with a hand-held electrode or an electrode array. The maps establish the mechanism responsible for tachycardia, and an appropriate area of myocardium is subsequently ablated. Induction is attempted intraoperatively following ablation and at a postoperative study. In many patients, tachycardia is no longer inducible, but in our experience tachycardia noninducibility immediately after ablation is only a rough guide to prognosis.

Implantable Tachycardia-Terminating Devices

Several implantable electrical devices have been described for the termination of recurrent ventricular arrhythmias. These include burst pacemakers,[40,41] underdrive pacemakers,[41] an automatic defibrillator,[42] and a transvenous catheter capable of cardioversion.[43] Most are designed to discharge automatically after detection of the abnormal rhythm. Induction studies are required to ensure that the tachycardia is properly sensed and reliably terminated. Antiarrhythmic drugs are occasionally used along with these devices in order to decrease the frequency of tachycardia episodes or to alter tachycardia rate. In such cases, testing should be repeated during drug therapy.

There is a risk of tachycardia acceleration by implantable devices, particularly burst pacemakers. Such a device should not be considered in patients with known tachycardia acceleration by ventricular burst pacing, which occurred in 39 percent of our patients in whom sus-

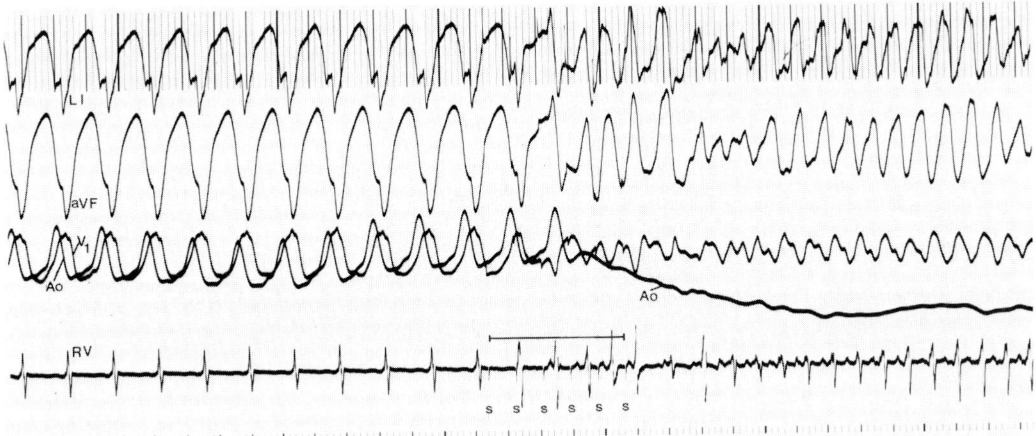

Figure 4. This ECG shows acceleration of ventricular tachycardia by ventricular burst pacing. Hemodynamically well-tolerated ventricular tachycardia with cycle length 290 msec is accelerated to a cycle length of 155 msec by a short burst of rapid ventricular pacing, with subsequent hemodynamic deterioration. s = pacing stimuli. Other abbreviations as in Figure 1. (From Mason, JW, and Winkle, RA,[4] with permission of the American Heart Association, Inc.)

tained ventricular tachycardia was induced[34] (Fig. 4). However, even extensive testing of burst pacemakers during induction study may not ensure long-term safety and efficacy.[44]

ROLE OF INDUCTION STUDIES IN SPECIFIC CLINICAL SETTINGS

Sustained Ventricular Tachycardia

Ventricular arrhythmia induction was first performed in patients with recurrent ventricular tachycardia, and the role of induction studies is most firmly established in this set of patients. The incidence of arrhythmia induction, 71 to 95 percent, is greatest in these patients (see Table 2), and in many cases induced tachycardia can be shown to be similar in morphology and rate to the clinical arrhythmia. Most of the data supporting the predictive value of invasive drug testing derives from patients with sustained ventricular tachycardia. Furthermore, activation sequence mapping is currently best limited to these patients.

Frequently there is a question as to whether a spontaneous, wide-complex tachycardia is ventricular tachycardia or supraventricular tachycardia with aberrant conduction. There are criteria based on arrhythmia morphology in the 12-lead electrocardiogram that favor one diagnosis or the other, but these criteria are frequently inapplicable or misleading.[45] Reproduction of the arrhythmia at induction study will nearly always establish the nature of the tachycardia. Atrioventricular dissociation during tachycardia strongly suggests a ventricular origin (see Figure 3), although it does not rule out the rare instance of atrioventricular nodal re-entry or junctional tachycardia with aberrant conduction and dissociated atrial activity. These possibilities can be eliminated only by observing dissociation between the ventricular electrogram and the His bundle electrogram. Conversely, a His bundle electrogram preceding each ventricular electrogram, with an HV interval identical to or slightly longer than that during sinus rhythm, establishes with near certainty the supraventricular origin of the tachycardia (Fig. 5).

Alternative approaches to therapy in patients with sustained ventricular tachycardia are limited. In most patients, tachycardia episodes are sufficiently sporadic that a protracted hospitalization would be required to establish efficacy of empiric drug trials. Empiric drug trials conducted on an outpatient basis are risky because of the life-threatening nature of the

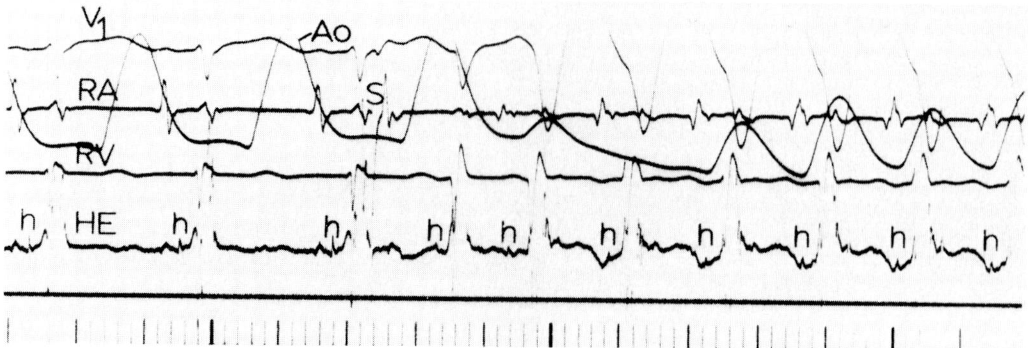

Figure 5. This ECG shows supraventricular tachycardia with aberrant conduction induced by atrial stimulation. A single atrial extrastimulus delivered during sinus rhythm induces a wide-complex tachycardia. His bundle depolarizations precede ventricular electrograms during tachycardia with an HV interval slightly longer than that during sinus rhythm, indicating a supraventricular origin of the tachycardia. S = paced atrial extrastimulus; h = His bundle depolarizations. Other abbreviations as in Figure 1.

arrhythmia. Hence some form of acute drug testing is desirable. One alternative to invasive arrhythmia induction studies is attempted suppression of spontaneous and exercise-provoked, complex ventricular premature beats, success with which Graboys and coworkers[46] have found to be predictive of a good prognosis. However, this approach is limited to patients exhibiting frequent complex ventricular premature beats, which many patients with recurrent ventricular tachycardia do not have.

Ventricular Fibrillation

Ventricular fibrillation is the only documented arrhythmia in most patients with out-of-hospital cardiac arrest. In survivors of out-of-hospital ventricular fibrillation not associated with acute myocardial infarction, Schaffer and Cobb[47] have shown a 30 percent recurrence rate over two years. Empiric therapy with antiarrhythmic drugs or coronary artery bypass surgery has been advocated,[48,49] but efficacy is unproven. Indeed, most patients with recurrent ventricular fibrillation are taking antiarrhythmic drugs at the time of recurrence.[47]

The incidence of arrhythmia inducibility in patients with a history of ventricular fibrillation is lower than in patients with ventricular tachycardia (see Table 2). It has been suggested that survivors of out-of-hospital cardiac arrest without inducible tachyarrhythmias have a low risk of recurrence even when not treated with antiarrhythmic drugs.[22–26] However, others have challenged these results.[50,51] Many of the patients without inducible arrhythmias were treated with antianginal drugs or coronary artery surgery on the assumption that their arrest resulted from myocardial ischemia. More information is needed on the mechanism of arrhythmias in these patients and on their prognosis before any treatment guidelines can be established on the basis of arrhythmia noninducibility.

When arrhythmias are induced in patients with prior ventricular fibrillation, approximately half of the induced arrhythmias are ventricular tachycardia and half are ventricular fibrillation (refer to Table 2 and Josephson, et al[52]). In neither case is it possible to compare morphologies of the clinical and induced arrhythmias. When ventricular fibrillation is induced, cardioversion is almost always necessary, adding to the morbidity of the induction study. Nonetheless, induction studies have been useful in guiding therapy with drugs and the implantable defibrillator in patients with ventricular fibrillation, and few alternative approaches exist. Graboys and coworkers[46] have used suppression of spontaneous or exercise-provoked ventricular premature beats as a therapeutic endpoint in patients with ventricular fibrillation, but many of these patients, like patients with recurrent ventricular tachycardia, do not have frequent spontaneous extrasystoles.

Unsustained Ventricular Tachycardia

We have found ventricular arrhythmia induction studies of limited value in patients with unsustained ventricular tachycardia. Arrhythmias were inducible in only 62 percent of these patients, and in many cases the induced arrhythmia was not unsustained ventricular tachycardia (see Table 2). Although acutely effective drugs could be found for nearly one third of the cases tested (see Table 5), this finding did not correlate significantly with long-term outcome, because it was excellent for the entire group.[53] Our experience contrasts with that of Schoenfeld and associates,[54] who have reported more success with induction studies in the treatment of these patients. Differing criteria for unsustained and sustained ventricular tachycardia could account for these results. Our current approach in patients with unsustained ventricular tachycardia is to guide drug therapy by suppression of spontaneous tachycardia as detected with ambulatory monitoring.

Syncope of Unknown Etiology

Intracardiac electrophysiologic study, including ventricular arrhythmia induction attempts, suggests a cardiac etiology for syncope in some patients in whom noninvasive cardiac and neurologic evaluations were nondiagnostic.[55–59] Ventricular arrhythmias were induced in 11 to 46 percent of the patients tested. Antiarrhythmic therapy, guided by acute testing, was successful in preventing further episodes of syncope in most of those patients. It should be noted that many of them had known underlying structural heart disease, abnormal electrocardiograms, or both. Other studies in patients with syncope but without known heart disease[60] or electrocardiographic abnormalities[61] have shown no inducible ventricular arrhythmias. Thus the yield of ventricular arrhythmia induction studies in patients with unexplained syncope varies with patient selection.

Prediction of Sudden Death in High-Risk Patients

It is well known that among patients surviving myocardial infarction the risk of sudden death is greatest in those with poor left ventricular function and in those who have complex ventricular ectopy (bigeminy, multiform or early coupled extrasystoles, runs of two or more) on ambulatory monitoring.[62,63] In order further to define patients at risk, ventricular arrhythmia induction studies have recently been performed in several cohorts of patients.[7,8,64] An increased risk of sudden death has been found in patients from each cohort who had inducible arrhythmias. However, the stimulation protocol and the criterion for a positive response differ among the studies. For example, Greene and colleagues[64] found that one or more repetitive responses to a single ventricular extrastimulus delivered during atrial pacing predicted sudden death in patients surviving myocardial infarction. However, Mason[65] and Ruskin and coworkers[66] found that a repetitive ventricular response, as defined by Greene and colleagues, occurred in only a small fraction of patients with spontaneous ventricular tachycardia or fibrillation and that it did not predict subsequent sudden death. More recently, Hamer[7] and Richards[8] and their associates have used more aggressive stimulation protocols in survivors of acute myocardial infarction and have found induction of sustained or unsustained ($\geq$5 beats) ventricular tachycardia to predict risk of sudden death. Similarly, among patients with myocardial disease or coronary artery disease, but not necessarily a prior myocardial infarction, Breithardt and coworkers[67] found that the risk of sudden death rose with increasing numbers of beats induced during ventricular arrhythmia induction study. Whether the predictive value of arrhythmia induction study in these patients is independent of other established predictors is uncertain. Furthermore, in patients identified by induction study to be at high risk for sudden death, it remains to be established which intervention, if any, can lower this risk.

The predictive value of ventricular arrhythmia induction studies in other patients at excess risk of sudden death, such as those with long QT syndromes or a family history of sudden death, has not been systematically examined. Patients with idiopathic hypertrophic subaortic stenosis or valvular aortic stenosis, though at risk for sudden death, should probably not be subjected to ventricular arrhythmia induction study because arrhythmias are poorly tolerated in these conditions.

COMPLICATIONS AND CONTRAINDICATIONS

Morbidity of ventricular arrhythmia induction studies most commonly results from induced arrhythmias that cannot be terminated or are accelerated by pacing techniques. Hemodynamic collapse with loss of consciousness ensues, and external cardioversion is required. At our institution, at least one cardioversion was required during serial study in 152 of 311 consecutive patients (49 percent).[34] There is almost always amnesia for the cardioversion but frequently not for the loss of consciousness that precedes. Infrequently, a patient requires multiple cardioversions for termination of a tachyarrhythmia or for those occurring spontaneously after a cardioversion. Less common sources of morbidity are vascular complications (hematoma, arteriovenous fistula, deep venous thrombosis, pulmonary embolism), pneumothorax, infection, and drug toxicity.[68]

In our institution no deaths, myocardial infarctions, or permanent neurologic sequelae have resulted from over 1500 ventricular arrhythmia induction studies. This is in large part attributable to a staff well trained in cardiopulmonary resuscitation, external cardioversion, and the use of emergency cardiac medications. In addition, studies are avoided in patients with significant obstruction of the left main coronary artery, unstable angina, severe heart failure, idiopathic hypertrophic subaortic stenosis, aortic stenosis, or known resistance to cardioversion. However, patients with severe coronary artery disease, even if anatomically diffuse, or moderate left ventricular dysfunction are commonly studied.

CONCLUSIONS

Despite continuing controversy, ventricular arrhythmia induction studies are widely used to establish diagnosis and to direct therapy in patients with known or suspected ventricular arrhythmias. New investigational antiarrhythmic drugs are now regularly evaluated by induction studies. Other therapies, such as surgery guided by activation sequence maps, have become feasible only with the advent of arrhythmia induction techniques. It is likely that induction studies will play a major role in the future growth and refinement of therapy for ventricular arrhythmias.

More widespread, perhaps routine, use of ventricular arrhythmia induction study to assess prognosis following myocardial infarction is possible. Empiric trials of beta-adrenergic antagonists have shown that mortality after myocardial infarction can be somewhat reduced by pharmacologic intervention.[69] However, the mechanism by which these drugs reduce mortality is unknown, and the residual mortality is still substantial. Future use of ventricular arrhythmia induction studies may identify patients likely to benefit from antiarrhythmic drug therapy after myocardial infarction.

REFERENCES

1. Wellens, HJ, Schuilenburg, RM, and Durrer, D: *Electrical stimulation of the heart in patients with ventricular tachycardia.* Circulation 46:216, 1972.
2. Fisher, JD, Cohen, HL, Mehra, R, et al: *Cardiac pacing and pacemakers II. Serial electrophysiologic-pharmacologic testing for control of recurrent tachyarrhythmias.* Am Heart J 93:658, 1977.
3. Hartzler, GO, and Maloney, JD: *Programmed ventricular stimulation in management of recurrent ventricular tachycardia.* Mayo Clin Proc 52:731, 1977.

4. Mason, JW, and Winkle, RA: *Electrode-catheter arrhythmia induction in the selection and assessment of antiarrhythmic drug therapy for recurrent ventricular tachycardia.* Circulation 58:971, 1978.

5. Horowitz, LN, Josephson, ME, Farshidi, A, et al: *Recurrent sustained ventricular tachycardia 3. Role of the electrophysiologic study in selection of antiarrhythmic regimens.* Circulation 58:986, 1978.

6. Mason, JW, and Winkle, RA: *Accuracy of the ventricular tachycardia-induction study for predicting long-term efficacy and inefficacy of antiarrhythmic drugs.* N Engl J Med 303:1073, 1980.

7. Hamer, A, Vohra, J, Hunt, D, et al: *Prediction of sudden death by electrophysiologic studies in high risk patients surviving acute myocardial infarction.* Am J Cardiol 50:223, 1982.

8. Richards, DA, Cody, DV, Denniss, AR, et al; *Ventricular electrical instability: A predictor of death after myocardial infarction.* Am J Cardiol 51:75, 1983.

9. Naccarelli, GV, Prystowsky, EN, Jackman, WM, et al: *Role of electrophysiologic testing in managing patients who have ventricular tachycardia unrelated to coronary artery disease.* Am J Cardiol 50:165, 1982.

10. Livelli, FD Jr, Bigger, JT, Gang, ES, et al: *Response to programmed ventricular stimulation: Sensitivity, specificity and relation to heart disease.* Am J Cardiol 50:452, 1982.

11. Farshidi, A, Tyndall, T, and Batsford, WP: *Inducibility of recurrent sustained ventricular tachycardia. Role of stimulation mode.* Circulation 62:III-261, 1980.

12. Swerdlow, CD, Blum, J, Winkle, RA, et al: *Decreased incidence of antiarrhythmic drug efficacy at electrophysiologic study associated with the use of a third extrastimulus.* Am Heart J 104:1004, 1982.

13. Wellens, HJJ, Duren, DR, and Lie, KI: *Observations on mechanisms of ventricular tachycardia in man.* Circulation 54:237, 1976.

14. Prystowsky, EN, Naccarelli, GV, Rahilly, GT, et al: *Electrophysiologic and anatomic characteristics associated with ventricular tachycardia induced at the right ventricular outflow tract but not at the apex.* Am J Cardiol 49:959, 1982.

15. Robertson, JF, Cain, ME, Horowitz, LN, et al: *Anatomic and electrophysiologic correlates of ventricular tachycardia requiring left ventricular stimulation.* Am J Cardiol 48:263, 1981.

16. Morady, F, Hess, D, and Scheinman, MM: *Electrophysiologic drug testing in patients with malignant ventricular arrhythmias: Importance of stimulation at more than one ventricular site.* Am J Cardiol 50:1055, 1982.

17. Reddy, CP, and Gettes, LS: *Use of isoproterenol as an aid to electric induction of chronic recurrent ventricular tachycardia.* Am J Cardiol 44:705, 1979.

18. Freedman, RA, Swerdlow, CD, Winkle, RA, et al: *Isoproterenol facilitation of ventricular tachycardia induction.* J Am Coll Cardiol 1:671, 1983.

19. Reddy, CP, and Sartini, JC: *Nonclinical polymorphic ventricular tachycardia induced by programmed cardiac stimulation: Incidence, mechanisms and clinical significance.* Circulation 62:988, 1980.

20. Untereker, WJ, Waxman, HL, Waspe, LE, et al: *Programmed electrical stimulation in patients without clinical ventricular tachycardia.* Circulation 66:II-147, 1982.

21. Spielman, SR, Schwartz, JS, McCarthy, DM, et al: *Predictors of the success or failure of medical therapy in patients with chronic recurrent sustained ventricular tachycardia: A discriminant analysis.* J Am Coll Cardiol 1:401, 1983.

22. Ruskin, JN, DiMarco, JP, and Garan, H: *Out-of-hospital cardiac arrest.* N Engl J Med 303:607, 1980.

23. Morady, F, Scheinman, MM, Hess, DS, et al: *Electrophysiologic testing in the management of survivors of out-of-hospital cardiac arrest.* Am J Cardiol 51:85, 1983.

24. Ruskin, JN, Garan, H, DiMarco, JP, et al: *Electrophysiologic testing in survivors of prehospital cardiac arrest: Therapy and long-term follow-up.* Am J Cardiol 49:958, 1982.

25. Tommaso, C, Kehoe, R, and Zheutlin, T: *Survivors of ischemic mediated sudden death—clinical, angiographic and electrophysiologic features and response to therapy.* Circulation 66:II-25, 1982.

26. Schoenfeld, MH, McGovern, B, Garan, H, et al: *Long-term follow-up of patients with ventricular tachycardia or fibrillation with no inducible arrhythmia during programmed cardiac stimulation.* J Am Coll Cardiol 1:606, 1983.

27. DiMarco, J, Garan, H, and Ruskin, J: *Partial suppression of induced arrhythmias during serial electrophysiologic testing.* Circulation 62:III-261, 1980.

28. Swerdlow, CD, Winkle, RA, and Mason, JW: *Prognostic significance of the number of induced ventricular complexes during assessment of antiarrhythmic therapy for ventricular tachyarrhythmias.* Circulation 68:400, 1983.

29. Swiryn, S, Bauernfeind, RA, Strasberg, B, et al: *Prediction of response to class I antiarrhythmic drugs during electrophysiologic study of ventricular tachycardia.* Am Heart J 104:43, 1982.

30. Swerdlow, CD, Gong, G, Echt, DS, et al: *Clinical factors predicting successful electrophysiologic-pharmacologic study in patients with ventricular tachycardia.* J Am Coll Cardiol 1:409, 1983.

31. Waxman, HL, Buxton, AE, Sadowski, LM, et al: *The response to procainamide during electrophysiologic study for sustained ventricular tachyarrhythmias predicts the response to other medications.* Circulation 67:30, 1983.

32. Ross, DL, Sze, DY, Keefe, DL, et al: *Antiarrhythmic drug combinations in the treatment of ventricular tachycardia.* Circulation 66:1205, 1982.

33. Waxman, HL, Sadowski, LM, Horowitz, LN, et al: *Electrophysiologic study to guide medical and surgical therapy of sustained ventricular tachycardia: Long-term predictive value.* Circulation 64:IV-240, 1981.

34. Mason, JW, Winkle, RA, Ross, DL, et al: *Ventricular tachyarrhythmia induction for drug selection: Experience with 311 patients.* In Lucchesi, BR, Dingell, JV, and Schwarz (eds): *Clinical Pharmacology of Antiarrhythmic Therapy.* Raven Press, New York, 1982.

35. Hamer, AW, Finerman, WB, Peter, T, et al: *Disparity between the clinical and electrophysiologic effects of amiodarone in the treatment of recurrent ventricular tachyarrhythmias.* Am Heart J 102:992, 1981.

36. Heger, JJ, Prystowsky, EN, Jackman, WM, et al: *Amiodarone. Clinical efficacy and electrophysiology during long-term therapy for recurrent ventricular tachycardia or ventricular fibrillation.* N Engl J Med 305:539, 1981.

37. Waxman, HL, Groh, WC, Marchlinski, FE, et al: *Amiodarone for control of sustained ventricular tachyarrhythmia: Clinical and electrophysiologic effects in 51 patients.* Am J Cardiol 50:1066, 1982.

38. Mason, JW, Stinson, EB, Winkle, RA, et al: *Surgery for ventricular tachycardia: Efficacy of left ventricular aneurysm resection compared with operation guided by electrical activation mapping.* Circulation 65:1148, 1982.

39. Josephson, ME, Harken, AH, and Horowitz, LN: *Long-term results of endocardial resection for sustained ventricular tachycardia in coronary disease patients.* Am Heart J 104:51, 1982.

40. Griffin, JC, Mason, JW, Ross, DL, et al: *The treatment of ventricular tachycardia using an automatic tachycardia terminating pacemaker.* PACE 4:582, 1981.

41. Fisher, JD, Kim, SG, Furman, S, et al: *Role of implantable pacemakers in control of recurrent ventricular tachycardia.* Am J Cardiol 49:194, 1982.

42. Mirowski, M, Reid, PR, Watkins, K, et al: *Clinical treatment of life-threatening ventricular tachyarrhythmias with the automatic implantable defibrillator.* Am Heart J 102:265, 1981.

43. Zipes, DP, Jackman, WM, Heger, JJ, et al: *Clinical transvenous cardioversion of recurrent life-threatening ventricular tachyarrhythmias: Low energy synchronized cardioversion of ventricular tachycardia and termination of ventricular fibrillation in patients using a catheter electrode.* Am Heart J 103:789, 1982.

44. Freedman, RA, Griffin, JC, Rothman, MT, et al: *Safety and efficacy of an automatic tachycardia-terminating device.* Circulation 66:II-217, 1982.

45. Wellens, HJJ, Bar, FWHM, and Lie, KI: *The value of the electrocardiogram in the differential diagnosis of a tachycardia with a widened QRS complex.* Am J Med 64:27, 1978.

46. Graboys, TB, Lown, B, Podid, PJ, et al: *Long-term survival of patients with malignant ventricular arrhythmia treated with antiarrhythmic drugs.* Am J Cardiol 50:437, 1982.

47. Schaffer, WA and Cobb, LA: *Recurrent ventricular fibrillation and modes of death in survivors of out-of-hospital ventricular fibrillation.* N Engl J Med 293:259, 1975.

48. Myerburg, RJ, Ghahramani, A, Mallon, SM, et al: *Coronary revascularization in patients surviving unexpected ventricular fibrillation.* Circulation (Suppl.) 51, 52:III-219, 1975.

49. Myerburg, RJ, Conde, C, Sheps, DS, et al: *Antiarrhythmic drug therapy in survivors of prehospital cardiac arrest: Comparison of effects on chronic ventricular arrhythmias and recurrent cardiac arrest.* Circulation 59:855, 1979.

50. Benson, DW Jr, Hession, WT, Zavoral, JH, et al: *Sudden cardiac arrest in young adults: Clinical and electrophysiological findings.* Am J Cardiol 49:928, 1982.

51. Roy, D, Waxman, HL, Lenzle, MG, et al: *Clinical characteristics and long term followup in survivors of cardiac arrest: Relation to inducibility at electrophysiologic evaluation.* Circulation 66:II-25, 1982.

52. Josephson, ME, Horowitz, LN, Spielman, SR, et al: *Electrophysiologic and hemodynamic studies in patients resuscitated from cardiac arrest.* Am J Cardiol 46:948, 1980.

53. Swerdlow, CD, Echt, DS, Soderholm-Difatte, V, et al: *Limited value of programmed stimulation in patients with unsustained VT.* Circulation 66:II-145, 1982.

54. Schoenfeld, MH, McGovern, B, Garan, H, et al: *The role of programmed cardiac stimulation in patients with nonsustained ventricular tachycardia.* J Am Coll Cardiol 1:607, 1983.

55. DiMarco, JP, Garan, H, Harthorne, JW, et al: *Intracardiac electrophysiologic techniques in recurrent syncope of unknown cause.* Ann Intern Med 95:542, 1981.

56. Wellens, HJJ, Bar, FWHM, Vanagt, E, et al: *Results of programmed stimulation in 80 patients having a history but no electrocardiographic documentation of tachycardia.* Am J Cardiol 47:433, 1981.

57. Brandenburg, RO, Holmes, DR, and Hartzler, GO: *The electrophysiologic assessment of patients with syncope.* Am J Cardiol 47:433, 1981.
58. Hess, DS, Morady, F, and Scheinman, MM: *Electrophysiologic testing in the evaluation of patients with syncope of undetermined origin.* Am J Cardiol 50:1309, 1982.
59. McAnulty, J, Morton, M, Schutz, R, et al: *Evaluation of syncope in patients with heart disease.* Clin Res 30:15A, 1982.
60. Li, CK, McAnulty, JH, Morton, M, et al: *Are electrophysiologic studies in patients with syncope without heart disease of diagnostic value?* J Am Coll Cardiol 1:607, 1983.
61. Prystowsky, EN, Klein, GK, Naccarelli, GV, et al: *Electrophysiologic study in patients with syncope and normal resting electrocardiograms.* Clin Res 29:697A, 1981.
62. Ruberman, W, Weinblatt, E, Goldberg, JD, et al: *Ventricular premature complexes and sudden death after myocardial infarction.* Circulation 64:297, 1981.
63. Bigger, JT, Weld, FM, and Rolnitzky, LM: *Which postinfarction ventricular arrhythmias should be treated?* Am Heart J 103:660, 1982.
64. Greene, HL, Reid, PR, and Schaeffer, AH: *The repetitive ventricular response in man.* N Engl J Med 299:729, 1978.
65. Mason, JW: *Repetitive beating after single ventricular extrastimuli: Incidence and prognostic significance in patients with recurrent ventricular tachycardia.* Am J Cardiol 45:1126, 1980.
66. Ruskin, JN, DiMarco, JP, and Garan, H: *Repetitive responses to single ventricular extrastimuli in patients with serious ventricular arrhythmias: Incidence and clinical significance.* Circulation 63:767, 1981.
67. Breithardt, G, Seipel, L, Meyer, T, et al: *Prognostic significance of repetitive ventricular response during programmed ventricular stimulation.* Am J Cardiol 49:693, 1982.
68. DiMarco, JP, Garan, H, and Ruskin, JN: *Morbidity associated with electrophysiologic procedures.* Am J Cardiol 49:959, 1982.
69. Staessen, J, Bulpitt, C, Cattaert, A, et al: *Secondary prevention with beta-adrenoceptor blockers in post-myocardial infarction patients.* Am Heart J 104:1395, 1982.
70. Vandepol, CJ, Farshidi, A, Spielman, SR, et al: *Incidence and clinical significance of induced ventricular tachycardia.* Am J Cardiol 45:725, 1980.
71. Kehoe, RF, Moran, JM, Zheutlin, T, et al: *Electrophysiological study to direct therapy in survivors of pre-hospital ventricular fibrillation.* Am J Cardiol 49:928, 1982.
72. Kowey, PR, Folland, ED, Parisi, AF, et al: *Programmed electrical stimulation of the heart in coronary artery disease.* Am J Cardiol 51:531, 1983.
73. Swerdlow, CD, Winkle, RA, and Mason, JW: *Determinants of survival in patients with ventricular tachycardia.* N Engl J Med 308:1436, 1983.

Physiologic Temporary Pacing: Techniques and Indications

Philip O. Littleford, M.D.

Temporary ventricular pacing has been available since 1957, and usage of the temporary endocardial electrode was first described by Furman in 1958. Since the late 1960s, temporary pacing has been a routine part of the cardiologist's therapeutic armamentarium. It has been used in the management of a wide variety of ventricular and atrial bradyarrhythmias and tachyarrhythmias. The most common form has been ventricular pacing, generally in the setting of heart block complicating acute myocardial infarction. However, temporary atrial and atrioventricular (AV) pacing has been used with increasing frequency in the intensive care units in association with a multipurpose Swan-Ganz catheter,[1] and recently there has been a marked increase in the use of temporary epicardial leads following open heart surgery.[2] The use of atrial as well as ventricular epicardial leads has produced an enhanced awareness of the hemodynamic and antiarrhythmic benefits of "physiologic" pacing, that is, maintaining AV synchrony under all pacing conditions.[3]

Because of advances in electrode design, improvement in venous access techniques,[4] and, most recently, the development of a multiprogrammable microprocessor-based pulse generator, physiologic pacing on a temporary as well as permanent basis is not only possible but practical and easily accomplished.

This chapter will describe in detail: (1) newer venous access techniques, particularly the subclavian and jugular routes; (2) the new temporary atrial and ventricular electrode systems and their method of insertion; (3) their adaptation to the new "universal" or permanent DDD pacing systems; and (4) their indications for use.

VENOUS ACCESS TECHNIQUES

In recent years, central venous access has become increasingly important as the hospital physician's therapeutic armamentarium has expanded to encompass parenteral nutrition, central venous pressure monitoring, Swan-Ganz catheterization, and multiple pacemaker lead insertions, both temporary and permanent. Nonetheless, for the uninitiated, the venture into the "central vein stick" causes all sorts of problems, both real and imagined. These concerns can be overcome, and central vein catheterization can be a safe, quick, and extremely useful procedure if a few key principles are followed.

It is absolutely essential that the vein be distended prior to needle insertion. Just as it is impossible either to withdraw blood or to insert an IV into a flat antecubital vein, it is likewise nearly impossible to cannulate a nondistended central vein.

A J wire and a small- or medium-bore thin-wall needle combination should be used. This is most commonly a 0.035, 50 cm J wire and a 6 to 7 cm 18 gauge, thin-wall needle.

Central vein access allows the rapid insertion of one or more temporary electrodes in a fashion that permits easy manipulation and a stable postinsertion position.

Subclavian Vein Catheterization

In the world of pacing, the use of the subclavian vein and the peel-away sheath introducer system has had a dramatic effect on the types of permanent pacemakers that are used.[4] The traditional cephalic cutdown techniques made it difficult to insert large or unusual electrodes, and rarely more than one electrode could be inserted through the cephalic vein. The sheath introducer system circumvents these problems, and two or more permanent electrodes can be inserted through the same subclavian vein at the same site. These same principles apply to temporary lead insertions.

Widely recognized complications of subclavian vein catheterization are pneumothorax, air embolism, subclavian artery puncture, hemothorax, and brachial plexus injury.[5] In the hands of the experienced operator, these complications are very infrequent.

Anatomy

The subclavian vein is the medial extension of the axillary vein as it courses behind the major pectoralis muscle group, arching over the first rib and thoracic cavity just lateral to the fibrous attachment joining the clavicle to the first rib. The proximal one half of the clavicle covers the subclavian vein.

Procedure

The right or left subclavian area is prepped and draped in the usual manner. The patient is placed in the Trendelenburg position, or the feet are elevated 30° to 45° with a foam wedge to increase the venous pressure and to distend the vein. A towel or rolled sheet placed between the shoulder blades tends to throw the shoulder back, raising the clavicle and allowing easier access to the subclavian vein.

The 18 gauge thin-wall needle with the 50 cm J wire can be used for the insertion, generally in combination with a peel-away sheath introducer system.* The insertion site is just lateral to the ligament that connects the clavicle to the first rib (Fig. 1). There is a general tendency for the inexperienced to go to the midclavicular area or beyond, and this is usually too far in the lateral direction.

In Figure 1, the route of the vein and the range of needle aims are illustrated by arrows A and B. In general, one should aim the needle toward a point below and behind the cricoid cartilage (Fig. 2). If a person is big-chested and husky, a deeper and more posterior orientation is used, as illustrated by position B. If the patient is thin-chested or especially if the patient is emphysematous, position A more accurately reflects the appropriate aim.

Once venous blood is freely drawn into the syringe (often the operator can feel a slight release of pressure as the vein is punctured), the needle is firmly stabilized, the syringe removed, and the 50 cm J wire inserted through the needle into the subclavian vein. As this is done, the patient is asked to turn the head toward the shoulder of the side being cannulated. This tends to make the angle between the jugular vein and the subclavian more acute, and passage into the superior vena cava is smoother. If the guide wire does not pass smoothly, it may have gone into the jugular vein, and usually the patient will complain of a rather unpleasant sensation in the region of the ipsilateral ear. If it moves without difficulty during the entire passage, in all likelihood it is in the superior vena cava or right atrium. If it does not pass at

*Permanent Lead Introducer System, 8, 10.5, and 12 French, Cordis Corporation, Miami, Florida

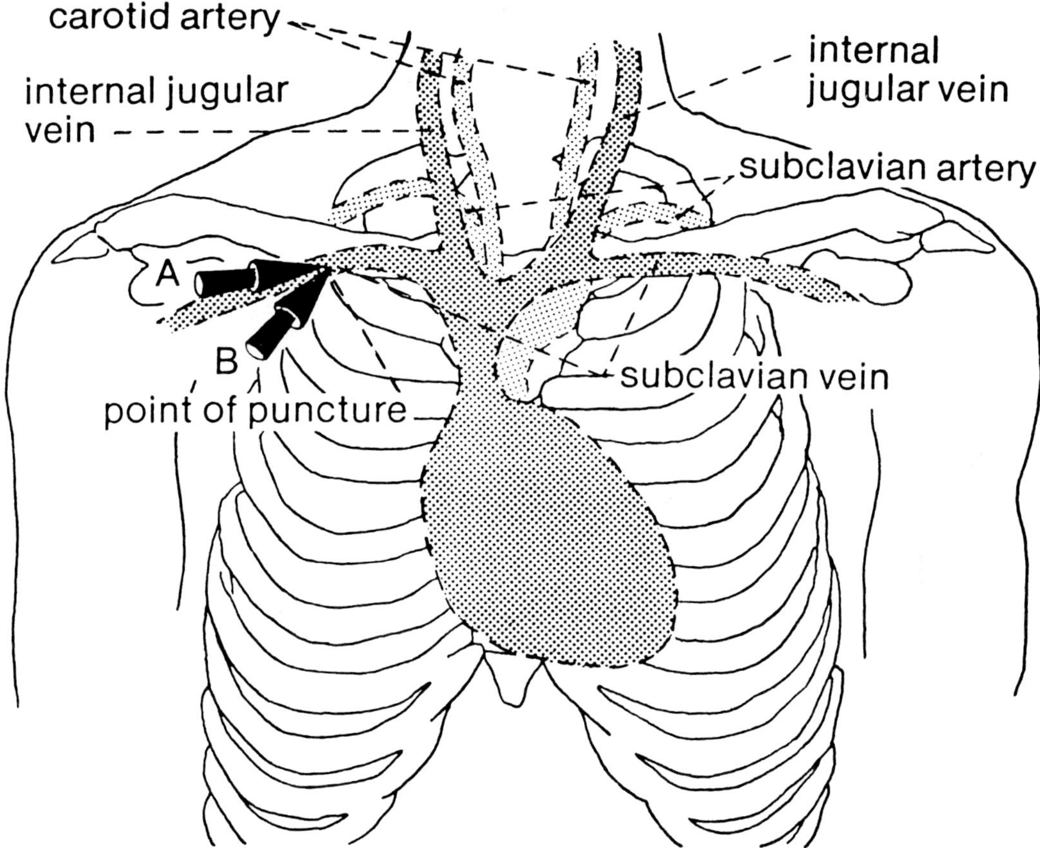

Figure 1. Diagram of the appropriate insertion sites for the subclavian vein and the various aims used (A, B).

all, a slow turning of the needle and the J wire will sometimes allow passage into the vein. If this is unsuccessful, another needle puncture should be tried with a slightly different orientation and insertion point. If bright red blood is aspirated and is pulsatile, one has struck the subclavian artery. The needle should be removed and firm hand pressure applied to the area for several minutes, and a more medial insertion site should be utilized. If air is aspirated, one has perforated the pleural space and penetration has been too lateral or too deep. At this point, the operator must make a decision whether to (1) continue to attempt the insertion on the same side; (2) go to the other side; or (3) abandon the subclavian access altogether.

Generally, in an otherwise healthy person, one pleural puncture with an 18 gauge thin-wall needle will often be innocuous. However, if there is some chronic obstructive lung disease, significant pneumothorax may occur and no further attempt should be made. If it is the operator's decision to continue on with the subclavian puncture and air is aspirated the second time, the procedure should be completely abandoned and another method of venous access attempted.

A small incision with a #11 blade allows the easy passage of the sheath introducer system over the guide wire into the vein. Its insertion requires some force (Fig. 3). If the angle between the subclavian vein and superior vena cava is too acute (this is especially likely from the right side), the introducer system may have some difficulty in "traversing the corner." In this case, raising the shoulder and turning the chin toward the ipsilateral shoulder will sometimes make the angle less acute and allow easier passage. The smaller the system, for exam-

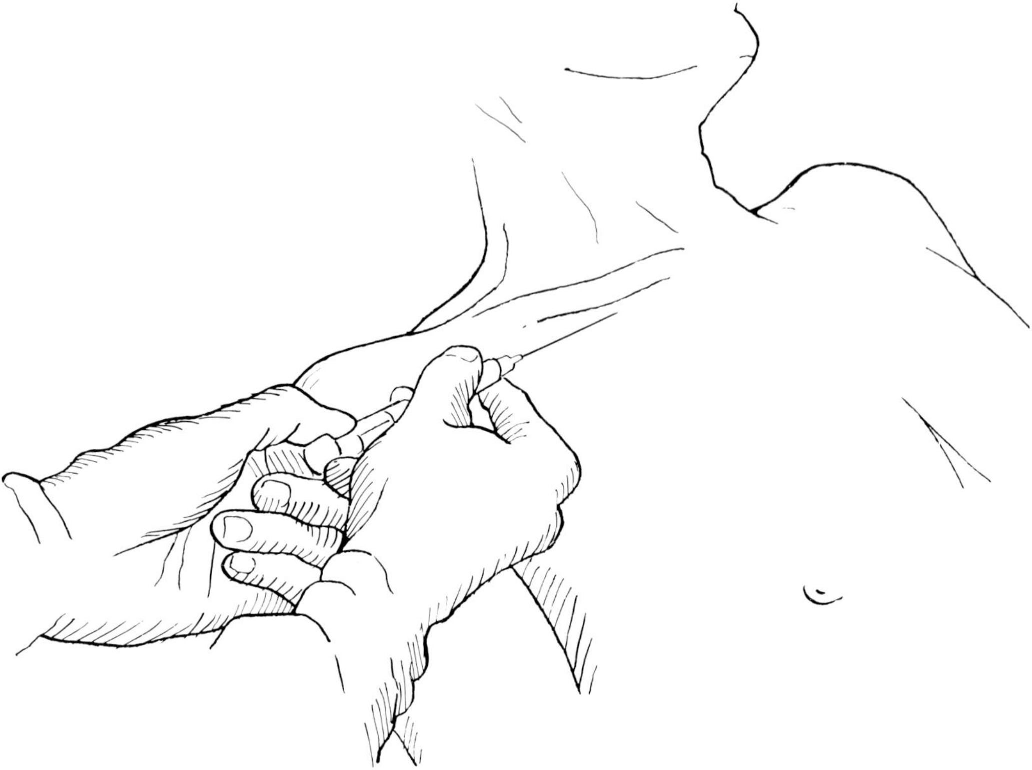

Figure 2. Insertion of the needle into the subclavian vein is shown here.

ple, 8 French versus 10.5 French, the more easily the acute angle between the subclavian vein and superior vena cava can be traversed.

The lead is then prepared for insertion, the vessel dilator and guide wire removed (Fig. 4), and great care taken to pinch off the sheath as the vessel dilator is pulled out to prevent any aspiration of air or excessive leakage of blood. With the forefinger and thumb being used as

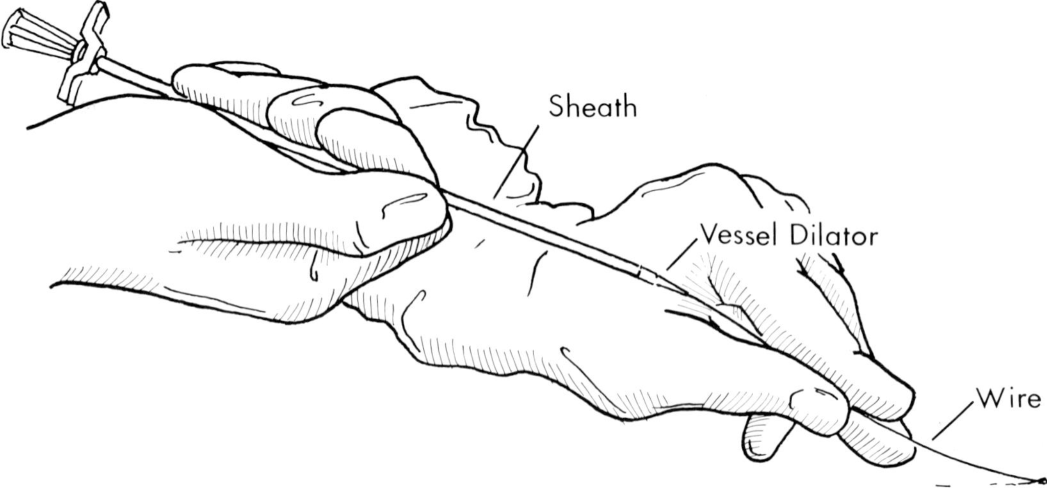

Figure 3. Insertion of the sheath/vessel dilator combination over the guide wire is shown here.

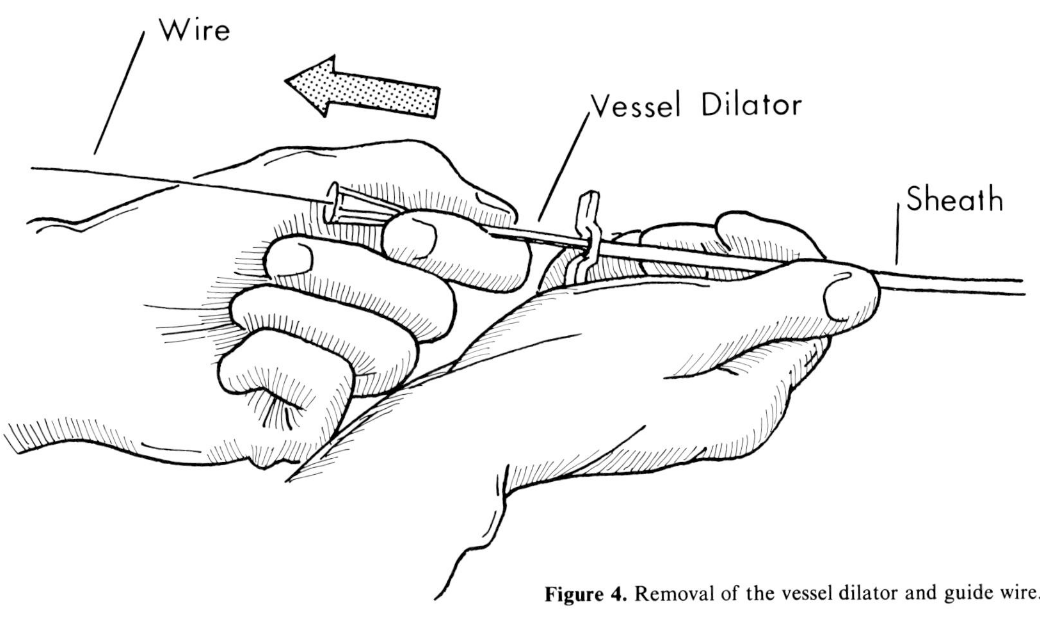

Figure 4. Removal of the vessel dilator and guide wire.

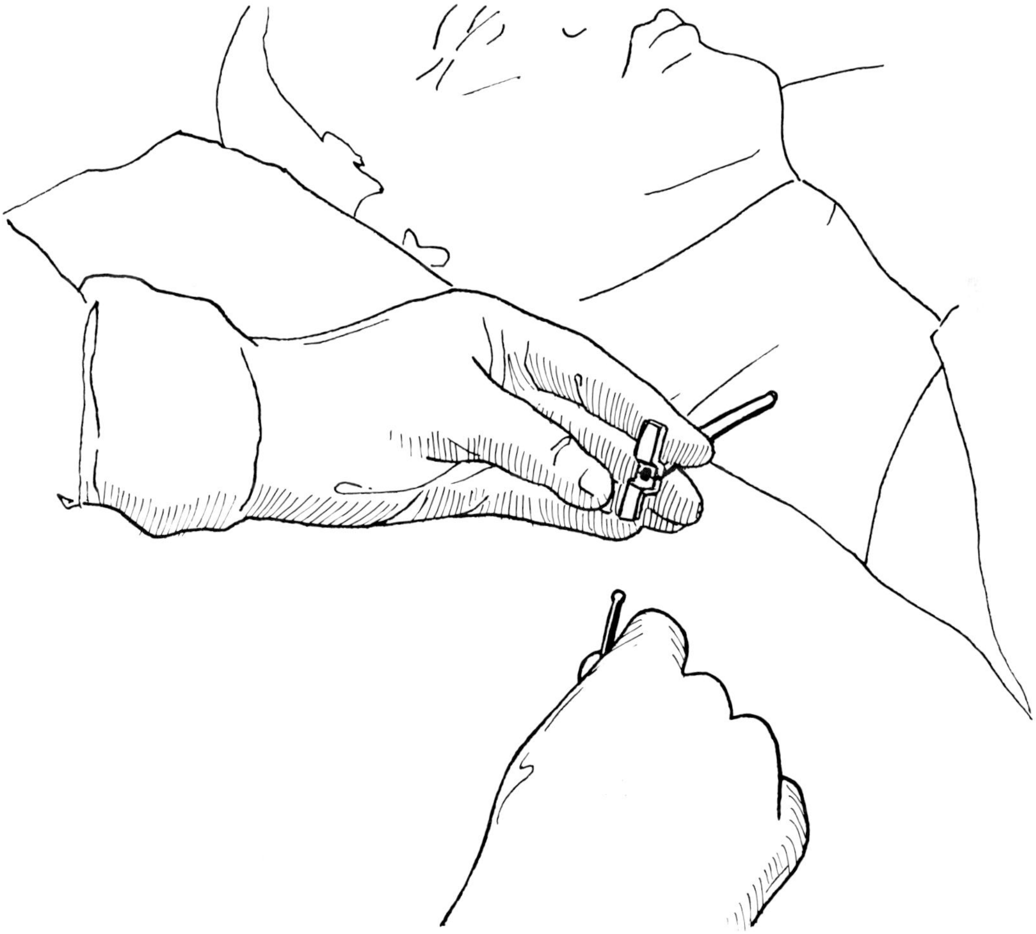

Figure 5. Insertion of the lead using the fingers to act as a pinch valve to prevent aspiration of air or excessive blood loss.

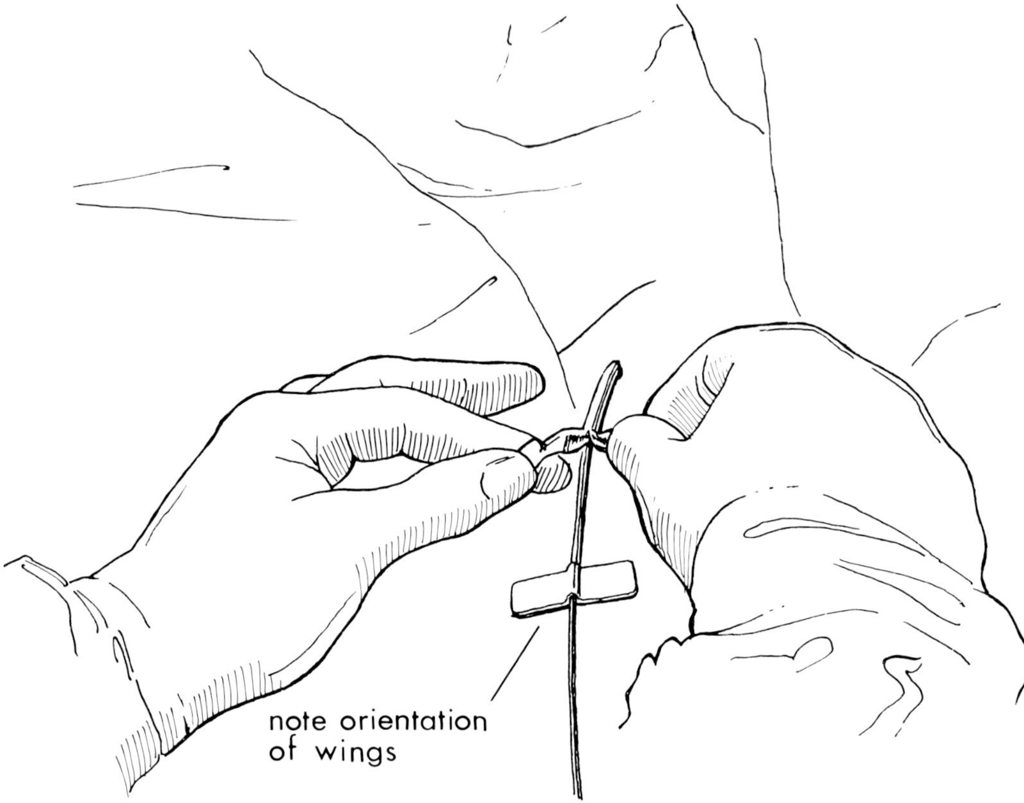

Figure 6. The peel-away operation. In the case of the temporary atrial lead, the skin side of the wings is down.

pinch valves on the sheath, the lead is inserted (Fig. 5) and the fingers are released to allow passage through the sheath into the superior vena cava. The lead is stabilized, and the sheath is carefully peeled away, making sure that the lead does not "snake" backward out of the superior vena cava as the peel-away operation is being accomplished (Fig. 6).

If this is a two-lead insertion, one can (a) use two needle punctures side by side and insert two guide wires; (b) use one needle puncture with a large sheath introducer system, inserting both electrodes through the same sheath (Fig. 7); or (c) insert one guide wire, then an introducer system, followed by removal of the vessel dilator alone, and the insertion of a second guide wire through the intact sheath, pulling the untorn sheath back, and leaving the two guide wires in place. The two guide wires will then provide the basis for two sheath introducer insertions.

Internal Jugular Vein Catheterization

The cannulation of the internal jugular vein has the great advantage of being generally free from serious complications. The two potential problems are striking the carotid artery (with attendant neck bleeding) and air embolism. There is very little chance of pleural space puncture, and, in the hands of the unskilled, it is generally considered a much safer technique than subclavian vein puncture. It has the disadvantage in pacemaker therapy of requiring a neck insertion of an electrode. In the case of a temporary lead, the electrode would have to be stabilized in the neck, which is intrinsically a more unstable position compared with the subclavian.

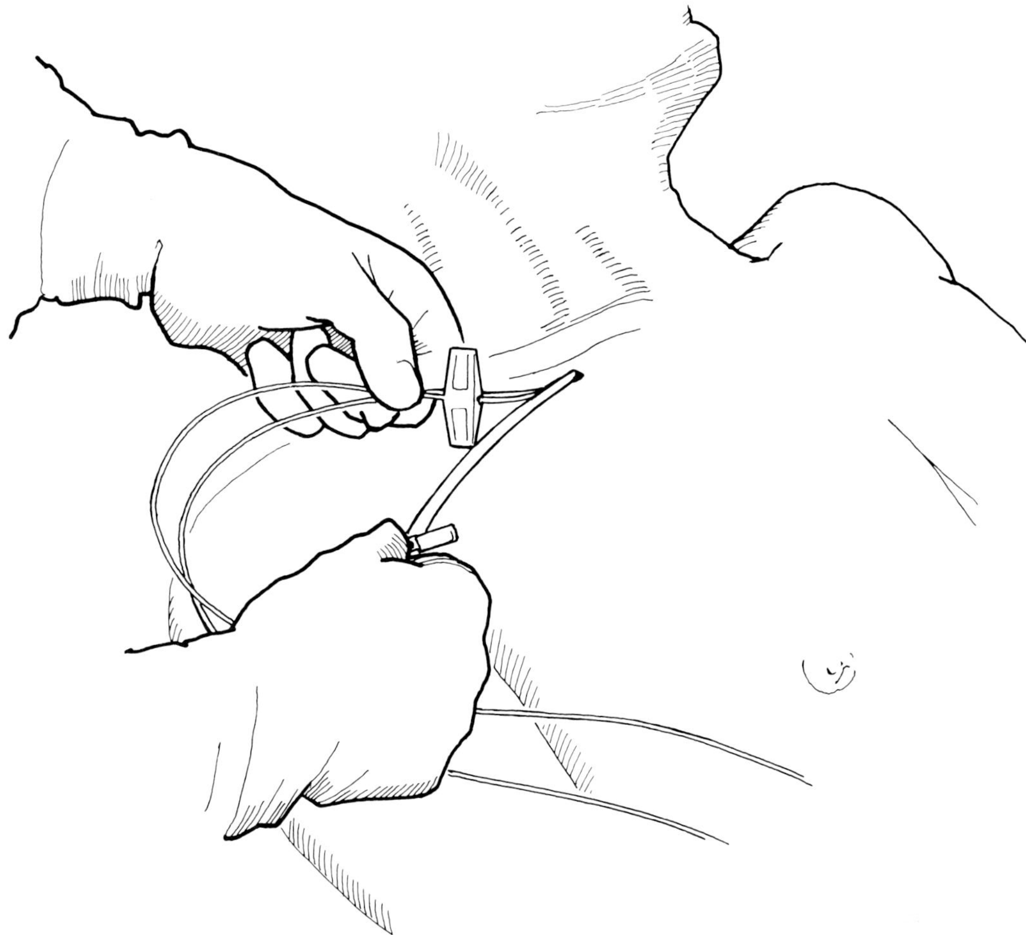

Figure 7. Insertion of two electrodes through one sheath.

Anatomy

The internal jugular vein lies behind the clavicular head of the sternocleidomastoid muscle. It is surrounded by the carotid sheath and is located just anterior and lateral to the carotid artery. If it is distended by Valsalva maneuver or Trendelenburg position, it is often almost 2 cm in diameter.

Procedure

The head of the patient is rotated to the opposite side. Skin preparation and draping are accomplished in the usual manner. A puncture site is located approximately 5 cm above the clavicle and 1 cm within the lateral border of the sternocleidomastoid muscle (Fig. 8). The needle is aligned so that it is parallel to the anterior border of the muscle. The operator's hand is elevated, directing the needle approximately 30° posterior to the coronal plane. This method directs the needle through the muscle "belly" into the vein and lateral to the carotid artery.

As aspiration yields dark venous blood, the needle is stabilized, the syringe disconnected, the 50 cm J wire inserted, and the lead insertion accomplished as noted above in the section on subclavian vein catheterization.

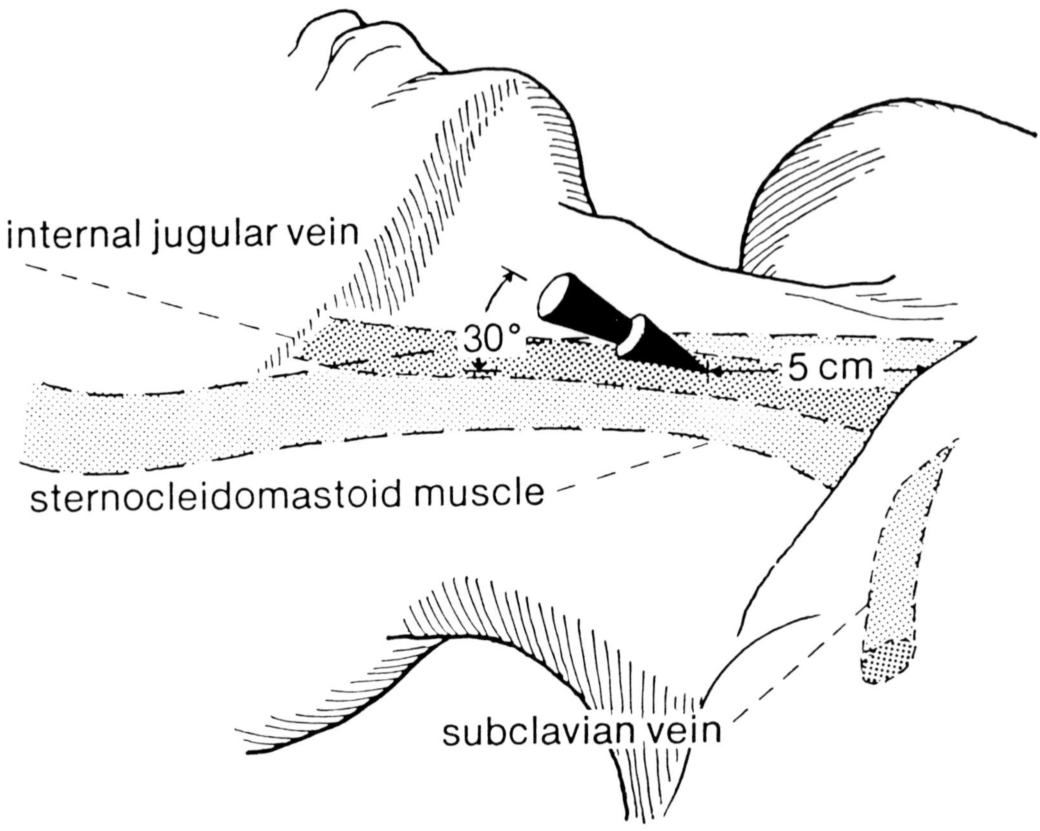

Figure 8. The internal jugular venous puncture site and appropriate aim of the needle.

Femoral Vein Catheterization

The femoral vein can be very useful for temporary lead insertion, both atrial and ventricular. It is difficult to accomplish in a "blind" or nonfluoroscopic manner and, of course, it is totally inappropriate for permanent leads. If the patient is bedfast, it is a reasonably stable position and can be useful when other approaches are difficult.

The distention of the vein is critical. This is easily done by a Valsalva maneuver, and this technique makes cannulation generally quite easy. The insertion site is just below the inguinal ligament at a point 1½ fingerbreadths medial to the arterial pulse (Fig. 9). The aim is approximately 30° to 45° off the plane of the body and very slightly in the medial direction. It is best to undertake the insertion with a glass syringe and needle combination, and the force of the Valsalva maneuver will often force the dark venous blood into the syringe in a sometimes dramatic manner. The J wire introducer sheath insertion techniques are identical to those noted above.

As with all surgical techniques, frequency of use improves skill. A sense for the anatomy, the general aim of the needle, and the limits of the procedures will all come with time. Again, there cannot be too much emphasis placed on the importance of using the appropriate needle and J wire combination and cannulating the vein while it is distended.

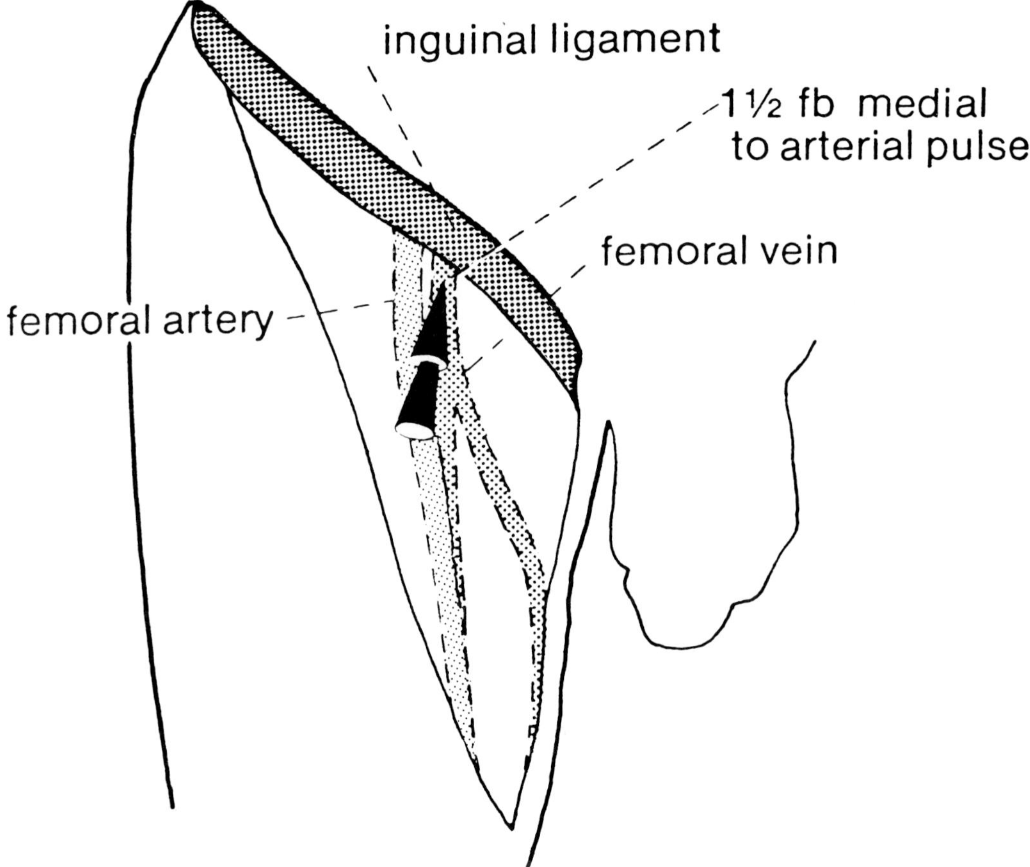

Figure 9. The insertion site of the femoral vein.

TEMPORARY LEAD SYSTEMS AND METHODS OF INSERTION

Temporary Atrial Lead Insertion

Temporary atrial pacing has been hampered by lack of a suitable catheter or electrode system that could provide reliable and effective capture for extended periods, whether the patient was supine or ambulatory. This mode of pacing has been largely limited to the very short-term use in the catheterization laboratory utilizing simple, non-preformed bipolar electrode pacing catheters. These standard catheters are introduced via the femoral vein and manipulated into either the atrial appendage or coronary sinus. Atrial stimulation is accomplished, but thresholds are sometimes quite high, enhancing the possibility of phrenic stimulation; and, in addition, P wave sensing is frequently poor.

Because the right atrial chamber lacks a structure against which the traditional straight pacing catheters can permanently rest, other investigators have attempted to circumvent this problem and have suggested different electrode configurations, with limited success. Berens and coworkers described a pacing loop that can be inserted from above or below by a Teflon catheter.[6] As the catheter is withdrawn, the loop expands to meet the wall of the right atrium, but consistent atrial pacing is difficult to achieve for extended periods of time. More recently, temporary atrial pacing has been attempted using a multipurpose flow-directed type of pul-

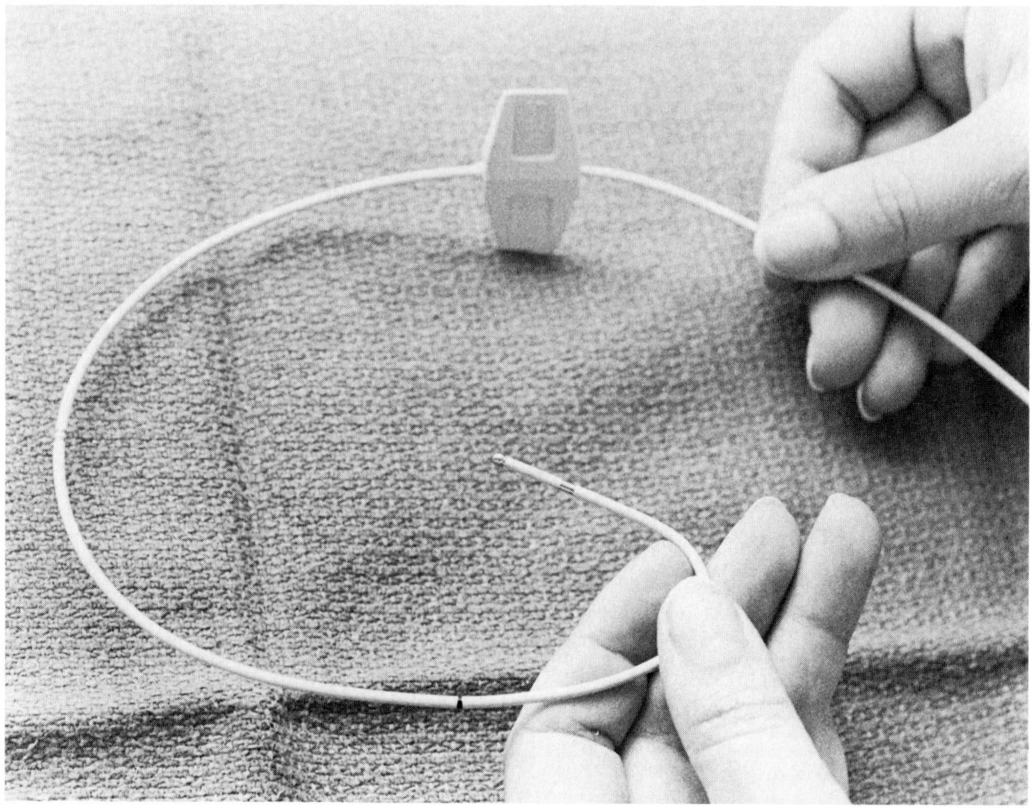

Figure 10. Winged atrial lead showing the "J" shaped bend, the ball tip and the wings perpendicular to the "J" of the lead.

monary arterial catheter (Swan-Ganz) with pacing electrode ring situated proximally.[1] The catheter can provide high-quality atrial electrograms and, for short periods, stable atrial and ventricular pacing in most patients; however, this catheter is used with lumens for hemodynamic monitoring and this, of course, limits its use to the bedfast patient.

The temporary pervenous atrial J system with orienting wings described below is a reliable atrial pacing system that can be used over long periods with low thresholds and adequate P wave sensing and that can be inserted at the bedside without fluoroscopy. It has the advantage of not requiring the presence of an atrial appendage for stable position.[7]

The catheter is a 6 French electrode with an 8 French ball cathodal tip, and a stainless steel anodal ring is positioned 2 cm from the spherical tip electrode. A pair of semirigid 1 cm × 2 cm polyurethane orienting wings are bonded 31 cm from the tip. The J shaped distal segment is approximately 3 cm in diameter with an outward bend and is nearly perpendicular to the plane of the wings (Fig. 10). The "skin side" of the wings is always facing the same direction as the J.* To maintain torque control, the catheter is fabricated from braided polyurethane material similar to that used for coronary angiography.

Catheter insertion technique is accomplished using the peel-away sheath introducer system as described above. The catheter's J distal-shaped segment is straightened by hand and inserted directly into the sheath with the skin side down and positioned in the superior vena

*Available from Cordis Corporation, Miami, Florida

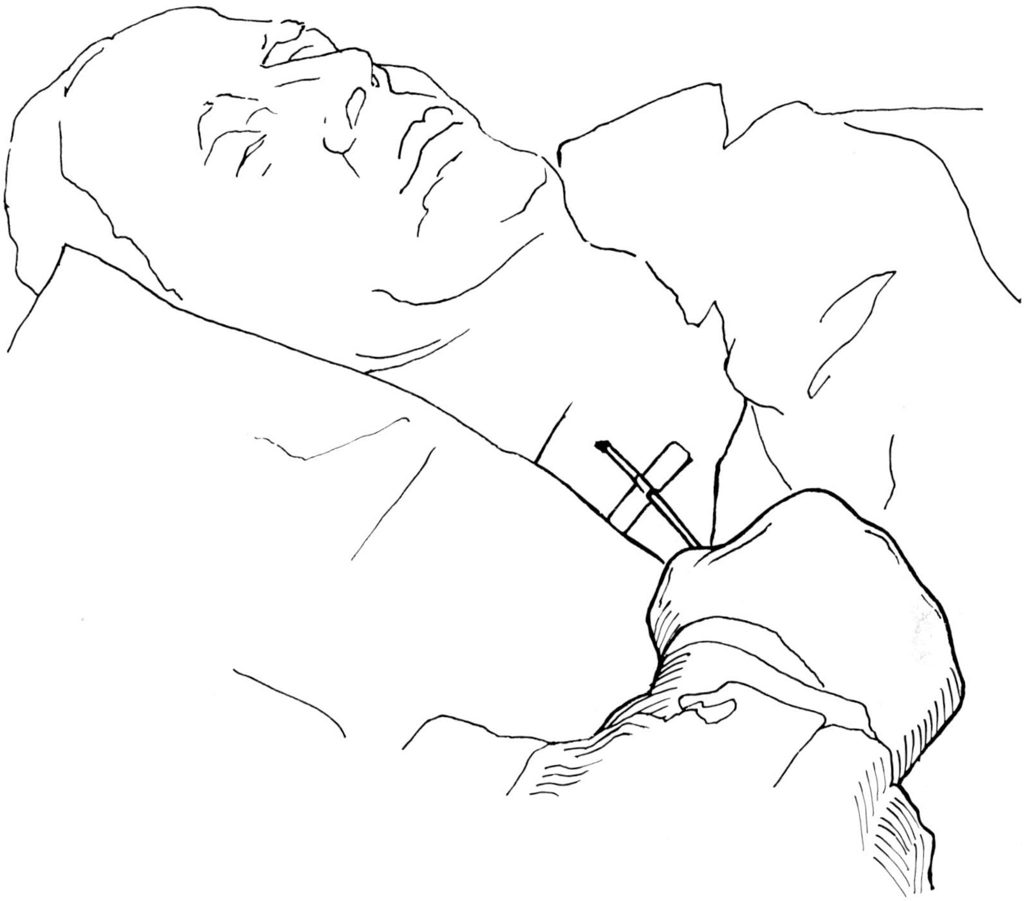

Figure 11. Placing the skin side of the wings down against the chest.

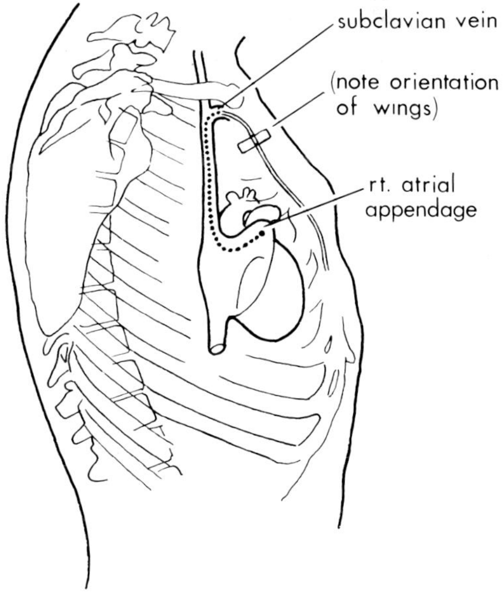

Figure 12. Sagittal view showing the orientation of the wings and the distal J tip in the atrial appendage.

cava (see Figures 5, 6). After the sheath is peeled away, the orienting wings are pushed all the way to the insertion site with the skin side oriented against the skin. The pacemaker is attached, turned on, and the lead is slowly withdrawn until capture is obtained—usually this is a distance of 1 cm to 6 cm. The wings are then taped flat to the skin, and skin sutures are placed fore and aft of the wing (Figs. 11, 12).

The catheter can be kept in place, with occlusive dressing techniques for sterility, anywhere from 1 to 14 days as dictated by the patient's clinical needs. Sensing is generally quite good, often ranging between 1 and 3 millivolts. Complete capture thresholds at 1 msec pulse widths are generally less than 6 milliamps. Insertion time is minimal in the hands of the experienced physician, often taking less than 3 or 4 minutes. As noted above, it can be done at the bedside from the right subclavian or jugular vein. The patient can be ambulatory, and the presence of the atrial appendage is not necessary for stability or capture.[7]

Temporary Ventricular Lead Insertion

It has been our practice to use the "remote anode" temporary lead, which is available in a 4 French and 6 French variety.* This electrode, first described by Preston,[8] is a pacing lead in which the cathode is the distal tip and the anode is 23 cm back, putting it in the superior vena cava. This lead has two advantages over the conventional bipolar temporary pacing catheter: (1) There is a consistently greater detected voltage for any type of ventricular depolarization and, therefore, improved sensing; and (2) there is a lessened chance of pacemaker-induced ventricular arrhythmias should the pacemaker stimulus fall during the vulnerable period of the preceding ventricular depolarization. There has been strong evidence that pacemaker-induced excitation during the vulnerable period occurs much more commonly with anodal stimulation than with cathodal stimulation.[9,10]

This lead also has the advantage, described below, of adapting a permanent unipolar dual lead DDD pulse generator to a temporary lead system by providing a remote anode.

The lead is inserted through the subclavian or jugular vein as described above and positioned fluoroscopically in the right ventricular apex in the usual manner.

If the ventricular lead insertion is approached from the left side, the natural curve of the lead will often place it directly into the right ventricle. If it is approached from the right side, the tip of the lead can be often "hooked" at the junction between the right atrium and inferior vena cava and turned in an anterior and medial manner and flipped across the tricuspid valve into the right ventricle. If one is viewing the heart in the anterioposterior (AP) position, quite often it is helpful to put the lead out into the pulmonary artery to ensure that it is not in the coronary sinus. If the patient can be rotated to the right anterior oblique position, the coronary sinus position is in the AV groove and posterior, and the right ventricular apex is anterior.

Once a proper position in the right ventricular apex is obtained with enough curve in the right atrium to ensure a stable support for the lead against the right atrial wall, it is then "twice sutured" to the skin.

EXTERNAL DDD PACING UNIT

Since the advent of the microprocessor-based DDD pacemaker, there has been a widespread and growing use of the DDD or "universal" pacemaker. We have adapted these internal permanent units for external use by employing the "Preston lead" and using its remote anode as the common anode for both the atrial and the ventricular leads. With its distance back from the tip of the ventricular lead, the remote anode is located high in the superior

*Cordis Corporation, Miami, Florida

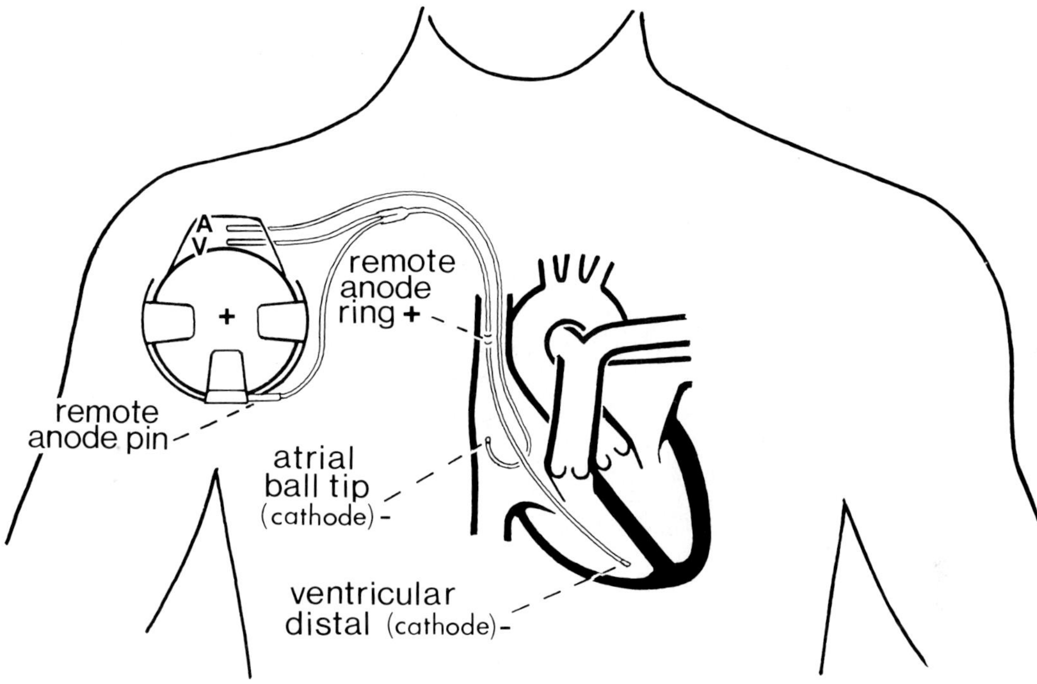

Figure 13. Remote anode ventricular lead with the attachment of the anode to the bracket holding the pacemaker case, and the attachments of the atrial and ventricular cathodes in the appropriate receptacles.

vena cava. The connector pin of this remote anode is attached to the clamp that in turn holds the case of the pacemaker (Fig. 13).

The cathode pins of the atrial and ventricular leads are connected into the atrial and ventricular receptacles, respectively. The anode of the atrial lead is covered with the small plastic glove and is nonfunctional. Thus, we have a unipolar temporary DDD pacemaker (Fig. 14).

Our experience with this unit has been considerable, and we have found that it provides reliable DDD pacing in both bedfast and ambulatory patients. The average time of use has been 4½ days. Of the 13 patients reported upon,[11] 7 have gone on to have permanent pacemakers. There were two temporary pacemaker failures because of ventricular lead displacement. Nine of the patients were ambulatory.

INDICATIONS FOR TEMPORARY PACING

Bradyarrhythmias

In general, temporary pacing should be considered when the patient is symptomatic (syncope, near syncope, dizziness, weakness, congestive heart failure), no matter what the etiology, and/or when the heart rate drops below 45 beats per minute.[12] Temporary pacing is especially appropriate when these conditions develop acutely. When the bradyarrhythmias are chronic and the patient is relatively asymptomatic, permanent pacing on an elective basis is generally satisfactory.

Physiologic pacing of the bradyarrhythmias can best be viewed by defining three general categories: (1) those in which the sinus mechanism is depressed and the AV node is intact; (2) those in which there is an element of heart block, that is, AV nodal or His bundle dysfunction; and (3) those in which there are elements of both (1) and (2).

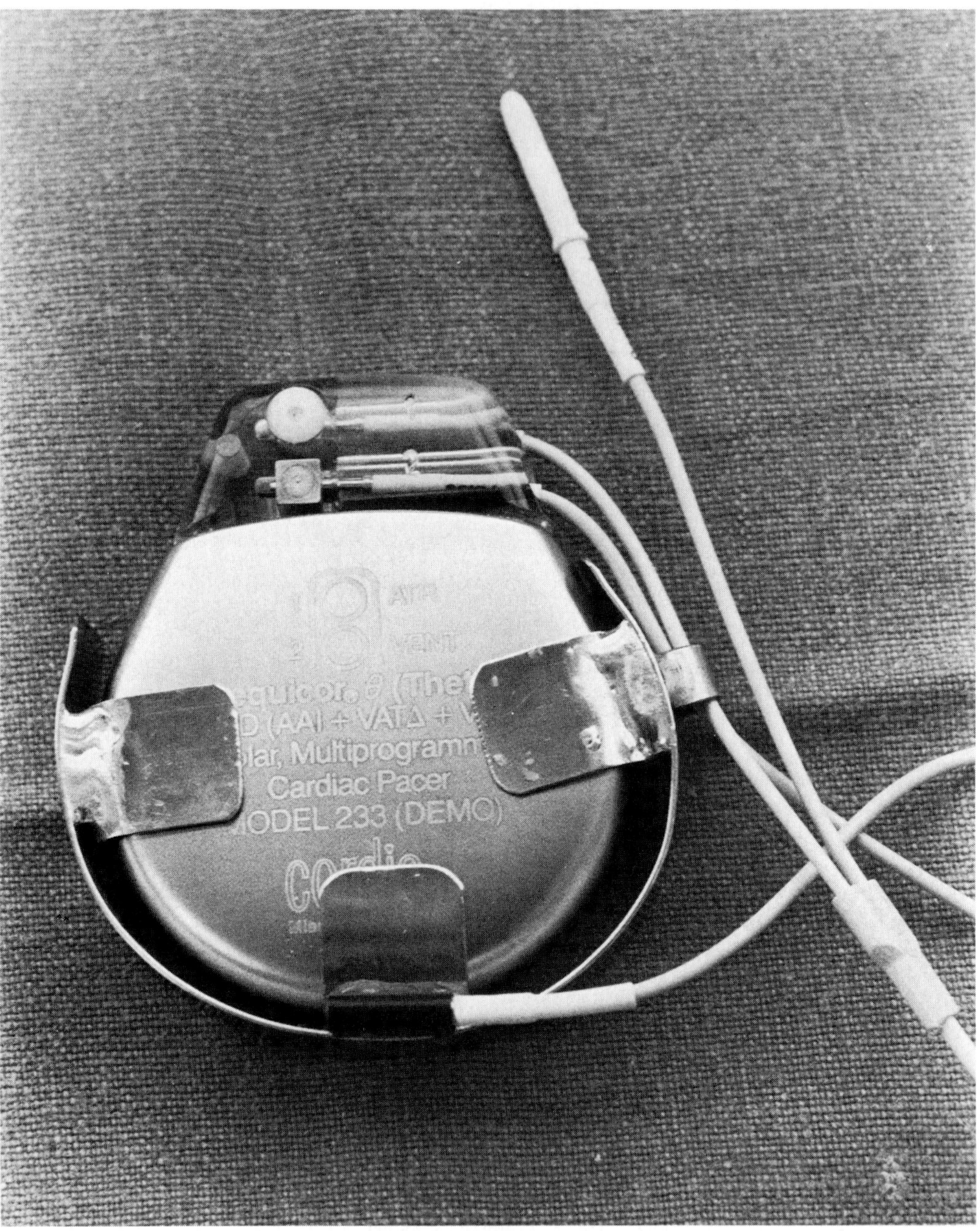

Figure 14. A close-up view of the case showing the connections of the remote anode to the bracket holding the case and the pins in the atrial and ventricular receptacles of the pulse generator.

Temporary Atrial Pacing

Sinus bradycardia or nodal bradycardia, whether on the basis of drugs, intrinsic disease, or both, can often be treated simply and efficiently with a temporary atrial pacemaker. In our experience, this indication often occurs in the setting of beta blockade in an elderly person with unstable angina or when using antiarrhythmic drugs in the setting of sick sinus syndrome.[7]

Nodal bradycardia, sinus bradycardia, or sinus arrest is not infrequently encountered following open heart surgery and is remarkably well managed with atrial pacing. This pacing is generally done using epicardial wires, but these have a short useful life.[13,14] Should the epicardial wires fail, the winged temporary atrial lead functions extremely well even when the patient is up and about.[7]

The use of the atrial pacemaker assumes the presence of an intact AV node. In our experience, if atrial pacing can conduct 1:1 to the ventricle with rates up to 125 beats per minute, the AV node is intact for purposes of treatment of the bradyarrhythmia and one need not be unduly concerned about AV conduction.

Very often there is a question as to the appropriateness of permanent atrial pacing in clinical situations such as mild bradycardia associated with bouts of atrial tachycardia, bradycardia in a setting of severe angina requiring large doses of beta blockade, or other bradyarrhythmias related to drug therapy. These clinical questions can be answered quite nicely by a short clinical trial of temporary atrial pacing followed by a period of observation with the pacer on and off, with the patient ambulatory and monitored.

Temporary Ventricular Pacing

Traditional temporary ventricular pacing is still the generally accepted form of therapy for the hospitalized patient with bradyarrhythmias. In our hands, we tend to limit this type of pacing to a patient with intractable atrial fibrillation and a slow ventricular response or when a patient, for whatever reason, needs temporary coverage for episodes of very transient bradycardia or heart block.

Temporary AV Sequential Pacing

Temporary AV sequential pacemakers have been available for some time and are now widely used in postoperative open heart units.[13,15]

Pacing of the atrium and ventricle in a sequential fashion is best used in a situation where there is both a deficiency in the sinus node and an element of heart block. This particular mode of pacing does not sense the atrium but does sense and is inhibited by the ventricle. It often is useful in the setting of drug therapy or drug excess in combination with diffuse conduction system disease as well as in the immediate postoperative open heart surgery.

Sick sinus syndrome not infrequently has an element of heart block, and atrial pacing at normal rates (65 to 90 beats per minute) will result in an unduly long AV interval (0.24 to 0.36 second). In this circumstance, temporary AV pacing is preferred.

In the cardiac care unit (CCU) setting, an acute inferior myocardial infarction, especially if it involves occlusion of the right coronary artery proximal to the sinoatrial (SA) node artery, will often result in marked bradycardia as well as heart block (usually Mobitz I); and if unresponsive to atropine, temporary AV pacing is indicated.

Temporary DDD Pacing

The DDD or "universal" pacemaker can sense and pace in both the atrium and ventricle. Its microprocessor circuits allow programming of a wide variety of minimal heart rates, AV intervals, maximum heart rates, currents, and sensitivities. The microprocessor can maintain AV synchrony in all conditions, hence the word "universal," but it is especially appropriate for the case of heart block with an intact or mildly diseased sinus mechanism. Thus, in a situation in which the sinus rate is above the minimum programmed rate, pacing of the ventricle will follow each detected P wave, that is, in a P wave synchronous fashion. If the sinus rate falls to the minimal programmed rate, AV sequential pacing will ensue (Fig. 15).

Use of a temporary DDD pacemaker would be especially appropriate with complete heart block following open heart surgery in the setting of acute myocardial infarction (Fig. 16).

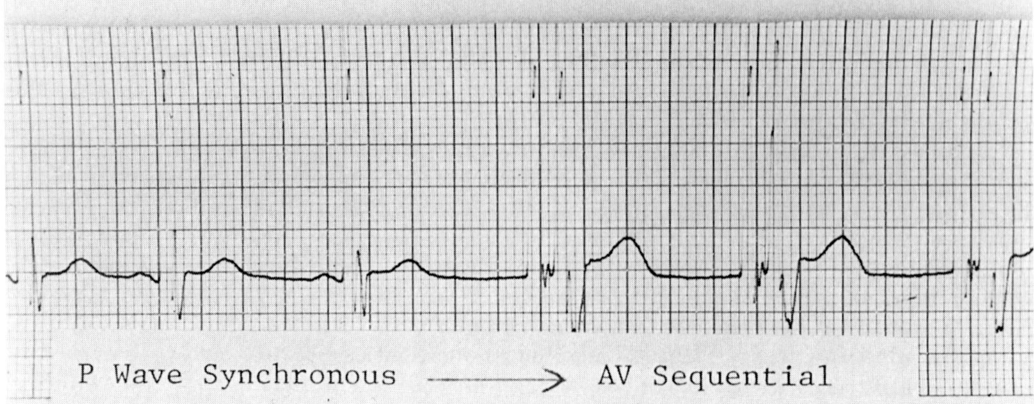

Figure 15. P wave synchronous pacing reverting to AV sequential pacing when the sinus rate drops to the minimum programmed rate.

Should the infarct be extensive and especially if there is major concern regarding maintenance of hemodynamics, this method of pacing can be of significant benefit. Furthermore, it provides the possible use of overdrive AV pacing for control of ventricular arrhythmias resistant to medication.

The temporary DDD pacemaker would also be valuable in a therapeutic trial, with a possible permanent pacer in mind, to determine the appropriateness of the DDD pacer in a patient with diffuse conduction system disease. Determinations can be made as to the appropriateness of mode (for example, atrial pacing versus AV sequential pacing versus DDD pacing), the appropriate minimal heart rate and AV intervals to optimize the antiarrhythmic and hemodynamic qualities of the pacemaker, and the correct atrial refractory period to avoid pacemaker-mediated tachycardias.

With the device and electrodes described above, there is no difficulty with the patient being ambulatory. It functions in a perfectly normal manner, as would a permanent DDD pacer.

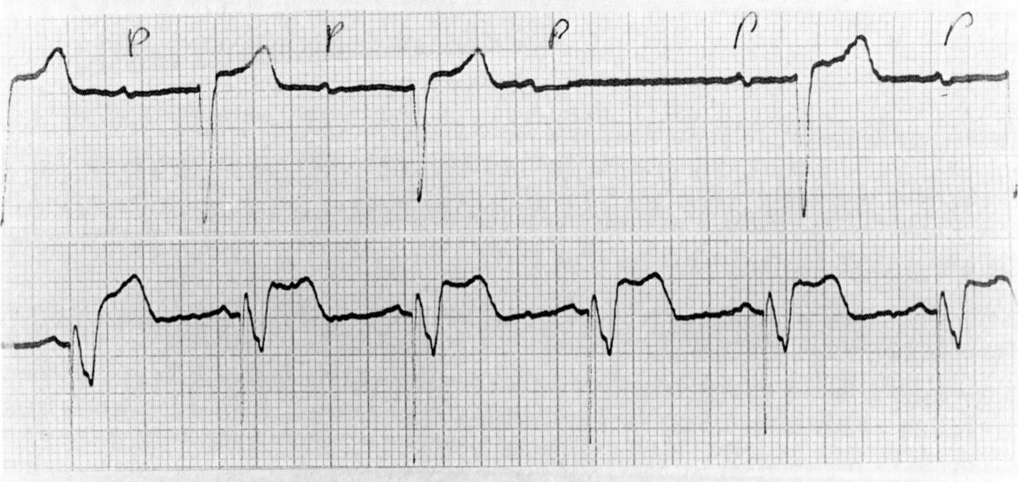

Figure 16. Heart block in the upper panel and P wave synchronous pacing in the lower panel following insertion of a temporary DDD pacemaker.

Tachyarrhythmias

It has long been appreciated that the tachyarrhythmias, atrial and ventricular, when resistant to medications alone, can often be controlled by overdrive pacing of the atria[16] or of atria and ventricles in sequence.[17]

Temporary Atrial Pacing

Atrial pacing is especially effective in the tachy-brady variant of sick sinus syndrome, or in other atrial arrhythmias including supraventricular tachycardia (Fig. 17), atrial flutter, or even intermittent atrial fibrillation resistant to medications. The use of overdrive atrial pacing (rate 90 to 120 beats per minute) in combination with beta blockade and antiarrhythmic drugs can be a very effective method of rhythm control in an intensive care setting or in a monitored ambulatory patient.

Insertion of a temporary atrial pacer set to overdrive rates prior to cardioversion can often avoid the brady-tachy pattern encountered immediately following the electrical shock.

Atrial pacing can frequently be used for controlling various ventricular arrhythmias including premature ventricular beats in an isolated or coupled fashion and ventricular tachycardias whether induced by drugs or ischemia.[17] Often fairly rapid overdrive rates are required; and should the AV node be compromised, AV sequential pacing would be indicated (see below).

Temporary AV Sequential Pacing

This form of pacing is particularly useful for the atrial arrhythmias (supraventricular tachycardia, atrial flutter, intermittent atrial fibrillation) in which there exists some element of heart block. Quite long AV intervals with atrial pacing alone at overdrive rates tend to reduce hemodynamic and antiarrhythmic effectiveness, and in these cases pacing both the atria and ventricles in sequence is indicated. The same can be said for the ventricular arrhythmias as noted above.

Temporary Ventricular Pacing

This approach should be avoided at overdrive rates, particularly if there is retrograde VA conduction. Pacing the ventricle at high rates with VA conduction and functioning atria can lead to significant hemodynamic compromise.[18] If the atria are nonfunctional, that is, fibril-

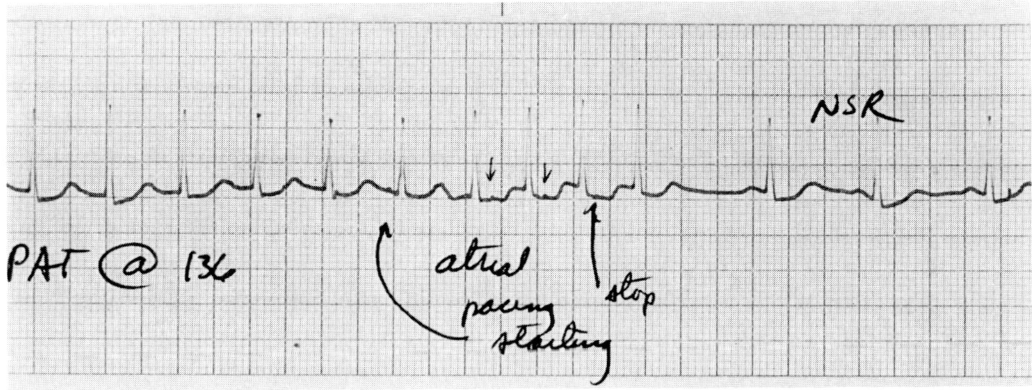

Figure 17. Paroxysmal atrial tachycardia (PAT) being converted by rapid atrial pacing using a temporary atrial pacemaker.

lating, and the purpose is to control ventricular arrhythmias, there would be no use for atrial or AV sequential pacing, and only ventricular pacing is indicated.

Temporary DDD Pacing

The temporary DDD unit used in an overdrive fashion will function in an AV sequential mode and, other than size, offers little advantage over the standard AV sequential pacemaker. The size differences are marked, however, and if the patient is to be ambulatory, one may prefer the much smaller DDD unit (Figs. 18, 19, 20, 21).

In our practice, we have found that we are making ever greater use of physiologic overdrive pacing in the control of a host of tachyarrhythmias.

Table 1 is a summary of methods and indications for temporary physiologic pacing. This summary provides a practical overview of where our technology is leading us and how best to use it. Mastery of the techniques described above can be a potent tool in the hands of the hospital cardiologist.

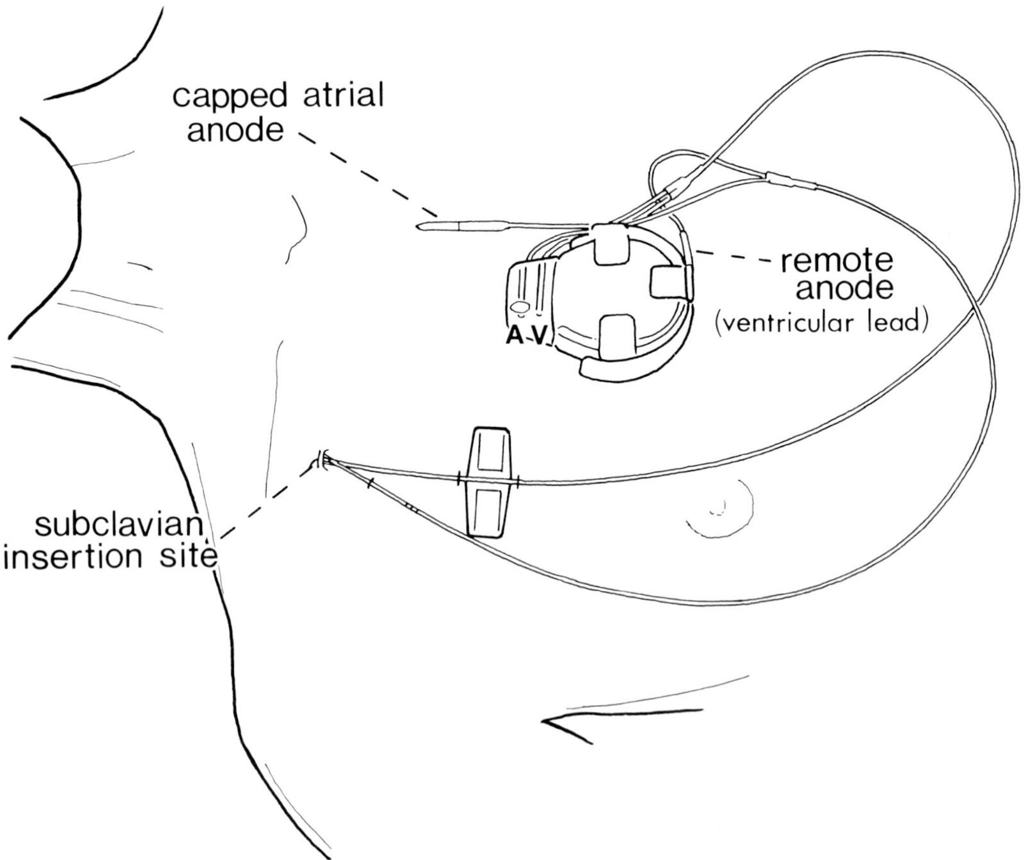

Figure 18. This drawing shows the two leads through the right subclavian vein attached to the temporary DDD pacemaker.

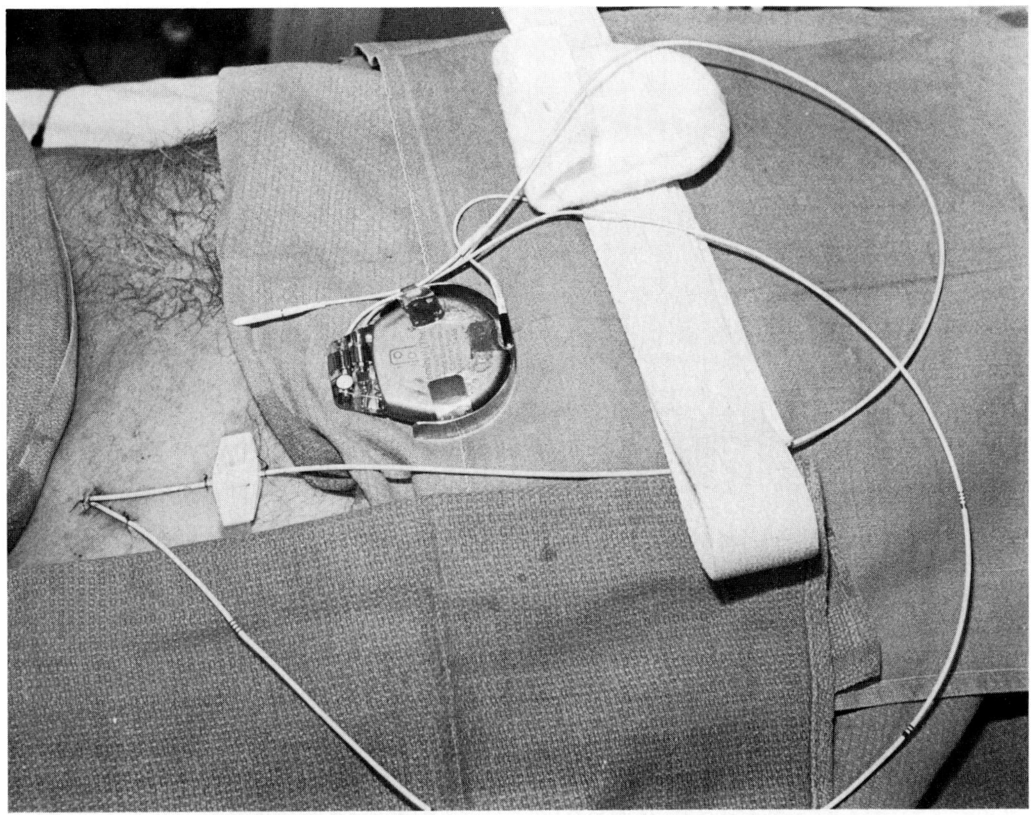

Figure 19. This is a photograph of the two-lead insertion with attachment to the DDD pacemaker.

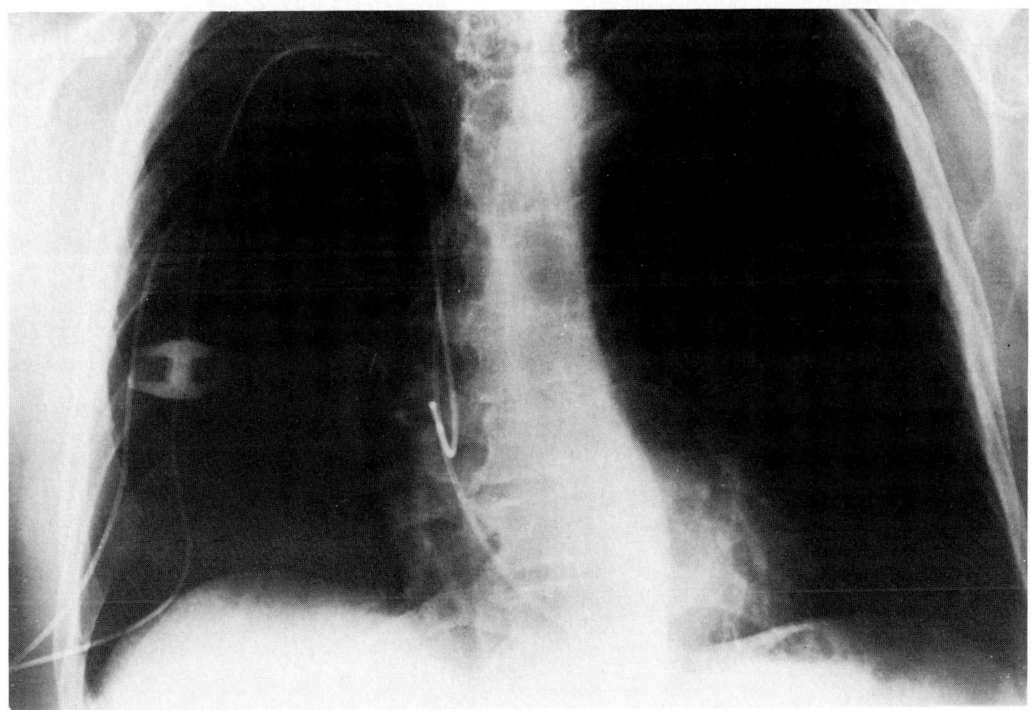

Figure 20. PA chest x-ray film showing the temporary atrial and ventricular leads in place.

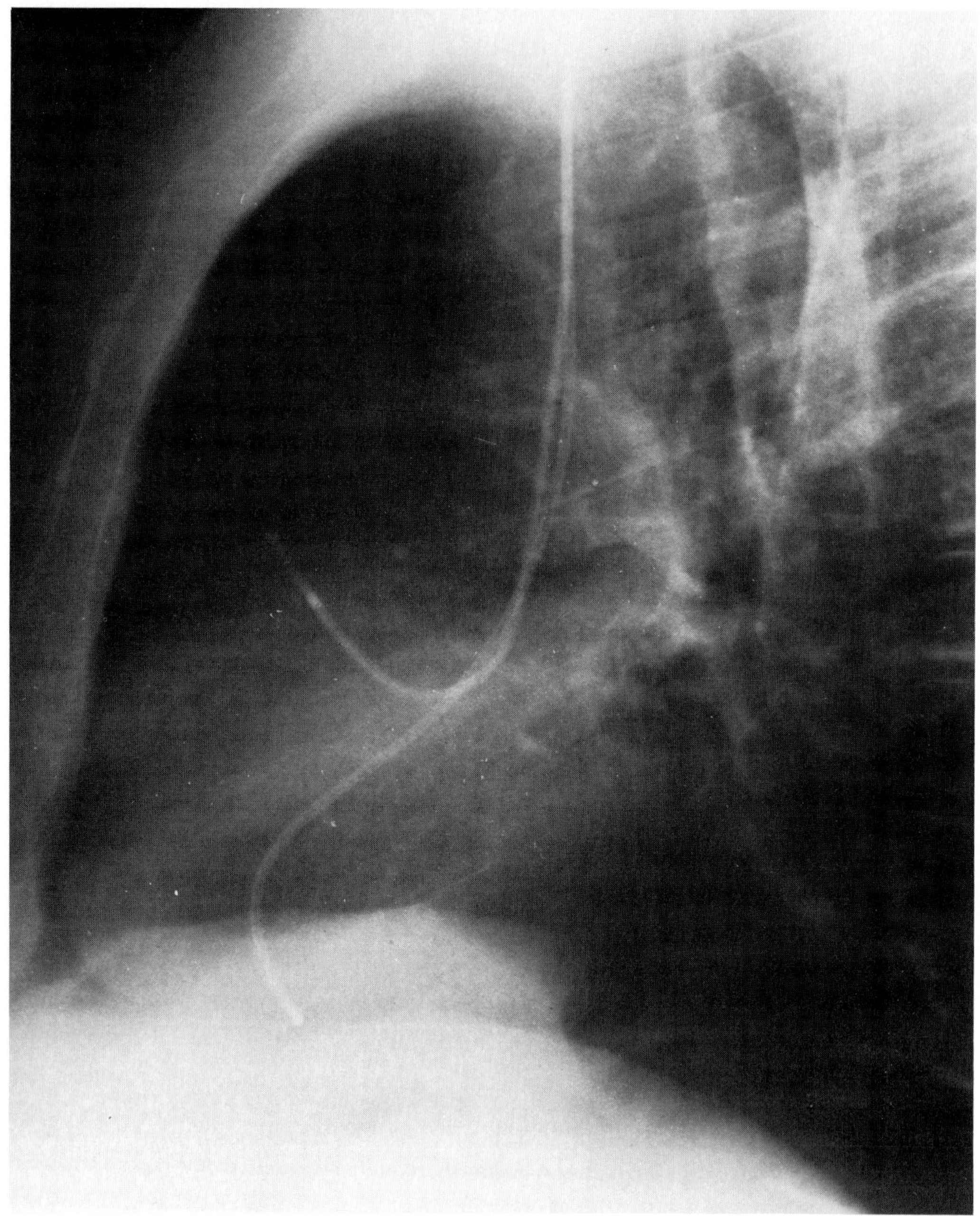

Figure 21. Lateral chest x-ray film showing temporary atrial and ventricular leads in place.

Table 1. Summary of indications

- I. Bradyarrhythmias
  - A. Temporary atrial pacing (assumes AV node intact—1:1 pacing up to 125 beats per minute)
    - 1. Acute treatment
      - a. Sinus bradycardia
      - b. Nodal bradycardia
      - c. Sinus arrest

        (on the basis of beta blockade, antiarrhythmics, ischemia, or open heart surgery)
    - 2. Clinical trial with reference to possible permanent pacemaker implantation
  - B. Temporary ventricular pacing
    - 1. Atrial fibrillation with slow ventricular response
    - 2. Acute coverage for very transient episodes of bradycardia whatever the cause
  - C. Temporary AV sequential pacing (assumes AV node is not intact or AV conduction is prolonged)
    - 1. Acute treatment
      - a. Sinus bradycardia
      - b. Nodal bradycardia
      - c. Sinus arrest

        (on whatever basis: beta blockade, antiarrhythmics, ischemia, infarction, open heart surgery)
  - D. Temporary DDD or "universal" pacing
    - 1. AV node dysfunction with intact or mildly diseased sinus node on whatever basis
    - 2. All bradycardias in which the atria are functional (nonfibrillating)
    - 3. Clinical trial
      - a. Appropriateness of pacing mode
      - b. Optimization of minimum heart rate and AV intervals
      - c. Reentry pacemaker-mediated tachycardias, observation and control

- II. Tachyarrhythmias
  - A. Atrial pacing at rates of 90 to 120 beats per minute (assumes an intact AV node)
    - 1. Tachy-brady syndrome
    - 2. Supraventricular tachycardia
    - 3. Atrial flutter
    - 4. Intermittent atrial fibrillation
    - 5. Immediately following cardioversion
    - 6. Ventricular arrhythmias
  - B. Temporary AV sequential pacing (assumes AV node dysfunction)
    - 1. Tachy-brady syndrome
    - 2. Supraventricular tachycardia
    - 3. Atrial flutter
    - 4. Intermittent atrial fibrillation
    - 5. Immediately following cardioversion
    - 6. Ventricular arrhythmias
  - C. Temporary ventricular overdrive pacing (pacing rates of 90 to 130 beats per minute)

    (ventricular arrhythmias with nonfunctioning [fibrillating] atria)
    - 1. Ventricular irritability
    - 2. Ventricular tachycardias

    DO NOT USE IF ATRIA ARE FUNCTIONAL AND VA (RETROGRADE) CONDUCTION IS PRESENT
  - D. Temporary DDD pacing (use at overdrive rates would be in AV sequential mode); advantage of size

REFERENCES

1. Mantle, JA, Massing, GK, James, TN, et al: *A multipurpose catheter for electrophysiologic and hemodynamic monitoring plus atrial pacing.* Chest 72:285, 1977.
2. Morin, JE, Wynands, JE, et al: *Temporary cardiac pacing following open-heart surgery.* Canad J Surg 25:128, 1982.
3. Hartzler, GO, Maloney, JD, Curtis, JJ, et al: *Hemodynamic benefits of atrial-ventricular sequential pacing after cardiac surgery.* Am J Cardiol 40:232, 1977.

4. LITTLEFORD, PO AND SPECTOR, SD: *Device for the rapid insertion of permanent endocardial electrode through the subclavian vein.* Ann Thorac Surg 27:265, 1979.
5. LINOS, DA, MUCHA, P, AND VAN HEERDEN, JA: *Subclavian vein, a golden route.* Mayo Clin Proc 55:315, 1980.
6. BERENS, SC, KOLIN, A, MACALPIN, RN: *New stable temporary atrial pacing loop.* Am J Cardiol 34:325, 1974.
7. LITTLEFORD, PO AND PEPINE, CJ: *A new temporary atrial pacing catheter inserted percutaneously into the subclavian vein without fluoroscopy.* PACE 4:458, 1981.
8. PRESTON, TA: *A new temporary pacing catheter with improved sensing and safety characteristics.* Am Heart J 88:289, 1974.
9. PRESTON, TA: *Anodal stimulation as the cause of pacemaker induced ventricular fibrillation.* Am Heart J 86:366, 1973.
10. MERX, W, HAN, J, AND YOON, M: *Effects of unipolar cathodal and bipolar stimulation on vulnerability of ischemic ventricles to fibrillation.* Am J Cardiol 35:37, 1975.
11. LITTLEFORD, PO AND PEPINE, CJ: *A temporary (external) DDD pacing unit.* Am J Cardiol, April 1984.
12. CHUNG, EK (ED): *Artificial Cardiac Pacing: Practical Approach.* Williams & Wilkins, Baltimore, 1978, p 161.
13. WISHEART, JD, WRIGHT, JEC, ROSENFELDT, FL, ET AL: *Atrial and ventricular pacing after open heart surgery.* Thorax 28:9, 1973.
14. MACLEAN, WA AND COOPER, TB: *Use of temporarily placed epicardial atrial wire electrodes for the diagnosis and treatment of cardiac arrhythmias following open heart surgery.* J Thorac Cardiovasc Surg 76:500, 1978.
15. FIELDS, J, BERKOVITZ, BV, AND MATLOFF, JM: *Surgical experience with temporary and permanent AV sequential demand pacing.* J Thorac Cardiovasc Surg 66:865, 1973.
16. DESANCTIS, RW: *Diagnostic and therapeutic use of atrial pacing.* Circulation 43:748, 1971.
17. DREIFUS, LS, BERKOVITS, BV, ET AL: *Use of atrial and bifocal cardiac pacemakers for treating resistant dysrhythmias.* Europ J Cardiol 3:257, 1976.
18. CURTIS, JJ, MALONEY, JD, BARNHORST, DA, ET AL: *A critical look at temporary ventricular pacing following cardiac surgery.* Surgery 82:888, 1977.

Bedside Hemodynamic Monitoring in the Cardiac Care Unit

Kanu Chatterjee, M.B., F.R.C.P.

The development of balloon flotation catheters[1] represents a major contribution to the management of critically ill cardiac patients because they permit the physician to identify the cause and appropriate management of low output state. The greatest amount of experience has been attained by studying patients with acute myocardial infarction; however, in recent years, bedside hemodynamic monitoring has been used with increasing frequency for the diagnosis and management of chronic heart failure. The ability to measure cardiac output, and right atrial, pulmonary capillary wedge, pulmonary artery, and systemic pressures at the bedside not only allows assessment of the severity of hemodynamic compromise but also permits evaluation of the effectiveness of a particular therapeutic intervention. Furthermore, determination of hemodynamics allows evaluation of prognosis of patients in certain clinical circumstances.

The hemodynamic variables that provide the most useful information and need to be monitored during the management of critically ill cardiac patients are heart rate and rhythm, arterial pressure, left ventricular filling pressure (pulmonary capillary wedge or pulmonary artery end-diastolic pressure), right ventricular filling pressure (right atrial pressure), pulmonary artery pressure, and cardiac output. From these measurements, several hemodynamic parameters, such as stroke volume and stroke work, and pulmonary and systemic vascular resistances can be derived. Determination of these derived hemodynamic parameters is useful for the evaluation of the cause and severity of right and left ventricular failure and also for appropriate therapy.

Direct determinations of arterial pressure by inserting an intra-arterial cannula is preferable in patients with low output state, particularly in the presence of hypotension, because a significant disparity exists between cuff pressure and intra-arterial pressure in these circumstances. In patients with severe peripheral vasoconstriction, central rather than peripheral arterial pressure should be monitored; therefore, femoral or brachial artery cannulation is preferable to radial artery cannulation in patients with cardiogenic shock.

Assessment of right and left ventricular function at the bedside during hemodynamic monitoring relies on the measurement of right atrial and pulmonary capillary wedge pressures and cardiac output. Right atrial pressure reflects the diastolic pressure of the right ventricle, and pulmonary capillary wedge pressure reflects the left ventricular diastolic pressure. Ventricular end-diastolic pressures in most circumstances can be used as their filling pressures. From the relationship between ventricular filling pressures and any index of its function, such as cardiac output, stroke volume, or stroke work, ventricular systolic function can be assessed. With the availability of triple lumen balloon flotation thermodilution catheters, which allow measurements of right atrial and pulmonary capillary wedge pressures and cardiac output,[2] simultaneous evaluation of right and left ventricular function can be made at the bedside.

Although in most clinical conditions pulmonary artery occluded (wedge) pressure closely reflects mean left atrial and left ventricular diastolic pressures and, therefore, can be used as left ventricular filling pressure, significant discrepancy between pulmonary capillary wedge pressure and left atrial and left ventricular diastolic pressures can occur in certain clinical situations. In patients with mitral valve obstruction (mitral stenosis, left atrial myxoma), left atrial and pulmonary capillary wedge pressures are higher than left ventricular diastolic pressures, and, therefore, in these patients pulmonary capillary wedge pressure cannot be used as left ventricular filling pressure.

Alteration in left ventricular diastolic compliance might also produce a significant discrepancy between mean pulmonary capillary wedge or left atrial pressure and left ventricular end-diastolic pressure. With decreased left ventricular diastolic compliance (severe left ventricular hypertrophy, restrictive cardiomyopathy), mean pulmonary capillary wedge pressure is significantly lower than left ventricular end-diastolic pressure. Furthermore, when left ventricular diastolic pressure is markedly elevated (exceeding 25 mm Hg), the difference between mean pulmonary capillary wedge and left ventricular end-diastolic pressure is greater and may exceed 20 mm Hg. This disparity is due to the differences in left ventricular, left atrial, and pulmonary venous compliances; the left atrium and pulmonary veins are more compliant structures than the left ventricle.

Increased intrathoracic and intrapericardial pressures are associated with elevated ventricular diastolic pressures. In these circumstances, however, neither the left ventricular end-diastolic pressure nor the pulmonary capillary wedge pressure represents the left ventricular filling pressure. Transmural pressure (left ventricular diastolic pressure-intrapericardial pressure) is the true left ventricular filling pressure. In the presence of increased intrapericardial pressure, the left ventricular diastolic pressure increases proportionately to the increase in intrapericardial pressure, although transmural pressure may not change. Thus, in cardiac tamponade or acute right ventricular dilatation—the conditions in which intrapericardial pressure is elevated[3]—pulmonary capillary wedge pressure cannot be used as the left ventricular filling pressure. In these conditions, right atrial pressure also does not reflect right ventricular filling pressure. Increased intrathoracic pressures (for example, positive pressure ventilation and tension pneumothorax) alter the relation between ventricular diastolic pressure and transmural pressure in the same way as the increased intrapericardial pressure and prevent the use of pulmonary capillary wedge pressure and right atrial pressure from representing left and right ventricular filling pressures, respectively. Furthermore, when intra-alveolar pressure is increased (as during positive pressure ventilation), a considerable difference is observed between pulmonary capillary wedge and left atrial pressure, particularly at a lower left atrial pressure.[4] However, when left atrial pressure is high (above 20 cm H_2O), this difference is minimal. The clinical situations where pulmonary capillary wedge pressure does not represent ventricular filling pressure are summarized in Table 1.

Pulmonary artery end-diastolic, mean pulmonary capillary wedge, and left ventricular end-diastolic pressures are virtually identical in patients with normal pulmonary vascular resistance. During prolonged hemodynamic monitoring, therefore, pulmonary artery end-diastolic pressure can be used instead of pulmonary capillary wedge pressure to represent left ventricular filling pressure.[5] If one uses pulmonary artery end-diastolic pressure, the potential complications associated with repeated balloon inflations to determine pulmonary artery occluded pressure can be avoided. However, in certain clinical situations, a significant difference between pulmonary artery end-diastolic pressure and pulmonary capillary wedge pressure exists, precluding the use of pulmonary artery diastolic pressure as left ventricular filling pressure. In the presence of elevated pulmonary vascular resistance, irrespective of the etiology, pulmonary artery end-diastolic pressure is significantly higher than the mean pulmonary capillary wedge pressure. In patients with primary pulmonary hypertension, cor pulmonale, thrombo-embolic pulmonary hypertension, and Eisenmenger's syndrome, the difference between pulmonary artery diastolic pressure and pulmonary capillary wedge pressure is considerable and far exceeds the normal expected difference of 1 to 3 mm Hg.

Table 1. The clinical conditions in which pulmonary capillary wedge pressure does not represent left ventricular filling pressure (transmural pressure)

1. *Mitral valve obstruction*
   Mitral stenosis; left atrial myxoma; ball valve thrombus; cor triatriatum
2. *When pulmonary venous pressure is higher than left atrial pressure*
   Congenital and acquired pulmonary veno-occlusive disease; total anomalous pulmonary venous drainage
3. *Increased intrapericardial pressure*
   Cardiac tamponade; acute right ventricular dilatation (right ventricular infarction, massive pulmonary embolism, acute severe tricuspid regurgitation)

DIAGNOSIS OF PATHOLOGIC CONDITIONS

Bedside hemodynamic monitoring aids in the diagnosis of a number of pathologic conditions encountered in the cardiac care unit (Table 2). One of the frequent clinical problems is to identify the mechanism of low systemic output in critically ill cardiac patients. Absolute or relative hypovolemia, predominant right ventricular failure, and predominant left ventricular failure are associated with decreased cardiac output. Determination of right atrial and pulmonary capillary wedge pressures allows the diagnosis of these conditions associated with low systemic output. The characteristic hemodynamic abnormalities of hypovolemic shock are decreased right atrial and pulmonary capillary wedge pressures in addition to decreased cardiac output and hypotension (Fig. 1). In contrast, in patients with left ventricular pump failure and cardiogenic shock, pulmonary capillary wedge pressure is elevated (more than 15 mm Hg) and higher than right atrial pressure, which may be normal or elevated, depending on whether or not right ventricular failure coexists (Fig. 2). Predominant right ventricular failure, irrespective of etiology, is associated with low systemic output. Acute right ventricular infarction, acute massive pulmonary embolism, primary severe tricuspid regurgitation, and severe precapillary pulmonary hypertension all can precipitate predominant right ventricular failure. The hemodynamic abnormalities in predominant right ventricular failure are disproportionate elevation of right atrial pressure in relation to pulmonary capillary wedge pressure and low systemic output. Depressed right ventricular systolic function may be evident from the decreased right ventricular stroke work index despite elevated right atrial pressure. The etiology of right ventricular failure can also be suspected from the associated hemodynamic abnormalities. Not only is precapillary pulmonary hypertension, such as pulmonary embolism, associated with elevated pulmonary artery pressure, but also the pulmonary artery diastolic pressure is significantly higher than the mean pulmonary capillary wedge pressure, and the calculated pulmonary vascular resistance is higher than normal. In contrast, in primary

Table 2. Pathologic conditions associated with low systemic output that can be diagnosed by bedside hemodynamic monitoring

- Hypovolemic shock
- Severe left ventricular failure and cardiogenic shock
- Severe mitral regurgitation
- Ventricular septal rupture
- Severe right ventricular failure
  - Right ventricular infarction
  - Severe primary tricuspid regurgitation
  - Precapillary pulmonary hypertension
- Noncardiac pulmonary edema
- Subsets of acute myocardial infarction

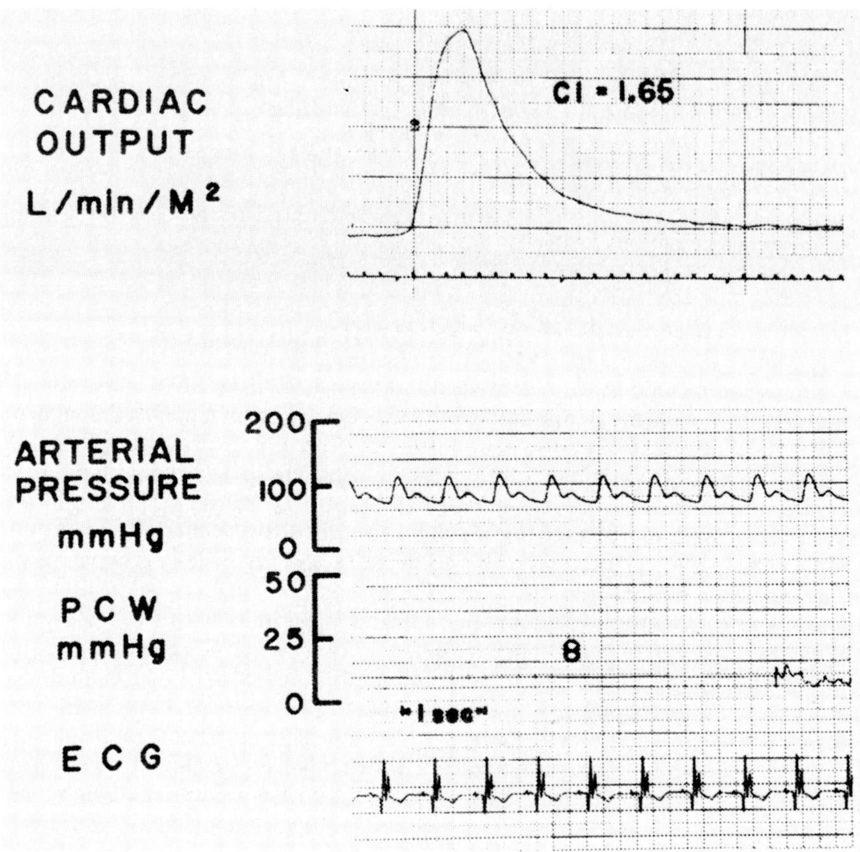

Figure 1. Hemodynamic findings in a patient with hypovolemic shock. Normal or low pulmonary capillary wedge pressure (PCW) and reduced cardiac index (CI) indicate relative hypovolemia. (From Chatterjee, K,[8] with permission.)

tricuspid regurgitation or acute right ventricular infarct, pulmonary artery pressure and pulmonary vascular resistance are normal or minimally elevated and the pulmonary artery diastolic and pulmonary capillary wedge pressures are similar. Severe tricuspid regurgitation can be recognized from the ventricularization of right atrial pressure, with an early and markedly increased amplitude of the regurgitant V wave in the right atrial pressure tracing. In severe right ventricular infarction, on the other hand, the morphology of the pulmonary artery pressure pulse is distorted owing to accentuated reflected A wave, associated with atrial systole (Fig. 3). Thus, careful attention to the changes in the right atrial, right ventricular, and pulmonary arterial pressure wave forms can provide important clues for the diagnosis of the etiology of right ventricular failure.

In patients with severe right ventricular infarction, equalization of right and left ventricular diastolic pressures can occur (see Fig. 3) owing to acute marked dilatation of the right ventricle, which increases the intrapericardial pressure from the encroachment of the limited intrapericardial space within the confinement of the infarct pericardium.[3] Thus, the hemodynamic abnormalities of severe right ventricular infarct simulate cardiac tamponade and constrictive pericarditis. Marked right atrial and right ventricular dilatation owing to severe tricuspid regurgitation may also cause equalization of the diastolic pressures of the intrapericardial cardiac chambers caused by a similar pathophysiologic mechanism (Table 3). It is

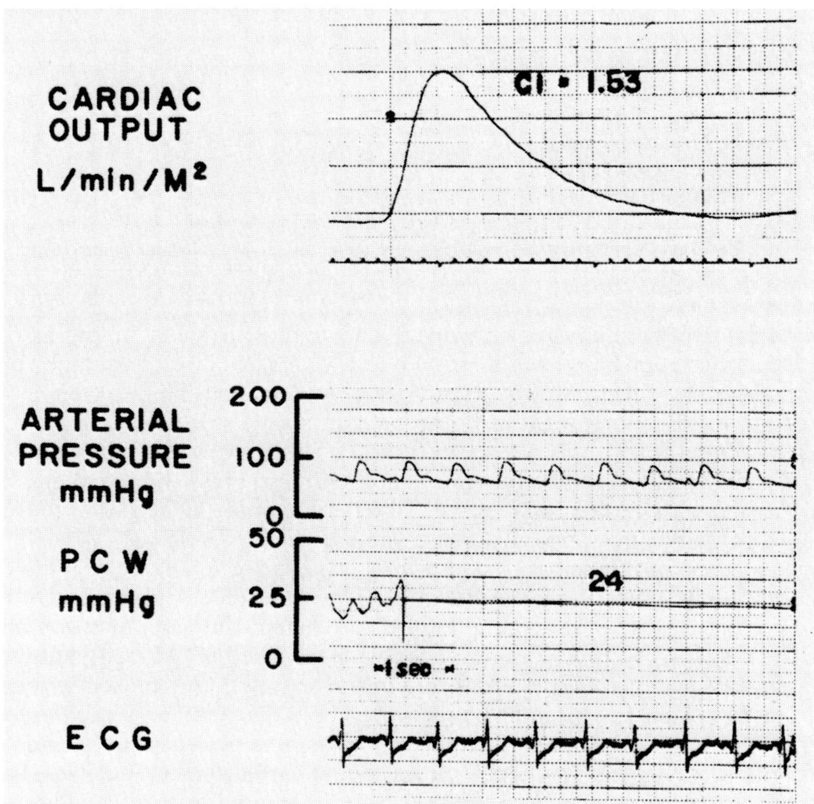

Figure 2. Hemodynamic findings in a patient with cardiogenic shock. Elevated pulmonary capillary wedge pressure (PCW) and reduced cardiac index (CI) indicate pump failure. (From Chatterjee, K, [8] with permission.)

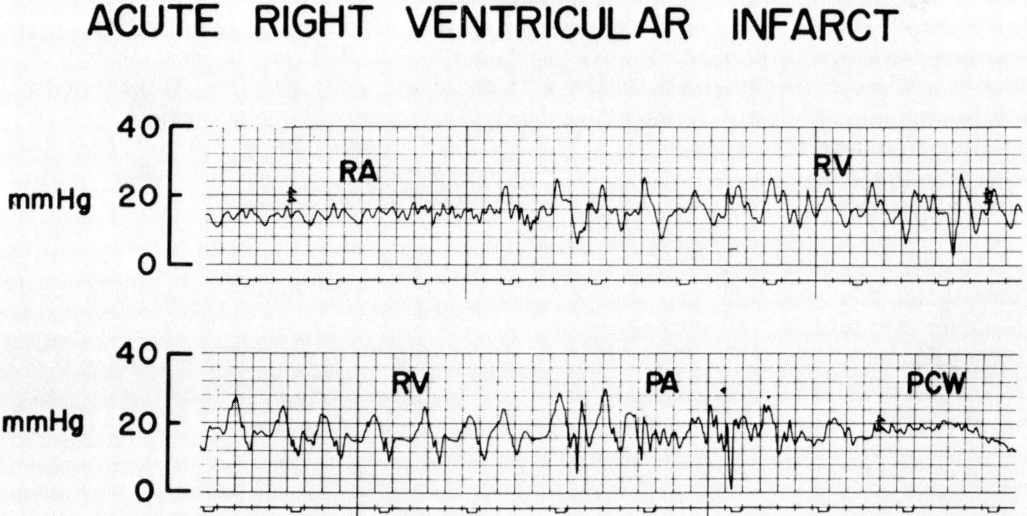

Figure 3. Hemodynamic findings in a patient with acute right ventricular infarct. Disproportionate elevation of right atrial (RA) and right ventricular (RV) end-diastolic pressures in relation to pulmonary capillary wedge (PCW) pressure suggests predominantly right ventricular failure. Right atrial and pulmonary capillary wedge pressures are similar, indicating equalization of diastolic pressures. (From Chatterjee, K,[8] with permission.)

Table 3. Hemodynamics in a patient with severe tricuspid regurgitation with dilated right ventricle and right atrium

Mean Right Atrial Pressure (mm Hg)	32
Mean Pulmonary Capillary Wedge Pressure (mm Hg)	32
Pulmonary Artery Diastolic Pressure (mm Hg)	29
Pulmonary Vascular Resistance (dynes sec cm^{-5})	106
Mean Pulmonary Artery Pressure (mm Hg)	36

Equalization of the diastolic pressures was noted without pericardial effusion. Normal pulmonary vascular resistance and modest elevation of pulmonary arterial pressure indicate primary tricuspid regurgitation.

difficult to differentiate between cardiac tamponade and right ventricular failure associated with right ventricular dilatation based on the hemodynamic abnormalities. Evaluation of right ventricular size and systolic function by echocardiography or scintigraphy is often necessary for the precise diagnosis.[7] Echocardiograms in cardiac tamponade reveal not only pericardial effusion but also right ventricular failure. In predominant right ventricular failure, right ventricular size is increased and its systolic function is depressed, whereas these findings are not encountered in patients with cardiac tamponade. Differentiation of the causes of low output syndrome based on hemodynamic abnormalities is summarized in Table 4.

Both papillary muscle infarct and ventricular septal rupture are relatively uncommon but catastrophic complications of acute myocardial infarction. The sudden appearance of a pansystolic murmur associated with severe pump failure may herald the onset of either of these complications. The diagnosis of these disorders can be established at the bedside by hemodynamic monitoring. In patients with acute severe mitral regurgitation caused by papillary muscle infarct, a giant V wave (regurgitant wave) is present in the pulmonary capillary wedge pressure tracing (Fig. 4). Mean pulmonary capillary wedge pressure, pulmonary artery pressure, and right atrial pressures are frequently elevated, and cardiac output declines. It needs to be emphasized that the presence of a giant V wave in the pulmonary capillary wedge pressure tracing is not pathognomonic of acute mitral regurgitation; increased venous return to the left atrium, as occurs in patients with ventricular septal rupture with large left-to-right intracardiac shunt, may increase the amplitude of the V wave. In the latter instance, this accentuated V wave may simulate the regurgitant wave of mitral regurgitation.[7] However, determination of the onset of the V wave in relation to the QRS complex in the electrocardiogram can be useful in differentiating between the regurgitant wave of mitral regurgitation and the accentuated V wave caused by increased venous return to the left atrium. In severe mitral regurgitation, regurgitation begins with the onset of isovolumic systole, and, therefore, the onset of the regurgitant wave coincides with the QRS complex. The onset of the V wave in ventricular septal rupture is delayed and occurs after the QRS complex.

Table 4. Hemodynamic differentiation of causes of low systemic output commonly encountered in cardiac care units

	RAP	*PCWP*	*Equalization of Diastolic Pressures*	*PADP vs PCWP*
Hypovolemic shock	low	low	absent	PADP = PCWP
Cardiogenic shock	normal or high	high	absent	PADP = PCWP
Right ventricular infarct	high	normal or high	may be present	PADP = PCWP
Precapillary hypertension	high	normal	absent	PADP > PCWP
Cardiac tamponade	high	high	present	PADP = PCWP

PADP = pulmonary arterial diastolic pressure
PCWP = pulmonary capillary wedge pressure

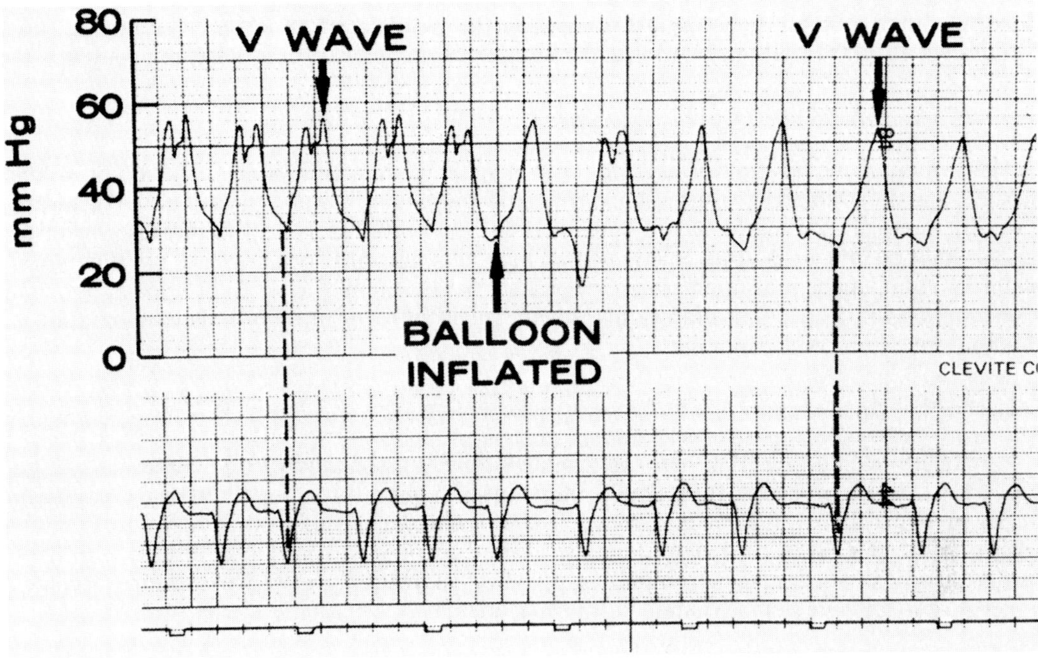

Figure 4. Giant V wave in the pulmonary capillary wedge pressure tracing indicates mitral regurgitation. Reflected V wave in the pulmonary artery pressure tracing can also be recognized. (From Chatterjee, K,[8] with permission.)

In patients with ventricular septal rupture, determinations of oxygen saturations in pulmonary artery and right atrial blood samples aid in the diagnosis; oxygen saturation of the pulmonary arterial blood is significantly higher than that of right atrial blood, owing to left-to-right shunt through the ventricular septal defect (Fig. 5). Caution needs to be exercised, however, to ensure that the tip of the catheter is in the central pulmonary artery and not in

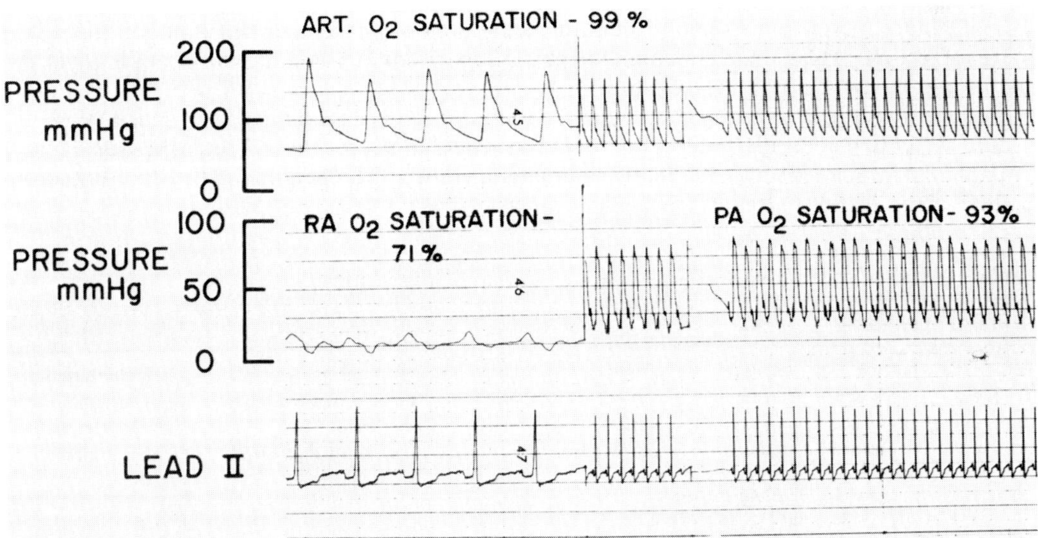

Figure 5. Diagnosis of ventricular septal rupture in a patient with acute myocardial infarction. Oxygen saturation in the pulmonary arterial blood (PA) was significantly higher than that in right atrial blood (RA). (From Chatterjee, K,[8] with permission.)

the distal small pulmonary artery branches or in the wedge position while blood samples are withdrawn. Blood samples drawn from the wedge position have a higher oxygen content.

Cardiac Tamponade

The hemodynamic feature of cardiac tamponade is equalization of the diastolic pressures of right and left ventricles; thus, right atrial and pulmonary capillary wedge pressures are virtually identical. Intracardiac pressures increase proportionately to the increase in intrapericardial pressure. It is apparent that these hemodynamic abnormalities are not diagnostic of cardiac tamponade inasmuch as similar hemodynamic changes can be observed in patients with severe right ventricular infarction or severe tricuspid regurgitation. Echocardiography is essential for the correct diagnosis.

Non-Cardiac Pulmonary Edema

Pulmonary edema caused by left ventricular failure is associated with an abnormally high pulmonary capillary wedge (usually 25 mm Hg or higher) pressure. Pulmonary capillary wedge pressure, however, is normal in non-cardiac pulmonary edema, such as occurs in adult respiratory distress syndrome. In patients with pre-existing left ventricular disease with non-cardiac pulmonary edema, determination of pulmonary capillary wedge pressure becomes imperative to exclude hemodynamic pulmonary edema.

Hemodynamic Subsets in Acute Myocardial Infarction

Bedside hemodynamic measurements allow relatively accurate assessment of left ventricular function in patients with acute myocardial infarction.[8–12] Determinations of specific hemodynamic deficits in individual patients are essential for the diagnosis of hemodynamic subsets and, thus, for delivery of rational therapy to the patients. Ideally, for the evaluation of left ventricular pump function from the hemodynamic measurements, it is desirable to determine an index of left ventricular systolic function (stroke work index, stroke volume, or cardiac output) at various levels of left ventricular filling pressure (LVFP). However, in practice, the relationship of left ventricular stroke work index (LVSWI) to LVFP, compared with normal ranges, permits reasonably accurate assessment of left ventricular function following acute infarction. Based on such hemodynamic comparisons, several subsets of acute myocardial infarction can be identified (Table 5).

Besides these broad subsets, hemodynamic monitoring permits diagnosis of special complications of acute myocardial infarction—right ventricular infarct, mitral regurgitation caused by papillary muscle infarct, and ventricular septal rupture. The hemodynamic differentiation of these complications already has been outlined.

Table 5. Hemodynamic subsets in acute myocardial infarction

LVFP	*LVSWI*	*CI*	*HR*	*AP*	*Subset*
normal	normal	normal	normal	normal	compensated
decreased	increased	normal	normal or increased	normal or elevated	hyperdynamic
decreased	decreased	decreased	increased	decreased	hypovolemia
increased	decreased	decreased	increased	normal or decreased	pump failure

LVFP = left ventricular filling pressure
LVSWI = left ventricular stroke work index
CI = cardiac index
HR = heart rate
AP = arterial pressure

Table 6. Suggested therapeutic measures in relation to hemodynamic subsets

Hemodynamic Subsets	*Suggested Therapy*
compensated	observation
hypovolemia	volume expansion
hyperdynamic	beta-adrenergic blocking agents
pump failure	afterload reducing agents; diuretics; inotropic agents; mechanical circulatory assistance

HEMODYNAMIC MONITORING DURING THERAPEUTIC INTERVENTIONS

In patients with acute myocardial infarction, hemodynamic monitoring not only permits identification of hemodynamic subsets but helps provide a rational therapeutic approach (Table 6).

Compensated or Hyperdynamic Left Ventricular Function

In these conditions, no specific therapeutic intervention is necessary except close observation for the development of any complications. In some patients with initially compensated left ventricular function, pump failure may supervene, owing to extension of the infarct or other complications. Hemodynamic monitoring may be useful to detect early deterioration of left ventricular function, thereby resulting in prompt implementation of therapy.

Hypovolemia

In patients with hypovolemic shock, intravenous fluid therapy usually improves cardiac performance. During fluid infusion, monitoring of pulmonary capillary wedge pressure and cardiac output helps determine the optimal filling pressure. In most patients with recent myocardial infarction with relatively normal left ventricular volume, optimal filling pressure in terms of stroke output is 14 to 18 mm Hg.[13] Further increase in pulmonary capillary wedge pressure enhances the risk of precipitating pulmonary edema. In some patients who initially appear hypovolemic, maintenance of optimal filling pressure with fluid administration is not accompanied by a significant improvement in left ventricular function. In such patients, concomitant left ventricular pump failure exists, and therapy for pump failure is indicated, while maintaining the optimal filling pressure.

Left Ventricular Failure

Vasodilator therapy has gained widespread acceptance in the management of pump failure complicating myocardial infarction.[14,15] However, determination of initial hemodynamics is required for the appropriate choice of the vasodilator agent. Sodium nitroprusside and nitroglycerin are the two vasodilator drugs most frequently used in the management of pump failure complicating myocardial infarction. There are, however, significant differences in the hemodynamic effects of sodium nitroprusside and nitroglycerin.[14] Nitroglycerin and other organic nitrates are predominantly venodilators. The most consistent hemodynamic effect of nitroglycerin is reduction of pulmonary capillary wedge and right atrial pressures, with little or no change in heart rate. The changes in cardiac output and stroke volume are variable; in patients with elevated pulmonary capillary wedge pressure, stroke volume and cardiac output either remain unchanged or increase modestly. In patients with normal pulmonary capillary wedge pressure, or when pulmonary capillary wedge pressure decreases to a very low level, stroke volume and cardiac output may decrease. In these patients, hypotension and reflex tachycardia may also occur. Thus, nitroglycerin is most appropriate for those patients with symptoms of pulmonary venous hypertension (pulmonary edema) but with adequate peripheral perfusion (normal or slightly decreased cardiac output).

Sodium nitroprusside is a potent vasodilator and causes direct smooth muscle relaxation of both the arteriolar and the venous beds. The hemodynamic effects of sodium nitroprusside in heart failure are characterized by a significant increase in cardiac output and stroke volume and a decrease in pulmonary capillary wedge and right atrial pressures. Systemic and pulmonary vascular resistances and pulmonary artery pressure decrease in the majority of patients. Tachycardia usually does not develop in patients with heart failure, despite some reduction in arterial pressure. In patients without heart failure, however, such a beneficial response may not be observed. In patients with normal left ventricular filling pressures, sodium nitroprusside may cause a decrease in stroke volume and cardiac output with a further decrease in filling pressure;[14] tachycardia and hypotension may occur in these circumstances. If filling pressure decreases to a very low level (less than 10 mm Hg) during nitroprusside therapy, stroke volume and cardiac output tend to decrease. It is apparent that the determination of initial filling pressure is necessary before institution of nitroglycerin or nitroprusside therapy. In patients with normal filling pressure, vasodilator therapy may not improve left ventricular function, and vasodilator therapy should be avoided.

Nitroprusside is most effective in patients with decreased cardiac output and elevated systemic vascular resistance. Thus, determination of initial systemic vascular resistance is helpful before nitroprusside therapy. Furthermore, to avoid significant hypotension during vasodilator therapy, monitoring the changes in cardiac output and systemic vascular resistance is desirable. The major objective of vasodilator therapy for the treatment of pump failure is to increase cardiac output by decreasing left ventricular afterload (systemic vascular resistance). If the increase in cardiac output is proportional to the decrease in systemic vascular resistance, mean arterial pressure remains unchanged. Thus, monitoring the changes in cardiac output, arterial pressure, left ventricular filling pressure, and systemic vascular resistance is preferable during vasodilator therapy. In some patients with left ventricular failure, arterial pressure decreases before there are any changes in cardiac output or pulmonary capillary wedge pressures. In these patients, vasodilator therapy should be discontinued. The general guidelines for vasodilator therapy for pump failure complicating myocardial infarction are outlined in Table 7.[16]

In patients with hypotension and markedly depressed left ventricular function, vasodilator therapy does not appear to improve immediate prognosis; vasodilator therapy in these patients may produce further hypotension and enhance myocardial ischemia, thereby causing further

Table 7. Guidelines for intravenous vasodilator therapy in acute pump failure

1. Determine initial hemodynamics for selection of vasodilator
2. Start therapy with low initial dosage (nitroprusside, 15 μg/min; phentolamine, 0.1 mg/min; nitroglycerin, 10 μg/min)
3. Gradual increase in infusion rate (every 5–15 min)
4. Monitor changes in blood pressure, heart rate, left ventricular filling pressure, cardiac output, systemic vascular resistance
5. If cardiac output increases, with a decrease in systemic vascular resistance and left ventricular filling pressure, and little change in blood pressure, maintain same infusion rate
6. If blood pressure decreases without change in cardiac output or left ventricular filling pressure, discontinue vasodilator or add inotropic agent

Table 8. Hemodynamic subsets in acute myocardial infarction

Subset	*Clinical Signs**	*SWI g − m/m²*	*LVFP mm Hg*	*Appropriate Therapy*
I	none	≥40	≤15	none necessary
II	none or ↓ perfusion	<40	≤15	volume expansion
III	pulmonary congestion	>20	>15	diuretics, venodilators
IVA	pulmonary congestion, ↓ perfusion	10–20	>15	combined arteriolar and venodilators
IVB	shock	≤10	>15	vasodilators, mechanical assist devices, inotropes

*Most common clinical signs, but these findings may not be present

deterioration in left ventricular function. Vasopressor agents and intra-aortic balloon counterpulsation are required to increase arterial pressure before vasodilator therapy can be instituted. The therapeutic interventions, according to the hemodynamic abnormalities and the severity of left ventricular failure in patients with acute myocardial infarction, are outlined in Table 8.[18]

Right Ventricular Infarct

Hemodynamic monitoring is essential during management of low output state associated with acute right ventricular failure following predominant right ventricular infarct. The principal mechanism for the decreased systemic output in severe primary right ventricular failure is decreased left ventricular preload.[3] Decreased left ventricular preload appears to be related to reduced right ventricular stroke volume (venous return to the left ventricle) and constraint on left ventricular filling owing to increased intrapericardial pressure. Systemic output increases with increased left ventricular preload during intravenous fluid administration. Monitoring the changes in right atrial and pulmonary capillary wedge pressures and cardiac output is required during intravenous fluid therapy in order to avoid excessive dilatation of the right ventricle, which is manifested by marked increase in right atrial pressure (25 mm Hg or more). Marked right ventricular dilatation may compromise left ventricular filling owing to further increase of intrapericardial pressure. It is desirable to maintain right atrial pressure less than 25 mm Hg during intravenous fluid therapy in patients with acute right ventricular infarct and low systemic output.

Vasodilator drugs such as nitroglycerin or nitroprusside are used along with intravenous fluid therapy to increase right ventricular stroke volume and, hence, left ventricular preload. The mechanism for the beneficial effect of these vasodilator agents in patients with predominant right ventricular failure is probably related to reduction of pulmonary vascular resistance (that is, right ventricular afterload). Monitoring the changes in pulmonary artery pressure and pulmonary vascular resistance is, therefore, preferable during vasodilator therapy in right ventricular failure.

Mitral Regurgitation and Ventricular Septal Rupture

Determination of hemodynamics is necessary not only for the precise diagnosis of severe mitral regurgitation and ventricular septal rupture complicating acute myocardial infarction but also to assess the response to therapy. Sodium nitroprusside produces beneficial hemodynamic and clinical effects in patients with severe mitral regurgitation.[19] Forward stroke volume and cardiac output increase along with decreased regurgitant fraction. Decreased regurgitant volume is associated with decreased magnitude of regurgitant V wave and mean

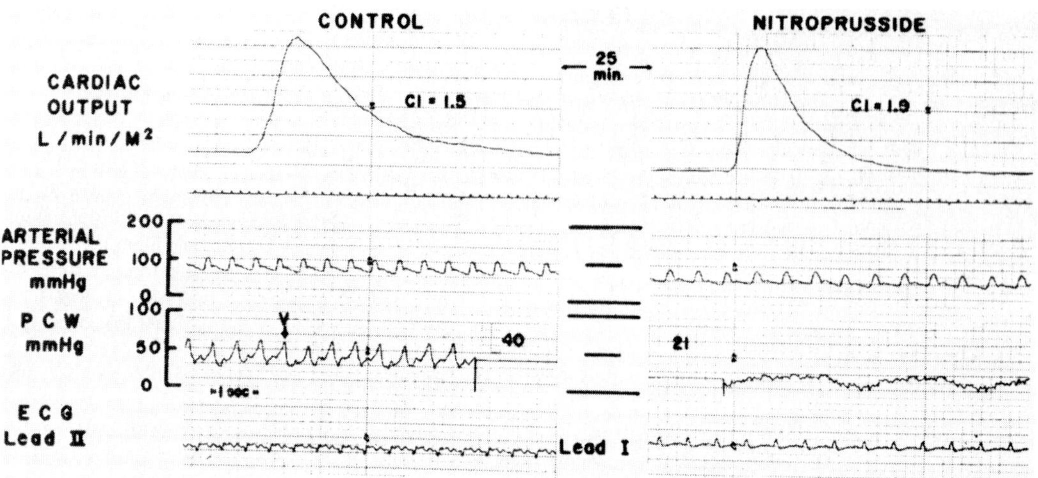

Figure 6. Beneficial hemodynamic effects of vasodilator therapy with sodium nitroprusside in a patient with severe mitral regurgitation complicating acute myocardial infarction. During nitroprusside infusion, cardiac index (CI) increased, and the mean pulmonary capillary wedge (PCW) pressure and the magnitude of the peak V wave decreased. There was only a slight decrease in arterial pressure. (From Chatterjee, K,[8] with permission.)

pulmonary capillary wedge pressure (Fig. 6). Changes in regurgitant V wave indirectly reflect changes in regurgitant volume. Thus, monitoring the pulmonary capillary wedge pressure and regurgitant V wave provides important clues to the beneficial effects of sodium nitroprusside in patients with severe mitral regurgitation. Sodium nitroprusside appears to be more effective in the presence of elevated systemic vascular resistance and in the absence of hypotension. In patients with significant hypotension and with normal or minimally elevated systemic vascular resistance, combined inotropic and vasodilator therapy—with or without intra-aortic balloon counterpulsation—is preferable to vasodilator therapy alone.

Although vasodilator drugs like isosorbide dinitrate and sodium nitroprusside decrease the magnitude of left-to-right shunt and increase systemic output in occasional patients with ventricular septal rupture, potential exists for increasing left-to-right shunt and hemodynamic deterioration during vasodilator therapy. The magnitude of left-to-right shunt in ventricular septal defect is related to the size of the defect and the ratio of the pulmonary vascular resistance to systemic vascular resistance. When the ventricular septal defect is very large, the magnitude of left-to-right shunt is largely determined by the ratio of pulmonary vascular resistance to systemic vascular resistance, inasmuch as the defect itself offers little resistance to left-to-right shunt. In patients with ventricular septal rupture complicating myocardial infarction, the defect is usually very large. Thus, vasodilator agents that potentially can decrease pulmonary vascular resistance more than systemic vascular resistance can enhance left-to-right shunt. Changes in left-to-right shunt and systemic output can be detected by monitoring pulmonary arterial and right atrial oxygen saturations. Increased systemic output and decreased left-to-right shunt is associated with decreased pulmonary arterial oxygen saturation and increased right atrial oxygen saturation; reduction in systemic output, however, is reflected in decreased right atrial oxygen saturation. It is apparent that hemodynamic monitoring is imperative during vasodilator therapy of low output state in patients with ventricular septal rupture. It needs to be emphasized that in the presence of left-to-right shunt, systemic output cannot be determined by right heart thermodilution technique.

Chronic Left Ventricular Failure

Determination of initial hemodynamics and cardiac output is helpful not only to assess the severity of chronic left ventricular failure but also to provide appropriate therapy. Knowledge

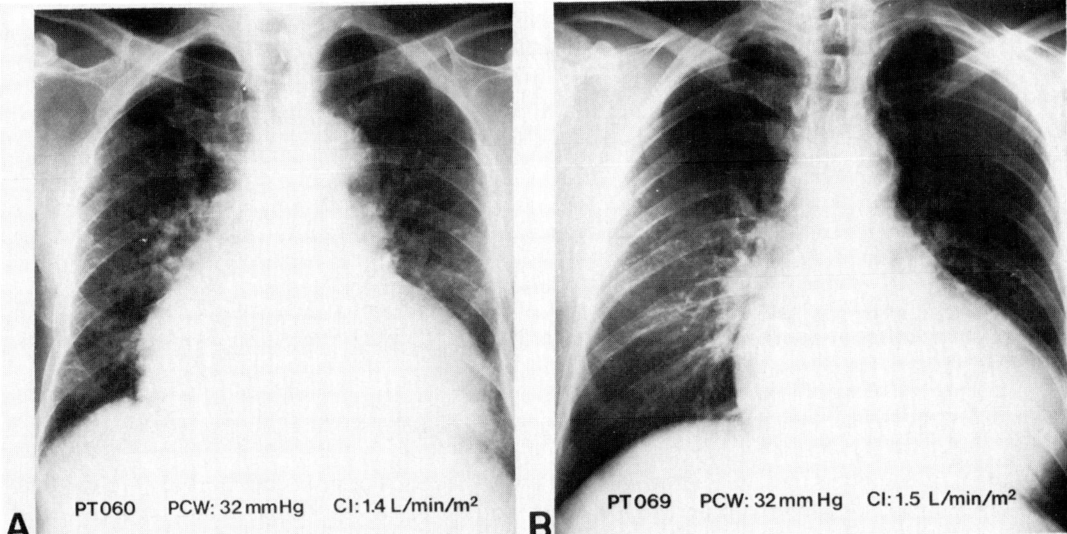

Figure 7. Shown are chest radiographs from two patients with identical hemodynamics and different radiographic findings. In patient A, alveolar edema was present; in patient B, no radiologic signs of pulmonary venous hypertension were detectable despite markedly elevated pulmonary capillary wedge pressure. (From Dash, H, et al,[22] with permission.)

of the level of pulmonary capillary wedge pressure is particularly informative regarding the choice of vasodilator and newer inotropic agents for the management of patients with chronic left ventricular failure. Although the presence of ventricular gallop indicates elevated left ventricular diastolic pressure, the sensitivity of this abnormal physical finding is low. Similarly, the radiologic findings of pulmonary venous hypertension are frequently absent in patients with chronic left ventricular failure with markedly elevated pulmonary capillary wedge pressure (Fig. 7).[22] Although alveolar edema is highly specific for elevated pulmonary capillary wedge pressure ($\geq$25 mm Hg), it only occurs in approximately 30 percent of patients with markedly elevated pulmonary venous pressure. The sensitivity of other radiologic "fluid abnormalities"—such as venous redistribution, interstitial edema, and pleural effusion—for the diagnosis of elevated pulmonary capillary wedge pressure appears to be low in patients with chronic left ventricular failure. Thus, hemodynamic monitoring is frequently necessary to determine the level of pulmonary capillary wedge pressure in these patients.

PROGNOSTIC INDICES

Prognosis of patients with acute myocardial infarction can be determined from the hemodynamic indices. In a number of investigations, various hemodynamic indices have been used to evaluate the immediate prognosis of patients with acute myocardial infarction. If left ventricular filling pressure remains normal during the acute phase of myocardial infarction, the immediate prognosis is excellent, whereas the prognosis becomes progressively worse with worsening left ventricular function. Ratshin and coworkers[20] reported 100 percent mortality when the cardiac index was less than 2.3 liters per minute per m^2 and left ventricular filling pressure 20 mm Hg or more. Scheidt and associates[21] reported that the hospital mortality exceeds 70 percent when left ventricular stroke work index is 20 g $-$ m/m^2 or less. A fairly accurate assessment of prognosis can be made by relating left ventricular filling pressure and stroke work index in patients with acute myocardial infarction. The hospital mortality is low in patients with normal left ventricular filling pressure. It is approximately 26 percent when the left ventricular filling pressure is elevated but left ventricular stroke work index is more

Table 9. Relationship between hemodynamic findings and hospital mortality following acute myocardial infarction

Left Ventricular Stroke Work Index ($g - m/m^2$)	*Left Ventricular Filling Pressure (mm Hg)*	*Hospital Mortality (%)*
30–60	15 or less	5.8
21 or more	16 or less	26
20 or less	16 or more	80

than 20 $g - m/m^2$. Hospital mortality is close to 80 percent in patients with elevated left ventricular filling pressure and markedly decreased stroke work index (20 $g - m/m^2$ or less) (Table 9).[9]

COMPLICATIONS

Potential complications associated with the use of balloon flotation catheters are (1) cardiac arrhythmias, (2) balloon rupture, (3) catheter knotting, (4) thrombus formation, (5) pulmonary infarct, and (6) perforation of the pulmonary artery.

During insertion of the catheters, ventricular premature beats occur frequently; however, sustained ventricular tachycardia is rare. If it does occur, the catheter should be withdrawn. Once the tip of the catheter is in the pulmonary artery, ventricular arrhythmias are not observed even when the catheter is left in position for several days. In patients with preexisting left bundle branch block, manipulation of the catheter in the right ventricle can precipitate complete AV block from catheter-induced trauma to the right bundle branch. This complication is always transient, and normal AV conduction returns within a few hours in almost all patients. Although insertion of a temporary right ventricular pacing electrode prior to the placement of balloon catheter will prevent ventricular asystole, such a practice is rarely necessary if catheter manipulation in the right ventricle is avoided.

Balloon rupture may be encountered during prolonged hemodynamic monitoring. Balloon rupture is diagnosed by loss of resistance during deflation and inflation of the balloon; and occasionally blood leaks through the balloon lumen. With ruptured balloon, pulmonary artery occluded pressure cannot be obtained; however, pulmonary artery end-diastolic pressure can be used for left ventricular filling pressure. Ruptured balloon may contribute to thrombus formation around the tip of the catheter; therefore, a catheter with ruptured balloon should not be kept in situ for any length of time.

Thrombus formation around the catheter is frequent, but subsequent pulmonary embolism occurs only rarely. With the introduction of heparin-impregnated catheters, this complication has declined.

Pulmonary infarction owing to the migration of the catheter to the wedge position is a potential complication of prolonged hemodynamic monitoring (Fig. 8). There is a natural tendency of the balloon flotation catheters to migrate to the distal pulmonary artery branches. This position can be recognized if the pressure recorded resembles pulmonary capillary wedge or damped pulmonary artery pressures. In such circumstances, the catheter should be withdrawn until undamped pulmonary artery pressure is recorded.

Pulmonary arterial perforation, although rare, is a potentially fatal complication and tends to occur in patients with severe pulmonary hypertension. Such complications can be avoided if the balloon is kept inflated for a minimum period to minimize the stress on the wall of the pulmonary artery. The balloon should not be inflated with fluid. Rupture of the pulmonary artery branches can occur from overdistention during balloon inflation. This complication tends to occur when the catheter tip migrates to the small pulmonary artery branches. After initial passage of the catheter, balloon inflation should be done slowly and with a small volume

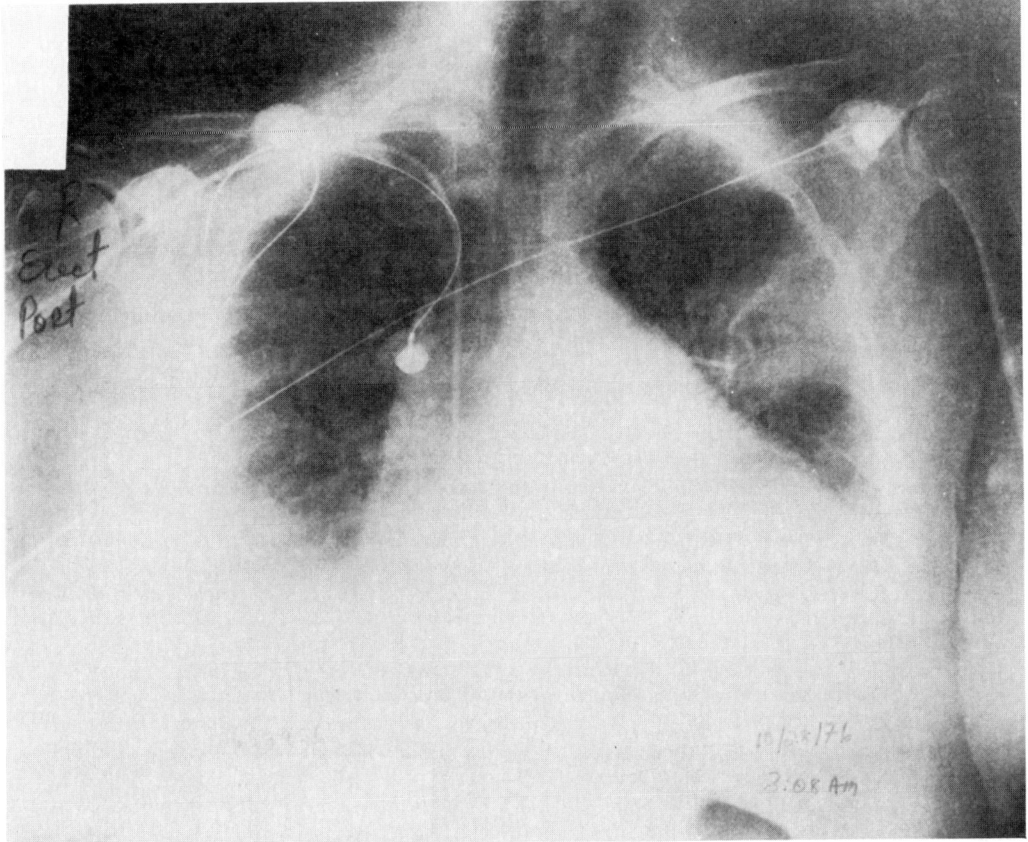

Figure 8. Pulmonary infarct during hemodynamic monitoring with a balloon flotation catheter. The tip of the catheter remained in the wedge position undetected for a prolonged period of time. (From Chatterjee, K,[8] with permission.)

of air. Small inflation volume (0.5 cc or less) to obtain pulmonary capillary wedge pressure suggests migration of the catheter tip to small pulmonary artery branches; in such circumstances, the catheter should be withdrawn to the central pulmonary artery branches.

Thrombophlebitis, infection, catheter knotting, and septicemia are uncommon complications. Repeated manipulations of the catheter and prolonged hemodynamic monitoring predispose to septicemia. Routine change of the catheter every fourth day and proper aseptic techniques during insertion and manipulation of the catheter prevent infection and sepsis.

SUMMARY

Bedside hemodynamic monitoring provides useful information regarding the differential diagnosis of the various pathologic mechanisms of low output syndrome. It also allows recognition of hemodynamic subsets of patients with acute myocardial infarction. Furthermore, hemodynamic monitoring is necessary for prompt evaluation of the response to therapeutic interventions in patients with low output syndrome. In patients with acute myocardial infarction, hemodynamic indices can also be used for evaluation of immediate prognosis. Because bedside hemodynamic monitoring is relatively safe, and with proper precautionary measures the potential complications can be avoided, hemodynamic monitoring should be considered in the management of all critically ill cardiac patients.

REFERENCES

1. Swan, HJC, Ganz, W, Forrester, J, et al: *Catheterization of the heart with use of a flow-directed balloon-tipped catheter.* N Engl J Med 283:447, 1970.
2. Forrester, JS, Ganz, W, Diamond, G, et al: *Thermodilution cardiac output determination with a single flow directed catheter.* Am Heart J 83:306, 1972.
3. Goldstein, JA, Vlahakes, GJ, Verrier, ED, et al: *The role of right ventricular systolic dysfunction and elevated intrapericardial pressure in the genesis of low output in experimental right ventricular infarction.* Circulation 65:513, 1982.
4. Butler, J, Culver, BH, Huseby, J, et al: *The hemodynamics of pulmonary edema.* Am Rev Resp Dis 25:173, 1977.
5. Rackley, CE, Russell, RO Jr, and Mantle, JS: *Clinical considerations of hemodynamic measurements and left ventricular function in myocardial infarction.* In Russell, RO and Rackley, CE (eds): *Hemodynamic Monitoring in a Coronary Intensive Care Unit.* Futura, Mt. Kisco, New York, 1974, p 173.
6. Sharpe, DN, Botvinick, EH, Shames, DM, et al: *The noninvasive diagnosis of right ventricular infarction.* Circulation 57:483, 1978.
7. Bethea, CF, Peter, RH, Behar, VS, et al: *The hemodynamic simulation of mitral regurgitation in ventricular septal defect after acute myocardial infarction.* Cath Cardiovasc Diag 2:97, 1976.
8. Chatterjee, K: *Bedside hemodynamic monitoring.* In Bolooki, H (ed): *Clinical Applications of Intra-Aortic Balloon Pump.* Futura, Mt Kisco, New York, 1977, pp 197–220.
9. Chatterjee, K and Swan, HJC: *Hemodynamic profile of acute myocardial infarction.* In Corday, E and Swan, HJC (eds): *Myocardial Infarction.* Williams & Wilkins, Baltimore, 1973, pp 51–61.
10. Swan, HJC, Chatterjee, K, and Ganz, W: *Hemodynamic measurements in the choice and evaluation of therapeutic interventions.* In Russek, HI (ed): *Cardiovascular Disease.* University Park Press, Baltimore, 1974, pp 133–141.
11. Parmley, WW and Chatterjee, K: *Evaluation of cardiac function in the coronary care unit.* In Donoso, E and Lipski, J (eds): *Acute Myocardial Infarction.* Stratton Intercontinental, New York, 1978, pp 86–98.
12. Chatterjee, K: *Acute heart failure.* In *Critical Care Manual.* Little, Brown & Co, Boston, 1976.
13. Crexells, C, Chatterjee, K, Forrester, JS, et al: *Optimal level of left-heart filling pressures in acute myocardial infarction.* N Engl J Med 290:1263, 1973.
14. Chatterjee, K and Parmley, WW: *The role of vasodilator therapy in heart failure.* Prog Cardiovasc Dis 19:301, 1977.
15. Chatterjee, K, Swan, HJC, Kaushik, VS, et al: *Effects of vasodilator therapy for severe pump failure in acute myocardial infarction on short term and late prognosis.* Circulation 53:797, 1976.
16. Massie, BM and Chatterjee, K: *Vasodilator therapy of pump failure complicating acute myocardial infarction.* Med Clin North Am 63:25, 1979.
17. Chatterjee, K: *Digitalis versus newer inotropic agents: Which to use.* Drug Therapy 12:83, 1982.
18. Chatterjee, K, Doyle, B, and Avakian, D: *Vasodilator therapy for heart failure.* In Pollack-Latham, C and Canobbio, MM (eds): *Current Concepts in Cardiac Care.* Aspen, Rockville, MD, 1982, pp 97–108.
19. Chatterjee, K, Parmley, WW, Swan, HJC, et al: *Beneficial effects of vasodilator agents in severe mitral regurgitation due to subvalvular apparatus.* Circulation 48:684, 1973.
20. Ratshin, RA, Rackley, CE, and Russell, RO Jr: *Hemodynamic evaluation of left ventricular function in shock complicating myocardial infarction.* Circulation 45:127, 1972.
21. Scheidt, S, Wilner, G, Fillmore, S, et al: *Objective hemodynamic assessment after acute myocardial infarction.* Br Heart J 35:908-916, 1973.
22. Dash, H, Lipton, MJ, Chatterjee, K, et al: *Estimation of pulmonary wedge pressure from chest radiograph in patients with chronic congestive cardiomyopathy and ischaemic cardiomyopathy.* Br Heart J 44:322, 1980.

Pericardiocentesis Using Echocardiography

Bruce C. Berger, M.D.

Pericardiocentesis is most often performed to relieve cardiac tamponade by removing fluid or for diagnostic purposes to obtain fluid for cytologic, bacteriologic, and chemical analyses. When performed to relieve cardiac tamponade, pericardiocentesis can be a life-saving procedure. Diagnostic pericardiocentesis may provide vital information and eliminate the need for an open surgical procedure.

However, pericardiocentesis is not without risk. Complications include arrhythmia, infection, ventricular puncture, hemopericardium and tamponade, vasovagal reactions causing hypotension, bradycardia or cardiac arrest, and, occasionally, death. Thus, it is obvious that pericardiocentesis must be done cautiously and should not be undertaken when the risk of complications is excessive.

Echocardiography has proven extremely valuable in the detection of pericardial fluid. Recently, several studies have demonstrated some echocardiographic findings useful in diagnosing cardiac tamponade.[1–3] The development of two-dimensional echocardiography has improved the quantitative assessment and localization of pericardial fluid. Other investigators have successfully used echocardiography to reduce the risk of planned pericardiocentesis as well as to monitor the actual procedure.[4–6]

EVALUATION BEFORE PERICARDIOCENTESIS

Echocardiography has significantly reduced the risk of diagnostic pericardiocentesis by improving the selection of patients. Its role in the diagnosis of pericardial effusion has been established.[7–9] Although the accuracy of the diagnosis is generally excellent, false-positive diagnoses can be caused by tumors,[10] mitral annular calcification,[11] pleural effusions, and the descending thoracic aorta.[12] Two-dimensional echocardiography has further improved the accuracy of the diagnosis of pericardial effusion and provides additional information on the amount and location of the fluid present.[4,12]

Wong and colleagues[5] evaluated the risk of pericardiocentesis in a series of 52 procedures performed between 1972 and 1978. Fifteen procedures were nonproductive (no fluid aspirated), and there were eight complications. All complications occurred in the course of nonproductive procedures. Surgical or postmortem followup demonstrated no pericardial effusion in 11 of the nonproductive procedures. Additionally, the incidence of complications in the last three years of the study (25 percent) was significantly lower than in the first three years (48 percent), which coincided with the increased use of echocardiography in the evaluation of patients before pericardiocentesis.

In another study,[6] fluid was obtained from more than 90 percent of patients in whom echocardiography showed pericardial effusion considered large and/or located both anteriorly and

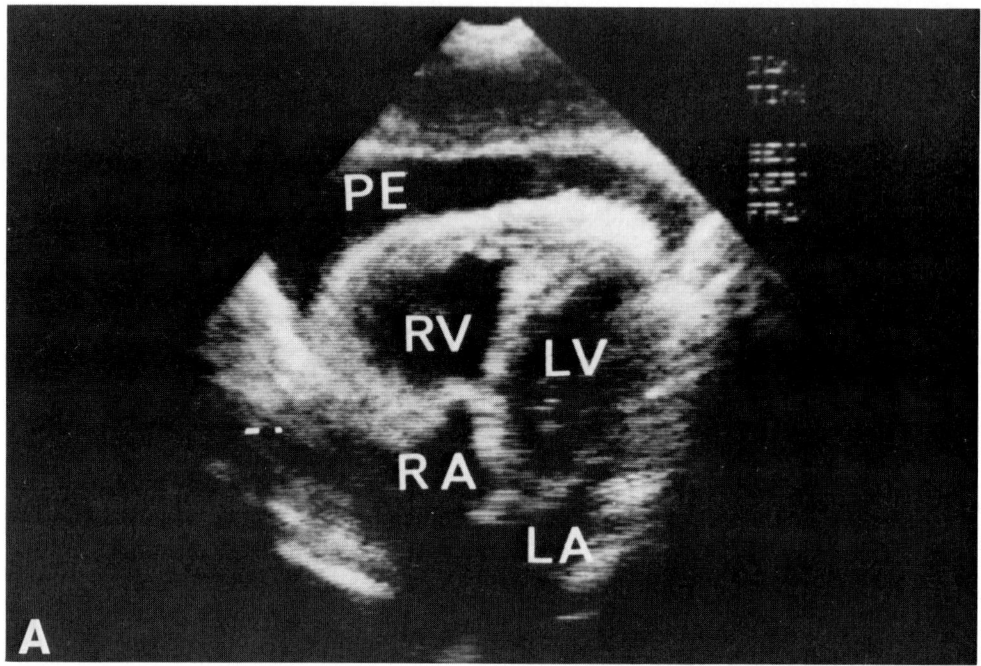

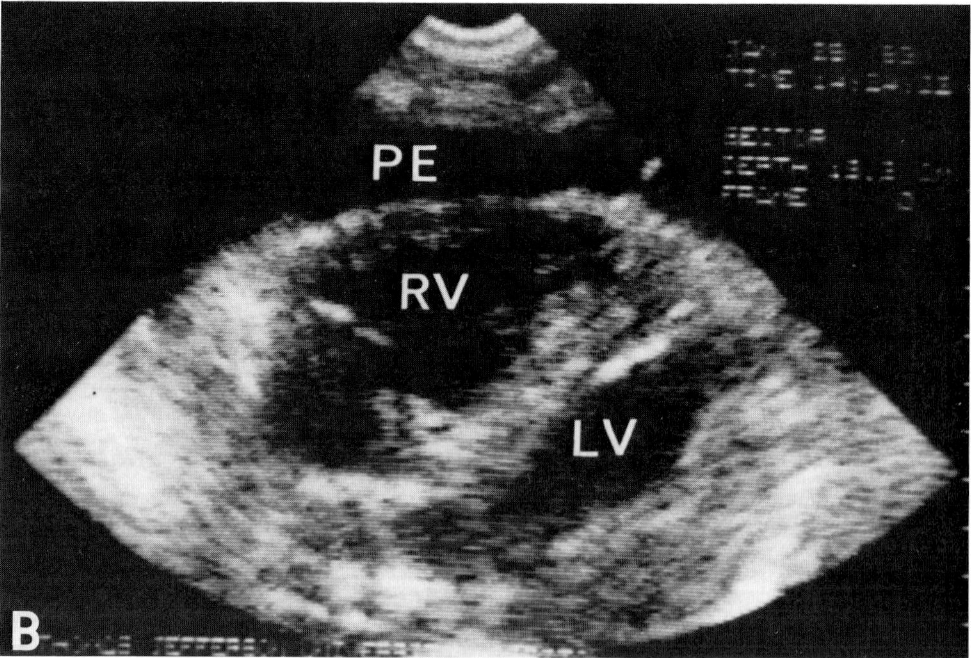

Figure 1. *A*, *B*, These are stop frame two-dimensional echocardiographic images from two patients obtained before pericardiocentesis using the subxiphoid approach. Long axis views show an anterior pericardial effusion. LA = left atrium; LV = left ventricle; PE = pericardial effusion; RA = right atrium; RV = right ventricle.

posteriorly. Pericardial tap was successful in only 50 percent of the cases when the echo showed only a small anterior effusion or only posterior fluid.

Although M-mode echocardiography is very useful in the evaluation of pericardial effusion, Martin and colleagues[4] showed that M-mode studies may overestimate the amount of fluid present when the effusion is small. Two-dimensional echocardiography was better able to quantify the amount of fluid present. Additionally, they were able to demonstrate the postural redistribution of pericardial fluid to the apical areas when the patient assumed the sitting position. This finding proved useful in excluding loculation of fluid. The authors postulated that this shift could explain the improved yield of pericardiocentesis in the sitting position.

For these reasons, all patients in whom pericardiocentesis is planned should have an echocardiogram performed prior to the procedure. Ideally, both M-mode and two-dimensional echocardiography should be done to evaluate quantity and location of fluid better. Because most pericardiocenteses are performed via the subxiphoid route in a semirecumbent position, we have found it quite useful to perform subxiphoid two-dimensional echocardiography in this position to document the presence of anterior fluid. When fluid is demonstrated in this view, the tap is usually productive and technically less difficult. Figure 1 shows subxiphoid two-dimensional echocardiograms from two patients obtained prior to diagnostic pericardiocentesis. In both patients, a large anterior effusion was present, and subxiphoid pericardiocentesis was uncomplicated.

PERICARDIAL TAMPONADE

Although echocardiography is extremely sensitive and can detect as little as 15 ml of pericardial fluid,[13] it is very difficult to determine the hemodynamic significance of a pericardial effusion by echocardiography. Cardiac tamponade has remained a clinical diagnosis that is confirmed by hemodynamic monitoring.[14] Many M-mode echocardiographic abnormalities have been reported in cardiac tamponade. These alterations include right ventricular compression,[15] respiratory variation in ventricular size,[16] and abnormalities of mitral valve motion.[16,17] However, these findings are not specific for cardiac tamponade or may require serial studies to be useful.[15,18–20]

Recently, a new echocardiographic sign has been found to be more sensitive and more specific for the diagnosis of cardiac tamponade. Several studies[1–3] have demonstrated an abnormal posterior motion of the right ventricular free wall in diastole. Shiina and coworkers[1] noted posterior right ventricular wall motion in early and mid-diastole, with anterior motion only in late diastole in patients with "impending tamponade." Armstrong and colleagues[2] found this sign in 14 of 17 patients with cardiac tamponade. Wall motion reverted to normal after pericardiocentesis in all cases. Only 7 of 69 patients without tamponade had abnormal right ventricular wall motion. Using two-dimensional echocardiography, they demonstrated that the abnormal right ventricular wall motion represented collapse of the right ventricular cavity in early diastole.

Engel and associates[3] demonstrated posterior motion of the right ventricular endocardium at 0.05 second or longer after opening of the mitral valve in 17 of 21 patients with cardiac tamponade. This finding was absent in 16 of 17 patients with large pericardial effusions without tamponade.

Figure 2 shows an M-mode echocardiogram that illustrates the abnormal posterior motion of the right ventricle in early diastole (point B), with anterior motion occurring only late in diastole (point C) in a patient with cardiac tamponade. Figure 3 illustrates the same patient's two-dimensional study and demonstrates diastolic collapse of the right ventricular free wall at the level of the outflow tract.

Thus, it appears that these new echocardiographic findings are relatively sensitive and specific for cardiac tamponade, or impending tamponade. Their absence suggests that an effusion is not compromising cardiac function. Serial studies may allow detection of tamponade physiology before acute hemodynamic compromise occurs.

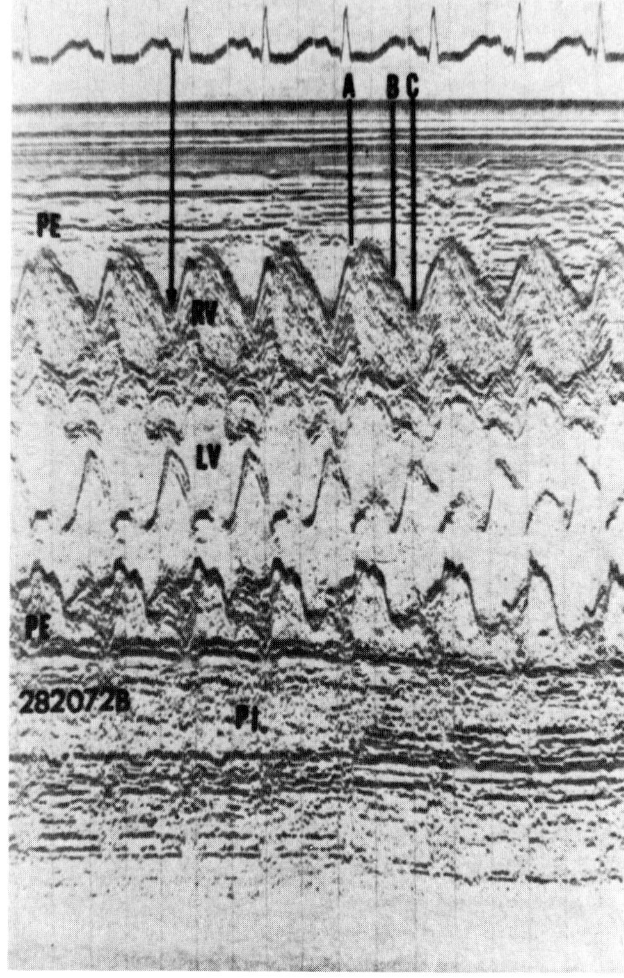

Figure 2. This is an M-mode echocardiogram demonstrating abnormal motion of the right ventricular wall in a patient with a malignant pericardial effusion and clinical evidence of cardiac tamponade. Point A represents end-diastole, point B end-systole, and point C the abnormal posterior motion of the right ventricle wall in early diastole. Anterior motion *(arrow)* occurs after atrial systole. Pl = pleural effusion; other abbreviations as in Figure 1. (From Armstrong, WF, et al,[2] with permission of the American Heart Association, Inc.)

When cardiac tamponade is suspected, and if the patient's clinical situation is not extreme, echocardiography should be performed to document the presence of pericardial fluid. If a significant effusion is present and the echo findings noted above are present, pericardiocentesis should be performed. A pulmonary artery catheter may be placed (if the situation permits) for hemodynamic monitoring to confirm the diagnosis as well as to document the drop in pressure with drainage of fluid. When the echocardiographic findings are equivocal, or if a diagnostic study cannot be obtained, hemodynamic monitoring should be used to make the diagnosis of tamponade and to monitor the pericardiocentesis.

ECHOCARDIOGRAPHY DURING PERICARDIOCENTESIS

In addition to improving the sensitivity and specificity of the diagnosis of pericardial effusion and tamponade before pericardiocentesis, echocardiography can be useful when performed during pericardiocentesis.

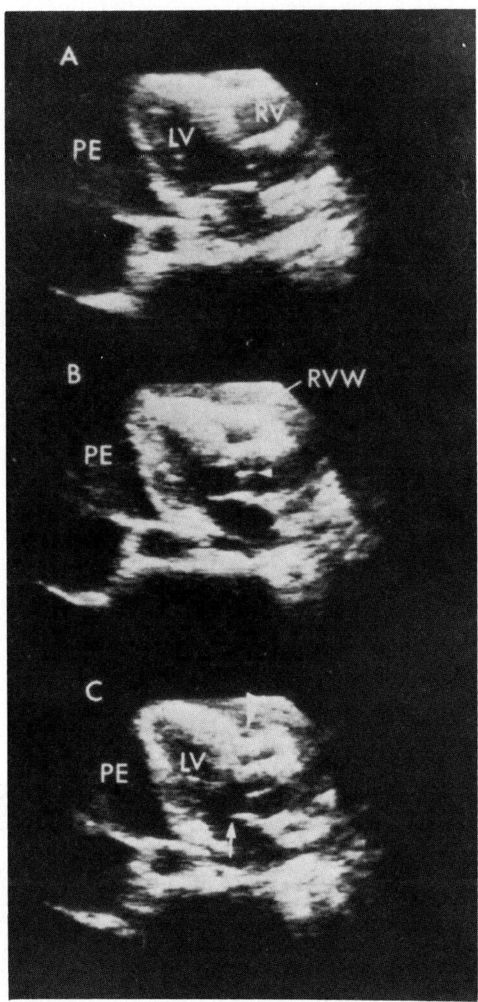

Figure 3. This is a parasternal long-axis, two-dimensional echocardiographic study from the same patient as in Figure 2. Frames *A, B,* and *C* correspond to the timing of points A, B and C in Figure 2. *A,* In end-diastole, both the right and left ventricles have a normal diastolic configuration, and both the aortic and mitral valves are closed. *B,* In end-systole, the aortic valve has just closed *(small arrowhead),* and all chambers have a normal systolic configuration. *C,* In early diastole, the mitral valve has just opened *(white arrow),* and a collapse of the right ventricle has occurred *(large arrowhead).* RVW = right ventricular wall; other abbreviations as in Figure 1. (From Armstrong, WF, et al,[2] with permission of the American Heart Association, Inc.)

Most pericardiocenteses are now performed using the subxiphoid approach[21] and using electrocardiographic monitoring.[22] Using the apical two-dimensional echo window, simultaneous echocardiography may allow one to visualize the size and location of the pericardial effusion during pericardiocentesis and to assist in assessing the amount of fluid remaining as the procedure progresses.[4] Figure 4 shows serial stop frame two-dimensional echocardiographic images obtained in the apical four-chamber view during a subxiphoid pericardiocentesis. The pericardial effusion became progressively smaller during the procedure, which was terminated when ventricular ectopy developed and no effusion could be demonstrated at the apex.

At times, the pericardiocentesis needle may also be visualized by echocardiography.[4] Recently, using a new needle guide that attaches to the transducer head of a mechanical sector scanner, we have performed simultaneous subxiphoid pericardiocentesis and echocardiography. We have been able to guide the insertion of the pericardiocentesis needle and to visualize the needle in the anterior pericardial space. However, this method has been useful only in relatively thin individuals with large effusions, inasmuch as mobility of the needle is limited by the transducer and because the needle guide decreases the length of needle available for insertion. This method should not be used to determine exact needle position or proximity to the myocardium, because the needle tip is not always well visualized. We have noted

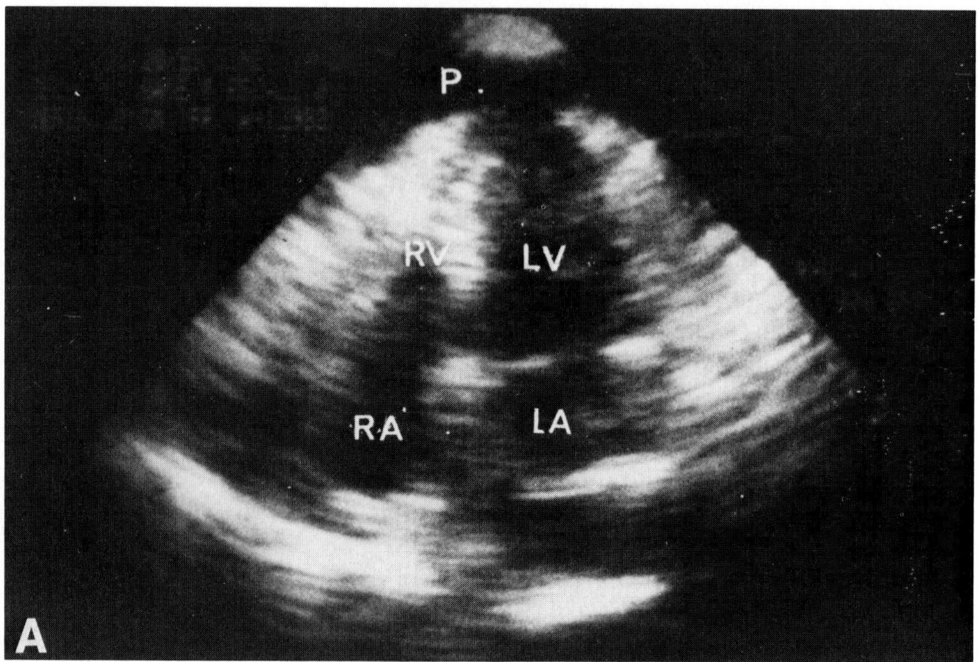

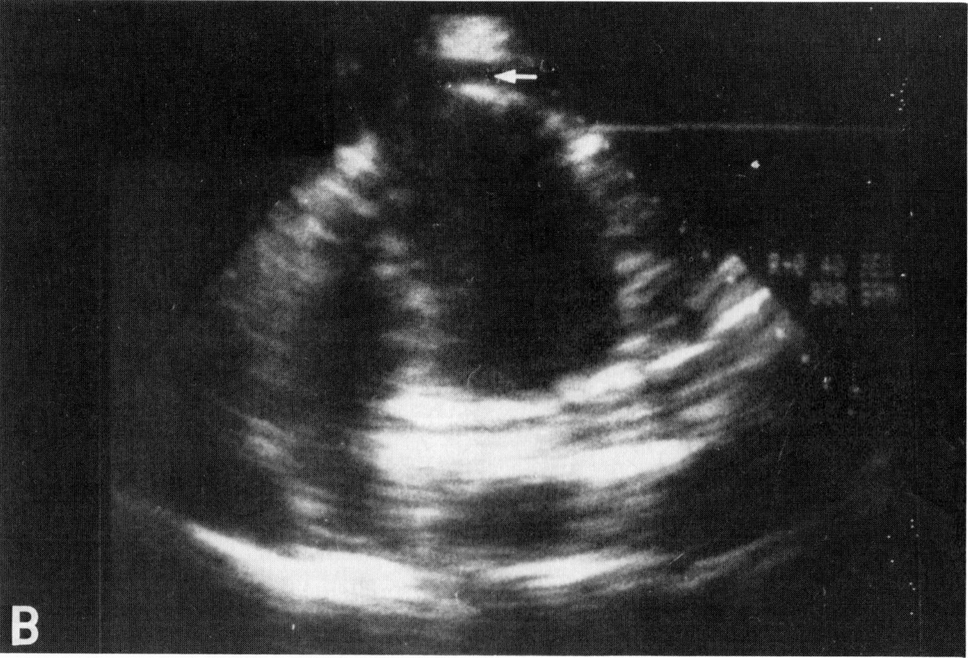

Figure 4. These are serial apical 4-chamber views obtained during subxiphoid pericardiocentesis. The apical pericardial effusion noted in *A* becomes smaller in *B (white arrow)* and is absent in *C (white arrow)* when the procedure was terminated. Abbreviations are the same as in Figure 1.

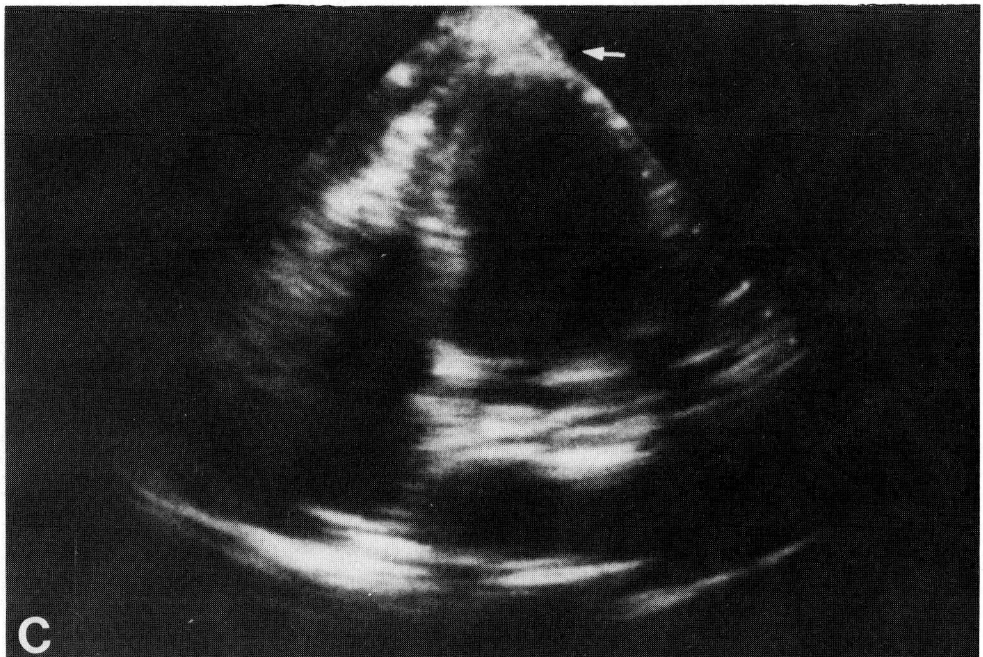

Figure 4. *Continued.*

ST segment elevation indicative of epicardial contact during electrocardiographic monitoring, even though the needle did not appear to be touching the myocardium on echocardiography. Figure 5 is an example of simultaneous subxiphoid two-dimensional echocardiography and pericardiocentesis obtained using a transducer and needle guide. Figure 5A shows the transducer and pericardiocentesis needle in the needle guide. Figure 5B demonstrates the anterior pericardial effusion. In Figure 5C, the white arrow points to the bright echo produced by the needle in the pericardial space. Obviously it is quite difficult to localize the position of the needle tip.

Occasionally, penetration into the right ventricular cavity during pericardiocentesis may occur without electrocardiographic changes. The differentiation between hemopericardium and intracardiac blood may be difficult. Determining the hematocrit of the aspirate is not always helpful and takes time. Waiting to see if the aspirate clots also takes time, particularly if anticoagulants are present. Chandraratna and coworkers[23] were able to determine the location of the tip of the pericardiocentesis needle by performing contrast echocardiography. Saline was flushed through the pericardiocentesis needle while recording the echocardiogram. A cloud of contrast echoes in the pericardial space indicated that the bloody aspirate was pericardial fluid. Contrast echoes in the right ventricle indicated intraventricular needle position. Figure 6 illustrates the cloud of echoes in the pericardial space seen when saline was flushed through the pericardiocentesis needle.

We have also found this technique useful when it becomes difficult to aspirate fluid during pericardiocentesis, or when ventricular ectopy occurs. We perform apical two-dimensional echocardiography in the four-chamber view during the procedure and inject saline when the needle position is in question. Although we do not always see the contrast in the pericardial space, the absence of right ventricular cavity echoes usually rules out an intracavitary needle position.

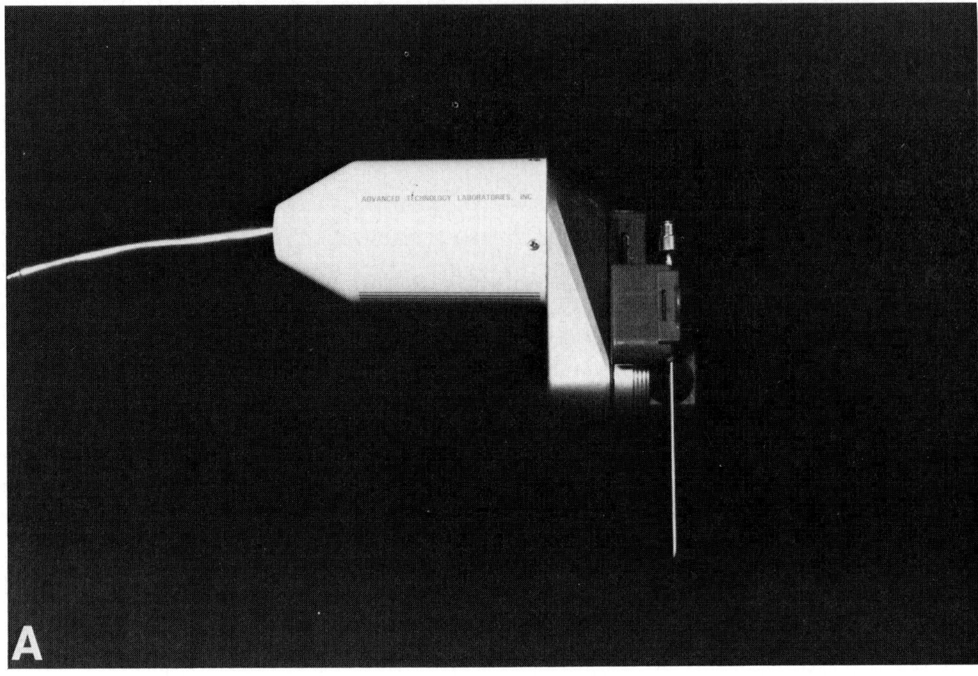

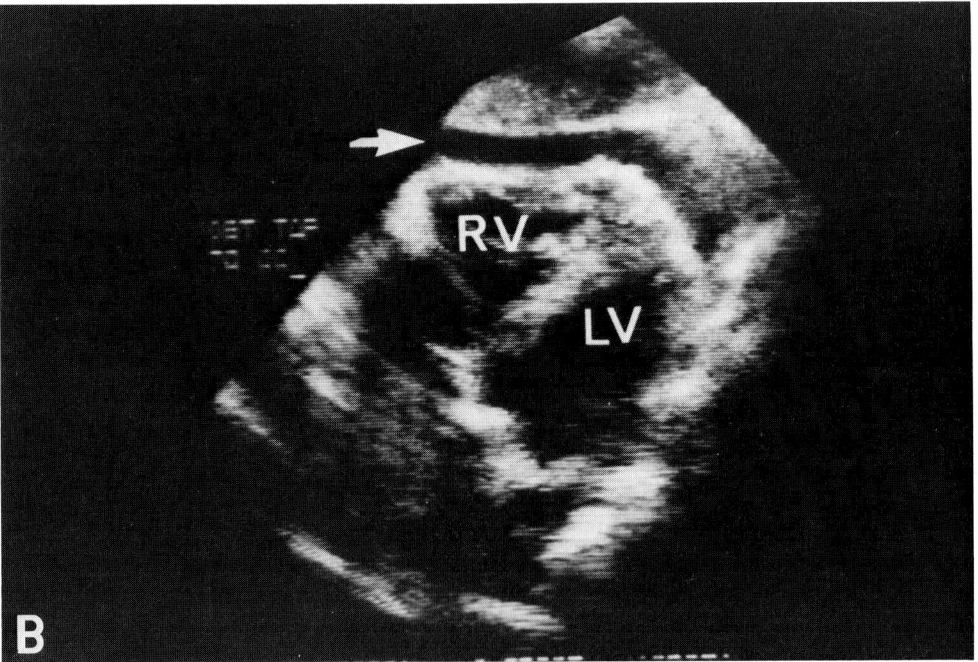

Figure 5. *A*, This is a two-dimensional echocardiography transducer with pericardiocentesis needle in needle guide. *B*, This subxiphoid long-axis view demonstrates the anterior pericardial effusion *(white arrow)*.

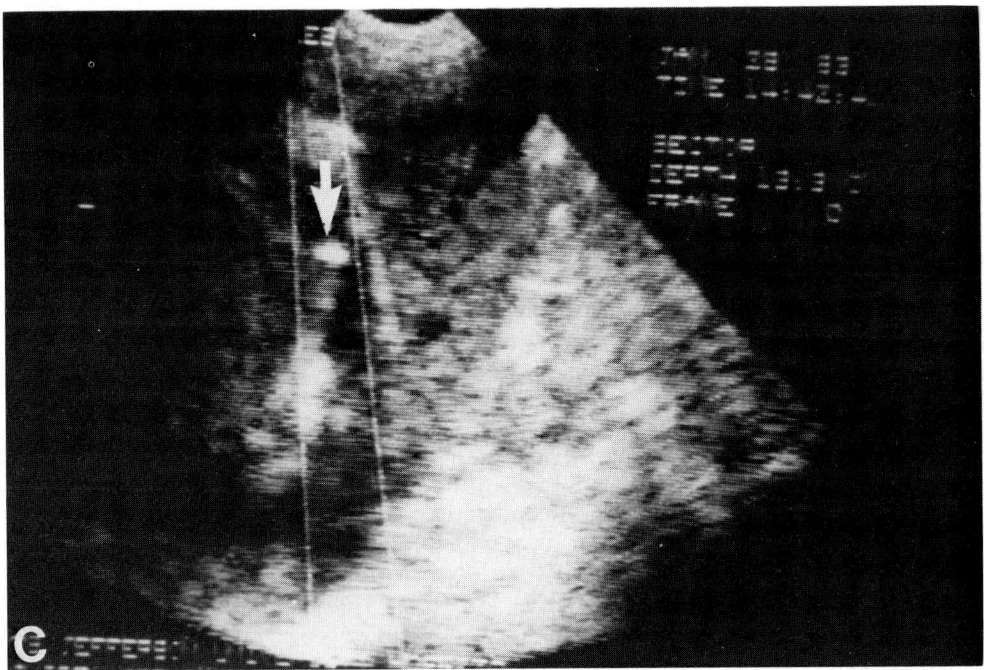

Figure 5. *Continued. C,* White arrow points to the bright echo produced by the needle in the pericardial space.

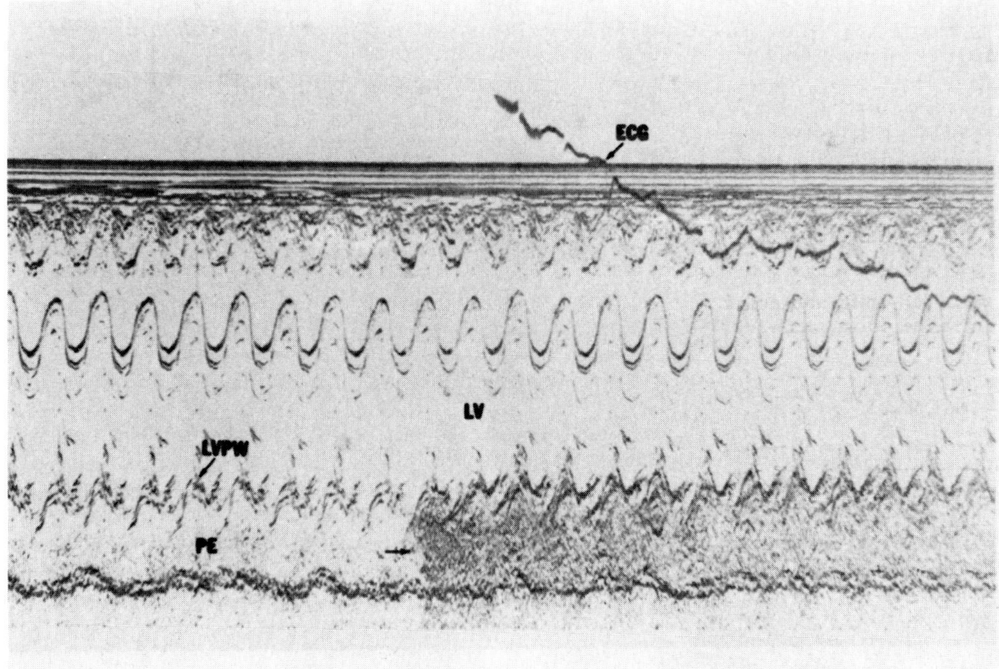

Figure 6. This echocardiogram was performed during pericardiocentesis, with saline injection through the pericardiocentesis needle. Dense echoes *(horizontal arrow)* are seen in the pericardial space. ECG = electrocardiogram; LVPW = left ventricular posterior wall; other abbreviations as in Figure 1. (From Chandraratna, PAN, et al,[23] with permission.)

SUMMARY

Echocardiography is the procedure of choice for the detection and localization of pericardial effusion. It should be performed in all patients prior to elective pericardiocentesis to confirm the diagnosis and to determine the size and location of the effusion in order to minimize the risk and to maximize the yield of pericardiocentesis.

When pericardial tamponade is suspected, echocardiography should be performed, time permitting, to document the presence of effusion, because other clinical entities, such as right ventricular failure, may mimic tamponade. Additionally, the finding of diastolic posterior motion of the right ventricular wall, or "diastolic collapse" of the right ventricle, is further evidence for the presence of tamponade and, at times, may eliminate the need for invasive hemodynamic diagnosis.

Echocardiography is also useful when performed during pericardiocentesis, to evaluate the size and location of the effusion as the procedure progresses. Contrast echocardiography can determine the position of the pericardiocentesis needle quickly and safely.

Thus the appropriate use of echocardiography has increased the safety and improved the yield of diagnostic and therapeutic pericardiocentesis.

ACKNOWLEDGMENT

I wish to express my appreciation to Karen Goldsmith for typing the manuscript.

REFERENCES

1. Shiina, A, Yaginuma, T, Kordo, K, et al: *Echocardiographic evaluation of impending tamponade.* J Cardiography 9:555, 1979.
2. Armstrong, WF, Schilt, BF, Helper, DJ, et al: *Diastolic collapse of the right ventricle with cardiac tamponade: An echocardiographic study.* Circulation 65:1491, 1982.
3. Engel, PJ, Hon, H, Fowler, NO, et al: *Echocardiographic study of right ventricular wall motion in cardiac tamponade.* Am J Cardiol 50:1018, 1982.
4. Martin, RP, Rakowski, H, French, J, et al: *Localization of pericardial effusion with wide angle phased array echocardiography.* Am J Cardiol 42:904, 1978.
5. Wong, B, Murphy, J, Chang, CJ, et al: *The risk of pericardiocentesis.* Am J Cardiol 44:1110, 1979.
6. Krikorian, JG and Hancock, EW: *Pericardiocentesis.* Am J Med 65:808, 1978.
7. Feigenbaum, H, Waldhausen, JA, and Hyde, LP: *Ultrasound diagnosis of pericardial effusion.* JAMA 191:711, 1965.
8. Feigenbaum, H, Zaky, A, and Waldhausen, JA: *Use of ultrasound in the diagnosis of pericardial effusion.* Ann Intern Med 65:443, 1966.
9. Feigenbaum, H: *Echocardiographic diagnosis of pericardial effusion.* Am J Cardiol 26:475, 1970.
10. Come, PC, Riley, MF, and Fortuin, NJ: *Echocardiographic mimicry of pericardial effusion.* Am J Cardiol 47:365, 1981.
11. D'Cruz, IA, Cohen, HA, Prabhu, R, et al: *Clinical manifestations of mitral annulus calcification, with emphasis on its echocardiographic features.* Am Heart J 94:367, 1977.
12. Haaz, WS, Mintz, GS, Kotler, MN, et al: *Two-dimensional echocardiographic recognition of the descending thoracic aorta: Value in differentiating pericardial from pleural effusions.* Am J Cardiol 46:739, 1980.
13. Horowitz, MS, Schultz, CS, Stinson, EB, et al: *Sensitivity and specificity of echocardiographic diagnosis of pericardial effusion.* Circulation 50:239, 1974.
14. Shabetai, R, Fowler, NO, and Guntheroth, WG: *Hemodynamics of cardiac tamponade and constrictive pericarditis.* Am J Cardiol 26:480, 1970.
15. Shiller, NB and Botvinick, EH: *Right ventricular compression as a sign of cardiac tamponade. An analysis of echocardiographic ventricular dimensions and their implications.* Circulation 56:774, 1977.
16. Settle, HP, Adolph, RJ, Fowler, NO, et al: *Echocardiographic study of cardiac tamponade.* Circulation 56:951, 1977.

17. D'Cruz, IA, Cohen, HC, Prabhu, R, et al: *Diagnosis of cardiac tamponade by echocardiography. Changes in mitral valve motion and ventricular dimensions with special reference to paradoxical pulse.* Circulation 52:460, 1975.

18. Martins, JB and Kerber, RE: *Can cardiac tamponade be diagnosed by echocardiography: Experimental studies.* Circulation 60:737, 1979.

19. Winer, H, Kronzon, I, and Glassman, E: *Echocardiographic findings in severe paradoxical pulse due to pulmonary embolization.* Am J Cardiol 40:808, 1977.

20. Brenner, JI and Waugh, RA: *Effect of phasic respiration on left ventricular dimension and performance in a normal population. An echocardiographic study.* Circulation 57:122, 1978.

21. Santos, GH and Frater, RWM: *The subxiphoid approach in the treatment of pericardial effusion.* Ann Thorac Surg 23:467, 1977.

22. Bishop, LH, Estes, EH Jr, and McIntosh, HD: *The electrocardiogram as a safeguard in pericardiocentesis.* JAMA 162:264, 1956.

23. Chandraratna, PAN, First, J, Langeven, E, et al: *Echocardiographic contrast studies during pericardiocentesis.* Ann Intern Med 87:199, 1977.

Percutaneous Intra-aortic Balloon Counterpulsation

Victoria M. Kusiak, M.D., and Sheldon Goldberg, M.D.

Supportive treatment for left ventricular power failure has undergone important changes over the past 20 years. Initially, medical therapy was employed using coronary vasodilatory drugs to improve myocardial oxygen supply, digitalis to improve left ventricular contractility, and vasoactive drugs to alter peripheral resistance and thereby to aid the failing ventricle.

Since 1961, with the development of counterpulsation[1] and its adaptation by Moulopaulus and colleagues[2] to include intra-aortic balloon pumping, a potent new therapy has been made available for the treatment of left ventricular power failure. From its first clinical use in 1968 by Kantrowitz and coworkers[3] in cardiogenic shock, to its use in 1973 by Buckley and colleagues[4] in patients unable to be weaned from cardiopulmonary bypass, to its fascinating application by Leinbach and associates[5] to preserve myocardium in anterior infarction, the intra-aortic balloon pump has proven its efficacy in supporting the left ventricle in a variety of clinical situations.

In 1979 the intra-aortic balloon pump was adapted for percutaneous insertion by Bregman and Casarella.[6] This meant that the balloon could be placed quickly, safely, and efficaciously in a large number of patients without vascular surgery. Since the initial experiences, more than 50,000 intra-aortic balloon devices have been inserted percutaneously, and the balloon has become an important adjunct to the treatment of ischemic heart disease and to the support of the failing left ventricle.

INTRA-AORTIC BALLOON COUNTERPULSATION: A REVIEW OF PHYSIOLOGIC PRINCIPLES

The principles of counterpulsation include augmentation of coronary perfusion pressure (arterial diastolic pressure) and reduction in the impedance to left ventricular ejection, and thus a reduction in heart work. The application of these two basic principles allows for a decrease in myocardial oxygen demand and a concomitant increase in myocardial oxygen supply, thereby creating the most favorable circumstances for amelioration of ischemic myocardium.

The intra-aortic balloon is a 40 to 50 ml polyurethane balloon attached to a central core, which is in turn connected to an external console that contains triggering circuitry and a driving gas mechanism (Fig. 1). The intra-aortic balloon can be positioned surgically in the descending thoracic aorta through a Dacron graft anastomosed end-to-side to the femoral artery, or it can be inserted percutaneously through a sheath placed in the femoral artery by the modified Seldinger technique (Fig. 2).

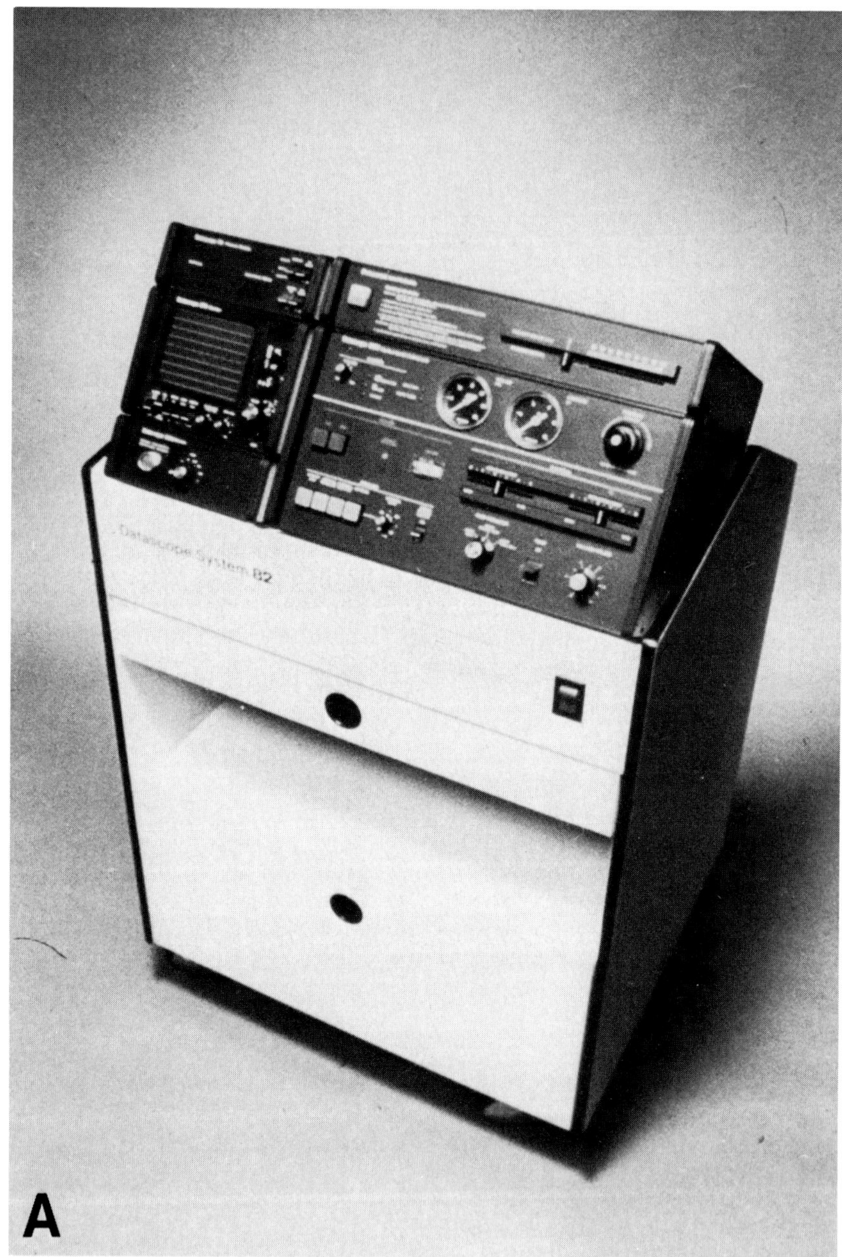

Figure 1. *A*, This is an intra-aortic balloon console.

Balloon inflation is timed to begin at aortic valve closure and end just prior to aortic valve opening, thus increasing coronary artery perfusion pressure during diastole (inflation) and decreasing afterload (left ventricular impedance) during systole (deflation) (Fig. 3).

The augmentation in coronary artery perfusion pressure that occurs with the intra-aortic balloon depends upon the magnitude and duration of augmentation of the mean aortic root diastolic pressure, which in turn depends on several physical variables of the balloon, its place-

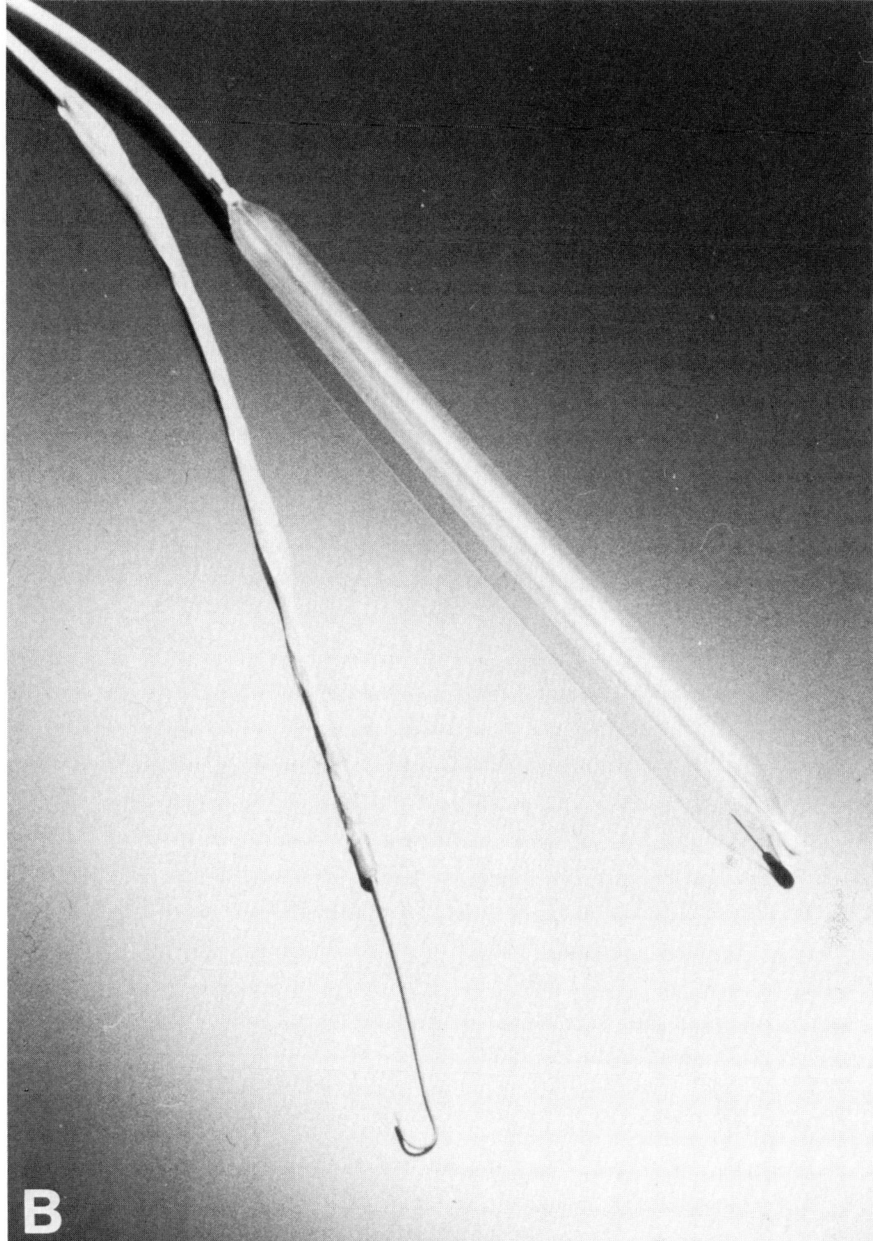

Figure 1. *Continued. B,* Intra-aortic balloon catheter is shown inflated *(right)* and wrapped for insertion with guide wire technique *(left).*

ment, and timing[7] (Table 1). Likewise, the decrease in impedance to left ventricular ejection is dependent upon the same variables. The amount of blood displaced by the intra-aortic balloon into the peripheral circulation during inflation will reduce aortic end-diastolic volume and decrease the impedance to ejection during the following contraction. The ventricle is thus unloaded, ventricular work is decreased, and myocardial oxygen consumption ($M\dot{V}O_2$) is reduced.

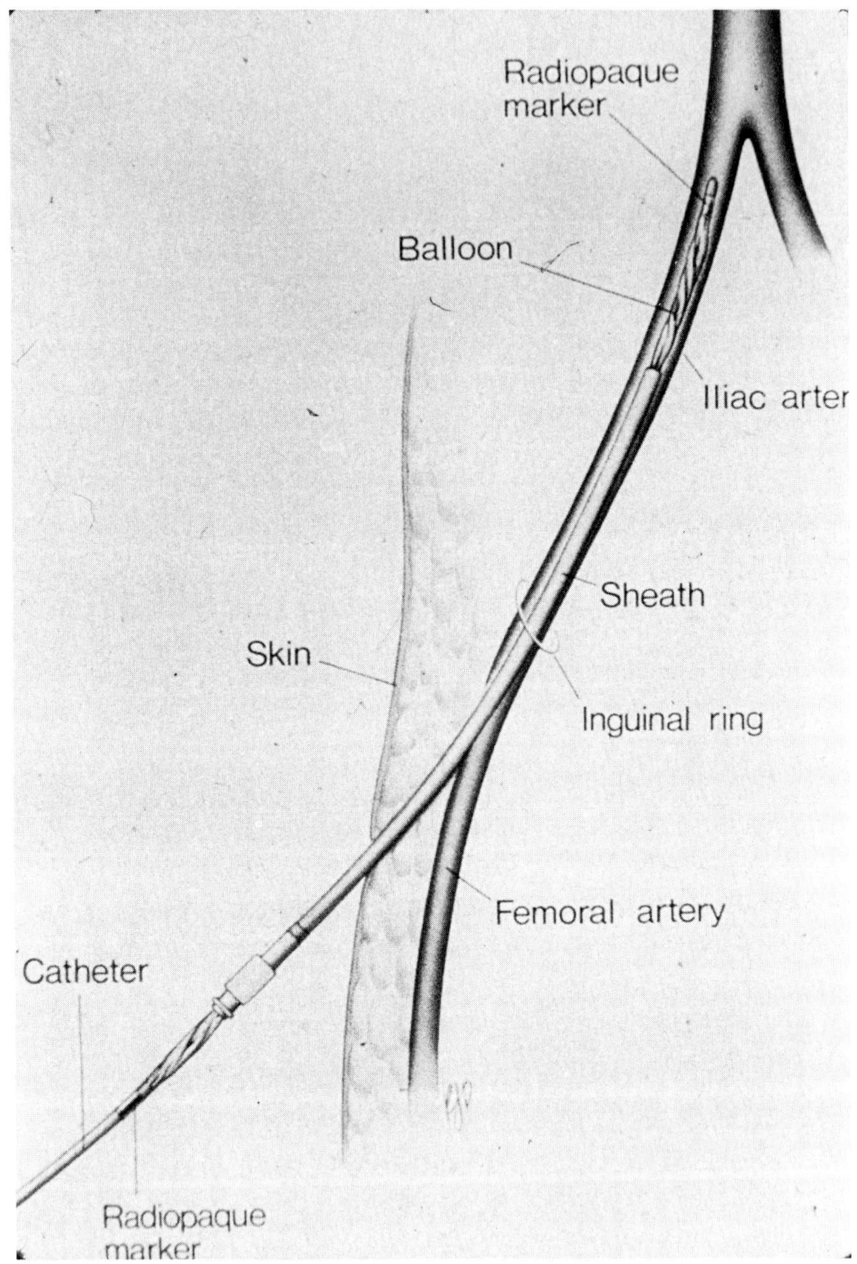

Figure 2. This is a schematic drawing of the technique of percutaneous intra-aortic balloon insertion through sheath.

Correct placement and precise timing of the intra-aortic balloon are necessary to maintain the desirable relationship between myocardial oxygen supply and demand. Improper timing may result in increased ventricular impedance and increased myocardial work (Fig. 4).

Whereas intra-aortic balloon pumping has been shown to improve hemodynamics,[8,9] to enhance impaired contractility,[10] and to increase myocardial perfusion,[11–14] studies of

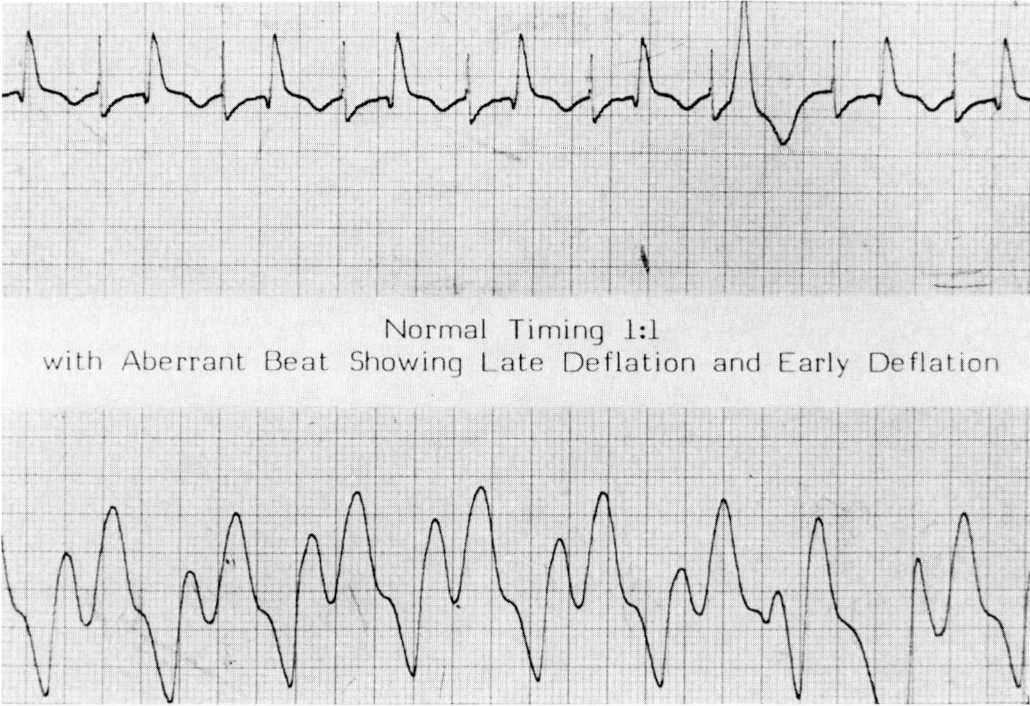

Figure 3. ECG *(top)* and arterial pressure trace *(bottom)* showing proper timing of inflation and deflation, resulting in augmentation of coronary perfusion pressure and systolic unloading.

Table 1. Variables influencing IAB counterpulsation*

	Variables	
Purpose of Counterpulsation	*Physical (IAB)*	*Biological*
Diastolic pressure augmentation	Position Volume Diameter Occlusivity Configuration Driving gas Timing	Arterial pressure Heart rate Aortic pressure-volume relation
Impedance and work reduction	Volume Occlusivity Inflation duration	Arterial pressure Heart rate Aortic pressure-volume relation Afterload reduction Preload reduction Augmented shortening

*From Weber, KT, and Janicki, JS,[7] with permission.

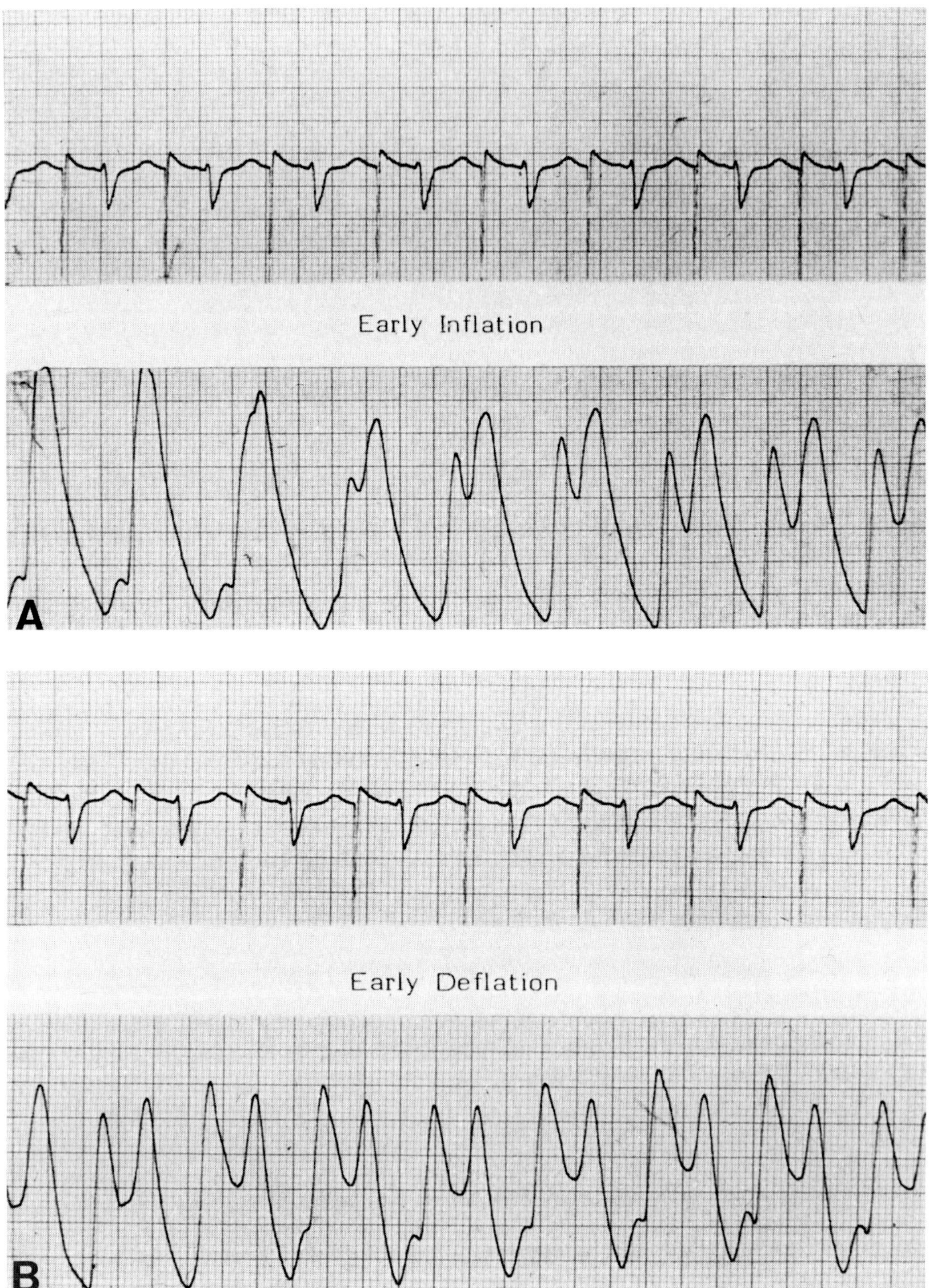

Figure 4. *A*, Improper timing with inflation occurring while aortic valve is open (note relation to dicrotic notch). *B*, Improper timing; deflation is occurring too early.

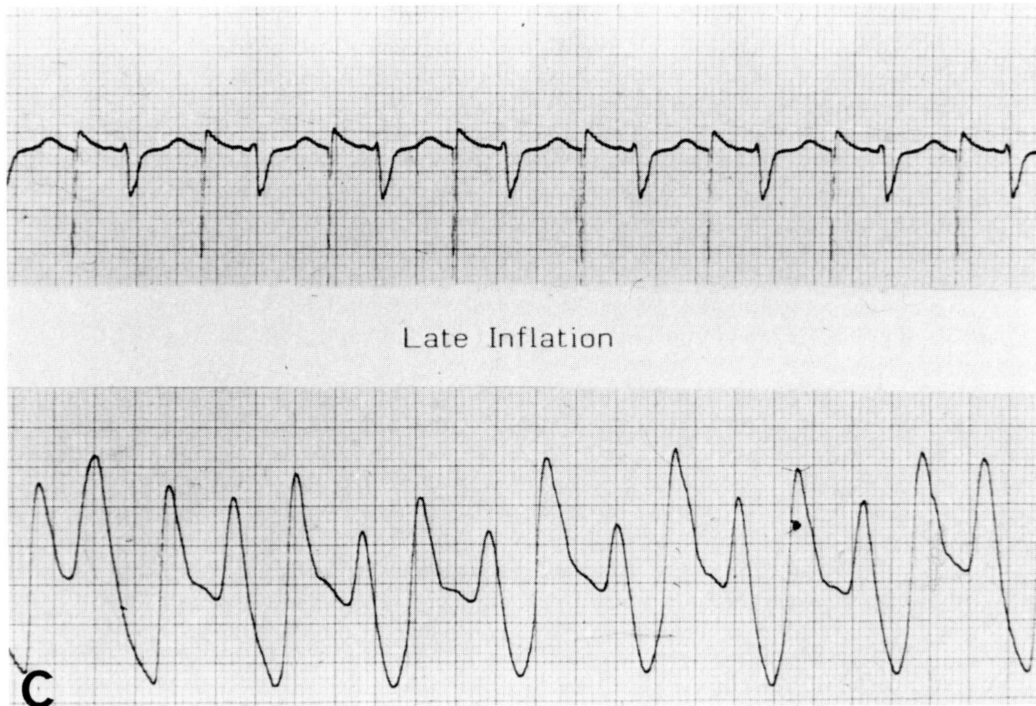

Figure 4. *Continued. C,* Improper timing, late inflation; note augmentation far too late after dicrotic notch.

changes in myocardial blood flow have been inconclusive. In several reports,[11,15] no change in perfusion of ischemic areas was observed with intra-aortic balloon pumping instituted within 1 hour of experimental coronary artery ligation, whereas other studies[12–14] have shown an increase in perfusion of the ischemic region.

The effect of the intra-aortic balloon on coronary blood flow and perfusion of ischemic myocardium depends in part on the baseline hemodynamic status of the patient. Mueller and coworkers[16] studied 12 patients in profound cardiogenic shock secondary to acute myocardial infarction. All patients had severe hypotension (systolic blood pressure less than 80 mm Hg), decreased mental status, decreased urine output (less than 25 ml per hour), and electrocardiographic evidence of acute myocardial infarction. All 12 patients were studied with and without intra-aortic balloon pump support, after having been stabilized with intubation, vasoactive agents, and volume correction to a pulmonary capillary wedge pressure of 10 to 14 mm Hg. Vasoactive agents were discontinued for 20 minutes prior to measurement of hemodynamic and metabolic parameters. Arterial and central venous pressures, arterial pH, and oxygen and carbon dioxide tensions were monitored and measurements made in steady state. Cardiac output, coronary blood flow, and samples of arterial and coronary sinus blood were obtained while recordings of arterial and central venous pressures and heart rate were made. These measurements were made in the baseline state, and after 4 to 6 hours of intra-aortic balloon counterpulsation. After 4 to 6 hours of continuous intra-aortic balloon pumping, 10 patients demonstrated a fall in peak systolic pressure from an average of 79 to 60 mm Hg, and diastolic and mean arterial pressures rose from 52 and 58 to 103 and 72 mm Hg during intra-aortic counterpulsation. Heart rate decreased from an average of 104 to 90 beats per minute, and stroke index rose from 13 to 20 ml per minute per m^2. Cardiac index increased from 1.22 to 1.69 liters per minute per m^2. Mean left ventricular outflow resistance decreased in all patients. Increases in systolic ejection rate and decreases in time-tension index per minute were statistically significant. Arterial lactate content decreased from a mean of 5.08 to 2.98 mmoles per liter, and urine output increased from 18 to 60 ml per hour. Coronary blood flow increased in all patients from a mean of 68 to 91 ml per 100 g per minute, and myocardial oxygen extraction decreased from 79 to 61 percent, whereas coronary sinus oxygen tension increased from 20 to 26 mm Hg. Myocardial oxygen consumption did not change significantly with intra-aortic balloon pumping. In 7 of these 10 patients, lactate was produced by the myocardium before intra-aortic balloon pumping, and lactate extraction was significantly reduced in three others. During intra-aortic balloon pumping, all patients extracted lactate an average of 15 percent. Thus in patients with profound shock following myocardial infarction, coronary blood flow increased, myocardial oxygen demand remained unchanged, and myocardial lactate production converted to extraction in all patients who were able to be studied serially.

Leinbach and associates[17] studied 10 patients with myocardial infarction and various degrees of circulatory collapse in a similar fashion but with somewhat different findings. All patients had a history of myocardial infarction and some degree of circulatory impairment. Heart rate, arterial and central venous pressures, left ventricular and pulmonary arterial pressures, coronary sinus and systemic arterial pO_2, pCO_2, pH, lactate and O_2 content, and coronary blood flow were measured as well as cardiac output. All patients were on vasoactive agents, and all measurements were performed during assist and after an average of 18 minutes without assist. As in the previous study, systolic pressure fell in all but one patient from an average of 95 mm Hg to 84 mm Hg without a change in the mean arterial pressure (70 to 69 mm Hg). Mean diastolic pressure was uniformly elevated (62 to 70 mm Hg). Cardiac output was not affected (3.81 per minute to 4.0 per min), and central venous pressure was unchanged. No significant changes were observed in arterial or coronary sinus pO_2, pCO_2, or pH. Coronary blood flow fell in seven patients, was unchanged in three, and rose in only four. Myocardial oxygen consumption paralleled coronary flow. Lactate metabolism was not consistently altered by intra-aortic balloon pumping.

The failure to observe a uniform increase in coronary blood flow in these patients may be explained in part by the technical limitations of the method used to measure coronary blood flow. The thermodilution coronary sinus catheter that was employed measures total flow and is unable to detect regional changes in coronary blood flow and metabolism. In those patients in whom coronary blood flow and $M\dot{V}O_2$ decreased, it can be postulated that the reduced systolic pressure diminished oxidative requirements and caused autoregulating vasoconstriction and a reduction in coronary blood flow that outweighed any increase in flow to ischemic areas. In patients with no change in coronary blood flow, it is possible that the increase in flow to ischemic areas was cancelled out by the reduction in flow to the normal myocardium. The technique used to measure coronary blood flow was insensitive to the regional changes. In those patients in whom total left coronary blood flow and $M\dot{V}O_2$ increased, profound shock (arterial pressure 57/34 mm Hg) was present and the increase in coronary blood flow most likely represents total lack of autoregulation and a coronary flow-limited situation. This subgroup of patients is similar to those patients studied by Mueller.

In summary, in patients in profound cardiogenic shock secondary to acute myocardial infarction, intra-aortic balloon pumping decreases peak systolic pressure but increases diastolic pressure (coronary artery perfusion pressure). Heart rate decreases as well as left ventricular outflow resistance. Predictable increases in total coronary blood flow are observed only in those patients so profoundly ischemic as to have lost all autoregulatory mechanisms. The inability to show increases in total coronary blood flow with intra-aortic counterpulsation in those patients not in profound shock may represent a failure of the technique used in measuring coronary blood flow to detect *regional* differences in blood flow in those patients with intact autoregulatory mechanisms.

SURGICAL VERSUS PERCUTANEOUS APPROACH TO THE INTRA-AORTIC BALLOON PUMP

The first intra-aortic balloons were inserted surgically into the common femoral artery. Surgical exposure of the common femoral artery is required, and a prosthetic graft is anastomosed to the vessel end-to-side. The intra-aortic balloon is then inserted through the graft and advanced retrograde to the descending thoracic aorta with or without the aid of fluoroscopy. The procedure requires a surgeon with vascular experience and takes 20 to 40 minutes to complete. Removal of the balloon necessitates a second surgical procedure that involves either oversewing or removal of the prosthetic graft. Several studies have evaluated the complication rate of intra-aortic balloon pumping and estimated a 20 percent incidence of complications using the surgical technique.[18–27]

Isner and associates,[28] in a pathology study, evaluated the incidence of complications and suggested a much higher rate, indicating that most of the complications occurred at the time of device insertion. Forty-five patients who died after insertion of an intra-aortic balloon device were studied at necropsy. Sixteen (36 percent) were found to have one or more complications (total 20) related to the use of the balloon. The twenty complications consisted of dissection of the aorta or branches (nine), arterial perforation (three), arterial emboli (three), arterial thrombi (three), limb ischemia (one), and local wound infection (one). None of the dissections were suspected before necropsy, and, indeed, of the entire 20 complications, only 4 (20 percent) were suspected before death (Table 2). Most complications of the balloon appear to result from device insertion (that is, dissection or arterial perforation). Patients with complications were not distinguished from patients without complications by the indication for insertion, by the underlying cardiac disorder, or by the ease of insertion.

In an effort to minimize the rate of complications, a percutaneous balloon system was developed. The percutaneous device is a modification of the original intra-aortic balloon in which the catheter section in the balloon membrane is replaced by a straight wire that allows the balloon membrane to be wrapped tightly around the wire and inserted through a 12 French sheath placed percutaneously in the common femoral artery. The sheath can be placed in a matter of minutes and the wrapped balloon quickly advanced to the descending thoracic aorta. After the balloon is in place in the descending thoracic aorta, it is unwrapped by twisting the wrapping knob in the opposite direction to that in which it was wrapped. Pumping can then proceed. This approach has greatly facilitated both the insertion and the removal of the intra-aortic balloon.

Table 2. Complications observed at necropsy in 16 patients after intra-aortic balloon insertion*

Complication	*Total*	*Due to insertion*	*Suspected before death*	*Balloon insertion* "Easy"	*Balloon insertion* "Hard"
Arterial dissection	9	9	0	4	5
Aorta and peripheral artery	6	6	0	4	2
Peripheral artery only	3	3	0	0	3
Arterial perforation	3	3	2	0	3
Arterial thrombi	3	0	1	0	0
Arterial emboli	3	0	0	0	0
Ischemic limb	1	0	1	0	0
Local sepsis	1	0	0	0	0
Total	20	12	4	8	8

*From Isner, JM, et al,[28] with permission.

The technique for percutaneous insertion is as follows: Whenever possible, insertion is performed in the cardiac catheterization laboratory under fluoroscopic guidance. After appropriate skin preparation and administration of local anesthesia, a soft J-tipped guide wire is inserted by standard percutaneous technique into the common femoral artery and advanced to the thoracic aorta. If the wire cannot be passed, or extreme tortuosity is encountered, an attempt may be made on the contralateral side. If the wire passes without difficulty, a 12 French 11-inch dilator-sheath introducer is inserted. The balloon membrane is then wrapped around the catheter either manually (in older devices) or by twisting the wrapping knob in self-wrap devices. After negative pressure is applied to the membrane, the dilator is removed from the sheath and blood flow controlled by pinching the sheath. The wrapped balloon is then inserted through the sheath and advanced under fluoroscopy to the descending thoracic aorta just distal to the takeoff of the left subclavian artery. Care must be taken so that the entire balloon exits the long sheath—this can be assured by measuring the balloon against the sheath before insertion. The balloon is then unwrapped by twisting the knob in the direction opposite to that in which it was wrapped. Pumping then can ensue. The balloon must then be fixed to the sheath so that it cannot slip back, and the entire system must be secured to the patient.

Removal of the intra-aortic balloon may be equally simple. After separating stay sutures, a vacuum is applied to the balloon membrane, the balloon is withdrawn until it contacts the sheath, and the entire balloon and sheath system is removed as a unit. Manual compression of the groin for 30 minutes usually achieves hemostasis. The patient must stay in bed without moving the involved extremity for 24 hours.

The entire insertion can be accomplished percutaneously in 5 minutes, allowing for rapid institution of balloon support for critically ill patients. In addition, because the J wire is passed under fluoroscopic guidance before sheath or balloon insertion is attempted, the patient is spared attempted insertion of the stiffer balloon device in the event of severe vascular disease or tortuosity. Finally, removal of the device does not usually require a surgical procedure and can be rapidly and safely accomplished at the bedside without undue patient discomfort.[6,29–31]

Recent modifications of the original percutaneous balloon represent attempts to make the device easier and safer to use. The size of the catheter has been reduced from 12 to 10.5 French, which allows use of an 11 French sheath in patients with small vessels or peripheral vascular disease. Balloon devices with a central lumen allow a guide wire to be placed through the balloon catheter itself to facilitate insertion; and, after removal of the wire, the lumen may serve as an arterial line for immediate monitoring and adjustment of intra-aortic balloon timing. Therefore, within the 5 minutes usually required for balloon insertion, properly timed external support can be provided for the critically impaired patient. Longer sheaths are also available for patients with tortuous vessels, thereby allowing easier placement of the balloon. A particularly beneficial modification of the system has been a change from the hand-wrapped devices to a self-wrapping system. With manually wrapped models, it is possible to wrap the membrane too tightly so that it does not unfold to allow for efficient pumping. With the self-wrapping system, which allows the operator to twist a wrapping knob rather than physically to wrap the balloon itself, it is easier to achieve a uniform wrap, and problems with unwrapping are less frequently encountered.

Thus far, thousands of intra-aortic balloons have been placed percutaneously, and the clinical experience with this technique for placement has borne out the initial promise of a rapid yet safe method for instituting pumping.

Subramanian and coworkers[29] described the clinical experience with percutaneous intra-aortic balloon placement in 37 patients, aged 45 to 79 years. The failure rate of passage was 10.8 percent (4 of 37). The average insertion time was 4 minutes. Hemodynamic changes with the percutaneous catheter balloon were similar to those with the standard intra-aortic balloon. Immediate complications, both major and minor, included balloon malposition in two patients, persistent bleeding with hematoma formation at the attempted insertion site in one

Table 3. Complications observed with percutaneous intra-aortic balloon placement*

	n
Minor	
Malposition into the ascending aorta	2
Delay or difficulty in unwrapping of the balloon in aorta	2
Transient bacteremia	1
Loss of dorsalis pedis after percutaneous removal	2
Major	
Bleeding at attempted puncture site	1
Renal embolism	1
Dissection of aorta(?)	1
Ischemic extremities	0
Related death	0

*From Subramanian, VA, et al,[29] with permission.

patient, transient bacteremia in one patient, loss of dorsalis pedis pulse after percutaneous removal with no symptoms in two patients, transient delay in balloon unwrapping in two patients, coincidental renal emboli in one patient, and aortic dissection in one patient (Table 3). This represents a major complication rate of 9 percent (3 of 33), as compared with the 20 percent major complication rate with surgically placed balloons, and a minor complication rate of 21 percent (7 of 33).

A study reported by Goldman and associates[32] allows direct comparison of complication rates in surgically versus percutaneously placed balloons. The complications associated with balloon insertion were reviewed in 389 patients; 299 balloons were placed surgically, and 90 were placed percutaneously. The percutaneous placements included the initial experience of the operators with the technique. Inability to insert the balloon was encountered in 5.7 percent of the surgical attempts and 4.4 percent of the percutaneous attempts. Vascular complications including dissection of the aorta, perforation of the aorta, bleeding, iliac or femoral occlusion, thromboembolism, and limb ischemia occurred in 14.6 percent of surgical attempts and 16 percent of the percutaneous attempts; however, 10 percent of the vascular complications in the percutaneous group were limb ischemia that reversed after removal of the balloon. It was believed that a surgical balloon could not have been passed in these patients. In addition, infection occurred in 17 percent of the surgical group and systemic bacteremia in 7 percent. The percutaneous group had no infectious complications (Table 4).

Goldman's group believed that the percutaneous rate of complications was falsely high in their series because the statistics included the learning phase of the operators. Even with inclusion of this learning phase and the incidence of reversible limb ischemia, overall complication rate in the percutaneous group was 20 percent, as opposed to 29 percent for the surgical group. The use of fluoroscopy with every percutaneous insertion and the use of the smaller French size balloon in patients with vascular disease may decrease this complication rate further.

The findings of Alcan and colleagues[33] suggest that percutaneous intra-aortic balloon placement is a highly successful and rapid means of initiating intra-aortic balloon pumping. When the percutaneous method of insertion was compared with surgical insertion, the complication rate was 15.2 percent versus 15.6 percent (p ns). Percutaneous placement was attempted in 51 patients with a success rate of 90.2 percent, whereas surgical placement was attempted in 100 patients with a success rate of 90 percent. The indications for placement were diverse. The major complications [total 7 (15.2 percent)] using the percutaneous technique included thromboembolic occlusion (six) and hematoma/bleeding (one). Using the sur-

Table 4. Complication rates in surgically versus percutaneously placed balloons*

Complication	Insertion: Surgical, no. (%) (n = 299)	Insertion: Percutaneous, no. (%) (n = 90)
Inability to insert	17 (5.7)	4 (4.4)
Vascular		
Dissection of aorta	4 (1.3)	2 (2.2)
Perforation of aorta, iliac arteries	1 (0.3)	2 (2.2)
Bleeding at insertion site	7 (2.3)	1 (1.1)
Iliac or femoral occlusion	3 (1.0)	1 (1.1)
Distal thromboembolism	13 (4.3)	0
Limb ischemia or gangrene	16 (5.4)	9 (10.0)
Infection		
Local, at insertion site	17 (5.7)	0
Systemic bacteremia	7 (2.3)	0

*From Goldman, BS, et al,[32] with permission.

gical method, the major complications [total 14 (15.6 percent)] included thromboembolic occlusion (ten), hematoma/bleeding (two), bacteremia (two), and aortic dissection (one). In the surgical group, two of the thromboembolic complications necessitated amputations, and the aortic dissection resulted in death.

Thus we conclude that the percutaneous method of intra-aortic balloon placement is highly efficacious, but we do not believe that the indications for placement have been increased by the technique, as the overall complication rate is comparable with the surgical technique. Careful weighing of the risk-benefit ratio with consideration of the overall plan of management is necessary to select candidates for placement and to minimize the duration of balloon pumping.

INDICATIONS FOR INTRA-AORTIC BALLOON PUMPING

Surgical Indications

The role of the intra-aortic balloon pump in cardiac surgical patients is evolving, and the frequency of its use varies from institution to institution and may depend on the expertise of the surgical and anesthesia team, especially in regard to the elective preoperative use of the balloon. Although initially developed for use in the medically unstable patient with severe left ventricular power failure, the balloon has found an important application in allowing patients to be weaned from cardiopulmonary bypass intraoperatively.[4,34,35–38]

The advent of the percutaneous technique for balloon placement has allowed rapid placement of the device in the operating room when it becomes apparent that medical therapy with pressors and afterload reducers is inadequate to wean the patient from bypass.

The elective preoperative use of the intra-aortic balloon pump in patients is more controversial. Some authors have recommended its use for patients with (1) left main coronary artery disease, (2) pre-infarction or unstable angina, or (3) moderately to severely depressed left ventricular function.[18,39–41] The reasons for these applications are that the induction of anesthesia and the process of weaning from bypass are considered less hazardous with the intra-aortic balloon pump in place.

Cooper and coworkers[18] followed a group of 65 patients with left main disease (greater than 50 percent stenosis), preinfarction angina (unstable electrocardiogram with pain) and poor left ventricular function (ejection fraction less than 50 percent) who underwent elective intra-aortic balloon pump placement preoperatively. Sixty-three patients survived. Although induction of anesthesia was accompanied by a systolic pressure drop of greater than 25 percent in 33 patients and to less than 100 mm Hg in 25 patients, cardiac function remained stable in all but 6 patients. There was a noticeable absence of left ventricular power failure, with only two patients exhibiting persistent postoperative hypotension. These two patients eventually died and were found retrospectively to have sustained perioperative infarctions. Two balloon complications were noted in this series, one requiring thromboembolectomy of the femoral artery and the other requiring delayed repair for bleeding.

Other authors have disagreed with the need for elective preoperative balloon placement in hemodynamically stable patients, reasoning that the risk of balloon-related complications is too high to mandate use of the device for other than hemodynamic problems. Kaplan and associates[36] reviewed the operative use of the intra-aortic balloon pump. Two hundred and three patients with left main coronary disease were operated upon. The intra-aortic balloon pump was used in only 1 percent of patients (all after cardiopulmonary bypass) and the operative mortality was less than 3 percent, as was the peri-infarction rate. Similar acceptable mortality and morbidity were found in patients undergoing coronary artery bypass grafting with poor left ventricular function, although only two received the intra-aortic balloon pump preoperatively (one for refractory pulmonary edema, one for cardiogenic shock with left ventricular aneurysm). The authors concluded that prophylactic use of the intra-aortic balloon pump was not necessary in those with left main disease, poor left ventricular function, and unstable angina.

No controversy exists, however, in those patients with hemodynamic compromise secondary to the acute mechanical complications of myocardial infarction (that is, ventricular septal defect or acute, severe mitral regurgitation). These patients uniformly fare better with the hemodynamic support offered by intra-aortic balloon pumping, and such support should be instituted as soon as the diagnosis is secure.[43–46]

Several reports have also suggested the use of the intra-aortic balloon in high-risk cardiac patients requiring major noncardiac surgery.[47,48]

In conclusion, the preoperative efficacy of intra-aortic balloon pumping has been proven in those patients with hemodynamic compromise secondary to acute mechanical complications of myocardial infarction, or secondary to ischemic disease and poor left ventricular function. In those cases in which no hemodynamic compromise exists, the preoperative use of an intra-aortic balloon pump is more controversial, and decisions must be made on a case-to-case basis.

Medical Indications

The intra-aortic balloon pump was originally developed as a device to treat left ventricular pump failure in cardiogenic shock. To date it has been used in patients in cardiogenic shock following acute myocardial infarction and also in patients with medically refractory left ventricular failure. Studies report its efficacy in stabilizing the patient in shock following infarction.[19,23,49–51] There is, in the majority of cases (70 to 90 percent), stabilization of the arterial pressure, an increase in cardiac output, a decrease in the pulmonary capillary wedge pressure, and an increase in urine output.

In a study by Willerson and coworkers,[27] 27 patients (age 31 to 71 years) were supported with the intra-aortic balloon pump. Twenty-three were in cardiogenic shock (blood pressure less than 85 mm Hg, oliguria, confusion) and, of these, 20 had suffered acute myocardial infarctions. In addition two patients had medically refractory ventricular tachycardia, and two had severe left ventricular failure. Shock was reversed in 19 of the 27 patients. Nine of these patients were successfully weaned from assistance but only three survived hospitalization. Of the remaining 10 patients who were initially stabilized on the balloon but could not be weaned, eight underwent cardiac catheterization. Four patients had disease amenable to coronary artery bypass grafting and were operated upon, but only one survived hospitalization. Likewise, in a study by Scheidt and associates,[19] 87 patients with cardiogenic shock were treated with the intra-aortic balloon pump. Fifty-two patients could not be weaned and died during balloon assistance. Thirty-two patients were weaned, but only 15 survived to discharge and only 8 of these were alive one year later.

More recently, because of the disappointing results obtained with therapy for cardiogenic shock with the balloon alone, mechanical support with the balloon has been accompanied by early cardiac catheterization and myocardial revascularization where feasible.[16,23,27,49] In a study of 40 patients with cardiogenic shock secondary to acute myocardial infarction, shock was reversed in 31 patients. Twenty-five patients were treated with the intra-aortic balloon pump alone, but only four survived to be discharged. Two of these patients died within 12 months. Fifteen patients judged unable to survive off balloon support underwent emergency cardiac catheterization and subsequent coronary artery bypass grafting, with intra-aortic balloon counterpulsation continuing during the procedures. Six of these patients survived longer than 12 months.[23] Leinbach and colleagues[49] reported a similar experience with 11 patients who underwent selective coronary and left ventricular cineangiography during intra-aortic balloon pumping for acute myocardial infarction and cardiogenic shock when weaning could not be accomplished. Of these, three underwent coronary artery bypass grafting and two survived.

Thus, in severely ill patients, the percutaneous technique facilitates balloon insertion, and the device can be placed in the catheterization laboratory before coronary angiography as part of a systematic approach including intra-aortic balloon support, cardiac catheterization, and myocardial revascularization where indicated.[16,23,27,49] The results of this combined approach to cardiogenic shock in the setting of acute myocardial infarction are still somewhat disappointing, with only 50 percent of patients suitable for surgery surviving to discharge.

A particularly important application of the intra-aortic balloon is in the setting of unstable angina. Gold and coworkers[26] studied 55 patients with refractory rest angina who underwent intra-aortic balloon pumping, coronary angiography, and coronary bypass surgery. Of these, 25 patients had typical angina associated with ST segment depression during pain, 12 had variant angina, and 18 had post-infarction angina. All patients had monitoring of the electrocardiogram (ECG), and systemic and pulmonary artery pressures. Control hemodynamic and ECG measurements were obtained while on medical therapy prior to pain and were repeated during spontaneous ischemic attacks. In all patients, spontaneous episodes of pain were accompanied by an increase in heart rate, an increase in mean arterial pressure, and elevation in the pulmonary capillary wedge pressure as well as ST-T wave evidence of ischemia. After the intra-aortic balloon pump was inserted, drug therapy was unchanged for the first 24 hours. The effect of temporary discontinuance of intra-aortic balloon pumping was assessed in all patients. Temporary cessation of intra-aortic pumping resulted in a rapid recurrence of angina in 40 percent of patients. All patients who had recurrence of angina with cessation of balloon pumping demonstrated the same hemodynamic changes present during spontaneous episodes of pain, that is, elevation of the heart rate, mean arterial pressure, and pulmonary capillary wedge pressure. All demonstrated ST-T wave changes compatible with ischemia. Resumption of intra-aortic balloon pumping resulted in elimination of angina in all cases, with resolution of the hemodynamic and electrocardiographic changes. The interruption of the ischemic attack by the intra-aortic balloon pump provided for a nonischemic interval during which coronary angiography could be performed at low risk. All underwent selective coronary angiography and myocardial revascularization surgery. The overall mortality was 5.5 percent, with a 2 percent incidence of myocardial infarction.

Similarly, in a study by Langou and associates,[53] 194 consecutive patients with unstable angina pectoris were studied. The criteria for unstable angina were prolonged typical angina pain (greater than 20 min), pain at rest, pain not completely relieved by nitroglycerin, unstable ST-T wave changes in the electrocardiogram, and no evidence of acute infarction. Sixty-four (33 percent) responded to medical therapy and underwent elective cardiac catheterization and coronary surgery; 130 (67 percent) did not respond to medical therapy. Of these latter patients, 75 (58 percent) received an intra-aortic balloon pump and underwent emergency cardiac catheterization and bypass surgery. Fifty-five (42 percent) of the medical nonresponders were not treated with the intra-aortic balloon pump, either because the device was not available (48) or because technical difficulties interfered with its placement (7). These patients also underwent emergency cardiac catheterization and surgery. The overall operative mortality rate was 6.1 percent. Medical responders had no mortality; medical nonresponders with the intra-aortic balloon pump had an operative mortality of 5.3 percent, and medical nonresponders without the pump had an operative mortality of 14.5 percent. The overall incidence of perioperative infarction was 13 percent: 6 percent in responders, 6.6 percent in nonresponders with the intra-aortic balloon pump, and 29 percent in nonresponders without the balloon.

Thus, intra-aortic balloon counterpulsation can reduce perioperative complications in patients with unstable angina unresponsive to medical therapy. Intra-aortic balloon pumping can be established quickly and safely in the cardiac catheterization laboratory, providing a safety margin for diagnostic coronary angiography. Revascularization can then be undertaken, when necessary, with the intra-aortic balloon pump in place.

The role of the intra-aortic balloon pump in cardiogenic shock and in unstable angina has been relatively well defined. With the advent of the percutaneous technique for placement, indications have been expanded to include catheterization-related events. During coronary angiography and left ventriculography in patients with severe triple-vessel disease, severe left main disease, or some degree of left ventricular dysfunction, it is not uncommon to induce bouts of prolonged myocardial ischemia or hypotension. These events can be readily reversed by the percutaneous institution of intra-aortic balloon pumping. The myocardium can then be protected from further ischemia, the blood pressure can be stabilized, and the information necessary for further therapeutic decisions can be obtained at relatively low risk.

Extremely high-risk patients for cardiac catheterization including those with acute ventricular septal defect and acute mitral regurgitation secondary to myocardial infarction can be hemodynamically stabilized at the time of catheterization with the percutaneously placed balloon and catheterized at much lower risk. If the clinical decision is to wait for surgery until such time as the acute infarction has had more time to heal, the balloon can be left in place.

Thus, the risk of cardiac catheterization can be decreased in selected patients by precatheterization insertion of the intra-aortic balloon, and patients can be stabilized during the catheterization procedure itself, if necessary, by intra-aortic balloon placement after development of symptoms. This allows the study to be completed so that the diagnostic information is available for decisions regarding surgery.

New Indications for Percutaneous Intra-aortic Balloon Pumping

In 1971, Maroko and associates[54] proved that a variety of hemodynamic and pharmacologic factors influence the extent and severity of myocardial necrosis following coronary occlusion. Reasoning that infarct size is the most important determinant of the degree of residual left ventricular power failure, they attempted to limit infarct size in dogs by a variety of manipulations. It became clear that following coronary occlusion, interventions that increased myocardial oxygen consumption increased the quantity of necrosis, and that for some time following acute coronary occlusion there is no clear demarcation between irreversibly injured myocardium and myocardium at risk but potentially salvageable. This observation was supported by pathologic studies that showed spotty ischemic damage in the periphery of the injured zone following acute coronary occlusion.[55]

Since these initial studies, Maroko and associates[56] have expanded the concept of myocardial salvage and limitation of infarct size to include such diverse interventions as hyaluroni-

Table 5. Interventions that modify myocardial injury following coronary occlusion*

- I. Interventions that reduce myocardial injury
  - A. By decreasing myocardial oxygen demand
    - 1. propranolol
    - 2. practolol
    - 3. cardiac glycoside in the failing heart
    - 4. counterpulsation
      - a. intra-aortic balloon
      - b. external counterpulsation
    - 5. nitroglycerin
    - 6. by decreasing afterload in hypertensive individuals—Arfonad
    - 7. by inhibition of lipolysis—beta-pyridylcarbinol
  - B. By increasing myocardial oxygen supply
    - 1. directly
      - a. coronary artery reperfusion
      - b. elevating arterial pO_2
      - c. thrombolytic agents
    - 2. through collateral vessels
      - a. elevation of coronary perfusion pressure by methoxamine, neosynephrine, or norepinephrine
      - b. intra-aortic balloon counterpulsation
      - c. external counterpulsation
    - 3. by increasing plasma osmolality
      - a. mannitol
      - b. hypertonic glucose
  - C. By augmenting anaerobic metabolism (presumed)
    - 1. glucose-insulin-potassium
    - 2. hypertonic glucose
  - D. By enhancing transport to the ischemic zone of substrate utilized in energy production (presumed)—hyaluronidase
  - E. By protecting against autolytic and heterolytic processes (presumed)
    - 1. hydrocortisone
    - 2. cobra venom factor
- II. Interventions that increase myocardial injury
  - A. By increasing myocardial oxygen requirements
    - 1. isoproterenol
    - 2. glucagon
    - 3. ouabain
    - 4. bretylium tosylate
    - 5. tachycardia
  - B. By decreasing myocardial oxygen supply
    - 1. directly
      - a. hypoxemia
      - b. anemia
    - 2. through collateral vessels—reducing coronary perfusion pressure (hemorrhage)
  - C. By decreasing substrate availability—hypoglycemia

*From Maroko, PR, et al,[56] with permission.

dase, glucose-insulin-potassium, hypertonic mannitol, cobra venom factor, beta blockers, reduction of systemic arterial pressure, and—not surprisingly—intra-aortic balloon pumping (Table 5).

Using epicardial electrocardiographic techniques and evaluating changes in average ST segment elevation, Maroko and coworkers[57] showed that intra-aortic balloon counterpulsation reduced the magnitude and extent of myocardial ischemic injury after experimental coronary occlusion in dogs, both when the intra-aortic balloon was employed prior to and 3 hours following acute coronary occlusion (Figs. 5, 6, 7). In 1978, Leinbach and associates[5] reported

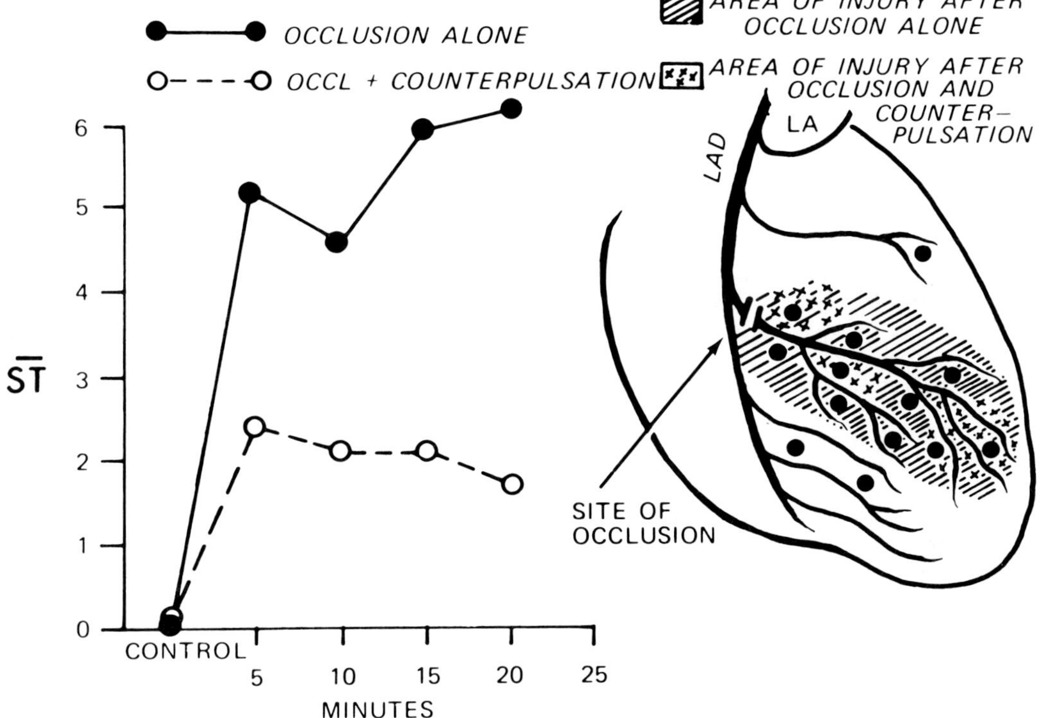

Figure 5. Illustrated here is reduction of zone of injury by intra-aortic balloon pumping. Epicardial mapping of ST segments in the control state and with 5, 10, 15, 20, and 25 minutes of coronary occlusion. With coronary occlusion alone, the mean ST elevation ($\overline{ST}$) is marked by a solid line; following 40 minutes of release of coronary occlusion, after ST segments have returned to baseline, occlusion is again performed, but this time with intra-aortic balloon counterpulsation functioning. There is marked reduction in injury current during coronary occlusion *(broken line)*. The zone of injury has been correspondingly decreased *(right panel)*.

on 11 patients with anterior infarctions less than 6 hours old without cardiogenic shock, in whom intra-aortic balloon pumping was undertaken in an attempt to control injury. Shock was excluded by hemodynamic measurements, and results were judged in comparison with a 1-hour pretreatment period. Standard precordial ECG leads and, in seven cases, 18 lead maps consisting of the standard leads and corresponding sites one interspace above and below were obtained. Five patients responded with an 84 percent fall in ST segment elevation in 1 hour, with preservation of R waves and good ventricular function. Six patients responded poorly, with only a 40 percent fall in ST elevation in 1 hour and Q wave development with poor residual left ventricular function. At coronary angiography it was discovered that the degree of response correlated with the presence or absence of residual left anterior descending artery (LAD) patency. Early use of the intra-aortic balloon interrupted injury and resulted in myocardial salvage only in those cases with residual LAD patency.

With the findings of Dewood and coworkers[58] that acute myocardial infarction is associated angiographically with complete coronary occlusion in 87 percent of patients studied within the first 4 hours of myocardial infarction, the clinical application of the balloon in this setting might appear limited; however, with the advent of myocardial reperfusion techniques[59] the combination of coronary reflow plus intra-aortic balloon pumping holds promise.

In addition to its potential benefit in myocardial salvage and limitation of infarct size, the intra-aortic balloon pump has considerable potential for use in the catheterization laboratory as the technique of percutaneous angioplasty becomes more widespread. Coronary artery dis-

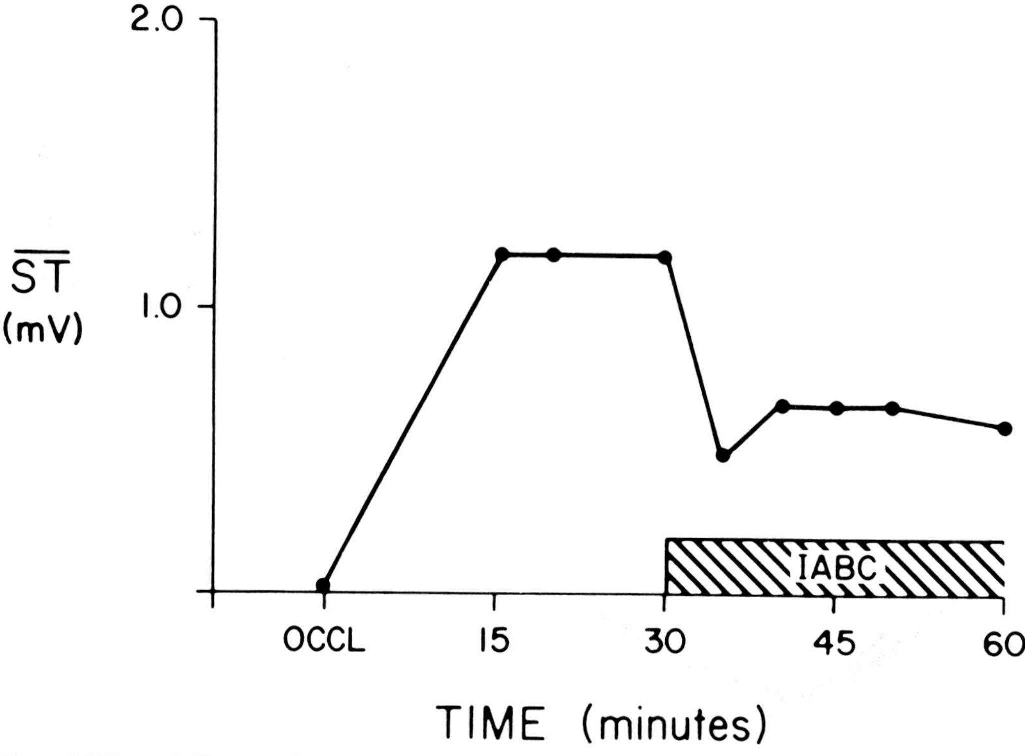

Figure 6. This graph illustrates similar animal experiments (see Figure 5). With coronary occlusion, ST elevation began in minutes and plateaued at 15 minutes. After 30 minutes of occlusion, intra-aortic balloon pumping dramatically reduced injury current.

section is a well-recognized complication associated with the use of subselective catheters, as is severe coronary artery spasm. In such events, coronary blood flow is acutely interrupted or obliterated. More often, decreased residual antegrade flow is apparent. In addition, there may be collateral circulation to the area fed by the involved coronary artery. When some residual flow or collateral flow is present, the rapid institution of intra-aortic balloon pumping may stabilize the patient and reverse the usual accompanying ST segment elevation, arrhythmias, and hypotension. As reported by Watson and associates,[60] when balloon pumping was begun immediately after ligation of the LAD in dogs, collateral coronary blood flow increased significantly. If pumping was delayed by 20 minutes, the collateral flow to the ischemic myocardium was unchanged by intra-aortic balloon pumping.

Fast, effective counterpulsation, as afforded by the percutaneous technique of intra-aortic balloon placement, may preserve ischemic myocardium in the setting of catheterization complications.

CONTRAINDICATIONS TO PERCUTANEOUS INTRA-AORTIC BALLOON PUMPING

The contraindications to percutaneous intra-aortic balloon pumping can be divided into absolute and relative contraindications. The balloon in most of its clinical applications is a stabilizing measure allowing time for definitive therapy to be initiated. It should always be used as part of a carefully organized plan of stabilization, diagnosis, and definitive therapy and should be avoided in a patient who is not a candidate for definitive therapy.

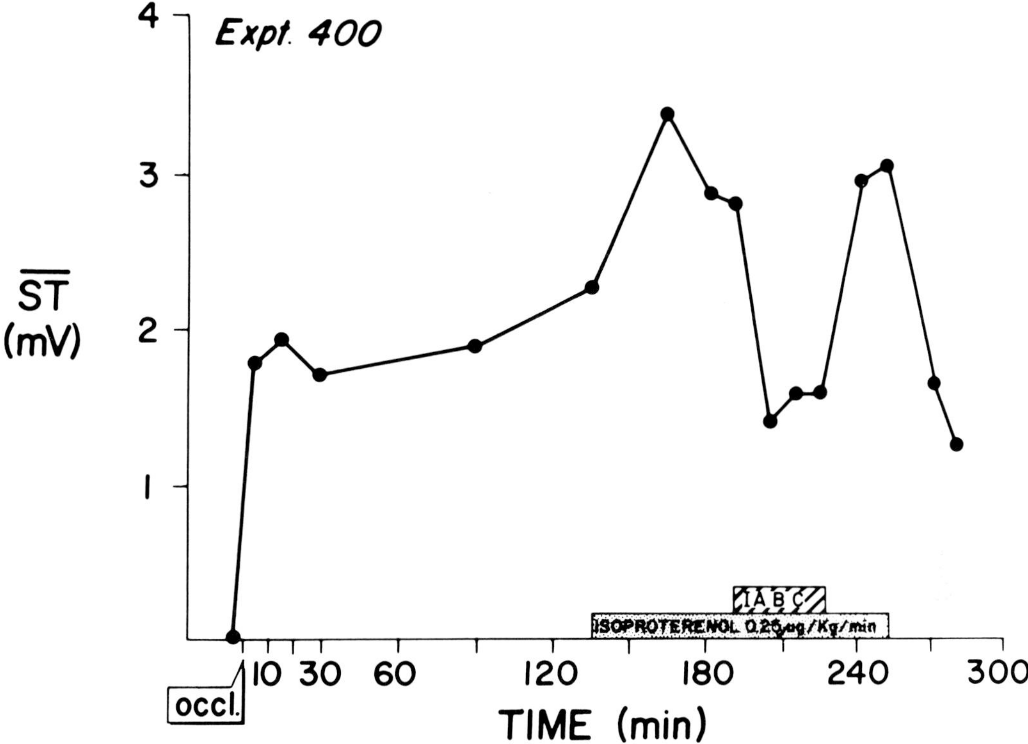

Figure 7. In a similar animal experiment (see Figure 5), epicardial ST elevation is marked at 5 minutes and is worsened by addition of isoproterenol. When intra-aortic balloon support begins, even after 180 minutes, there is reduction in injury current. When the balloon is turned off, injury current worsens.

Absolute contraindications to balloon insertion include:

1. underlying terminal illness that would preclude surgery or extreme support systems,
2. underlying brain death,
3. significant aortic insufficiency (AI) (balloon pumping in this instance would result in a marked increase in the AI secondary to balloon inflation in diastole; blood would be forced through the incompetent valve into the left ventricle in much greater volumes than at baseline),
4. known abdominal aortic aneurysm (this would be a contraindication, both because of the increased risk of balloon placement and the mechanical effects of balloon inflation on the severely diseased aortic wall).

Relative contraindications to intra-aortic balloon pumping include:

1. advanced age,
2. severe peripheral vascular disease,
3. associated unresolved intra-abdominal process,
4. known bleeding disorder.

CONCLUSIONS

The intra-aortic balloon pump is a powerful tool for stabilization of the hemodynamically compromised patient. Properly placed and timed, it increases cardiac output, increases coronary artery perfusion pressure, and decreases afterload on the left ventricle, thus increasing myocardial oxygen supply and decreasing myocardial oxygen consumption.

It is known to be life-saving in situations of hemodynamic collapse from acute mechanical complications of myocardial infarction (ventricular septal defect and mitral regurgitation) and in cardiogenic shock. Because of its effect on coronary perfusion dynamics, the balloon can be used to stabilize patients with unstable angina and impending myocardial infarction prior to cardiac catheterization and surgery. Perhaps its most clinically important use at present is in weaning patients from cardiopulmonary bypass intraoperatively. The percutaneous technique allows for rapid, safe institution of intra-aortic balloon counterpulsation in the operating room or catheterization laboratory setting and can stabilize those patients who suffer procedural complications.

The intra-aortic balloon pump should be used as a stabilizing therapy as part of an organized approach that includes definitive diagnosis and therapy. Therapeutic potential exists in the area of reduction of myocardial infarct size.

REFERENCES

1. Clauss, RH, Birtwell, WC, Albertal, G, et al: *Assisted circulation—The arterial counterpulsator.* J Thorac Cardiovasc Surg 41:447, 1961.
2. Moulopaulus, SD, Topoz, S, and Kolff, WJ: *Diastolic balloon pumping (with carbon dioxide) in the aorta: A mechanical assistance to the failing circulation.* Am Heart J 63:669, 1962.
3. Kantrowitz, A, Tjonneland, S, Freed, PS, et al: *Initial clinical experience with intra-aortic balloon pumping in cardiogenic shock.* JAMA 203:113, 1968.
4. Buckley, MJ, Craver, JM, Gold, HK, et al: *Intra-aortic balloon pump assist for cardiogenic shock after cardiopulmonary bypass.* Circulation 47-48:III-90, 1973.
5. Leinbach, RC, Gold, HK, Harper, RW, et al: *Early intra-aortic balloon pumping for anterior myocardial infarction without shock.* Circulation 58:204, 1978.
6. Bregman, D and Casarella, WJ: *Percutaneous intra-aortic balloon pumping: Initial clinical experience.* Ann Thorac Surg 29:153, 1979.
7. Weber, KT and Janicki, JS: *Intra-aortic balloon counterpulsation: A review of physiologic principles, clinical results and device safety.* Ann Thorac Surg 17:602, 1974.
8. Amsterdam, EA, Awan, NA, Lee, G, et al: *Intra-aortic balloon counterpulsation: Rationale, application and results.* In Rackley, C (ed): *Critical Care Cardiology.* Cardiovascular Clinics 11/3 FA Davis, Philadelphia, 1981.
9. Powell, JW, Daggett, WM, Negro, AE, et al: *Effects of intra-aortic balloon counterpulsation on cardiac performance, oxygen consumption and coronary blood flow in dogs.* Circ Res 26:754, 1970.
10. Sasayama, S, Osahoda, G, Tahabachi, M, et al: *Effects of intra-aortic balloon counterpulsation in regional myocardial function during acute coronary occlusion in the dog.* Am J Cardiol 43:59, 1979.
11. Watson, JT, Willerson, JT, Fixler, DE, et al: *Temporal changes in collateral coronary blood flow in ischemic myocardium during intra-aortic balloon pumping.* Ann Thorac Surg 16:445, 1973.
12. Gill, CC, Wechsler, AS, Newman, GE, et al: *Augmentation and redistribution of myocardial blood flow during acute ischemia by intra-aortic balloon pumping.* Ann Thorac Surg 16:445, 1973.
13. Limet, RR, Ross, JN, Hajevac, I, et al: *Effects of intra-aortic balloon counterpulsation (IABCP) in the distribution of coronary blood flow in experimental ischemic left ventricular failure.* J Cardiovasc Surg 13:305, 1972.
14. Saini, VK, Hood, WB, Hechtman, HB, et al: *Nutrient myocardial blood flow in experimental myocardial ischemia. Effects of intra-aortic balloon counterpulsation and coronary reperfusion.* Circulation 52:1086, 1975.
15. Shaw, J, Taylor, DR, and Pitt, B: *Effect of intra-aortic balloon counterpulsation on regional coronary blood flow in experimental myocardial infarction.* Am J Cardiol 34:552, 1974.
16. Mueller, H, Ayres, SM, Conklin, F, et al: *The effects of intra-aortic counterpulsation on cardiac performance and metabolism in shock associated with acute myocardial infarction.* J Clin Invest 50:1885, 1971.
17. Leinbach, RC, Buckley, JB, Austen, GW, et al: *Effects of intra-aortic balloon pumping on coronary flow and metabolism in man.* Circulation 43-44C:I77, 1971.
18. Cooper, GN, Singh, AK, Christien, FC, et al: *Pre-operative intra-aortic balloon support in surgery for left main coronary stenosis.* Ann Surg 185:242, 1977.

19. Scheidt, S, Wilner, G, Mueller, H, et al: *Intra-aortic balloon counterpulsation in cardiogenic shock: Report of a co-operative clinical trial.* N Engl J Med 288:979, 1973.
20. Lefemine, AA, Kosowsky, B, Madoff, I, et al: *Results and complications of intra-aortic balloon pumping in surgical and medical patients.* Am J Cardiol 40:416, 1977.
21. Beckman, CB, Geha, AS, Hammond, GL, et al: *Results and complications of intra-aortic balloon counterpulsation.* Ann Thorac Surg 24:550, 1977.
22. Cleveland, JC, LeFemine, AA, Malsro, F, et al: *The role of intra-aortic balloon counterpulsation in patients undergoing cardiac operations.* Ann Thorac Surg 20:652, 1975.
23. Dunkman, WG, Leinbach, RC, Buckley, MJ, et al: *Clinical and hemodynamic results of intra-aortic balloon pumping and surgery in cardiogenic shock.* Circulation 46:465, 1972.
24. Leinbach, RC, Gold, HK, Dinsmore, RE, et al: *The role of angiography in cardiogenic shock.* Circulation 47,48:95, 1973.
25. Wolfson, S, Karsh, DL, Langau, RA, et al: *Modifications of intra-aortic balloon catheter to permit introduction by cardiac catheterization techniques.* Am J Cardiol 41:733, 1978.
26. Gold, HK, Leinbach, RC, Buckley, MJ, et al: *Refractory angina pectoris: Follow-up after intra-aortic balloon pumping and surgery.* Circulation 54:III-41, 1976.
27. Willerson, JT, Curry, GC, Watson, JT, et al: *Intra-aortic balloon counterpulsation in patients in cardiogenic shock, medically refractory left ventricular failure and/or recurrent ventricular tachycardia.* Am J Med 58:183, 1975.
28. Isner, JM, Cohen, SR, Virmani, R, et al: *Complications of the intra-aortic balloon counterpulsation device: Clinical and morphologic observation in 45 necropsy patients.* Am J Cardiol 45:260, 1980.
29. Subramanian, VA, Goldstein, JE, Sos, TA, et al: *Preliminary clinical experience with percutaneous intra-aortic balloon pumping.* Circulation 62:I-123, 1980.
30. Vignola, PA, Swaye, PS, and Gosselin, AJ: *Guidelines for effective and safe percutaneous intra-aortic balloon pump insertion and removal.* Am J Cardiol 48:660, 1981.
31. Desilets, PT and Hoffman, R: *A new method of percutaneous catheterization.* Radiology 85:122, 1954.
32. Goldman, BS, Hill, TJ, Rosenthal, GA, et al: *Complications associated with use of the intra-aortic balloon pump.* Canad J Surg 25:153, 1982.
33. Alcan, KE, Stertzer, SH, Wallsh, E, et al: *Comparison of wire-guided percutaneous insertion and conventional surgical insertion of intra-aortic balloon pump in 151 patients.* Am J Med 75:24, 1983.
34. Bolooki, H, Williams, W, Thurer, RJ, et al: *Clinical and hemodynamic criteria for use of the intra-aortic balloon pump in patients requiring cardiac surgery.* J Thorac Cardiovasc Surg 72:756, 1976.
35. Stewart, S, Biddle, T, and Deweese, J: *Support of the myocardium with intra-aortic balloon counterpulsation following cardio-pulmonary bypass.* J Thorac Cardiovasc Surg 72:109, 1976.
36. Kaplan, JA, Craver, JM, Jones, EL, et al: *The role of the intra-aortic balloon in cardiac anesthesia and surgery.* Am Heart J 98:580, 1979.
37. Bregman, D, Cohen, SR, and Kaskel, PS: *Intra-aortic balloon pumping: Indications and benefits.* Primary Cardiology, October 1972.
38. McEnany, MT, Kay, HR, Buckley, MJ, et al: *Clinical experience with intra-aortic balloon pump support in 728 patients.* Circulation 58:I-124, 1978.
39. Garcia, JM, Mispireta, CA, Smyth, NPD, et al: *Surgical management of life-threatening coronary artery disease.* J Thorac Cardiovasc Surg 72:593, 1976.
40. Cooper, GN, Singh, AL, Vargas, LL, et al: *Preoperative intra-aortic balloon assist in high risk revascularization patients.* Am J Surg 133:463, 1977.
41. Goldman, BS, Walker, P, Gunstensen, J, et al: *Intra-aortic balloon pump assist: Adjunct to surgery for left ventricular dysfunction.* Canad J Surg 19:128, 1976.
42. Brundage, BH, Ullyat, DJ, Winahur, S, et al: *The role of aortic balloon pumping in post-infarction angina, a different perspective.* Circulation 62:119, 1980.
43. Gunstensen, J, Goldman, BS, Scully, HS, et al: *Evolving indications for preoperative intra-aortic balloon pump assistance.* Ann Thorac Surg 27:535, 1976.
44. Lappos, DG, Powell, WMJ Jr, and Daggett, WM: *Cardiac dysfunction in the perioperative period.* Anesthesiology 47:117, 1977.
45. Mundth, ED: *Preoperative intra-aortic balloon pump assistance.* Ann Thorac Surg 22:603, 1976.
46. Webb, WR, Parker, FB Jr, Neville, JF Jr, et al: *Acute mechanical complications of coronary arterial disease.* Arch Surg 109:25, 1974.
47. Miller, MG and Hall, SV: *Intra-aortic balloon counterpulsation in a high risk patient undergoing emergency gastrectomy.* Anesthesiology 42:103, 1975.

48. Baron, DW and O'Rourke, MF: *Long-term results of arterial counterpulsation in acute severe cardiac failure complicating myocardial infarction.* Br Heart J 38:285, 1976.

49. Leinbach, RC, Dinsmore, RE, Mundth, ED, et al: *Selective coronary and left ventricular cineangiography during intra-aortic balloon pumping for cardiogenic shock.* Circulation 45:845, 1972.

50. Buckley, MJ, Leinbach, RC, Kastor, JA, et al: *Hemodynamic evaluation of intra-aortic balloon pumping in man.* Circulation 41:II-130, 1970.

51. Hagemeijer, F, Laird, JD, Haalebos, MMP, et al: *Effectiveness of intra-aortic balloon pumping without cardiac surgery for patients with severe heart failure secondary to a recent myocardial infarction.* Am J Cardiol 40:951, 1977.

52. Gold, HK, Leinbach, RC, Sanders, CA, et al: *Intra-aortic balloon pumping for control of recurrent myocardial ischemia.* Circulation 47:1182, 1973.

53. Langou, RA, Geha, AS, Hammond, GL, et al: *Surgical approach for patients with unstable angina pectoris: Role of the response to initial medical therapy and intra-aortic balloon pumping in perioperative complications after aortocoronary bypass grafting.* Am J Cardiol 42:629, 1978.

54. Maroko, PR, Kjekshus, JK, Sobel, BE, et al: *Factors influencing infarct size following experimental coronary artery occlusions.* Circulation 43:67, 1971.

55. Page, DC, Caulfield, JB, Kastor, JA, et al: *Myocardial changes associated with cardiogenic shock.* N Engl J Med 285:133, 1971.

56. Maroko, PR and Braunwald, E: *The reduction of infarct size—An idea whose time (for testing) has come.* Circulation 50:206, 1974.

57. Maroko, PR, Bernstein, EF, Libby, P, et al: *Effects of intra-aortic balloon counterpulsation on the severity of myocardial ischemic injury following acute coronary occlusion.* Circulation 45:1151, 1972.

58. Dewood, MA, Spores, J, Notske, RN, et al: *Prevalence of total coronary occlusion during the early hours of transmural myocardial infarction.* N Engl J Med 303:897, 1980.

59. Rentrop, P, Blake, H, Kastering, K, et al: *Acute myocardial infarction: Intra-coronary application of nitroglycerin and streptokinase in combination with transluminal recanalization.* Clinical Cardiology 2:354, 1979.

60. Watson, JT, Willerson, JT, Fixler, DE, et al: *Temporal change in collateral coronary blood flow in ischemic myocardium during intra-aortic balloon pumping.* Circulation 49-50:II-58, 1974.

Interventional Cardiac Catheterization in Congenital Heart Disease*

William J. Rashkind, M.D., with the technical and editorial assistance of MaryAngela S. Tait, B.S.

Cardiac catheterization in man has achieved widespread use only in the last 30 years. The first attempt on a human subject was described in 1833. Because of the inaccessibility of the journal containing his work and the outmoded concepts in treatment he used, J. F. Dieffenbach's early studies on both animals and humans have been overlooked. He wrote that experiments on animals taught him that the introduction of foreign bodies into the large vessels and the heart "was tolerated in a wonderful way." He added that it was known that the external surface of the heart possessed a certain degree of insensibility to mechanical stimuli but that "this was also the case to a certain extent with its interior walls." He should certainly receive credit both for his early animal studies, in which he showed how well the introduction of foreign bodies into the heart could be tolerated, and for the first description of a human catheterization. The patient was moribund from cholera, which was considered to be a disease in which there was accumulation of blood in the heart, emptying the periphery and overloading the heart. Dieffenbach attempted to reach the heart to remove the "extra blood." "In an almost dying patient, I opened ... the brachial artery in its upper third. As not a drop of blood flowed, I introduced, as I had planned, an elastic catheter into the vessel approximately as far as the heart. No blood appeared through the catheter. The heart became clearer and more rapid, and I now withdrew the catheter.... It is greatly to be regretted that this operation of interest for all physiology was performed on a man who was so near to death and who shortly afterwards was seized by convulsions and rendered his soul." Dieffenbach's pioneering in human cardiac catheterization should not be downgraded because his theories were misguided.[1]

Although his were undoubtedly the first studies, there is serious doubt as to whether Dieffenbach actually reached the heart. The same criticism applies to the studies of Bleichroeder, Unger, and Loeb, who published descriptions of experiments performed in 1922 on animals and humans using catheterization techniques. Unger and Loeb catheterized Bleichroeder and reached the axillary vein and the inferior vena cava. During one such attempt, Bleichroeder complained of a stabbing pain in his chest, suggesting that the heart *may* have been reached.[2] None of these earlier studies should in any way detract credit for priority, courage, and significance from Forssmann's studies on himself, reported in 1929 as "Catheterization of the Right Heart," for he clearly was the first to *document* catheterization of the right heart in humans.[3] In a series of papers in the early 1940s, Cournand and his colleagues Richards, Ranges, and Riley gave credibility to cardiac catheterization. Cournand's studies with Bald-

*Supported in part by USPHS grant HL 12307, NHLBI, and grants from the American Heart Association, Southeastern Pennsylvania and Delaware chapters.

win and Himmelstein culminated in their volume, *Cardiac Catheterization in Congenital Heart Disease.*[4] The method soon achieved widespread use for physiologic studies in man and for making precise anatomic and physiologic analyses of congenital heart defects.

THERAPEUTIC USE OF CARDIAC CATHETERS

Rubeo-Alvarez and Limon-Lason described a single attempt at relief of pulmonic stenosis using a cardiac catheter method in 1950.[5] No subsequent reports have ever been published by them. In 1966, W. W. Miller and I reported a method for balloon atrioseptostomy, a technique that has had wide and continued application since that time.[6] Subsequently, a wide variety of procedures have been developed to expand the cardiac catheter from a solely investigational and diagnostic device to a therapeutic instrument. The following list describes various interventional cardiac catheterization procedures that have been reported to have been used in children:

1. balloon atrioseptostomy
2. blade atrioseptotomy
3. transvenous or transarterial pacemaker insertion (temporary or permanent)
4. retrieval of foreign bodies from the cardiovascular system
5. transcatheter patch atrial septal defect closure
6. transcatheter plug patent ductus arteriosus closure
7. occlusion of arteriovenous fistulae
8. occlusion of collateral vessels
9. occlusion of shunts, natural or surgical
10. transvalvar balloon angioplasty
11. transcoarctation balloon angioplasty
12. dilatation of stenosed and/or hypoplastic pulmonary arteries

The above list is relatively complete. Balloon dilatation of a variety of other strictures has also been reported and includes dilatation of pulmonary veins, obstructed aortico-pulmonary shunts, caval obstruction, and so on.

This chapter will be divided into two sections: the first will be a summary of our methods of balloon atrioseptostomy, patch closure of atrial septal defects, and patent ductus arteriosus occlusion;[7] the second will be a brief literature review of the remainder of the aforementioned procedures. Transvascular pacing will be omitted inasmuch as a full body of literature on this subject is extant.

BALLOON ATRIOSEPTOSTOMY

Our initial attempts, in animals, to produce an atrial septal defect with a catheter device took on several forms. The initial devices were as simple as a bent wire through a large catheter and as complicated as a miniaturized bronchoscopic snare. Devices of this sort did work in animals but were deemed unsafe because occasionally the atrial wall rather than the septum was opened. Ultimately, the decision was made to concentrate on balloon catheters. Early experiments on puppies were difficult because the puppy usually has a sealed atrial septum by the time it is big enough for experimentation. The Prince of Serendip must have been at my side when I found a litter of puppies all of whom had probe-patent foramina ovale. These puppies were subjected to septostomy, and serial autopsies over a four month period showed that all the defects remained open.

Clinically, a special balloon-tipped catheter is used for the procedure. Initially, a double-lumen catheter was employed to assist in localization of the balloon in the left atrium. However, the widespread availability of biplane fluoroscopy has obviated the need for a second lumen. The current equipment, therefore, is a single-lumen balloon-tipped catheter, generally 4.5 to 6 French, which can be introduced via a 6 French sheath. Cardiac catheterization is performed in the usual manner to achieve a complete diagnosis. After the diagnosis has been established, the balloon-tipped catheter is passed via the sheath into the inferior vena cava, to the right atrium, and across the foramen ovale into the left atrium. The balloon is slowly dilated with dilute radio-opaque material. If the balloon happens to be in a pulmonary vein, slow dilatation will result in the balloon being extruded to lie free in the left atrial chamber. Once the operator is certain that the catheter tip is in the left atrium, the balloon is inflated to a volume of approximately 2 ml, or to a diameter of approximately 15 mm. At this point, the operator must vigorously jerk the catheter through the atrial septum into the right atrium, being careful not to wedge it into the inferior cava. It is allowed to float free in the right atrial chamber while the balloon is deflated (Fig. 1). The success of the procedure is directly proportional to the *jerk* at the end of the catheter.

From May 1965 through April 1980, 307 patients have been treated by the balloon atrioseptostomy technique at The Children's Hospital of Philadelphia. This chapter describes the followup data on the first 300 of these patients. The most frequent lesion for which this method was used was d-transposition of the great arteries (d-TGA). There were 186 patients (62 percent) whose primary diagnosis was transposition. Seventy-four (40 percent) had isolated d-TGA (included in this group were patients with hemodynamically insignificant ventricular septal defect or patent ductus and patients with mild pulmonic stenosis with peak left ventricular to pulmonary artery systolic gradient of under 35 mm Hg); 30 (16 percent) had ventricular septal defects; and 14 (7 percent) had ventricular septal defect and pulmonic stenosis. In addition, 30 (10 percent) had d-TGA associated with extremely complex, additional cardiovascular anomalies. Of the remaining patients, the distribution by lesions was as fol-

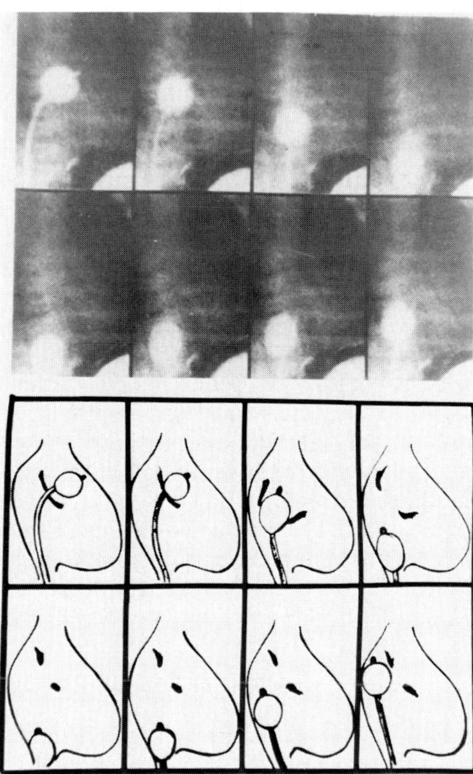

Figure 1. The upper half illustrates a septostomy in consecutive frames from a 30 per second cineangiogram, and the lower half is a diagrammatic representation of the same frames.

lows: pulmonary atresia with intact ventricular septum, 32 patients (11 percent); total anomalous pulmonary venous return, 31 patients (10 percent); tricuspid atresia, 28 patients (10 percent); left ventricular hypoplasia complexes, 16 patients (5 percent); and there were 5 patients (2 percent) with a variety of other congenital cardiac defects.

In the following description of the results of the use of this technique, the term effective palliation rate is defined as the rate of survival from the first admission to the present time or to *elective* surgical correction. In the group of transposition patients classified as isolated, and in the group with ventricular septal defect, 86 percent were discharged improved from their first admission, and 72 percent had effective palliation. (The long-term results of corrective surgery for these patients is beyond the scope of this chapter.) The presence of a hemodynamically significant patent ductus arteriosus, with or without a coexisting ventricular septal defect, was generally lethal. In the nontransposition group of patients, the best effective palliation rate was obtained in tricuspid atresia. Eighty percent of those patients were long-term survivors; all had additional treatment consisting of some type of aortic-pulmonary shunting. Three of that group died from left ventricular failure 10 years or more after initial palliation. In those patients with pulmonary atresia and intact ventricular septum, and in those with total anomalous pulmonary venous return, the effective palliation rate was approximately 60 percent. Many patients were successfully palliated for long-enough periods of time to facilitate total surgical correction.

Generally, the atrial septum is paper thin, and balloon atrioseptostomy may be performed easily. Occasionally, the atrial septum is too thick to permit production of an adequate atrial defect with a balloon catheter. Park and coworkers[8] have reported excellent results in such patients with a retractable blade catheter. We have employed their technique on a few patients with satisfactory results.

The largest group of patients for whom balloon atrioseptostomy will continue to be used is that with transposition of the great arteries. We have made some interesting ancillary observations about transposition in the past 15 years. There has been a striking change in the clinical profile of the infant presenting to us with transposition. In the first five years of septostomy, only half the patients appeared in the first week of life. In the last five years, almost *all* have appeared in the first week of life. Indeed, whereas only 13 percent arrived on the first day of life in the first five years, now nearly 70 percent are seen within the first 24 hours of life. We have also noticed a striking change in the occurrence of subpulmonic stenosis. In the first five years, less than 30 percent of the patients developed this complication. This has increased to an incidence of 62 percent in the most recent five-year period. In the last five years, 70 percent of the infants ballooned within the first 24 hours of life acquired pulmonic stenosis, many within the first few months after septostomy. Fortunately, our management of these patients currently is facilitated by the fact that Mustard's operation can be performed successfully in early infancy. Another observation of interest about transposition was made in our laboratory by Dennis Wood. In the normal infant, a short axis view of the heart shows that the cavity of the anterior right ventricle has the shape of a banana, and the cavity of the posterior left ventricle has the shape of a grapefruit. In transposition, the situation is reversed, and the anterior right ventricle has the shape of the grapefruit, and the posterior left ventricle, the shape of a banana. (The latter is well demonstrated on a short axis two-dimensional echocardiogram.) The grapefruit-banana shape relationship is sustained after Mustard's operation and provides an interesting comment on the biologic adaptability of human tissue. Moreover, it offers encouragement regarding the ability of the modified right ventricle to function as a systemic ventricle for a long period of time.

PATCH CLOSURE OF ATRIAL SEPTAL DEFECTS

The first successful closure of an atrial septal defect in a human by transcatheter technique was reported by King and coworkers in 1976.[9] Our studies at The Children's Hospital of

Philadelphia paralleled theirs but involved a different type of equipment. They have discontinued their clinical studies, but we are continuing both experimental and clinical testing.[7]

Methods and Materials

DEVELOPMENT OF A SIX-RIB, THREE-HOOK SYSTEM. The prosthesis consists of a six-rib skeleton. The arms are fashioned of 0.010 inch ribs fastened to a stainless steel hub. The ribs have helical turns at the hub end to permit proper recoil from a folded position. The outer end of each alternate rib terminates in a small barbed hook. In addition, small eyes are formed at the terminal ends of all six ribs to permit anchoring of the foam matrix. The hub is precisely machined to be an integral part of the delivery system. The ribs are covered by a fine mesh, open-cell, foam sheet disc sewed into place. Figure 2 shows a skeleton and the completed prosthesis.

The delivery system consists of a standard 6 French catheter with a locking tip at its distal end. The locking tip mechanism consists of an expanding sleeve (0.05 inch in diameter) that interlocks with the hub of the closure disc. The sleeve is expanded by means of a central helical guidewire. The catheter and closure disc, when threaded onto the guide wire, fix the disc hub to the locking tip while allowing free axial motion of the assembly along the guide wire. Removal of the guide wire allows the closure disc to be freed from the locking tip. The collapsed prosthesis fits into a thin-wall metal pod bound to the distal end of a catheter. It has the approximate caliber of 10 to 12 French. The proximal end is fitted with a double zero ring locking mechanism that surrounds the helical spring wire, and a side arm with a luer-lock tip that permits flushing of the entire system before, during, and after operation. The entire system is self-contained and prevents blood loss or air embolization. Figure 3 illustrates the delivery system.

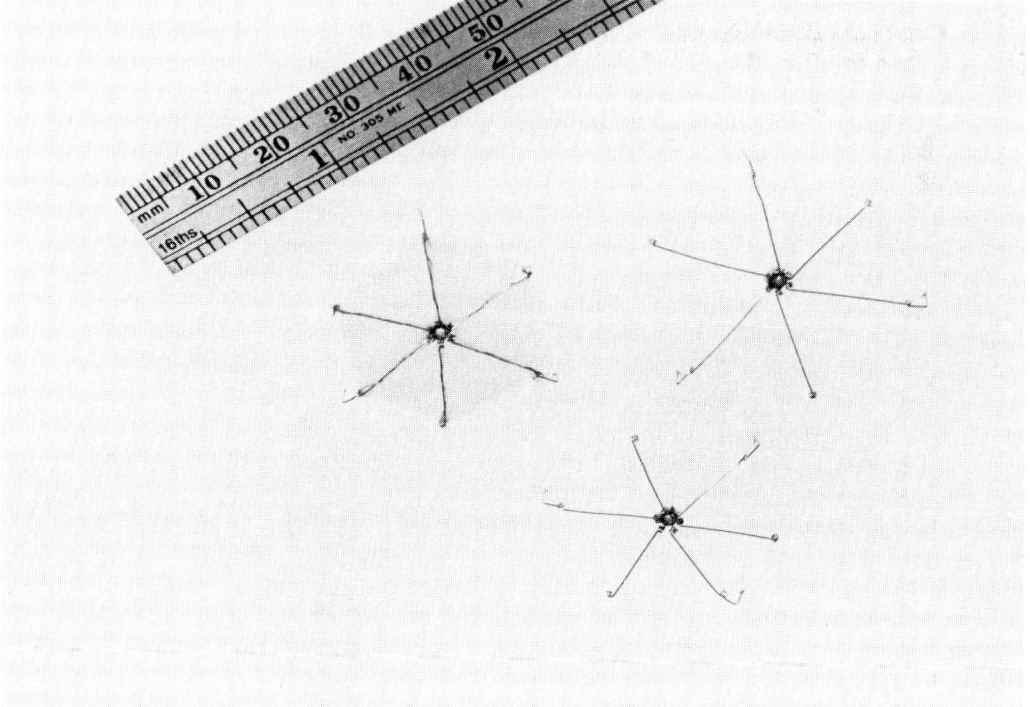

Figure 2. Illustrated are two atrial septal defect prosthesis skeletons and one covered prosthesis.

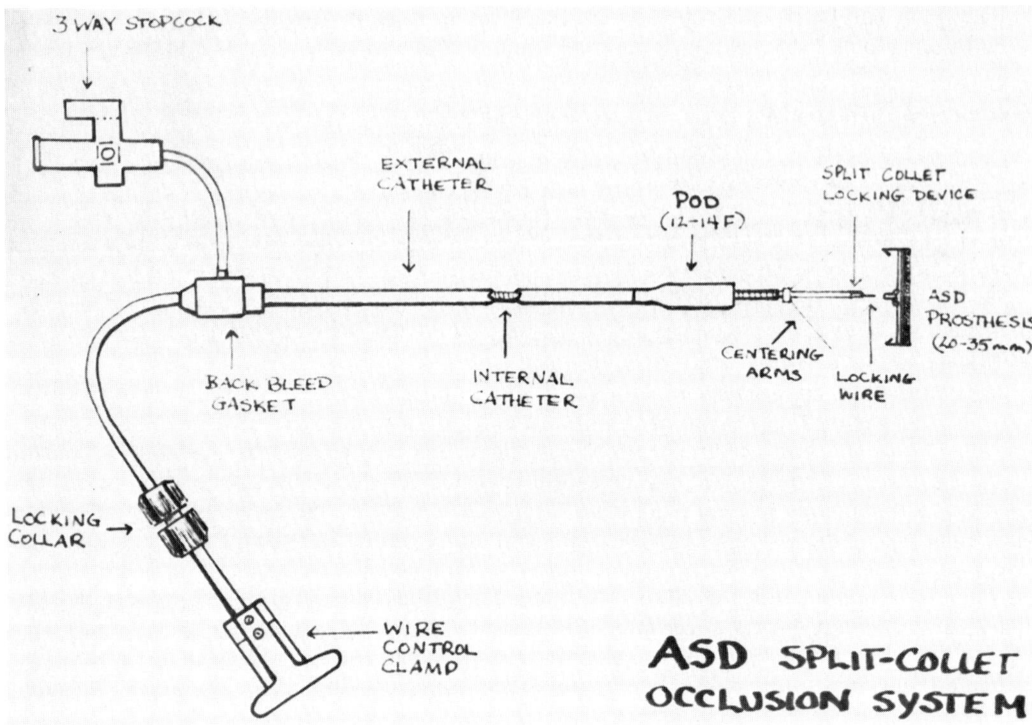

Figure 3. This is a diagrammatic illustration of the atrial septal defect occlusion system.

There is a centering mechanism that is fashioned in a similar manner to the skeleton of the prosthesis. A central stainless-steel hub is welded to the locking tip approximately 15 mm from the tip. It has five side arms bent into outward gentle curves. The portion near the hub is connected to it via a spring mechanism identical to that of the prosthesis. In operation, the arms are collapsed inside the carrying pod catheter. When extruded from the pod, they spring open and provide a funnel shape. On retraction of the entire system, the centering device funnels the prosthesis (which is just distal to it) over the atrial septal defect and permits anchoring of the hooks in the proper portion of the atrial septum (Fig. 4).

METHODS OF CLINICAL IMPLANTATION. The procedure is performed in the cardiac catheterization laboratory. The patient is sedated with morphine (0.1 mg per kg) and pentobarbital (4 mg per kg). Complete cardiac catheterization is done to determine the accuracy of the diagnosis and the location and size of the defect. In each patient, selective cineangiograms are obtained with contrast injection into the left atrium, with the patient in a 30° left anterior oblique position. This view has proved most satisfactory in placing the atrial septum on end and permits good visualization of the defect. Sizing of the defect is performed in the following manner. A balloon-tipped catheter is passed across the atrial septal defect and inflated in the left atrium with a dilute contrast solution. Gentle traction is applied until the balloon is impacted in the defect. The balloon is slowly deflated until it just passes through the defect. The residual volume of the contrast material in the balloon is carefully measured and recorded. The balloon-tipped catheter is then removed from the patient, reinflated with the exact same volume of solution, and the diameter of the balloon measured. The use of this latter maneuver permits not only accurate sizing of the defect but accurate location of the defect by recording a film strip with the inflated balloon in place in the defect. In addition, the possibility of anomalous pulmonary venous return to the right atrium is excluded. This determination is accomplished in two ways. First, every effort is made to explore both right

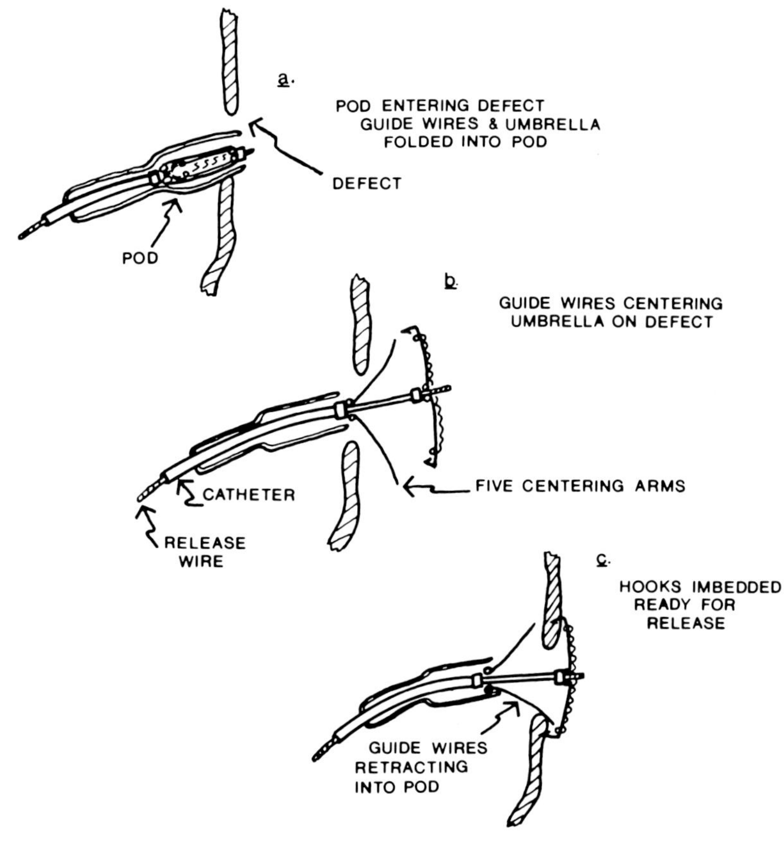

Figure 4. This is a diagrammatic illustration of the emplacement of the atrial septal defect occlusion prosthesis.

and left pulmonary veins with a catheter and to be sure that they connect directly with the left atrium. If there is any residual doubt after these maneuvers, a balloon-tipped catheter is used to occlude the atrial septal defect, and oxygen contents are measured in the superior vena cava, inferior vena cava, and right atrium. If there is no elevation in oxygen content in the right atrium, it may be assumed that anomalous pulmonary venous drainage through the right atrium has been excluded.

When satisfied that the defect is of appropriate size, shape, and location to warrant transcatheter closure, the entire system is introduced and delivered as described above. Figure 4 is a scheme of the implantation sequence. Light heparinization (50 mg per kg) is started immediately prior to the procedure and continued at the same dose every 6 hours for 48 hours. Anteroposterior and lateral chest films are obtained immediately after the patient leaves the cardiac catheterization laboratory and are repeated 24 and 72 hours later. The patient is discharged from the hospital usually on the third to fourth postprocedure day.

Results

The first six clinical implants were of a three-rib prosthesis type. Only 50 percent of these provided satisfactory closure. The remainder of the clinical implants have been of the six-rib, three-hook type. Overall, 22 patients have been admitted to the clinical atrial septal defect closure study. Four implantations were not attempted because the defects were too large, that is, by balloon sizing they measured larger than 25 mm in diameter. Three were not attempted because the defect was considered too small to warrant any risk. Nine have been adequately closed; and the results in five have been unsatisfactory. Four of the latter have had subsequent uneventful surgical closure.

TRANSCATHETER OCCLUSION OF PATENT DUCTUS ARTERIOSUS

In 1907, Munro proposed an operation for closing a ductus arteriosus and described the procedure in detail.[10] It was nearly 30 years before a bona fide attempt was made at surgical closure. Graybiel and his associates[11] intended to ligate the ductus in a 22-year-old girl with infectious endocarditis but were able only to apply plicating sutures and did not achieve a lasting success. In 1939, the modern era of surgery for congenital heart disease was inaugurated when Gross and coworkers[12] performed the first successful ductus ligation. Within a few years, many surgeons were duplicating this feat; and ductus surgery became commonplace, safe, and effective. Porstmann and associates[13] first proved the clinical applicability of transcatheter closure of the ductus in 1967 and have since successfully treated over 200 patients.[14] Their method is most applicable to young adults and older children. The purpose of the present communication is to report a technique for transcatheter closure of ductus arteriosus suitable for young children and infants and its successful application in children as young as 1 month and as small as 2.4 kg.[15]

Methods and Materials

DEVELOPMENT OF EQUIPMENT. The initial prosthesis was a small (1.0 to 1.5 mm diameter) disc of polyurethane foam bound to a three-rib, stainless-steel skeleton. Each rib was welded

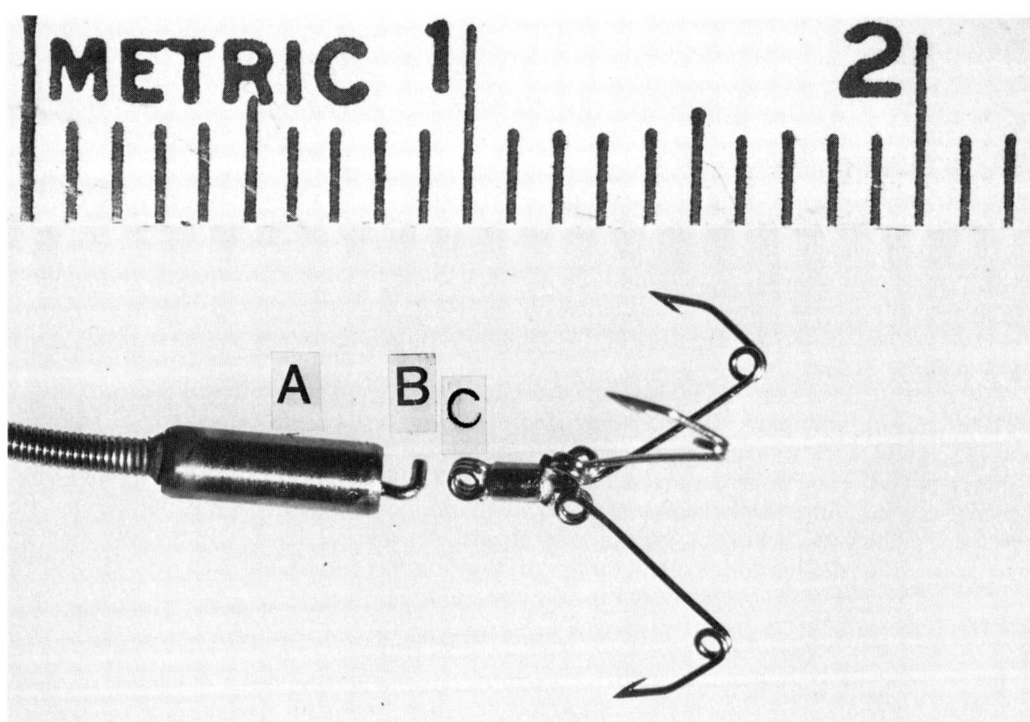

Figure 5. Illustrated is an uncovered skeleton of the hooked type of patent ductus occlusion prosthesis, showing a sleeve (A), pin (B), and eye (C) mechanism.

to a central hub and terminated in a minihook. It was a miniaturized version of the transcatheter atrial septal defect device described earlier in this chapter. It was modified to the following format, which is one of the two versions currently being used. The modified prosthesis consists of a miniature grappling-hook-shaped skeleton made of stainless-steel, which is filled with a cone of medical-grade polyurethane foam. Each of the three limbs of the grappling hook connects to the central hub by a spring, which permits the three arms to be collapsed against each other. Each arm also has a small joint near its hook end, which permits the end of each arm to be folded upon itself. In this manner, the entire device can be collapsed and carried in a sheath of approximately 8 French caliber. At the apex, the three arms are welded together and terminate in a small eye (Fig. 5).

Delivery System. The distal end of the system consists of a pin-sleeve mechanism. The pin is the terminus of a wire that traverses the entire delivery catheter complex and is welded to a proximal release mechanism. The sleeve is a stainless-steel cylinder welded to a helical wound coil wire that also traverses the entire delivery catheter system and is welded to another part of the release mechanism. This design permits the pin end of the central wire to slide in the coil wire. To engage the prosthesis, the pin is slid out of the sleeve and into the eye of the prosthesis. The eye and pin are then retracted into the sleeve and locked into place by the delivery mechanism. In this position it is impossible to detach the prosthesis from the pin-sleeve linkage. The two wires are carried within a catheter sheath with a 15 mm thin-wall metal tube pod at the tip. This pod serves as a receptacle for the collapsed prosthesis. The opposite end of the carrying catheter is sealed by a 0 ring and has a side arm that permits flushing of the carrying catheter to prevent air embolization and accumulation of blood in the system. Figure 6 is a schematic representation of the system.

Clinical Implantation. The procedure is performed in the cardiac catheterization laboratory. The patient is sedated with morphine (0.1 mg per kg) and pentobarbital (4 mg per kg). General anesthesia is *not* used. Biplane aortograms are obtained in the posteroanterior and lateral views to demonstrate the location, size, and shape of the ductus. Review of over 100 aortograms has shown that the ductus is almost always superimposed upon the tracheal

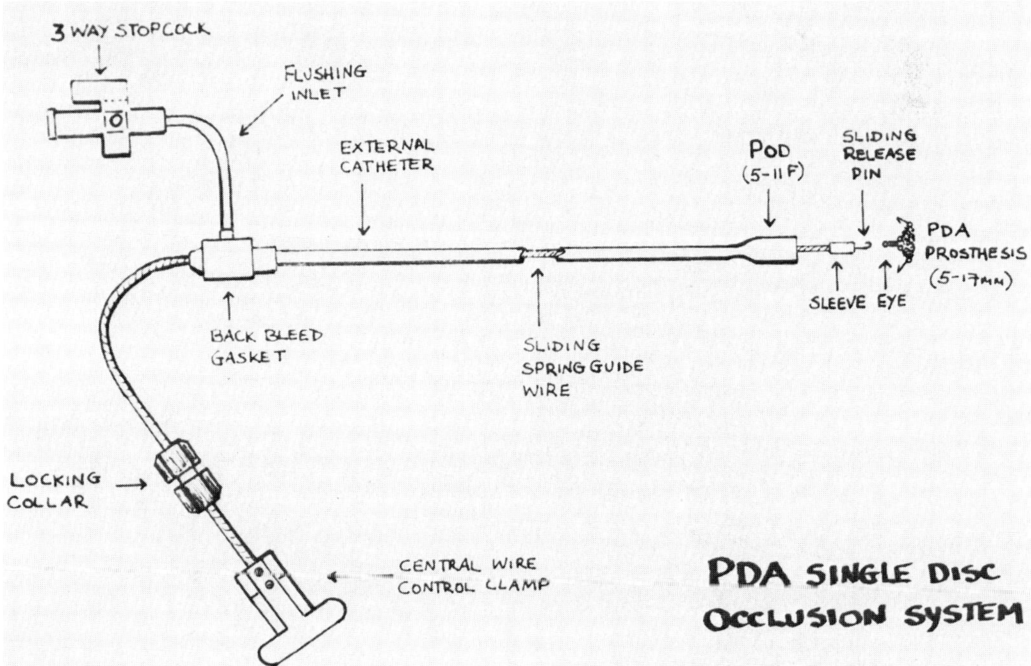

Figure 6. This is a diagrammatic illustration of the patent ductus arteriosus hooked prosthesis occlusion system.

shadow in the lateral view. Heparinization (50 mg per kg) is started. The prosthesis, inside the delivery system, is introduced into the femoral artery, passed retrograde into the thoracic aorta, and manipulated into the ductus arteriosus. The prosthesis is extruded from the catheter and allowed to expand in the ductus. Gentle but firm traction on the carrying device is used to imbed the hooks into the wall of the ductus. When the prosthesis is properly and firmly seated, the transporting catheter system is detached and removed from the femoral artery. Heparinization (50 mg per kg q6 h) is continued for 48 hours. Portable anteroposterior and lateral chest films are taken every 12 hours after the patient leaves the cardiac catheterization laboratory. The patient is discharged from the hospital usually on the third to fourth postprocedure day.

Results

Twenty patients were included in the study. No attempt was made on three of the patients, because sizing of their defects by balloon catheter indicated that they were too large to close by this method. There were seven failures or incomplete closures. Six of these patients have had uneventful surgical closure of their defects. Ten patients have had successful and com-

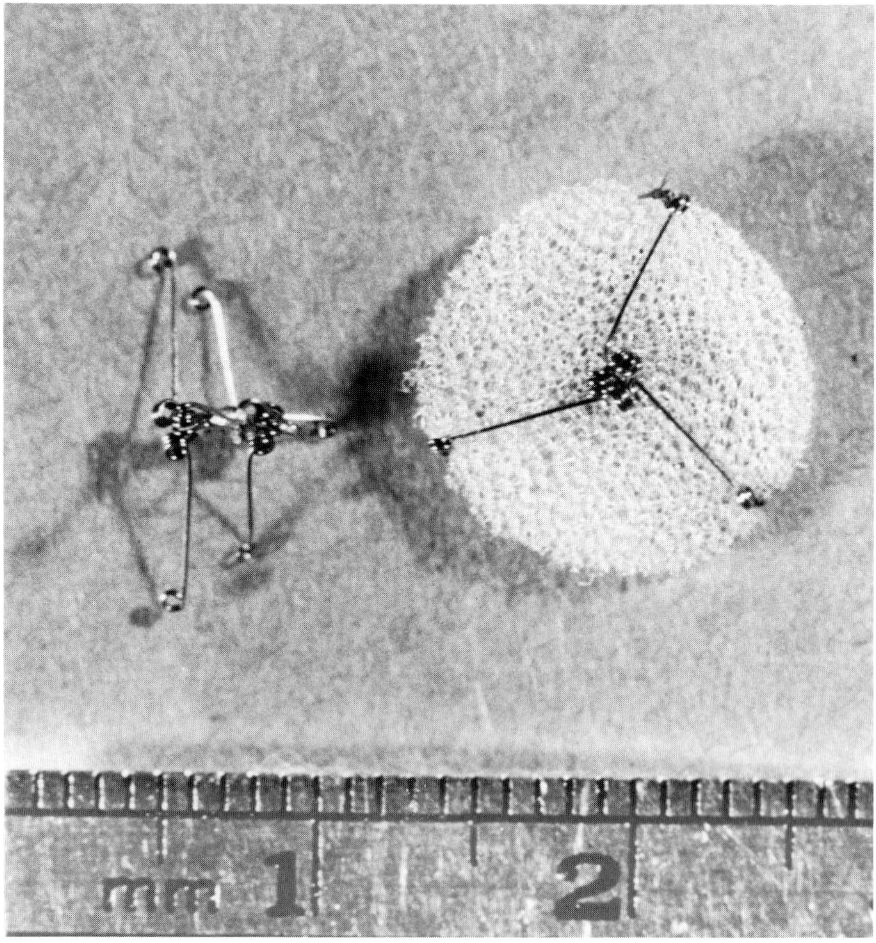

Figure 7. This is a photograph of two double-disc, hookless patent ductus arteriosus occlusion prostheses. On the left, in profile, a bare skeleton; and on the right, a foam disc-covered prosthesis.

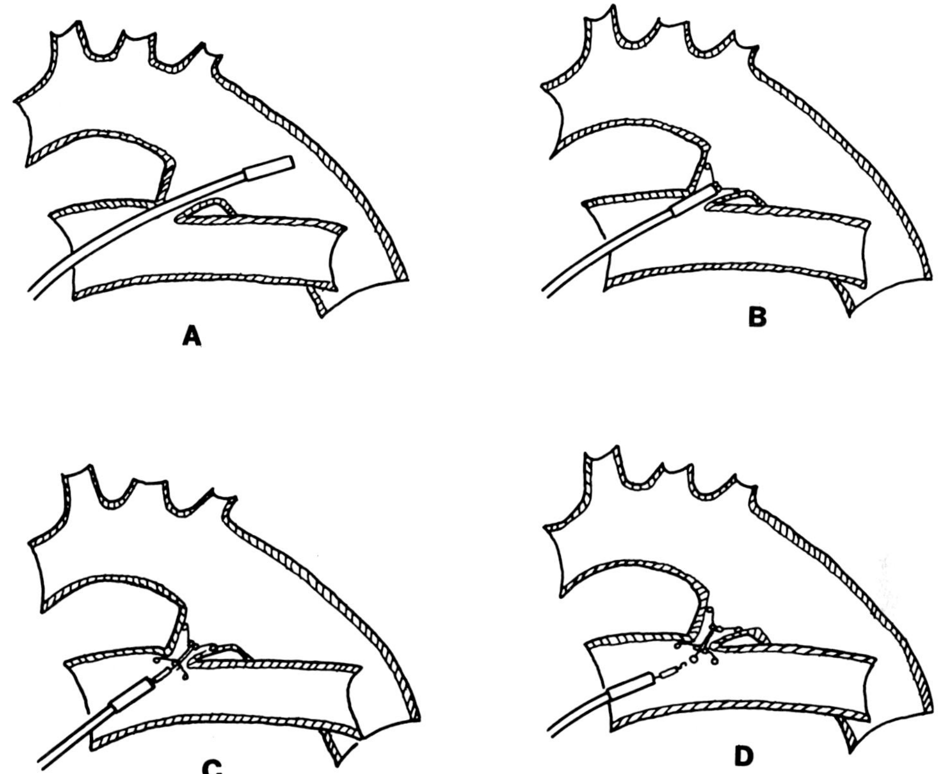

Figure 8. This is a diagrammatic illustration of the emplacement of the double-disc ductus occlusion prosthesis.

plete occlusion of their ductus by this technique. Thus, of the seventeen patients considered suitable for an attempt at transcatheter closure, the success rate has been 60 percent.

The system was redesigned to permit the use of the double-disc, nonhooked prosthesis that could be passed via the pulmonary artery into the aorta and anchored by extruding the first disc in the aorta, pulling it back until it bent on itself in the funnel-shaped ductus, then pulling the pod off the aftercoming disc until it anchored onto the pulmonary artery side of the ductus. The device (Fig. 7) could then be disconnected. This system has had complete animal testing, and early clinical trials are encouraging. Of eight patients admitted to the study, three were too large to attempt, four have been closed completely, and one has had incomplete closure. Figure 8 is a schematic representation of the implantation sequence.

The patients in the ductus study ranged in age from 1 month to 13 years. Their weights ranged from 2.4 kg to 40 kg.

BALLOON ANGIOPLASTY

Percutaneous transluminal dilatation (balloon angioplasty) techniques in the recanalization of arteriosclerotic obstructions and the dilatation of vascular stenosis have been applied to peripheral, coronary, renal, visceral, and vertebral arteries, and the abdominal aorta. First introduced by Dotter and Judkins in 1964[16] and later modified by Gruntzig in 1974[17] and again in 1979,[18] this procedure has become a recognized adjunct to the management of atheromatous disease, primarily in adults. Modifications of the technique have been applied to nonatherosclerotic disease, including congenital stenotic lesions, in adults and children. Martin and coworkers[19] reported the results of percutaneous transluminal angioplasty in 14 patients with various lesions such as fibromuscular dysplasia, Takayasu arteritis, neurofibromatosis, surgical anastomoses, and arteriovenous fistulae. The principal current usage in pediatrics is for dilation of pulmonic valve stenosis, recoarctation of the aorta, and peripheral pulmonary artery stenosis.

COARCTATION OF THE AORTA

Sos and associates[20] suggested application of the balloon angioplasty technique to the discrete type of coarctation of the aorta and tested it on postmortem specimens. Lock and colleagues[21] extended Sos's work to excised aortic coarctations from six children who underwent resections and reanastomoses. Dilatation was attempted within 2 hours of resection using a Gruntzig polyvinyl chloride catheter. Encouraged by their data on specimens, they created an animal model of coarctation and were successful in dilating these in vivo.[22] They and several other authors have found the method to be of dubious value in the primary treatment of coarctation but of definite help in patients with recoarctation. Lock suggests high inflation pressures are necessary, using a balloon with a maximum diameter up to 1.5 times the diameter of the aorta proximal to the coarctation.

PULMONIC STENOSIS

Kan and coworkers[23] reported the experimental basis for balloon valvoplasty for pulmonary valve stenosis. Kan and other coworkers[24,25] reported early clinical trials with very encouraging results. Other groups have performed the procedure and have described favorable results to me. At the time of this writing, the cases reported in the literature (primarily from Kan's Johns Hopkins group) and others reported by personal communication bring the total to about 25 patients.

PERIPHERAL PULMONIC STENOSIS AND HYPOPLASTIC PULMONARY ARTERIES

Lock and associates[26] have described the experimental approach to this problem. They created an animal model in the newborn lamb and achieved good results in dilating branch stenoses. They have also reported early clinical trials with satisfactory initial results.[27] In addition, they have had some fascinating success in dilating hypoplastic pulmonary arteries. A few of the vessels they have succeeded in dilating are past the hilum of the lung and therefore beyond surgical access. This technique offers some hope to children who currently are labelled inoperable.

EMBOLIZATION PROCEDURES

Early work in this area involved the injection of plastic spheres in an attempt to occlude inoperable cerebral arteriovenous malformations.[28] Silicone polymers, polyvinyl alcohol spheres, and detachable balloons were also tried for these defects. White and associates[29] have treated a wide variety of lesions with detachable balloons, with particular emphasis on pulmonary arteriovenous fistulae. In addition to the work of White and his Johns Hopkins group, many other investigators have performed vascular occlusions for pulmonary and peripheral systemic arteriovenous malformations, including cerebral, renal, pelvic, spinal, and abdominal lesions. Publications on these subjects have been far too numerous to recount here. Of particular interest in pediatric cardiology has been the occlusion of large aortico-pulmonary collaterals. White has used detachable balloons for this purpose. Zuberbuhler and associates[30] have described the instillation of methyl methacrylate, and several authors have used the steel coils originally described by Gianturco and coworkers.[31] Clearly, embolization methods—whether using detachable balloons, coils, polyvinyl alcohol pellets, methyl methacrylate, or other types of injectable or detachable materials—are being used with increasing frequency for a wide variety of lesions, either to simplify subsequent surgery or to eliminate the need for surgery completely.

FOREIGN BODY RETRIEVAL

The first description of retrieval of a foreign body from the cardiovascular system was by Thomas and colleagues[32] in 1964, using a special forceps. Massumi and Ross[33] used a simple catheter-wire snare device in 1967, and I described a simple modification for use in children in 1969.[34] Our group has subsequently used a ureteral basket snare to retrieve a variety of foreign bodies from the heart and great vessels in over 25 children. A complete review of the wide variety of devices used to retrieve all sorts of intravascular and intracardiac foreign bodies is beyond the scope of this chapter. An excellent and comprehensive summary has been provided by Bloomfield.[35]

SUMMARY

Cardiac catheterization has proved its value as a major tool in the diagnosis of congenital cardiac defects. The advent of noninvasive imaging of various sorts has altered the role of diagnostic catheterization. Within the past two decades, cardiac catheter instruments to provide therapy have been applied to many lesions. Improvements in design and methods will expand the use of therapeutic catheterization. It is inevitable that better results will be obtained for those defects currently being treated that way, and undoubtedly the method will be applied to other conditions. These developments should continue to cement the relationship between pediatric cardiologists and cardiovascular surgeons. As balloon atrioseptostomy led to more "corrective" operations for transposition patients, so these new techniques will lead to less frequent use of that regrettable term, *inoperable.*

REFERENCES

1. Dieffenbach, JF: *Physiologisch-Chirurgisch Beobachtigen die Cholera-Kraken.* Cholera Arch 1:86, 1832.
2. Bleichroeder, F, Unger, E, and Loeb, W: *Intraarterielle therapy.* Klin Wochenschr 49:1502, 1912.
3. Forssman, WTO: *Die sondierung des rechten Herzens.* Klin Wochenschr 8:2085, 1929.
4. Cournand, A, Baldwin, JS, and Himmelstein, A: *Cardiac Catheterization in Congenital Heart Disease.* The Commonwealth Fund, New York, 1949.
5. Rubeo-Alvarez, V and Limon-Lason: *Treatment of pulmonary valvular stenosis and tricuspid stenosis with a modified cardiac catheter.* Proc First National Conference on Cardiovascular Disease, Washington, D.C., 1950.
6. Rashkind, WJ and Miller, WW: *Creation of an atrial septal defect without thoracotomy.* JAMA 196:991 1966.
7. Rashkind, WJ: *Transcatheter treatment of congenital heart disease.* Circulation 67:711, 1983.
8. Park, SC, Neches, WH, Zuberbuhler, JR, et al: *Clinical use of blade atrial septostomy.* Circulation (Suppl. III):172, 1977.
9. King, TD, et al: *Secundum atrial septal defect: Non operative closure during cardiac catheterization.* JAMA 235:2506 1976.
10. Munro, JC: *Ligation of the ductus arteriosus.* Ann Surg 46:335, 1907.
11. Graybiel, A, Streider, JW, and Boyer, NH: *An attempt to obliterate patent ductus arteriosus; in patients with subacute bacterial endarteritis.* Am Heart J 15:621, 1938.
12. Gross, RE and Hubbard, JP: *Surgical ligation of a patent ductus arteriosus: Report of first successful case.* JAMA 112:729, 1939.
13. Porstmann, W, Wierny, L, and Warnke, H: *Closure of persistent ductus arteriosus without thoracotomy.* Thoraxchirurgie 15:199, 1967.
14. Porstmann, W: Personal communication, 1981.

15. Rashkind, WJ and Cuaso, CC: *Transcatheter closure of patent ductus arteriosus. Successful use in a 3.5 kilogram infant.* Pediatr Cardiol 1:3, 1979.

16. Dotter, CT and Judkins, MP. *Transluminal treatment of arteriosclerotic obstruction: Description of a new technic and a preliminary report of its application.*. Circulation 30:654, 1964.

17. Gruntzig, AR: *Die perkutane Rekanalisation chronischer arterieller Verschlusse (Dotter-Princip) met einem doppellumigen Dilatations-katheter.* Fortschr Rontgenstr 124:80, 1976.

18. Gruntzig, AR: *Perkutane dilatation von Coronarstenosen—Beschreibung eines neuen Kathetersystems.* Klin Wochenschr 54:543, 1976.

19. Martin, ED, Diamond, NG, and Casarella, WJ: *Percutaneous transluminal angioplasty in non-atherosclerotic disease.* Radiology 135:27, 1980.

20. Sos, T, Sniderman, KW, Rettek-Sos, B, et al: *Percutaneous transluminal dilatation of coarctation of thoracic aorta post mortem.* Lancet 2:970, 1979.

21. Lock, JE, Castaneda-Zuniga, WR, Bass, JF, et al: *Balloon dilatation of excised aortic coarctation.* Radiology 143:689, 1982.

22. Lock, JE, Niemi, T, Burke, BA, et al: *Transcutaneous angioplasty of experimental aortic coarctation.* Circulation 66:1280, 1982.

23. Kan, JS, Anderson, JH, and White, RI Jr: *Experimental basis for balloon valvuloplasty of congenital pulmonary valvular stenosis.* Proc Sect Cardiol Amer Acad Ped, New York, p 101A, October 1982.

24. Kan, JS, White, RI Jr, Mitchell, SE, et al: *Percutaneous balloon valvuloplasty: A new method for treating congenital pulmonary valve stenosis.* N Engl J Med 307:540, 1982.

25. Kan, JS, White, RI Jr, Mitchell, SE, et al: *Transluminal balloon valvuloplasty for the treatment of congenital pulmonary valve stenosis.* J Am Coll Cardiol 2:588, 1983.

26. Lock, JE, Neimi, BA, Einzig, S, et al: *Transvenous angioplasty of experimental branch pulmonary artery stenosis in newborn lambs.* Circulation 64:886, 1981.

27. Lock, JE, Castaneda-Zuniga, WF, Fuhrman, BP, et al: *Balloon dilation angioplasty of hypoplastic and stenotic pulmonary arteries.* J Am Coll Cardiol 2:588, 1983.

28. Luessenhop, AJ, Kachmann, R, Shevlin, W, et al: *Clinical evaluation of artificial embolization in the management of large cerebral arteriovenous malformations.* J Neurosurg 23:400, 1965.

29. White, RI Jr, ursic, TA, Kaufman, SL, et al: *Therapeutic embolization with detachable balloons.* Radiology 126:521, 1978.

30. Zuberbuhler, JR, Dankner, E, Zoltun, R, et al: *Tissue adhesive closure of aortic-pulmonary communications.* Am Heart J 88:41, 1974.

31. Gianturco, C, Anderson, JH, and Wallace, S: *Mechanical devices for arterial occlusion.* Am J Roentgenol 124:428, 1975.

32. Thomas, J, Sinclair-Smith, B, Bloomfield, D, et al: *Non-surgical retrieval of a broken segment of steel spring guide from the right atrium and inferior vena cava.* Circulation 30:106, 1964.

33. Massumi, RA and Ross, AM: *A traumatic, nonsurgical technic for removal of broken catheters from cardiac cavities.* N Engl J Med 277:195, 1967.

34. Rashkind, WJ: *A cardiac catheter device for removal of plastic catheter emboli from children's hearts.* J Pediatr 74:618, 1969.

35. Bloomfield, DA: *The nonsurgical retrieval of intracardiac foreign bodies—an international survey.* Cathet Cardiovasc Diagn 4:1, 1978.

Digital Subtraction Angiography in the Evaluation of Cardiac Disease

Edwin L. Alderman, M.D., and Diana F. Guthaner, M.D.

The use of temporal subtraction techniques in vascular diagnosis has been popular for image enhancement since the implementation of cut film techniques in the 1950s. Typically, a vascular structure, opacified with contrast, is obscured by overlying bony structures or soft tissue motion artifact. A mask, that is, an image without contrast (taken immediately prior to or after the contrast injection), can be subtracted from the contrast image. The resultant image recorded on film demonstrates substantially enhanced visualization of the contrast-filled vessel with cancellation of the relatively "noisy" background of overlapping heterogeneous tissue densities. However, misregistration of body structures because of involuntary motion such as swallowing or respiration which may occur during the time interval between the two images results in prominent artifacts.

Film subtraction offered little flexibility and could not deal with dynamically moving objects such as the heart. However, the development of digital systems allows the images to

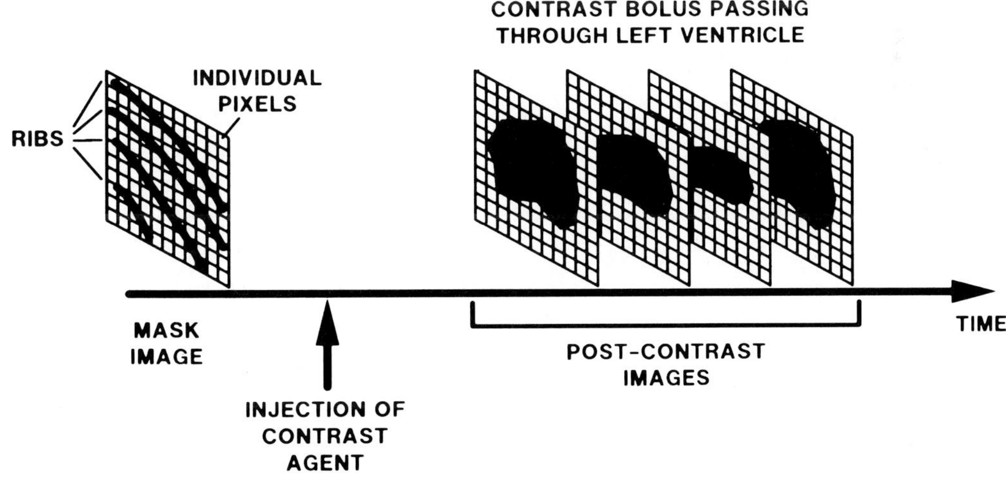

Figure 1. Digitized images are recorded in sub-units referred to as pixels. The mask image containing no contrast displays ribs as bone density and the heart as tissue (water) density. As an intravenously injected bolus of contrast passes through the left ventricle, the difference between the mask image and the sequence of post-contrast images eliminates overlying bone density, permitting visualization of the contrast-filled left ventricle.

be subdivided into a horizontal and vertical array of discrete picture elements called pixels. The brightness of each pixel is assigned a digital value for computer subtraction of the mask by the computer.[1,2] Figure 1 shows schematically how the contrast-filled left ventricle seen on a sequence of frames can be enhanced by serial subtraction of a mask image containing no contrast. Rapid subtraction is accomplished by a digital image processor that can store two or more digitized images, the corresponding pixels of which are arithmetically subtracted and the resultant image displayed. Image array processors require a substantial amount of digital memory, because a single image can be subdivided into 512 horizontal and 512 vertical pixels (512 × 512) necessitating 262,144 words of solid-state memory to store a single image. Over the past 10 years there has been an exponential increase in the number of bits of memory contained in a single memory chip, with current 64K (65,536) bit memory chips costing less than $10.00 each. It is largely the substantial and continuing reductions in cost and increasing capacity of solid-state and mass-memory devices that have permitted the rapid development of digital subtraction.

The advantages of digital subtraction angiography (DSA) over previous film subtraction methods are increased flexibility, accuracy and speed in the subtraction process, the ability to manipulate and to weight the subtraction process using complex algorithms, and the capability to make dimensional and densitometric measurements on individual or sequential images.

FUNCTIONAL COMPONENTS OF A DIGITAL SUBTRACTION ANGIOGRAPHY SYSTEM

The increasing sophistication of DSA systems for cardiac applications necessitates an understanding of its critical components. The radiographic system that provides images of the left ventricle and coronary arteries may be viewed as an imaging chain. Each component of

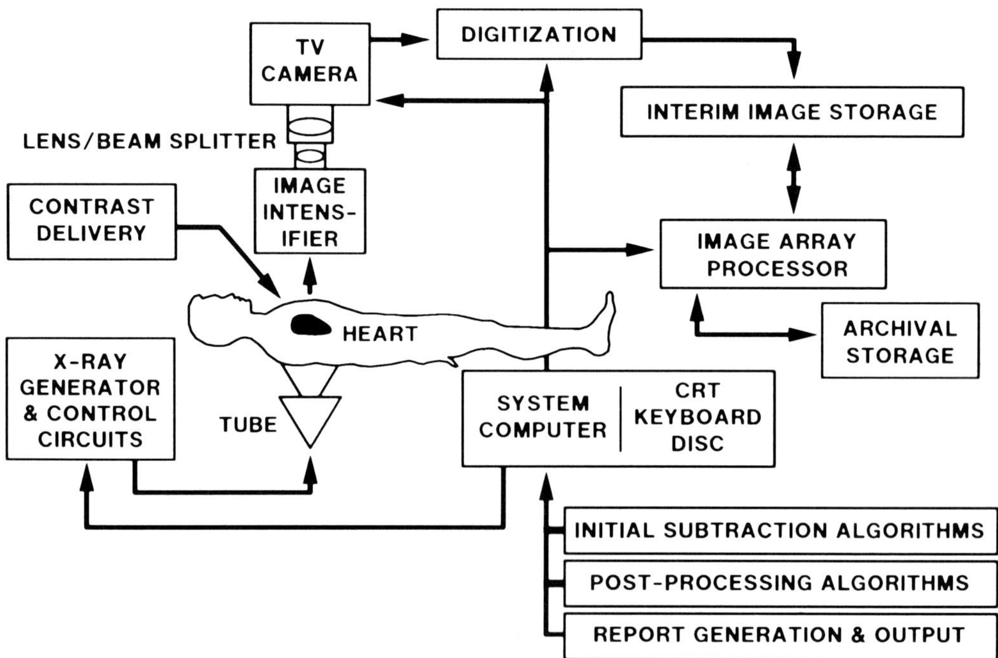

Figure 2. Each of the functional components required for digital subtraction angiography is shown in its diagrammatic relationship.

the chain is important. Any single weak link leads to degradation of the image quality. The modern-day radiographic chain includes the x-ray generator, control circuits, x-ray tube, table, the image intensifier, beam splitter, lens, cine camera, cine film, film processing, and finally, the cine projector. DSA requires the same radiographic imaging chain. However, cine film recording of the image is replaced by a video camera which allows processing using computer hardware, associated peripherals, and program logic (or software). Each of these components is diagrammed in Figure 2. Tables 1 to 6 enumerate the important features or design considerations that are applicable for cardiac DSA.

X-ray Generator, Controls, and Tube

Existing x-ray systems can operate in three modes (Table 1). Standard continuous fluoroscopy is limited by state and federal safety standards to relatively low level of x-ray exposure. However, the signal-to-noise ratio (that is, image structural content to random background noise) is known to be proportional to increases in x-ray dose. Thus, one potential operational mode for DSA systems is use of continuous fluoroscopy (normally 1 to 4 ma) but with boosted x-ray output, generally to the 15 to 20 ma range.

In the radiographic mode, x-ray pulses lasting $\frac{1}{20}$ to $\frac{1}{6}$ of a second are used to expose cut films which are rapidly replaced in automatic mechanical film-changing devices. The x-ray equipment control circuits for the radiographic mode are relatively uncomplicated relays permitting convenient interface with the DSA control computer. However, the duration and intensity of the x-ray pulses are such that most generators and x-ray tube heat capacities will not permit pulsing at rates greater than 6 to 10 per second.

For exposure of a 35 mm cine film (cine mode), 2 to 10 millisecond pulses are delivered to the x-ray tube at rates of 60 pulses per second or more. An image intensifier that electronically amplifies the x-ray image permits a substantially lower dose of x-rays per pulse than does the radiographic mode in which the x-ray photons directly expose the film. This mode would seem ideal for DSA. However, control circuits for cine pulse generators are much more

Table 1. DSA system components

X-RAY GENERATOR, CONTROLS AND TUBE
Choice of operational mode
Continuous boosted fluoroscopy
Radiographic mode
Cine pulse mode
Operates under DSA computer control
X-ray tube heat capacity (focal spot size)
Duration of x-ray pulse
Add-on vs dedicated system
Dual energy x-ray source (alternating generator)
CONTRAST DELIVERY
Site of contrast bolus delivery (intravenous; intra-arterial)
Dose and rate of administration
Contrast limitations—allergy; dose restrictions
Integrity of bolus—tricuspid regurgitation; heart failure
CARDIAC POSITION (misregistration artifacts)
Extraneous voluntary and involuntary motion
Thoracic motion (respiration; body motion; panning)
Cardiac motion (ECG gating)
Overlapping structures

complex than required in the radiographic mode. Because x-ray tube pulsing for cine film recording must be tightly linked to the motion of film through the cine camera, the system is relatively intolerant of externally imposed control and is thus difficult to link to DSA systems.

It is these and other aspects of existing radiographic systems that make the distinction between an "add on" DSA system versus a dedicated system. The necessity that a digital system control x-ray pulsing requires an electronic interface between the DSA computer and the x-ray control circuits. Although clearly there are cost advantages to adding a digital system to an existing radiographic chain, it is probable that dedicated systems in which the generator, x-ray tube, and imaging chain are designed primarily for digital processing will ultimately result in higher-quality images.

A potentially important development in x-ray generator and tube design is the production of two different x-ray photon energies (high and low kilovoltage [KV]) to generate two separate digitized images. Because the x-ray attenuation coefficients for air, fat, tissue, and bone are different for different x-ray photon energies, it is possible to compute, for each pixel location, its relative tissue composition and to create subtracted images that exclude either overlapping bone or soft tissue density from iodine density. This technique of dual energy subtraction necessitates a specialized alternating x-ray generator and is the subject of continuing academic and commercial investigation.

Contrast Delivery

The site, dose, and rate of contrast administration determine the concentration of contrast media that reaches the structure of interest (see Table 1). In the development of cardiac DSA

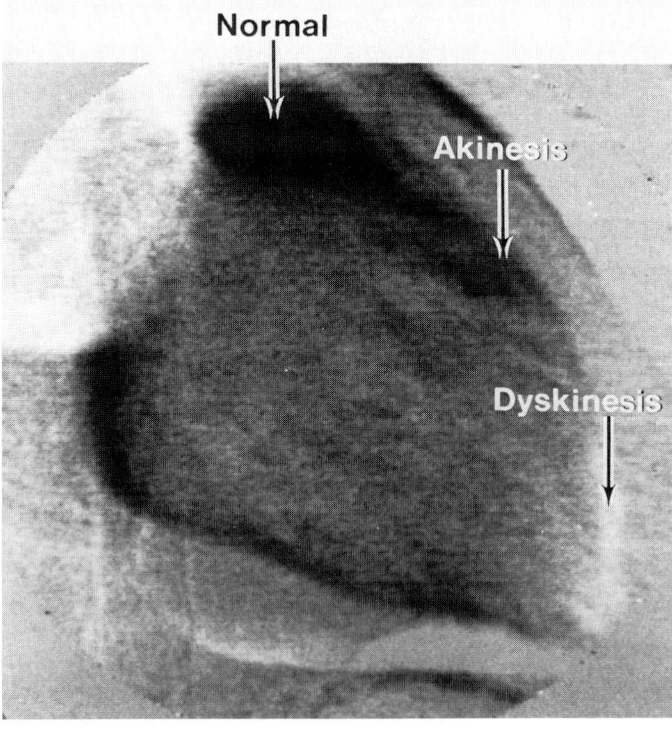

Figure 3. The technique of time-interval differencing is shown in a patient who received 40 ml of 76 percent contrast into the superior vena cava. During the levo phase adjacent end-diastolic and end-systolic frames were selected for differencing against each other. Systolic excursion of the left ventricular wall at the inferior and anterior basal portions of the ventricle produces a blackened area, whereas apical dyskinesis produces a white area. This technique helps amplify and visualize wall motion abnormalities.

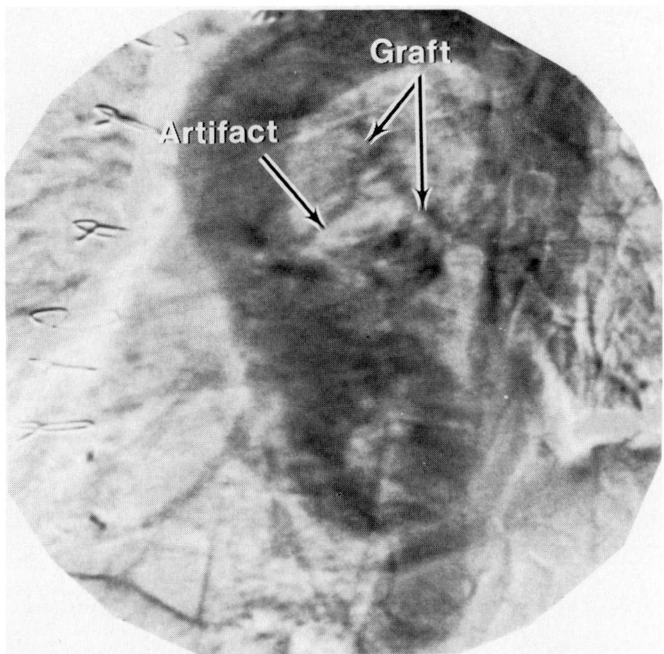

Figure 4. Forty ml of 76 percent Renografin was administered into the superior vena cava. Levo phase visualization of the aorta and mediastinum in the left anterior oblique projection displays the proximal portions of a graft supplying a diagonal artery. Additional grafts to the right coronary artery and the left anterior descending artery are only marginally visualized. Misregistration artifacts caused by minor motion of thoracic and pulmonary vascular structures are responsible for most of the linear densities.

as a "noninvasive" or outpatient screening test, contrast is typically administered via a small indwelling catheter into an antecubital vein, the superior vena cava, or inferior vena cava. Typically, for visualization of the left ventricle and aorta, 40 ml of 76 percent Renografin are injected over a span of 2 seconds (Figs. 3, 4). The use of side-hole or pigtail catheters avoids complications of extravasation and venous perforation.

However, the greater the distance of contrast administration from the left ventricle, the more dilute will become the bolus, thus decreasing opacification and necessitating higher doses for adequate visualization. Multiple boluses of contrast are necessitated if different projections are required or if the effect of interventions on left ventricular performance is to be assessed. Moreover, intravenous injections may be adversely affected by tricuspid regurgitation, advanced heart failure, and cardiomegaly, all of which tend to decrease the peak contrast concentration reaching the left ventricle.

Another approach is to use DSA as an adjunct to selective intra-arterial angiography. For example, selective visualization of the left ventricle or aortic root, which customarily necessitates 40 to 50 ml of contrast administered over 2 to 3 seconds, can be accomplished with as little as 10 to 15 ml of contrast diluted to an equivalent volume (40 to 50 ml) (Fig. 5). Thus, DSA as an adjunct to intra-arterial contrast administration offers the advantage of reducing contrast load.

Cardiac Position

It is a basic assumption of DSA that pixels to be subtracted will remain in spatial registration on adjacent frames. This is more easily accomplished for stationary peripheral arteries. However, a combination of thoracic and cardiac motion produces what are referred to as "misregistration artifacts" and constitutes the single most important factor degrading DSA

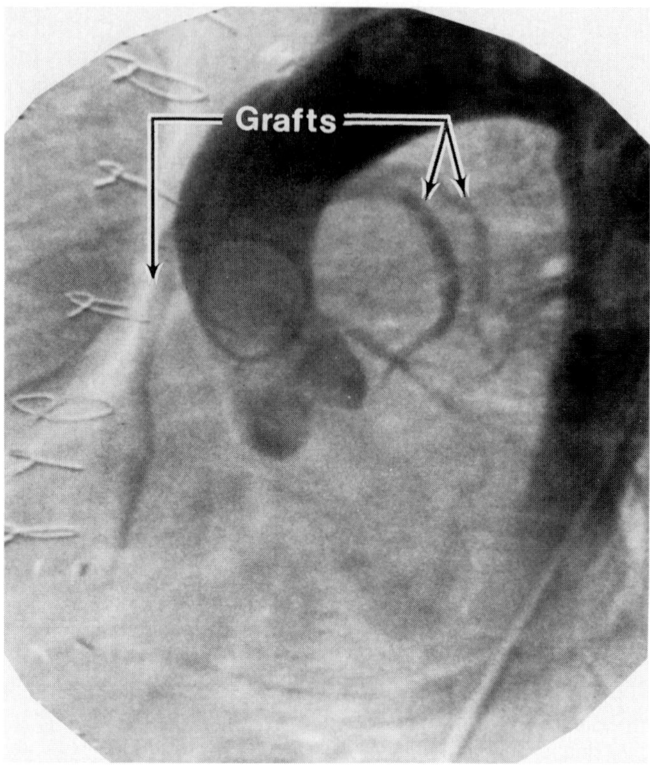

Figure 5. Forty ml of diluted contrast was administered via pigtail catheter into the aortic root of the same patient shown in Figure 4. Three grafts are readily visible. Image contrast was enhanced by subtraction using a blurred mask.

images of the chest (see Table 1). Figure 6 (*bottom*) shows slight misregistration of sternal sutures and the diaphragm resulting from slight motion of the thorax with respiration. Superimposed vascular and bony structures tend to move with body motion and respiration and, when subtracted on adjacent frames, lead to a variety of artifacts, that is, misregistration artifacts. The motion of an uncooperative patient or movement of the table in order to pan over structures of interest violates the requirement for a stationary object. Electrocardiogram (ECG) gating techniques are now being successfully applied in order to reduce the artifact produced by motion of the heart.

Image Intensifier

All DSA systems require an image intensifier of the highest possible contrast and spatial resolution (Table 2). Cesium iodide intensifiers have become standard in radiographic systems. The image area should be adequate to cover the field of interest. Because the DSA technique results in a substantial increase in the dynamic range between black and white portions of the picture, it is necessary to provide greater uniformity of image density in the non-contrast-containing image. Typically, filters (aluminum sheets of variable shapes and thicknesses) are carefully positioned over the x-ray port so as to attenuate "brightness" in or adjacent to the area of interest. This requirement, in part, results from expansion of the dynamic range resulting from the subtraction process. Areas of inadequate brightness and areas of too much brightness or oversaturation in the images acquired before subtraction will show loss of image content after subtraction.

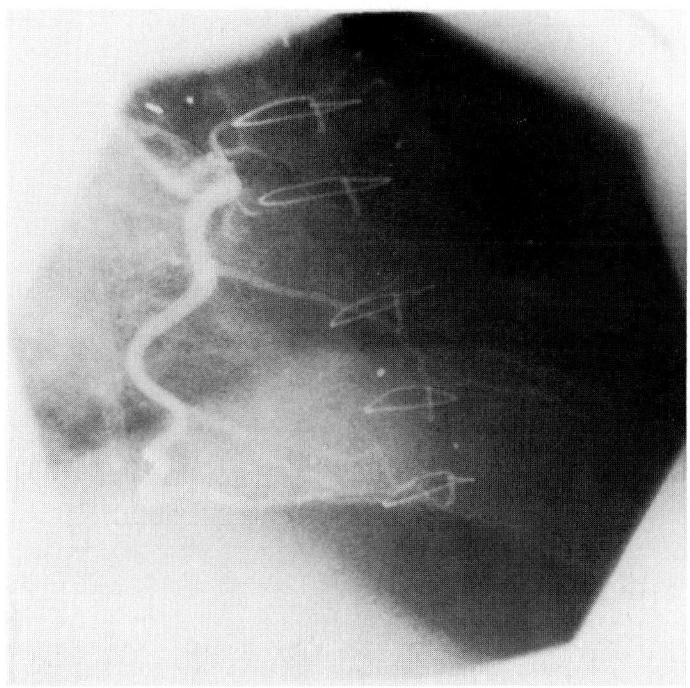

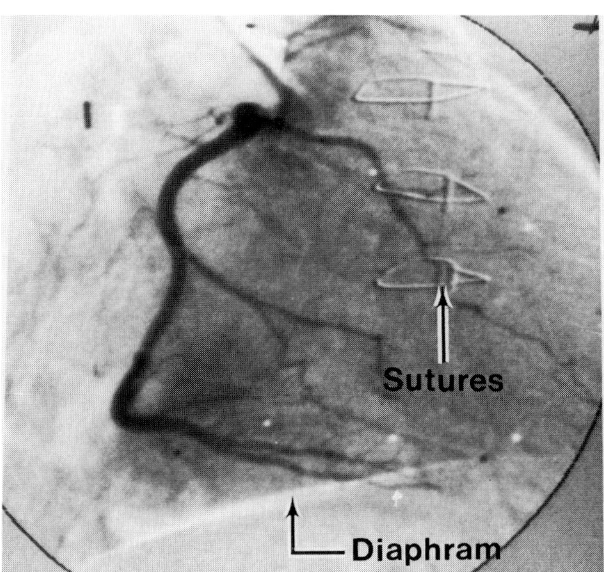

Figure 6. *Top*, This is a cine film recording of a selective right coronary artery injection using standard technique. *Bottom*, The result of an identical right coronary selective injection is shown; however, subtraction of a blurred mask obtained several cardiac cycles earlier has enhanced contrast of the vessel. Small misregistration artifacts associated with the metallic sternal sutures and diaphragm motion are apparent.

Table 2. DSA system components

IMAGE INTENSIFIER
High contrast, high spatial resolution
Adequate field of view
Uniformity of image density over area of interest
VIDEO CAMERA, LENS AND LIGHT DISTRIBUTOR
Lens and aperture control
Light distributor (beam splitter) control
High signal-to-noise ratio video camera (1000/1)
Composition and size of plumbicon target
Progressive scanning
Variable scanning rate
DIGITIZATION
Pixel density/spatial resolution (256 × 256; 512 × 512; 1024 × 1024)
Grey scale (number of significant bits)
Linear vs log amplification
Location in relation to video camera

Video Camera, Lens and Light Distributor

The light distributor, or beam splitter, in present catheterization/angiographic laboratories has been designed primarily with cine angiographic work in mind (see Table 2). Thus, during cine exposures, the mirrors contained within the light distributor send approximately 10 percent of the light to the video camera and 90 percent to the cine film camera. The implementation of a digital system is optimized by directing 100 percent of available light from the image intensifier to the video camera in order to maximize the signal-to-noise ratio. Moreover, radiographic systems include an aperture that regulates the light reaching the television camera. In order to ensure that images for digital subtraction are within the dynamic range of the video camera, the DSA system computer must have automatic control over the aperture in order to adjust the light intensity reaching the camera.

The television camera itself is of a special composition, typically a plumbicon-type target that is noted for high resolution and excellent signal-to-noise ratio. The typical video camera used for standard fluoroscopy and which is supplied by x-ray equipment manufacturers has a signal-to-noise ratio in the range of 200:1 to 500:1. More expensive, higher-quality plumbicon cameras with 1000:1 signal-to-noise ratios are customarily required for DSA. The resolution of the video camera depends upon not only the composition of the target that is scanned by the electron beam but also the size of the target. Scanning of this target is typically triggered by the DSA system computer which initiates progressive line-by-line scanning to follow the x-ray pulse at an appropriate interval. Standard video cameras typically scan alternate horizontal lines, filling in the intervening lines during a second pass (interlacing two fields to constitute a single frame). Because passage of a contrast bolus through a structure of interest would lead to different densities in the two interlaced fields, it is typically necessary to use a video camera that progressively scans all lines in sequence in order to generate a single-image frame. The scanning rate is adjusted to match the particular mode of x-ray pulsing.

Digitization

The conversion of each pixel from an analog gray scale level to digital bits can now be accomplished at sufficient speed to cope with pixel densities of 512 × 512 acquired at 30 frames per second (7.5 million pixel digitizations per second) (see Table 2). The quality of gray scale digitization is determined by the number of bits associated with each pixel; 8 bits can store 64 shades of gray, and 10 bits can provide 256 shades of gray. The number of horizontal and vertical pixels in conjunction with the size of the image intensifier field determines spatial resolution. The manner of digitization must also take into account the fact that tissue absorption of x-ray photons is not linearly but logarithmically proportional to the amount of tissue through which the x-ray has passed. An additional concern is the distance of the digitization process from the video camera, which may add artifact in electrically noisy environments.

Interim Storage

In order for the image processor, which does the actual subtraction, to function efficiently, an interim image storage device must be provided that has a very high-speed communication link with the image processor (Table 3). Storage of digitized images is very demanding in terms of total memory. There is general concurrence that present and future systems require recording capability that can absorb digital data at the high frame rates required for cardiac DSA. Table 4 summarizes image storage requirements for cardiac DSA systems. A 256 × 256 pixel frame requires 64,536 words of memory, which is 4 times the requirement for 128 × 128 pixel frames. Optimal visualization of the left ventricle during angiography usually necessitates a pixel matrix of 256 × 256. In order to resolve details of wall motion, imaging at 30 frames per second for a typical intra-arterial study lasting 8 seconds would require about 16 million words (16 megabytes) of memory for the single study. For intravenous contrast administration with the left ventricle as the area of interest, a 10-second exposure duration

Table 3. DSA system components

INTERIM STORAGE
Digital storage
Storage capacity
Record rate
Playback rate
Direct storage vs packing algorithm
Evolving disk technology (multihead, laser read/write)
IMAGE ARRAY PROCESSOR
Processing speed
Access time to interim image storage
Number of internal video frames accessible for mathematical processing
SYSTEM COMPUTER
Multi-task capability
CRT terminal with special function keys
System computer interfaces with x-ray system, contrast delivery, TV camera, digitization, image array processor, interim and archival image storage devices
User control over digital procedure functions
Ease of user interaction with system
Special devices (e.g., joy stick, track ball, and so forth)
Documentation
System reliability
Maintenance and service
Modularity of software components
Space, cooling and acoustic considerations

Table 4. Storage requirements and characteristics of cardiac imaging modalities

	Typical Frame Rate	*Typical Pixel Resolution*	*Spatial Resolution in Line Pairs/ mm† (unless specified)*	*Bytes of Storage per Frame (K bytes)**	*No. of Seconds for Typical Study*	*Total Bytes of Storage per Patient Study (M bytes)*
INTRAVENOUS STUDY						
LV angio	30 fps	256 × 256	0.6	64k	10 sec‡	20 M bytes
	30 fps	128 × 128	0.3	16k		5 M bytes
INTRA-ARTERIAL STUDY						
LV angio (single plane)	30 fps	256 × 256	0.6	64k	8 sec	16 M bytes
Coronary angios	8 fps	512 × 512	1.7	256k	6 runs at 6 sec each	144 M bytes
	8 fps	1024 × 1024	3.3	1024k		574 M bytes
Vascular study (carotid or graft study)	4 fps	512 × 512	1.1	256k	2 runs at 8 sec each	16 M bytes
CINE FILM						
LV or coronary§	30–60 fps	—	2.5–3.5	—	6–8 sec	—
ECHOCARDIOGRAPHY						
(phased array)¶	30 fps	640 × 480	1.5 mm depth 3.4 mm lateral	—	unlimited	—
RADIONUCLIDE IMAGING						
LV (^{99}Te blood pool)	16 fps (gated)	64 × 64	2–4 cm	4K	250 sec	—

*Assumes 1 byte per pixel, although this will vary depending upon number of bits of grey level per single pixel and use of packing algorithms.
†Based on intensifier image area of 9 inches for LV and vascular angiography and 6 inches for coronary angiography.
‡Assumes only levo phase recording.
§Limit of image intensifier resolution owing to superimposed quantum mottle and cine film/projection system optics.
¶Acoustic frame rate; display screen pixel resolution; spatial resolution at 7.5 cm depth.

may be required (if the right heart and pulmonary phases were not recorded) with the resultant acquisition of 20 megabytes of digitized data.

The precise requirements for adequate selective coronary artery imaging using DSA have not yet been accepted; however, 8 frames per second recordings made with a 512 × 512 pixel matrix yield a spatial resolution of approximately 1.7 line pairs per millimeter (see Table 4). This spatial resolution is below the 2.5 to 3.5 line pairs per millimeter capability of most current high-performance image intensifiers and cine film systems. Increasing spatial resolution to 3.3 line pairs per millimeter would require a pixel matrix of 1024 × 1024 leading to four-fold increase in digital storage requirements from 262,144 words per frame to 1,048,576 words per frame. A 512 × 512 pixel density presently would require 144 megabytes of memory for an average coronary arteriogram that included a total of 6 runs at 6 seconds each for a total of 36 seconds.

As Table 4 points out, for each complete left ventricular (LV) and coronary angiographic patient study, 160 to 200 megabytes of digital memory would be required. As recently as five years ago, digital disks of such size would be prohibitively expensive; however, Winchester (hard disk) technology and the use of efficient packing algorithms have made high-speed recording and playback of this large mass of digitized video data possible. Most digital data disks use a single head moving radially at high speed across a rapidly spinning disk. However, the development of disks with multiple heads and laser video disks with both read and write (record) capability will facilitate the ability to record, to store, and to play back large numbers of digitized video frames. In the future the declining cost of solid-state memory may permit large arrays of digital chips to substitute for digital disks as the interim image storage device.

Image Array Processor

The image processor is the device that rapidly performs mathematical manipulations on large arrays of data stored in solid-state memory (see Table 3). The access time of the image processor to the interim digital video storage files and the number of frames accessible within the image processor are important determinants of the speed and complexity of image-processing algorithms.

System Control Computer

The system computer is responsible for overall operation of the DSA system (see Table 3). Typically, the system computer must interface and control the radiographic system, contrast delivery, the video camera, image digitization, the array processor, and the interim and archival image storage devices. Different types of DSA procedures necessitate differing setup parameters that must be either preselected or individually controllable. Technicians and physicians interacting with the system typically use a terminal with video screen, keyboard, multiple special-function keys, and optional specialized-control devices such as joy sticks or track balls. System documentation, reliability and availability of maintenance and service are important considerations. Caution must be exercised to avoid failure of the digital subtraction computer system adversely affecting the basic radiographic imaging chain. It is helpful if the computer system has multitask capability so that archiving and other administrative tasks can be carried out in background at the same time that image processing continues under user direction.

Initial Subtraction Algorithms

There are a variety of basic subtraction algorithms, each of which may be applicable in special circumstances (Table 5). The most common and standard subtraction method is referred to as temporal subtraction, or mask mode. As shown in Figure 1, a mask image, devoid of contrast, is acquired either prior to or following transit of contrast bolus through the region of interest. The mask can be acquired as an average composite of multiple sequential frames or can be acquired as an ECG-gated mask at specific times in relation to the cardiac cycle. The image or images containing contrast may be averaged together or may be sequentially differenced against the mask.

Time-interval differencing continuously acquires new masks maintaining a relatively short interval between the mask and subsequent image so that the change in contrast density, as

Table 5. DSA system components

INITIAL SUBTRACTION ALGORITHMS
Timing of mask in relation to contrast bolus
Mask composition (number of frames, gated, and so forth)
Types of subtraction
Temporal subtraction (mask mode)
Time interval differencing (short-term changes)
Gated subtraction
Dual energy subtraction (variation in tissue attenuation as function of KV)
Bandpass techniques (dynamic temporal algorithms)
Hybrid subtraction (combined temporal and dual energy)
POST-PROCESSING ALGORITHMS
Contrast enhancement
Noise suppression
Selective frame averaging and subtraction
Realignment of mask and image
Linear (global or micro)
Complex
Densitometric analyses

the bolus passes through the structure of interest, is shown. Figure 3, which shows differences between end-diastolic and end-systolic frames, shows interval loss of contrast as black and incremental contrast as white.

Band-pass techniques take advantage of the fact that the gradual rise and fall in contrast concentration passing through a particular structure has distinctly different temporal dynamics from the more rapid pixel density shifts resulting from motion associated with the cardiac cycle. Thus, artifacts resulting from motion related to the cardiac cycle can be excluded.

Dual energy subtraction utilizes two different KV x-ray photon energies to compute relative tissue composition at each pixel location based upon differences in tissue attenuation as a function of KV^3 so that either bone or soft tissue may be effectively removed. Hybrid subtraction combines the advantages of temporal subtraction (bone subtraction) and dual energy subtraction (soft tissue motion artifact subtraction) techniques.

Post-Processing Algorithms

The distinct advantage of computer-driven DSA in comparison with film subtraction is the ability to utilize a variety of complex post-acquisition reprocessing algorithms[4] (see Table 5). A large body of knowledge in the field of computer image processing already exists, which permits application of algorithms for contrast enhancement, noise suppression, and edge finding. Selected frames may be averaged and subtracted so that, depending upon relative motion, an alternate mask can be obtained either before or after the contrast injection. It is also possible to make small adjustments in the alignment of the mask and contrast-filled image. Pixel-by-pixel linear and rotational shifts can be helpful in eliminating misregistration artifacts. It is also possible to realign only small portions of the mask and image. Complex realignment algorithms referred to as "rubber sheeting" may be necessary to accommodate for rib, pulmonary vascular, and cardiac motions which are inherently nonlinear and complex. An additional strength of DSA is the fact that the gray scale values for each pixel are available on a frame-by-frame basis, permitting densitometric types of analyses. This type of data is similar to that available from radionuclide angiography and is of use in calculating left ventricular ejection fraction and in demonstrating differences in myocardial perfusion. Although the accuracy of quantitative densitometric measurements is limited by scatter and veiling glare, relative differences can be readily appreciated.

Report Generation and Output

An important part of any DSA system is analyses of the subtracted processed pictures to extract quantitative, functional, or hemodynamic data which comprise the final report (Table 6). For left ventriculography, the typical analyses include measurement of ejection fraction and quantitative assessment of regional wall motion based on manual or semiautomated definition of the endocardial silhouette. DSA systems typically use previously developed geometric computer algorithms (for example, area-length calculation of left ventricular ejection fraction) which have been developed for quantitating wall motion in contrast ventriculography. However, the availability of digitized pixel information permits additional densitometric assessment of global and regional left ventricular function. Densitometric measurements obtained from DSA left ventriculograms provide data which are quite analogous to those obtained with technetium^{99} blood pool scans and lend themselves to similar processing.[5] In addition, phase and amplitude analyses can summarize in a single image the time to maximal rate of pixel change for each pixel within the left ventricular cavity.

The utility of DSA for interpreting and reporting coronary angiography is not yet well defined. Despite suspended respirations and ECG gating, it appears that selectively injected coronary artery segments do not consistently achieve precise superimposition from cardiac cycle to cardiac cycle. In part, this disparity results from the relatively small size of coronary

Table 6. DSA system components

REPORT GENERATION AND OUTPUT
Interpretive reports
- LV angiography
  - global and regional wall motion (geometric)
  - phase and amplitude analysis (summarizes peak wall motion)
  - densitometric
- Coronary angiography
  - ECG gating
  - blood flow and velocity
  - densitometry
  - myocardial perfusion and washout
- Report output
  - multi-format image cameras
  - video tape
  - graphic printer/plotter

ARCHIVAL STORAGE
Analog vs digital
Computer control
Compact and high density
Cost and logistics

vessels (1 to 4 mm diameter) compared to the greater motion of the epicardial surface of the heart which produces obscuring misregistration artifacts. In addition, failure of superimposition may reflect immediate changes in contractile state resulting from the intracoronary contrast itself.

Densitometric measurements over the myocardium may add substantial information to selective coronary arteriography. It is possible to measure the velocity of coronary blood flow by assessing the densitometric profile of the moving contrast bolus in sequential frames. Of greater potential interest is the utilization of the myocardial blush phase to assess relative perfusion of the myocardium and rates of subsequent contrast washout. This type of information is analogous to, but should not be considered physiologically synonymous with, thallium-201 perfusion scanning.

Final reports generated by a DSA system designed for cardiac work can include film output from multiformat imaging cameras. In addition, some systems may implement analog video tape as output devices for both raw and processed image sequences in a manner similar to modern echographic output which superimposes computer-generated cursors and graphics on the video image. A graphics printer/plotter provides capability for generating narrative description as well as diagrammatic representations of left ventricular wall motion and coronary anatomy.

Archival Storage

With image storage requirements approaching 200 megabytes per patient study, digital archival storage becomes a potentially costly problem (see Table 6). Digital tape, which has large capacity, has inherently slower record and replay rates compared with video disks. The availability of the system computer to process archival storage transactions as a background function permitting other system operations to continue becomes important. The degree of compactness of recorded data and cost must be considered in determining requirements for archival storage.

INTRAVENOUS DSA FOR CARDIAC DIAGNOSIS

The application of DSA in cardiac diagnosis can be subdivided into applications of intravenously administered or intra-arterially administered contrast (Table 7). Typically, intravenous contrast use implies an outpatient or screening procedure. In patients with cardiac disease, particularly coronary disease, there is often a requirement to assess the concomitant presence of cerebral, peripheral, or renal vascular disease because of bruits, history of TIAs, claudication, or hypertension. In addition, there are patients who because of prior extensive peripheral vascular disease or prior vascular graft surgery have severely restricted catheter access sites. Screening of such patients for femoral or axillary artery continuity and patency can reduce the amount of catheterization laboratory time and decrease patient discomfort associated with trial-and-error approaches to vascular entry.

Intravenous contrast administration has permitted visualization of aortocoronary grafts. Although the mediastinum is an area of multiple overlapping vessels, patent aortocoronary grafts can be seen with 50 to 80 percent certainty.[6] Typically, two separate projections are required. Anterior and lateral grafts (for example, left anterior descending, diagonal) are more readily seen than posterior and right grafts (circumflex, marginal). Inability to detect patent grafts (that is, false-negatives) occurs frequently and thus limits predictive accuracy of the technique. The point of graft insertion into native coronary vessels is poorly seen because of overlapping contrast in both pulmonary veins and the LV cavity. Although an unusual clinical occurrence, grafts that are patent at their origin and body but distally obstructed may visualize, giving the impression of patency. An additional limitation is the present inability of intravenous DSA graft visualization to detect significant graft stenoses or thrombus. Figure 4 shows visualization of the central portions of a graft to the left anterior descending artery. Vascular misregistration artifacts obscure identification of two other patent grafts seen in Figure 5.

Table 7. Digital subtraction angiography for cardiac diagnosis

INTRAVENOUS
Vascular angiography
Screen patients with known vascular disease for catheterization access
Assess concomitant cerebral, renal and peripheral vascular disease
Bypass graft patency
Coronary artery visualization (not possible at present)
LV angiography
Screening test for LV dysfunction—global and regional
Response of wall motion to interventions (e.g., atrial pacing, nitroglycerin, exercise)
Relative cost/risk/benefit analysis, vis-a-vis radionuclide and echographic techniques
Screening in complex congenital heart disease
INTRA-ARTERIAL
Vascular angiography
Road map for catheter manipulation through vascular anomalies and tortuosity
Locating aortocoronary and internal mammary graft ostia
Concurrent carotid or other vascular studies
Coronary angiography—selective and supra-aortic valvular injection
Enhance contrast
Functional analyses—perfusion and flow velocity analysis
LV angiography—selective injection
Contrast dose reduction
Densitometric analyses
Functional analyses—phase analysis
Technology transfer from cine film to video

Although hopes have been expressed that coronary arteries could be visualized from right-sided contrast injections, this has not been possible. The superimposition of contrast-filled pulmonary veins, left atrium and left ventricle over the relatively small coronary arteries prevents their visualization, much less lesions within them.

Left ventricular visualization from intravenous contrast administration can be used as a screening test for assessing global or regional left ventricular dysfunction or for assessing results of therapeutic interventions. Quantitative indices of left ventricular wall motion obtained from intravenous DSA studies compare favorably with selective left ventriculograms.[7] However, when one compares intravenous digital subtraction angiography with radionuclide and echographic techniques for left ventricular visualization, careful consideration must be given to relative cost/risk/benefit analysis. Caution must be exercised in this regard if a requirement for biplane LV views in conjunction with other peripheral vascular DSA studies leads to administration of considerable amounts of contrast in patients with known heart failure. DSA can also be used to assess the response of left ventricular wall motion to interventions such as atrial pacing, nitroglycerin administration, or exercise. However, each test necessitates an additional contrast injection. Intravenous contrast administration for cardiac chamber visualization has been used in patients with congenital heart disease.[8,9] A knowledge of the anatomic connections and shunts may facilitate subsequent catheterization and selective angiography.

INTRA-ARTERIAL DSA FOR CARDIAC DIAGNOSIS

During the course of a cardiac catheterization procedure, DSA is a useful adjunct in certain circumstances (see Table 7). Injection of small doses of contrast into the aortic root or arch may expedite locating coronary graft and internal mammary ostia for selective catheter cannulation. Performance of a supravalvular aortogram in the appropriate obliquity using DSA and diluted contrast in patients with multiple grafts can confirm patency or occlusion of grafts not selectively entered. Figure 5 shows visualization of the mid-portions of three grafts using DSA to enhance images obtained using 40 ml of 2:1 dilution of contrast administered into the aortic root.

The addition of DSA to standard catheterization/angiographic procedures permits more angiography than would customarily be done because of contrast dose restraints.[10] Patients having angiography of multiple grafts, native vessels, left ventricle, and carotid/arch vessels may approach the standard contrast dose limit of 5 ml per kg. Contrast limitations become particularly important for patients with heart failure, renal insufficiency, or diabetes mellitus. Patients for whom cardiac surgery is performed within 12 to 24 hours after extensive angiography sometimes exhibit transient postoperative renal impairment and thus would benefit from contrast dose reduction.

Coronary arteries can be visualized using DSA enhancement from supraaortic contrast injections. The utility of this procedure is not clear, although it may be helpful in screening for coronary ostial lesions in suspect patients or in obtaining perfusion studies. DSA as an adjunct to selective coronary angiography does provide excellent contrast pictures and permits contrast dilution by factors of 5- to 10-fold. Figure 6 shows coronary artery images obtained with standard selective contrast recorded by conventional cine techniques (6, *top*) and recorded using 512 $\times$512 matrix with subtraction of a blurred mask (6, *bottom*).

A critical issue is whether the selective coronary images recorded digitally, with or without subtraction, provide equivalent detail to that offered by cine film techniques. Table 4 points out that the theoretic resolution of digital recording is 1.7 line pairs per mm (512 $\times$ 512 pixel matrix) which is below the 2.5 to 3.5 line pair per mm resolution of cine film techniques. However, theoretic resolution limits are not the same as image conspicuity (that is, ability to discern anatomic detail), which is a function of multiple other factors including noise, image size, and contrast. It is a future possibility that a combination of higher pixel density (1024

$\times$ 1024) and the inherent contrast enhancing and noise suppression of DSA systems may lead to a change in standard recording techniques from cine film to digitized video images.

Although present DSA systems do not offer the coronary image resolution presently contained on cine film, the ability for functional analyses such as myocardial perfusion and coronary flow velocity may offer an important adjunct. Using color monitors one can display time of arrival and washout of contrast from the myocardium, thus permitting analysis of perfusion characteristics.

Digitally recorded 30 frames per second selective LV angiograms do provide adequate resolution (256 $\times$ 256) to extract the important diagnostic information. Lowered contrast requirements may permit two single-plane LV angiograms to be performed gaining additional diagnostic information, whereas in the past reluctance to give additional contrast boluses inhibited this practice in laboratories lacking biplane equipment. Moreover, digitally recorded and processed left ventriculography permits functional analyses of the dynamics of regional wall motion. Figure 3 shows an image made by differencing the end-diastolic and end-systolic contrast-filled left ventricle, emphasizing areas of ejection (black) and dyskinesis (white). In addition to standard geometric analyses of left ventricular performance based on the tracing of endocardial contours, densitometric measurements are possible. This permits a different type of measurement of ejection performance, including displays of rate of change and timing of LV ejection characteristics.

ADVANTAGES AND DISADVANTAGES OF INTRAVENOUS CARDIAC DIGITAL SUBTRACTION ANGIOGRAPHY

Intravenous DSA has established itself as an excellent tool for imaging peripheral vessels with elimination of overlying air, fat, or bone densities (Table 8). In general, spatial resolution for intravenous left ventriculography exceeds that of radionuclide techniques, as does temporal resolution. However, exercise interventions are more difficult with DSA (although pos-

Table 8. DSA: advantages and disadvantages

Intravenous cardiac digital subtraction angiography
ADVANTAGES
Excellent detail of stationary vessels with elimination of overlying air, fat or bone density
Image resolution for LV exceeds radionuclide techniques
Enhancement of detail using post-processing
DISADVANTAGES
Requirement for object stability to avoid motion artifacts
Multiple contrast boluses for different projections or to study effects of intervention
Limited duration of visualization compared to echocardiography or radionuclide imaging
Uses ionizing radiation
Intra-arterial cardiac digital subtraction angiography
ADVANTAGES
Requires less contrast for selective injections (lowers patient morbidity)
Facilitates catheterization procedure (road mapping; screening for grafts or vascular anomalies)
Potential logistic advantages of DSA image store, display and reporting vs cine film
DISADVANTAGES
Current systems are first generation
Optimal digital storage device not certain
Incremental cost vs reimbursement
Reduced spatial resolution compared to film
Artifacts difficult to exclude entirely

Table 9. Comparison of patient x-ray exposure

	Duration of Patient Exposure	*Roentgens per pt. Study*	*Total Absorbed Energy (ergs × 10^4)*
LV STUDY			
DSA-boost fluoro (iv)	10 sec	2.3	2.4
Cine-30 fps (LV selective)	8 sec	3.6	3.7
Cine-60 fps (LV selective)	8 sec	7.2	7.4
Radionuclide (^{99}Te)	—	—	140.0
CORONARY STUDY			
DSA-radiographic; 8 fps (ic)	6 sec	12.7	13.0
DSA-boost fluoro (ic)	6 sec	1.3	1.3
Cine-8 fps (ic)	6 sec	0.7	0.7
Cine-30 fps (ic)	6 sec	2.7	2.8

Cine 6 msec pulse duration: 72 KV for average 70 kg adult patient
DSA boost fluoro: 20 ma
DSA radiographic: 35 msec/frame
Radionuclide: 20 mCi ^{99}Te injected
X-ray exposures assume 7″ intensifier; 95% incident energy absorbed; effective energy as 40% of maximum energy
ic = intracoronary
iv = intravenous

sible) than with radionuclide techniques because of the requirements for thoracic stability. DSA, like radionuclide methods, has capability for complex post-processing of the recorded sequence of image frames showing the passage of the contrast bolus through the heart, thereby providing functional types of analyses to be performed.

The disadvantages of intravenous cardiac DSA include the requirement for object stability in order to avoid motion artifacts. If one is to obtain different projections or to study the effects of interventions, one must inject multiple contrast boluses, each typically containing 40 ml of 76 percent contrast. The duration of visualization is limited by contrast dose compared with echocardiography and radionuclide blood pool scanning which permit unlimited recording.

DSA does expose the patient to ionizing radiation. Table 9 compares patient x-ray exposure for typical LV and coronary examinations using DSA, conventional cine and radionuclide techniques. Although it is difficult to make these types of comparisons because of markedly different radiographic techniques involved, the incident energy absorbed can be computed in ergs. The results in Table 9 show that, in general, DSA techniques do not lessen x-ray exposure. In fact, some of the gain in image quality in DSA systems may be the result of increased x-ray dose. Reports of DSA results should always include x-ray exposure information so that reasonable comparisons with existing techniques can be made. It is possible that cardiac angiographers may accept slower frame rates for selective coronary angiography, compensating for increased x-ray dose per frame.

ADVANTAGES AND DISADVANTAGES OF INTRA-ARTERIAL CARDIAC DSA

Intra-arterial DSA reduces contrast requirements for selective peripheral vascular, aortic, left ventricular, and coronary injections (see Table 8). This, in turn, lowers patient morbidity, particularly for individuals in heart failure or with renal dysfunction. The presence of a DSA unit in a catheterization/angiographic laboratory may facilitate progress of an individual case by providing a "road mapping" function and as an adjunct for screening patients for other vascular disease.

In the future, there may be potential logistic advantages of a DSA system that utilizes entirely digital image storage, display and reporting mechanisms. This transfer of technology is not yet feasible, because of relative unavailability of extremely large capacity digital video disks, the unresolved issue of whether a 1024 × 1024 pixel matrix will be required for adequate coronary artery image resolution, and concerns about relying upon computer-based imaging with increased potential for hardware malfunctions.

The disadvantages of intra-arterial DSA are several. It should be recognized that all systems currently available reflect first-generation hardware and software. Multiple advances are being planned and implemented with increasing experience. An important consideration in the addition of a digital system to an existing catheterization laboratory is the incremental cost versus usefulness and the ability to achieve patient or third-party payer reimbursement. Whether one implements an all-digital system or adds a cardiac DSA system to existing radiographic equipment, the primary advantages at present result from noncardiac, intravenous vascular angiography and as an adjunct to conventional intra-arterial angiography. Cardiac DSA using intravenous contrast is limited by difficulties associated with motion artifacts and overlapping contrast-filled structures and, thus, is largely restricted to LV visualization.

CONCLUSIONS

Despite the complexity of a DSA system, it is evident that a very important contribution to the detection and assessment of peripheral, renal, and cerebral vascular disease has been developed. However, relatively stationary vascular structures lend themselves to far better quality imaging than cardiac structures. The motion of vascular structures, including pulsation within the lungs and mediastinum as well as cardiac motion, makes the problem of registration artifacts a formidable one. The use of intravenous digital subtraction angiography for screening of patients with suspected vascular or left ventricular lesions seems valuable. At the present time, intravenous DSA for visualization of the coronary arteries is not possible, and visualization of bypass grafts remains unreliable. DSA as an adjunct for invasive catheterization/angiographic procedures seems most useful in patients with advanced vascular disease or in those individuals who would most benefit from a reduction in contrast dose. Typically these are patients of advanced age who have substantial vascular disease, renal dysfunction, or overt heart failure. Thus, it seems likely that in a high-volume laboratory with a substantial population of patients who are at higher-than-average risk for procedural morbidity, the implementation of a cardiac DSA unit could be beneficial. However, rapid evolution of technology and presently ill-defined indications for use of intravenous DSA suggest caution before broadening implementation of this technique.

ACKNOWLEDGMENT

The authors gratefully acknowledge the assistance of Dr. Roland Finston in providing calculations of ionizing radiation exposures associated with the various imaging techniques.

REFERENCES

1. Kruger, RA, Mistretta, CA, Houk, TL, et al: *Computerized fluoroscopy in real time for noninvasive visualization of the cardiovascular system.* Radiology 130:49, 1979.
2. Meaney, TF, Weinstein, MA, Buonocore, E, et al: *Digital subtraction angiography of the human cardiovascular system.* AJR 135:1153, 1980.
3. Brody, WR, Cassel, DM, Sommer, FG, et al: *Dual energy projection radiography: Initial clinical experience.* AJR 137:201, 1981.
4. Nelson, JA, Miller, FJ, Mineau, DE, et al: *Clinical applications of digital filtration techniques.* In Heintzen, PH and Brennecke, R (eds): *Digital Imaging in Cardiovascular Radiology.* Thieme, New York, Thieme-Stratton, 1983, pp 183–192.

5. NALCIOGLU, O, SEIBERT, JA, ROECK, WW, ET AL: *Comparison of digital subtraction densitometry and area-length method in the determination of left ventricular ejection fraction.* Proc SPIE 314:294, 1981.

6. WHITING, JS, NIVATPUMIN, TH, PFAFF, M, ET AL: *Assessing the coronary circulation by digital angiography: Bypass graft and myocardial perfusion imaging.* In HEINTZEN, PH AND BRENNECKE, R (EDS): *Digital Imaging in Cardiovascular Radiology.* Thieme, New York, Thieme-Stratton, 1983, pp 205–211.

7. GOLDBERG, HL, BORER, JS, MOSES, JW, ET AL: *Digital subtraction intravenous left ventricular angiography: Comparison with conventional intraventricular angiography.* J Am Coll Cardiol 1:858, 1983.

8. BURSCH, JH, BRENNECKE, R, RADTKE, W, ET AL: *Digital fluoroscopy: Applications in congenital heart disease.* In HEINTZEN, PH AND BRENNECKE, R (EDS): *Digital Imaging in Cardiovascular Radiology.* Thieme, New York, Thieme-Stratton, 1983, pp 216–225.

9. BUONOCORE, E, PAVLICEK, W, MODIC, MT, ET AL: *Anatomic and functional imaging of congenital heart disease with digital subtraction angiography.* Radiology 147:647, 1983.

10. CRUMMY, AB, STIEGHORST, MF, TURSKI, PA, ET AL: *Digital subtraction arteriography (DSA).* In HEINTZEN, PH AND BRENNECKE, R (EDS): *Digital Imaging in Cardiovascular Radiology.* Thieme, New York, Thieme-Stratton, 1983, pp 175–183.

Index

A "t" following a page number indicates a table. A page number in *italics* indicates a figure.